KUMA

MEDICAL MANAGEMENT AND THERAPEUTICS

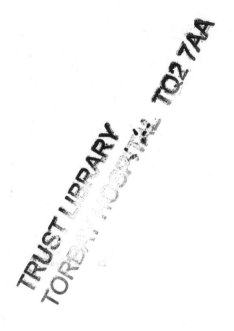

Commissioning Editor: *Pauline Graham*
Senior Development Editor: *Ailsa Laing*
Project Manager: *Kerrie-Anne McKinlay*
Designer: *Kirsteen Wright*
Illustrations Manager: *Merlyn Harvey*
Illustrator: *Ethan Danielson*

KUMAR & CLARK'S

MEDICAL MANAGEMENT AND THERAPEUTICS

Edited by

PROFESSOR PARVEEN KUMAR
CBE BSc MD DM(HC) FRCP(L&E) FRCPATH

Professor of Medicine and Education, Barts and The London School
of Medicine and Dentistry, Queen Mary University of London, and
Honorary Consultant Physician and Gastroenterologist, Barts and The
London NHS Trust and Homerton University Hospital NHS Foundation
Trust, London, UK

DR MICHAEL CLARK
MD FRCP

Honorary Senior Lecturer,
Barts and The London School of Medicine and Dentistry,
Queen Mary University of London, London, UK

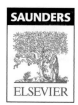

SAUNDERS

ELSEVIER

Edinburgh   London   New York   Oxford
Philadelphia   St Louis   Sydney   Toronto 2011

SAUNDERS
ELSEVIER

© 2011 Elsevier Ltd. All rights reserved.

ISBN 9780702027659

British Library Cataloguing in Publication Data
A catalogue record for this book is available from the British Library

Library of Congress Cataloging in Publication Data
A catalog record for this book is available from the Library of Congress

Notices

Knowledge and best practice in this field are constantly changing. As new research and experience broaden our understanding, changes in research methods, professional practices, or medical treatment may become necessary.

Practitioners and researchers must always rely on their own experience and knowledge in evaluating and using any information, methods, compounds, or experiments described herein. In using such information or methods they should be mindful of their own safety and the safety of others, including parties for whom they have a professional responsibility.

With respect to any drug or pharmaceutical products identified, readers are advised to check the most current information provided (i) on procedures featured or (ii) by the manufacturer of each product to be administered, to verify the recommended dose or formula, the method and duration of administration, and contraindications. It is the responsibility of practitioners, relying on their own experience and knowledge of their patients, to make diagnoses, to determine dosages and the best treatment for each individual patient, and to take all appropriate safety precautions.

To the fullest extent of the law, neither the Publisher nor the authors, contributors, or editors, assume any liability for any injury and/or damage to persons or property as a matter of products liability, negligence or otherwise, or from any use or operation of any methods, products, instructions, or ideas contained in the material herein.

Contents

Contents

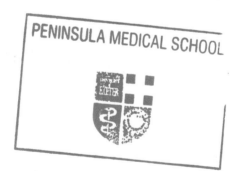

Contributors

Neil Ashman FRCP PhD
Consultant Nephrologist, Renal Unit, Royal London Hospital, London, UK

Jonathan Ball MRCP MSc EDIC MD FCCP
Consultant & Honorary Senior Lecturer in General & Neuro Intensive Care, St George's Hospital & Medical School, London, UK

Sally Bradberry BSc MD MRCP FAACT
Consultant Clinical Toxicologist, National Poisons Information Service, City Hospital, Birmingham, UK

Alistair Chesser MB BChir FRCP PhD
Consultant Nephrologist, Renal Unit, Royal London Hospital, London, UK

Michael Clark MD FRCP
Honorary Senior Lecturer, Barts and The London School of Medicine and Dentistry, Queen Mary University of London, London, UK

Jason Coppell MA MBBS MRCP FRCPath
Consultant Haematologist, Royal Devon & Exeter Hospital, Exeter, UK

Mehul Dhinoja MBBS MRCP(UK)
Consultant Cardiologist & Electrophysiologist, Arrhythmia Service, St Bartholomew's Hospital, London, UK

Vimal J Gokani BMedSci MB BS MSc MRCS
NIHR Academic Clinical Fellow, Department of Cardiovascular Sciences, University of Leicester, Leicester, UK

Philippa Hanson MBBS MRCP BMedSci MD
Consultant Physician, Diabetes Endocrinology and General Medicine, Newham University Hospitals Trust, London, UK

Paul Jarman MA MBBS(Hons) PhD
Consultant Neurologist, The National Hospital for Neurology and Neurosurgery, London, UK

Parveen Kumar CBE BSc MD DM(HC) FRCP FRCP(Edin)
Professor of Medicine and Education, Barts and the London School of Medicine and Dentistry, Queen Mary University of London, UK; Honorary Consultant Physician and Gastroenterologist, Barts and The London NHS Trust and Homerton University Hospital NHS Foundation Trust, London, UK

Susannah Leaver MBBS MRCP
Specialist Registrar, Respiratory Department, St George's Hospital, London, UK

Joel Mawdsley MRCP, MD
Consultant in Gastroenterology, West Middlesex University Hospital, Middlesex, UK

Sarah Ngan BMedSci MBBS MRCP PhD
Specialist Registrar, Medical Oncology, Hammersmith Hospital, London, UK

Timothy Planche MD MRCP FRCPath
Consultant Microbiologist/Hon Senior Lecturer, Department of Medical Microbiology, St George's Hospital, London, UK

Dev Pyne MBBS(Hons) MA FRCP
Consultant Rheumatologist/Lead Clinician, Barts and the Royal London Hospital, London, UK

Tony M Rahman MA DIC PhD FRCP
Consultant ICU Physician & Gastroenterologist, Department of Intensive Care Medicine & Gastroenterology, St George's NHS Trust, London

Peter A Riley MD FRCPath
Consultant Medical Microbiologist, Department of Medical Microbiology, St George's Hospital, London, UK

Arjune Sen MRCP, PhD
Specialist Registrar, Department of Clinical and Experimental Epilepsy, National Hospital for Neurology and Neurosurgery, London, UK

Chris Skene MB ChB MRCP
Specialist Registrar, Department of Cardiology, Royal Infirmary of Edinburgh, Edinburgh, UK

James E Thaventhiran MRCP Dip HIV Med
Clinical Research Fellow, Wellcome Trust Immunology Unit, University of Cambridge, Cambridge, UK

Allister Vale MD FRCP FRCPE FRCPG FFOM FAACT FBTS Hon FRCPSG
Director, National Poisons Information Service and West Midlands Poisons Unit, City Hospital, Birmingham; School of Biosciences and College of Medicine and Dentistry, University of Birmingham, Birmingham, UK

Mohini Varughese BSc(Hons) MBBS MRCP FRCR
Consultant Clinical Oncologist, Taunton and Somerset Foundation Trust, Taunton, Somerset, UK

Simon Michael Ward MB BS MRCP(UK)
Consultant Physician and Geratologist, Department of Medicine, Oxford Radcliffe NHS Trust, Oxford, UK

James Wilkinson PhD MRCP MB BS BSc(Hons)
Specialist Registrar, Cardiology Department, London Chest Hospital, London, UK

Preface

This book has been produced in response to readers of *Kumar & Clark's Clinical Medicine* who consistently requested a handbook with all the essentials for medical management and therapeutics for use at the bedside. Here it is; a portable handbook which covers the essential ground between the detailed descriptions and treatment of diseases found in *Kumar & Clark's Clinical Medicine* and the therapeutic lists found in standard formularies.

We have concentrated on the therapeutic side of what procedures to perform, how and — critically — why; what to prescribe when, how and why; supplying definitions and, to help the reader, we have added short paragraphs on how to investigate and diagnose various conditions.

The book covers all areas likely to be seen in acute general healthcare centres throughout the world. It has been written by young doctors who are at the forefront of healthcare delivery and is therefore very practical and up to date.

The order of the chapters coincides with those you are familiar with in *Kumar & Clark's Clinical Medicine*, which we hope will help you navigate your way around this new book.

Colour and ease of access to the information through a bulleted, algorithmic layout makes it easy to read and digest.

Key features:
- Portable
- Practical drug dosages
- Easy-to-read layout with colour
- Related to *Kumar & Clark's Clinical Medicine*
- Continuity of editorship, style and clarity
- Comprehensive

Parveen Kumar and Michael Clark

Abbreviations

Most abbreviations are explained at their first occurrence in the relevant chapter. Others that crop up across the book and are common medical currency are explained here.

ABGs	arterial blood gases
ACE	angiotensin-converting enzyme
ACTH	adrenocorticotrophic hormone
ADH	antidiuretic hormone
ADR	adverse drug reaction
AIDS	acquired immune deficiency syndrome
ALT	alanine aminotransferase
ANA	antinuclear antibodies
ANCA	antineutrophil cytoplasmic antibodies
ARB	angiotensin receptor blocker
ARDS	acute respiratory distress syndrome
AST	aspartate transaminase
BMI	body mass index
BMR	basal metabolic rate
BP	blood pressure
bpm	beats per minute
cAMP	cyclic adenosine monophosphate
CJD	Creutzfeld-Jakob disease
CNS	central nervous system
CPR	cardio-pulmonary resuscitation
CRP	C-reaction protein
CSF	cerebrospinal fluid
CT	computed tomography
CVP	central venous pressure
CXR	chest X-ray
DNAR	Do Not Attempt Resuscitate
dsDNA	double-stranded deoxyribonucleic acid
DVT	deep vein thrombosis
EBV	Epstein–Barr virus
ECG	electrocardiogram
EEG	electroencephalogram
ELISA	enzyme-linked immunosorbent assay
EMG	electromyogram
ESR	erythrocyte sedimentation rate
FBC	full blood count
FEV$_1$	forced expiratory volume in 1 second
FVC	forced vital capacity
GCS	Glasgow coma score
eGFR	estimated glomerular filtration rate
HAV	hepatitis A virus
Hb	haemoglobin
HBV	hepatitis B virus

HCAI	healthcare-acquired infection
HCV	hepatitis C virus
HDU	high-dependency unit
HIV	human immunodeficiency virus
HLA	human leucocyte antigen
HR	heart rate
HRT	hormone replacement therapy
ICU	intensive care unit
IFN	interferon
IM	intramuscular
INR	International Normalized Ratio
IV	intravenous
JVP	jugular venous pressure
LDH	lactate dehydrogenase
LFTs	liver function tests
MCV	mean cell volume
MRI	magnetic resonance imaging
MRSA	meticillin-resistant *Staphylococcus aureus*
NICE	National Institute for Health and Clinical Excellence
NSAIDs	non-steroidal anti-inflammatory drugs
PCR	polymerase chain reaction
PE	pulmonary embolism
PET	positron emission tomography
RCT	randomized controlled trial
Rh	Rhesus
SC	subcutaneous
SLE	systemic lupus erythematosus
STI	sexually transmitted infection
TB	tuberculosis
TIA	transient ischaemic attack
TNF	tumour necrosis factor
U&E	urea and electrolytes
US	ultrasound
vCJD	variant Creutzfeld-Jakob disease
VTE	venous thromboembolism
WHO	World Health Organization

Acknowledgements

The following features are from Kumar & Clark 2009 Clinical Medicine, 7th Edition, with permission:

Tables: 1.2, 1.3, 2.2, 2.3, 2.4, 2.5, 2.6, 3.1, 4.3, 5.3b, 6.1, 6.3, 8.1, 10.3, 11.1, 11.2, 13.4, 13.6, 15.1, 15.2, 15.3, 15.4, 16.4, 17.4 and 18.1.

Boxes 1.1, 2.1, 3.2, 4.1, 4.2, 4.3, 5.2, 5.3, 5.4, 6.2, 6.3, 7.1, 8.1, 15.1, 15.2, 15.3, 16.1, 16.2, 17.2, 17.4 and 18.1.

Figures 2.1, 5.1, 5.2, 6.1, 6.2, 7.1, 7.2, 7.3, 7.4, 7.5, 7.6, 9.1, 9.2, 9.3, 11.3, 11.4, 12.6, 12.12, 12.16, 12.17, 12.19, 12.20, 13.2, 13.3, 13.4, 13.5, 14.1, 15.1, 16.1, 16.2, 19.1, 20.1 and 20.14.

Inpatient medical care   1

GOOD MEDICAL PRACTICE

Providing good clinical care

Good medical care depends upon a good relationship between the doctor and the patient. The quality of care is improved with better patient communication, along with trust, honesty and openness about decisions that are made in partnership with the patient.

The General Medical Council in the UK has published guidance for doctors and outlines their duties of care (www.gmc-uk.org). National practices differ from country to country but all have similar regulatory bodies and guidance. Remember:

- Respect the views of your patients, including their ethnic and cultural background.
- Discuss their diagnosis, prognosis and treatment with them.
- Give them the necessary information to make their own decisions.

Doctors have a duty to keep up to date and to practise evidence-based medicine. Continuing professional development is necessary to achieve this. They must:

- recognize the limits of their competence
- prescribe drugs or treatment only with an adequate knowledge of the patient's health
- provide treatments based on the best available evidence
- respect the patient's right to ask for a second opinion
- seek consent for any procedure or treatment
- seek senior help or advice where appropriate
- respect confidentiality in practice
- respect autonomy in the treatment of vulnerable patients and those with psychiatric illness
- know the ethical and legal boundaries of the duty to protect life and health.

Clinical records

Records should be written with a pen and be dated and signed, with a printed name below the signature. They must be legible, clear and accurate.

They must include clinical findings, investigations and treatment(s) prescribed, the consent given, the decisions made and the information given to the patient, with details of follow-up or referrals. Records should be updated at the time of seeing the patient or soon after. The original record should never be altered but an additional note (signed and dated) should be made alongside any mistake. Records should be kept in a secure place. Computerized records are increasingly being used in some countries.

Assessment and general management

- Take a history, including psychological and social factors.
- Examine the patient.
- Arrange appropriate investigations.
- Arrange appropriate treatment with the patient's consent.

There are validated scoring systems that help assess how ill the patient is. An example is the Modified Early Warning Score.

Modifed Early Warning Score (MEWS)

This simple physiological scoring system (Table 1.1) can be used at the bedside in a medical admission unit. It identifies patients at risk of deterioration who will require a higher level of care in either an HDU or an ICU.

A nurse or healthcare worker can record six vital signs on a chart (heart rate, respiratory rate, blood pressure, conscious level, temperature and hourly urine output for the previous 2 hours). A score of between 1 and 3 is recorded for each vital sign. The sum of all the scores determines the MEWS score. A score of 4 and above will prompt the nurse to call the patient's doctor, and scores of 5 or more are associated with an increased risk of death and immediate admission to HDU or ICU.

Communication between handing-over teams can also be a problem in busy clinical environments. A suggested proforma that covers the essential factors in transferring patient care is SBAR (situation, background, assessment, recommendation — NHS Institute for Innovation and Improvement).

SBAR

This is a mechanism by which teams can clarify what information should be communicated between members of the team. It develops better

Table 1.1 Modified Early Warning Score (MEWS)

Score	3	2	1	0	1	2	3
Systolic BP (mmHg)	<70	71–80	81–100	101–199		>200	
Heart rate (bpm)	<40		41–50	51–100	101–110	111–129	130
Respiratory rate (bpm)		<9		9–14	15–20	21–29	30
Temperature (°C)	<35	34–35		35–38.4		>38.5	
AVPU score				Alert	Reacting to **v**oice	Reacting to **p**ain	Unresponsive

communication and teamwork, leading to increased patient safety. Standardized prompt questions in the four sections listed below are used to ensure that members of staff share concise and focused information with the correct level of detail. SBAR aids good communication and encourages prompt action on the part of the receiver.

● S Situation
  • Identify yourself and the site/unit you are calling from.
  • Identify the patient by name, consultant, patient location and vital signs. Give a reason for your report.
  • Describe your concern.
● B Background
  • Give the reason for the patient's admission.
  • Explain the significant medical history.
  • Give a brief summary of the background.
● A Assessment
  • Vital signs — heart rate, respiratory rate, oxygen saturations, BP, temperature, AVPU (**a**lert, responds to **v**oice, responds to **p**ain, **u**nresponsive; a patient responding to pain only is equivalent to a patient with a Glasgow coma score of <8).
  • MEWS score.
  • Clinical impression, severity of patient, additional concern.
● R Recommendation
  • Explain what you need — be specific about the request and time frame.
  • Make suggestions.
  • Clarify expectations.

PRE- AND PERI-OPERATIVE CARE AND ASSESSMENT

The aim of these assessments is to reduce the morbidity and mortality of patients undergoing surgery. Most units run pre-operative clinics prior to admission for surgery. Many procedures are performed as day cases, with local or spinal anaesthesia or short general anaesthetics.

The general condition of the patient is reviewed; cardiovascular and respiratory problems can often be addressed and treated prior to surgery. A commonly used five-point grading system has been developed by the American Society of Anesthesiologists (ASA):

● ASA I   Healthy patient
● ASA II   Mild systemic disease, no functional disability
● ASA III   Moderate systemic disease, functional disability
● ASA IV   Severe systemic disease, life-threatening
● ASA V   Moribund, unlikely to survive 24 hours with or without an operation.

Anaemia, malnutrition, and electrolyte and metabolic disturbances should also all be corrected prior to surgery, if possible. Evaluation by the anaesthetist is performed in patients with chronic disorders and in those who are at high risk, e.g. the acutely ill.

History and examination

A **full history** with co-morbidities (particularly in the elderly) should be documented and an examination performed.

Kumar & Clark's Medical Management and Therapeutics

Co-morbidities

- **Diabetes mellitus.** Management is described on p. 595.
- **Ischaemic heart disease.** The incidence of myocardial infarctions in patients with previous heart attacks is >25%, compared to 0.2% in the healthy. Elective procedures should be delayed for at least 6 months (urgent surgery for 3 months) after an infarct. Unstable angina constitutes a very high risk.
- **Hypertension.** This should be controlled, as untreated hypertension carries a higher risk for myocardial infarctions and cerebrovascular disorders.
- **Liver disorders.** The risks depend on the aetiology of the disorder. Defer surgery in jaundiced patients with abnormal coagulation until the jaundice has resolved; relieve any biliary obstruction by stenting and give vitamin K (10 mg slow IV injection). The Child–Pugh classification can be used for patients with chronic liver disease to predict their operative mortality: class A (up to 10%) to class C (50–70%). Drugs that are metabolized by the liver are contraindicated in these patients and should only be prescribed if absolutely essential. The nursing and medical staff should be informed if the patient is hepatitis B- or C-positive, or HIV-positive.
- **Respiratory problems.** Pre-operative evaluation will require an assessment of lung function — spirometry with ABGs if the spirometry is abnormal and patients have long-term respiratory problems.
- **Current medication.** This should be noted and decisions made about continuation of therapy, particularly if the patient is on anticoagulants or antiplatelet therapy.
- **Drug allergies/sensitivities.** These should be noted with the reaction to the drug in the clinical record and a red (instead of a white) armband attached to the patient's wrist.
- **Smoking.** Patients should be informed of the risks associated with smoking, and the benefits of stopping smoking prior to surgery must be emphasized. These include decreased sputum production, improved sputum clearance by cilia (often within 1–2 days of stopping smoking), increased oxygen-carrying capacity of the blood, reduced concentration of circulating nicotine (can cause vasoconstriction) and less bronchospasm.
- **Alcohol.** An assessment of alcohol intake should be made when taking the history. Patients may have alcohol-related chronic liver disease or develop acute alcohol withdrawal in the early post-operative period. Alcohol also causes an induction of the liver enzymes involved in the metabolism of some of anaesthetic drugs.

Elective surgery carries less risk of peri-operative problems than emergency surgery, in which there are often many co-morbidities and the patient is seriously ill.

Routine pre-operative tests

These are often not necessary in a patient undergoing minor or elective surgery.

- **FBC** — not unless there are co-morbidities or if more than a very small amount of blood is expected to be lost
- **Coagulation tests** — not necessary unless there is a bleeding disorder, the patient is on anticoagulants, or epidural anaesthesia is planned
- **LFTs, biochemistry and U&E** — not unless there are co-morbidities

- CXR — only for those with cardio-respiratory problems
- ECG — for the elderly or patients with a history of heart disease, or if examination revealed a cardio-respiratory problem
- Blood group and cross-matching — depending on the nature of the operation.

Prophylaxis for deep vein thrombosis

Anti-DVT/VTE measures include early ambulation, which reduces the risk of DVT/PE. Graduated compression stockings (unless patient has peripheral arterial disease) and **low-molecular-weight heparin** or oral anti-thrombotic agents e.g. **dabigatran** or **rivaroxaban** should be used. See p. 245 for details.

Beta-blockers

The current evidence supporting β-blocker therapy in non-cardiac surgery is poor and it should not be used, apart from in very 'high-risk' patients.

Post-operative care

The overall aim is to prevent complications or to detect them early, should they arise.

- Fluid and electrolyte balance — p. 369.
- Care of wounds, sutures and drains
- Pain control — p. 25.
- Early ambulation
- Physiotherapy — given particularly for chest, orthopaedic and peripheral vascular operations.
- Complications — treated as necessary, e.g. chest infections with antibiotics.
- Arrangements for discharge to home or convalescence — should be addressed early in the post-operative period so that arrangements can be made.

SPECIFIC INTERVIEWS

Obtaining consent

Doctors seeking consent for a particular procedure must have proper knowledge of how the procedure is performed and its possible complications.

- Consent must be 'informed' to an adequate standard.
- Patients must be competent to consent to treatment.
- Patients must not be coerced into accepting treatment against their wishes.
- The doctor and patient should both sign the consent form before the procedure.

Patients need to weigh up the pros and cons of proposed treatments. They cannot do so without the basic ability to reason about information concerning what is wrong with them, what their doctors propose to do about it, and what potential benefits and risks are involved in treatment. Common and serious potential adverse events should be discussed with the patient.

Breaking bad news

These interviews are often difficult. The aim is to make sure that the patient is enabled to understand and make the best of even very bad circumstances. These interviews should always be carried out in a quiet place and without interruption; if possible, patients should have someone with them. Explain your status and your responsibility to them.

It is always best to start off by finding out how much patients know about their condition and how they feel about their illness. Some indication should then be given by the clinician that the news is bad and possibly more serious than initially thought. Pause here to allow the patient to think. It might be worthwhile going through the results of investigations and explaining how the diagnosis has been confirmed. Give information in small chunks, being honest and not hedging about the diagnosis. Avoid technical terms and check that patients understand what you are telling them. Diagrams may be helpful.

Watch for the patient's reactions; if the patient is too upset, it may be that you will have to return to continue the interview. Talk about the treatments that are available to provide a good quality of life, e.g. dealing with pain and some other symptoms. Always provide some positive information and hope but do not be overly optimistic.

Responding to the patient's emotions can be very difficult. The patient may become very upset but the clinician may also be upset. Empathize as much as possible. Answer their questions. The patient might ask about the time frame of the illness. This is very difficult to give so do not provide a figure.

End with a date and time for a further interview (preferably soon) to answer questions and also to see other members of the family that the patient wishes you to see. Give a contact name and number, and also supply contact addresses of good support organizations. Write what you have told the patient and the patient's wishes clearly in the clinical records.

PATIENT SAFETY AND INFECTION CONTROL

Patients admitted to hospitals are in unfamiliar surroundings, are incapacitated and are susceptible to infections due to their illness, e.g. because of poor nutrition, as well as being exposed to hospital-acquired infections.

Approximately 10% of patients contract **healthcare-acquired infections** (HCAIs; previously called nosocomial infections). Risk factors for HCAIs include being on mechanical ventilation, trauma, prolonged length of stay in hospital and the presence of catheters (IV, urinary, naso-gastric tubes). Cross-infection is a problem, particularly with MRSA.

A safety culture must be fostered amongst all healthcare professionals, as preventable harm in healthcare is nearly always caused by medical errors and system failures. To do this, the awareness of possible problems must be raised and a safety culture of openness and learning ensured, along with sustained good risk management.

- Infection control measures. Poor infection control practice in hospitals and other healthcare environments can cause the transfer of infection from person to person. Transfer may be airborne, via fomites, or via a direct contact route. It is essential that all healthcare workers wash or clean their hands before and after patient contact; whenever necessary, they should wear gloves, aprons and other personal protective equipment. This is particularly necessary when performing invasive procedures or manipulating indwelling devices, such as cannulae. Indwelling lines must be checked regularly for signs of infection and this observation should be documented in the notes. Alcohol-based hand washes, which are freely available in the hospital, are a quick and easy alternative to hand washing but they do *not* prevent the spread of *Clostridium difficile*, which requires formal hand washing for physical removal of spores from the hands.

- *Air-borne transmission* prevention again relies on hand washing and also on the use of masks by patient and healthcare worker. Positive pressure isolation is used for patients having cancer chemotherapy treatments.
- *Isolation facilities* should always be available, e.g. for MRSA infection.

● Antibiotics. Antibiotics, particularly broad-spectrum ones, e.g. cephalosporins, should only be used when absolutely necessary, as hospital-acquired infections (particularly *C. difficile* and MRSA) have been linked to hospital over-prescribing. Many hospitals have their own antibiotic prescription policies based on local sensitivities and a reduction in the use of cephalosporins.

● Reduction of medical and procedural errors. Most hospitals have guidelines and protocols to avoid errors. All new personnel should be given an induction about the procedures to maintain patient safety and this should be followed up with continuing education.

● Patient nutrition. The Malnutrition Universal Screening Tool (MUST) has been used to assess the nutrition of patients entering hospitals (p. 123). Many hospital inpatients are malnourished. Patients should be provided with protected mealtimes, good hydration and good nutritional care with fact sheets. These are outlined in the Council of Europe's ten key characteristics of good nutritional care in hospital (www.bapen.org.uk).

● Radiation from medical imaging. The ordering of imaging procedures is increasing as technology advances. Document all exposures to ionizing radiation. For example, a patient undergoing myocardial perfusion imaging receives 15.6 millisieverts (mSv), CT abdomen 8–10 mSv and percutaneous coronary intervention 15 mSv, compared with a CXR, which is only 0.02 mSv. These doses of radiation may, in the long term, present a small risk for the development of cancer.

PRESCRIBING

Good prescribing requires a diversity of skills. Medicines should only be prescribed if they are really necessary and if the risks of *not* giving the drug outweigh the side-effects/harmful effects of the drug itself.

- Drugs should only be prescribed if an accurate diagnosis has been made. Exceptions would include pain relief and 'blind' antibiotics for severe sepsis.
- Co-morbidities should be documented, as some diseases may have an effect on the drug itself, e.g. its elimination.
- Polypharmacy should be avoided as far as possible and drug interactions checked before a new drug is added to the regimen.
- The decisions on therapy must be made with patients and they should be told exactly which drugs they are going to be given and why. This increases the likelihood of patients taking the drugs as prescribed, as they feel they are equal partners in the decision-making (concordance).
- Always look up the drug and its dosages and effects. This can either be done online, e.g. www.bnf.org, or from information in local hospital pharmacy booklets.

- The side-effects of treatment should be explained to patients in a language they understand prior to starting the medication.
- Allergies: Always document these fully in the notes with actual clinical reaction. A red name band should replace the usual white band on the patient's wrist.

The WHO *Guide to Good Prescribing* is a useful training programme to assist in prescribing medicines (http://whqlibdoc.who.int/hq/1994/WHO_DAP_94.11.pdf).

Drug metabolism

Pharmacokinetics (what the body does to the drug) and pharmacodynamics (what the drug does to the body)

Note that absorption, distribution, metabolism, and hepatic and renal elimination of drugs or their metabolites differ from person to person. Therefore the route of administration and the dose of the drug should be tailored to the patient's needs. This may involve changing the drug, increasing/decreasing the dosage or choosing another route of administration.

Many drugs are metabolized by the liver. The metabolism varies between individuals, often because of changes in the cytochrome p450 family of enzymes. Inhibition or induction of cytochrome p450 isoenzymes is a major cause of drug interaction. Some examples are given in Box 1.1. Thus, for example, warfarin is metabolized by CYP2C9. Between 2 and 10% of people are homozygous for an allele that results in low enzyme activity and this leads to higher plasma warfarin levels.

Box 1.1 Some inducers and inhibitors of cytochrome p450

Inducers
- Carbamazepine
- Hyperforin*
- Nifedipine
- Non-nucleoside reverse transcriptase inhibitors (NNRTIs)
- Omeprazole
- Paclitaxel
- Phenytoin
- Protease inhibitors, e.g. ritonavir

Inhibitors
- Allopurinol
- Cimetidine
- Macrolides, e.g. erythromycin, clarithromycin
- Grapefruit juice (contains flavinoids)
- Imidazoles, e.g. ketoconazole
- Quinolones, e.g. ciprofloxacin
- Quinidine
- Sulphonamides
- Clopidogrel

*Hyperforin is one of the ingredients of the herbal product known as St John's wort, used by herbalists to treat depression. Although it is marketed as a licensed medicine, it is a reminder that drug interactions can occur with alternative, as well as conventional, medicines.

The variability of a drug's action within the body is partly due to the drug receptor and the polymorphism of this receptor.

The interplay between pharmacokinetics and pharmacodynamics will influence drug selection and drug dosage.

Prescribing for the elderly

This may require changes in drug dosages in the presence of co-morbidities. It should be remembered that concordance diminishes as the number of prescribed drugs increases and also in the face of cognitive impairment.

- Rates of hepatic drug metabolism and renal excretion decline with age. Extrapolation of dosage regimens from younger adults could therefore lead to drug toxicity.
- Predisposition to toxicity can also occur with changes in drug distribution, a reduction of body mass, changes in body composition, and the preferential distribution of the cardiac output to the brain.
- Co-morbidity (and therefore often polypharmacy too) can lead to increased opportunities for drug interactions.
- Exaggerated pharmacodynamic effects of drugs acting on the cardiovascular system, CNS and gastrointestinal tract occur more commonly (Table 1.2).

Prescribing in pregnancy/breast feeding

Clinicians should be very cautious of prescribing any drug to pregnant women. Always consult the relevant literature for any drug prescribed to check its effects in women of childbearing age, in pregnancy and in nursing mothers.

Never prescribe a drug to pregnant women unless it is absolutely necessary and you have checked for possible teratogenic effects on the fetus.

Table 1.2 Common adverse effects of drugs in the elderly

Drug	Effect
β-Blockers (including eye drops) Digoxin	Bradycardia
Nitrates α-Adrenoceptor-blockers Diuretics	Postural hypotension
Diuretics (thiazides)	Glucose intolerance, gout
Antimuscarinic drugs Tricyclic antidepressants Neuroleptics Minor tranquillizers Anticonvulsants Hypnotics Opioids	Confusion, cognitive dysfunction
Bisphosphonates (mainly alendronic acid)	Oesophageal ulceration and stricture formation
NSAIDs	Gastric erosions Upper gastrointestinal bleeding Perforated peptic ulcer Renal impairment

Appendix A gives websites for drug use. If a known teratogenic drug is required during pregnancy (e.g. an anticonvulsant), always discuss the adverse effects on the fetus with the parents, preferably prior to conception.

Most drugs can be detected in breast milk, albeit in small amounts. A few drugs, e.g. aspirin and carbimazole, can cause harm to the infant if ingested in breast milk.

Writing a prescription

International non-proprietary names (INNs) of drugs should always be prescribed, as proprietary names can cause confusion and can be more expensive. There are rare exceptions where it is necessary to prescribe proprietary preparations, e.g. mesalazine (mesalamine), as the delivery characteristics of the product may vary.

- Write legibly (or use a computer).
- Give the name and address of the patient (if writing an outpatient prescription).
- Name the drug. Do not use abbreviations, e.g. GTN.
- State the dose required as mg or ml (or mL). Write 'micrograms' or 'units' out in full. Avoid decimal points, if possible, or write 0.5 mg rather than .5 mg, as this can lead to mistakes.
- State which route of administration you want the drug to be given by. The abbreviations IV (for intravenous), IM (for intramuscular) or SC (subcutaneous) are usually recognized. Write 'orally' rather than p.o. (by mouth).
- To state frequency, do *not* use Latin abbreviations, as many doctors do not learn Latin. Write once daily (or ×1 daily), twice daily (or ×2 daily), three times daily (×3 daily), four times daily (×4 daily), when required (but also spell out the minimum dose interval), or immediately (not stat).
- Give special information, if required, e.g. 'with food', 'on an empty stomach' or 'at night'. You must be familiar with the way certain drugs are given, e.g. bisphosphonates cause oesophageal damage and must be taken sitting or standing with plenty of water.
- State the amount you want dispensed. Drugs often come in packages to last days, weeks or months. Prescribe these, if possible, as fewer mistakes will be made in dispensing.
- **Sign**, write your name in **capitals** and **date** the prescription.

Prescribing controlled drugs

- Prescriptions must be written out in full, in legible hand-writing and in ink. Computer-based prescriptions should still be signed in ink. Write out the patient's name and address (or hospital ward). Do not use a sticker with the patient's name.
- State the name and strength of the formulation.
- State the type of formulation (e.g. oral liquid, suppository, modified-release capsule or tablet).
- State dose and frequency, e.g. twice daily.
- Write the total amount to be supplied in words as well as figures.
- Sign and date the prescription, e.g.

Patient: Mr AN Other, Ward 21. DOB 01-01-1950. Hospital no. 123456 Please dispense ten (10) times ten milligram (10 mg) MORPHINE SULPHATE modified release capsules to TOTAL one hundred milligrams (100 mg) only.

JB
Dr J BLOGGS Day, month, year

ADVERSE DRUG REACTIONS (ADRS)

The unwanted effects of drugs occurring under normal conditions of use are a significant cause of morbidity and mortality. About 5% of acute medical emergencies are admitted with ADRs. Between 10 and 20% of hospital inpatients suffer an ADR during their inpatient stay. Unwanted effects of drugs occur more frequently in the elderly, and the risk of an ADR rises sharply with polypharmacy.

Classification

Two types of ADR are recognized (Table 1.3):

Table 1.3 Examples of adverse drug reactions

Drug	Adverse reaction
Type A (augmented) Anticoagulants	Bleeding
Insulin	Hypoglycaemia
ACE inhibitors/antagonists	Hypotension
Antipsychotics	Acute dystonia and dyskinesia Parkinson's disease Tardive dyskinesia
Tricyclic antidepressants	Dry mouth
Amiodarone	Hyperthyroidism Hypothyroidism Pulmonary fibrosis
Cytotoxic agents	Bone marrow dyscrasias Cancer
Glucocorticoids	Osteoporosis
Type B (idiosyncratic) Benzylpenicillin	Anaphylaxis
Radiological contrast media	Anaphylaxis Nephrogenic systemic fibrosis, e.g. gadolinium
Amoxicillin	Maculopapular rash
Sulphonamides Lamotrigine	Toxic epidermal necrolysis
Volatile anaesthetics Suxamethonium	Malignant hyperthermia
Diclofenac Isoflurane, sevoflurane Isoniazid Rifampicin Phenytoin	Hepatotoxicity

- Type A (augmented) reactions, which are common, predictable, usually dose-dependent but occasionally serious. They can occur after a single dose (e.g. hypotension with ACE inhibitors) or can take place after months (e.g. amiodarone causing pulmonary fibrosis) or years (catatonic drugs causing cancer).
- Type B (idiosyncratic) reactions, which bear no resemblance to the recognized pharmacological or toxicological effects of the drug. They are therefore unpredictable, usually dose-independent, often serious but fortunately rare.

The following six characteristics can help distinguish an adverse reaction from an event due to some other cause:

- *Time interval.* E.g. minutes (acute anaphylaxis), months (aplastic anaemia) or years (drug-induced malignancy).
- *Nature of the reaction.* Some are typically iatrogenic, e.g. maculo-papular rashes, angio-oedema, fixed drug eruptions, toxic epidermal necrolysis.
- *Plausibility.* An event may be a manifestation of a known pharmacological property of the drug (type A). Recognition of type B reactions may be very difficult unless there is a previous report in the literature.
- *Exclusion of other possible causes*
- *Laboratory tests* e.g. plasma concentration, diagnostic histopathological features.
- *De-/rechallenge.* Results of dechallenge (withdrawal of the drug) and rechallenge (giving the drug again). The latter may be very hazardous and is seldom justified.

Management

- Type A reactions. Reduction in dosage usually helps.
- Type B reactions. The drug should be withdrawn (and never re-instituted).
- Specific therapy. This is sometimes required for ADRs such as bleeding with warfarin (vitamin K), acute dystonias (benzatropine) or acute anaphylaxis. See Emergencies in Medicine p.000.

Any adverse or unexpected drug reaction should be reported to a national authority. In the UK, this is done via a Yellow Card system to the Medicines and Healthcare Regulatory Authority (MHRA).

CLINICAL TRIALS

Evidence-based medicine is the systematic approach to justify the administration of a drug or treatment. Treatments should be used in routine clinical care only if they have been demonstrated to be effective in formal clinical trials. These trials need to be well designed with proper control groups, be properly randomized and have proper end-points. There should be similarity between groups that are being compared with defined entry criteria.

Randomized controlled trials (RCTs)

These can be performed as a 'parallel group design' study where patients with a particular condition are given one of two treatments, usually allocated randomly (**randomized controlled trial**).

- A 'single blind' trial is where the patient is unaware of the drug and a 'double blind' is where both the patient and the doctor are unaware — reducing the bias of both patient and doctor.
- Recruitment can be from several locations ('multicentre' trial).
- In a 'crossover trial' the patient receives both the active and the comparator drug in a random fashion.

Although a large, well-designed, double-blind RCT is the gold standard for obtaining best evidence, it is very expensive and other trials can also be useful.

Controlled observational trials can also be used to test the clinical effectiveness of therapeutic interventions; historical controlled trials, case-control studies and before-and-after studies can be used. The case-controlled trials compare patients who have a particular condition (the 'cases') with those who do not have that condition ('controls'). They are used to identify the 'risk factors' for specific conditions by the estimation of the odds ratio.

Odds/risk ratios and number needed to treat

The **odds ratio** (OR) is the probability of an event occurring, as opposed to the probability of the event not occurring. Thus, for an adverse event, the OR can be calculated as the number with the event (a), divided by the number without the event (b), divided by the odds of the event occurring in the placebo group, i.e. the number of controls with an adverse event (c), divided by the number without (d). Thus:

$$OR = (a/b) \text{ divided by } (c/d)$$

The **risk ratio** or **relative risk** (RR) is calculated by dividing the number with the adverse event (a) by the total number of the cases (a + b). This sum is then divided by the number of people in the placebo group who have an adverse event (c) by the total number in the placebo group (c + d).

$$RR = a/(a+b) \text{ divided by } c/(c+d)$$

If, for example, the total was 4, it would mean there was 4 times the risk.

The relative risk reduction would then be 1−RR.

The benefits or harm of drug therapy can be expressed as the **number needed to treat** (NNT) in order to prevent one adverse clinical event, e.g. a myocardial infarct, thus (NNTB) (benefit), or as the **number needed to treated for harm to occur** (NNTH) (harm). This is calculated as for relative risk but by subtracting instead of dividing. Thus:

$$a/(a+b) - c/(c+d) = A$$

$$NNT_H = 1/A$$

Interpretation of diagnostic tests

Diagnostic tests are interpreted according to their sensitivities and specificities and their predictive values. For example, if:

a = patients with disease who have a positive test
b = patients with no disease who have a positive test
c = patients with disease who have a negative test
d = patients with no disease who have a negative test

- **Sensitivity** is the proportion of patients with a particular disease who have a positive test, i.e. a/(a + c).

- **Specificity** is the proportion of patients who do not have the disease and have a negative test, i.e. $d/(c + d)$.
- **Positive predictive value** is the proportion of people with the disease who have a positive test, i.e. $a/(a + b)$.
- **Negative predictive value** is the proportion of people who do not have the disease and have a negative test, i.e. $d/(c + d)$.

Thus, when reviewing the results of a test, we can assess the likelihood of whether a test result (symptom or sign) would be expected in a patient with the disease compared to a patient without the disease. This **likelihood ratio** (LR) can be calculated from the equation

$$\text{sensitivity}/(1 - \text{specificity})$$

A high LR indicates that a particular disorder is more likely in people with a given result.

The **receiver operator characteristic (ROC) curve** also uses the sensitivity and specificity results to plot the discriminating power of a test. The opposite ends of the curve will show either high sensitivity and low specificity, or high specificity and low sensitivity. The area under the ROC curve also has the ability to discriminate between patients with and without a disease when two different tests are compared.

STATISTICAL ANALYSIS

The average

The 'average' value (or 'central tendency') can be expressed as follows:

- **Mean** — the average of a distribution of values that are grouped symmetrically around the central tendency
- **Median** — the middle value of a sample, used where the values in a sample are asymmetrically distributed around the average
- **Mode** — the interval that contains more values than any other in a frequency distribution of values.

In a symmetrically distributed population the mean, median and mode are the same.

In clinical studies the value of a particular variable (e.g. height, weight, BP, haemoglobin) may be described, quantitatively, in a sample of a defined population.

Confidence interval (CI)

This is the confidence that can placed on a sample 'average' truly reflecting the average value of a population. The CI describes the probability of a sample mean being a certain distance away from the population mean. If, for example, the mean systolic BP of 100 students is 124 mmHg with a CI of 95% of ± 15, then if one replicates the study 100 times, the value of the mean will be within the range of 109–139 mmHg on 95 occasions. Thus, the larger the sample is, the smaller will be the CI.

'p' value

An alternative to the CI is the probability (p value), which is used if the population has a normal distribution. The basic assumption is that there is no difference between two groups (i.e. the Null Hypothesis). Statistical tests are used to determine the probability that an observed difference is due to chance. By convention, if it is less than 1 in 20 ($p < 0.05$), it is described as being 'statistically significant' and is unlikely to be due to chance (i.e. rejecting the Null Hypothesis). If the p value is >0.05, there is no statistical difference between the two groups and the Null Hypothesis cannot be rejected.

Standard deviation (SD) v standard error (SE)

The SD gives an estimate of the variability of the population from which the sample was taken. If the population has a 'normal' distribution, i.e. exhibits a Gaussian 'bell-shaped curve', then 95% of people will have values within 2 SD above and below the mean.

The SE of the sample mean depends on both the SD and also the sample size, i.e.

SE = SD/square root (sample size)

The SE will fall as the sample size is increased, but the SD will not change.

The 95% confidence interval (see above) is:

mean $\pm 2 \times$ SE.

Correlation

- The degree of correlation between two ordinal variables can be investigated by calculating the **correlation coefficient** ('r'), which may range from 1 to –1. If r is 1, there is complete and direct concordance between the two variables; if r = –1, there is complete but inverse concordance; and where r = 0 there is no concordance. The correlation coefficient measures the degree of association between the two variables.
- Statistical tables can inform investigators as to the **probability** that 'r' is due to chance. If the probability is less than 1 in 20 (p < 0.05), then it is regarded as 'statistically significant'. However, it must be emphasized that the 1 in 20 rule does not exclude the possibility that a presumed association is due to chance. Also, the fact that there is an association between two variables does not necessarily mean that it is causal.

DO NOT ATTEMPT RESUSCITATE (DNAR) ORDERS

- The resuscitation status of every patient should be discussed by senior doctors at the time of admission and the decision documented in the notes.
- Many hospitals have specific DNAR forms. Deciding a person's resuscitation status is a careful balance of risk versus benefit. The patient's co-morbidities and pre-morbid quality of life should be taken into account.
- Involve the patient and family in this discussion, and explain the medical reasoning behind the decision. If the patient requests that CPR is not performed in the event of cardio-pulmonary arrest, those wishes should be respected.

Remember that a decision not to resuscitate a patient is not the same as the decision to withhold other treatments. A patient who is not for resuscitation may still be eligible for antibiotics, fluids, endoscopy and even surgery. Management should remain positive, allowing the patient to die free of distress and with dignity.

CARE OF THE DYING

A decision by a multidisciplinary that a patient is dying is agreed and should be recorded in the clinical record. This decision must be discussed with the carers and relatives of the patient. The National Institute for

Kumar & Clark's Medical Management and Therapeutics

Box 1.2 Best practice in the last hours and days of life

- Current medications are assessed and non-essentials discontinued
- 'As required' subcutaneous medication is prescribed according to an agreed protocol to manage pain, agitation, nausea and vomiting and respiratory tract secretions
- Decisions are taken to discontinue inappropriate interventions, including blood tests, intravenous fluids and observation of vital signs
- The ability of the patient, family and carers to communicate is assessed
- The insights of the patient, family and carers into the patient's condition are identified
- Religious and spiritual needs of the patient, family and carers are assessed
- Means of informing family and carers of the patient's impending death are identified
- The family and carers are given appropriate written information
- The GP practice is made aware of the patient's condition
- A plan of care is explained and discussed with the patient, family and carers

Source: National Institute for Clinical Excellence 2004 Guidance on Cancer Services. Improving Supportive and Palliative Care for Adults with Cancer.

Health and Clinical Excellence (2004) guidance on improving supportive and palliative care for adults is shown in Box 1.2.

The Liverpool Care pathway for the dying patient has been widely adopted and used in many general healthcare settings to support clinicians to make decisions about care of the dying.

Confirmation of death

Verification of death can be daunting. Ask relatives to leave the ward while you confirm the death.

There are a number of steps that should be carried out during this final examination in order to avoid mistakes. The approach is similar to any critically ill patient, with assessments of the A, B, C and D.

1. Check that the patient is unresponsive and that there are no signs of life. Look at the chest for movements, and at the throat for signs of swallowing.
2. Auscultate for breath sounds for 2 mins.
3. Check for absence of the carotid pulse.
4. Auscultate for heart sounds for 1 min.
5. Using a pen-torch, ensure that the pupils are not reactive, i.e. are fixed in diameter.
6. Some advocate checking the fundi for 'trucking' — the segmentation of the blood vessels.

Findings should be clearly documented in the medical notes, with the exact time of pronouncement of death. The presence or absence of a pacemaker and radioactive implant should be noted, as this may cause explosions if the body is cremated. The presence of other medical devices, such as cannulae, should be documented; these should not be removed. A death certificate should be filled out as soon as practicable.

Inform the nursing staff, the next of kin and the patient's primary care physician. Ensure that the patient's family are looked after and that they also have the opportunity to ask any questions.

Diagnostic tests for the confirmation of brainstem death

These are performed in intensive care situations when the patient is on a ventilator. (See page 561.)

SPECIFIC CLINICAL PROBLEMS

Allergy

- **Atopy.** Approximately one-third of the population is atopic, i.e. produce an exaggerated IgE response to normal environmental allergens. Clinically this response may manifest with eczema, hay fever or asthma (p. 496).
- **Allergic reactions.** These are increased in atopic persons but also occur in the rest of the population following sensitization to a particular allergen, e.g. drugs, blood transfusions, bee stings and other environmental factors. They are due to an IgE-mediated degranulation of the mast cells releasing mediators, e.g. histamine, which cause leakage of dermal and sub-dermal capillaries.

Clinical features of allergic reactions

Severe symptoms include urticaria, angio-oedema and anaphylaxis. Allergic reactions usually occur within minutes of exposure to an antigen, although sometimes this can be delayed. Establish the time lag between the exposure to a particular allergen and the onset of symptoms. A history of previous allergic symptoms, drugs taken (including complementary), possible allergens in the home or workplace (occupation), and a family history of allergic disorders may be helpful.

- **Urticaria** (hives, 'nettle rash') is common. Itchy weals or swellings develop acutely in the skin due to leaky dermal vessels. Acute urticaria lasts < 6 weeks but chronic persists longer than this. The 'trigger' can be food (e.g. strawberries, seafoods, food colourings), insect venom, a drug, physical factors (e.g. heat, cold, pressure) or vigorous exercise. Drugs include aspirin, NSAIDs, ACE inhibitors, opiates, antibiotics or radio-contrast media. Occasionally, urticaria can be secondary to viral or parasitic infections or may rarely occur with SLE. Often the cause is not found.
- **Angio-oedema** is a localized swelling of the subcutaneous tissues, presenting as a soft-tissue swelling around the eyes, mouth, lips and hands; it is rarely itchy. When it affects the larynx and tongue it can be a life-threatening emergency, as it causes obstruction of the airways. It can also affect the intestine and cause abdominal pain. It usually occurs with urticaria. Severe angio-oedema can lead to anaphylaxis (see below).
  - *Hereditary angio-oedema* is usually not associated with urticaria. It is recurrent and lasts from hours to days. It can be precipitated by trauma, even dental procedures.

Kumar & Clark's Medical Management and Therapeutics

- *Acute hereditary angio-oedema* is treated with C1 esterase concentrates or fresh frozen plasma. For maintenance treatment, anabolic steroids (e.g. **stanozol** or **danazol**) are used, as they stimulate an increase in hepatic synthesis of C1 esterase.

Investigations

History is usually the most useful factor in diagnosing urticaria. Investigations are unnecessary unless there are factors suggesting an underlying cause. The following can be useful in doubtful cases and for cases of angio-oedema:

- Blood tests include FBC (looking for non-specific eosinophilia — an absolute count of $> 1.5 \times 10^9/L$ suggests an atopic cause), C1 esterase inhibitor deficiency (<50% of normal) and complement (C3, C4, C1) inhibitor levels.
- Serum mast cell tryptase can be useful, as it peaks within 2 hours and remains raised for 24 hours or so.
- For some food allergies
  - Serum IgE and an IgE to a specific allergen (radioallergosorbent test, RAST).
  - Skin prick tests using a droplet of diluted standardized allergen on the forearm.
  - Challenge tests to allergens, e.g. food challenge; these should only be performed by specialists.

Treatment

- Antihistamines. Antihistamines, e.g. **cetirizine** 10 mg daily or 5 mg twice daily, **desloratadine** 5 mg daily, **fexofenadine** 120–180 mg (for chronic urticaria) daily, or **loratadine** 10 mg daily. **Chlorphenamine** 4 mg 4–6-hourly to a maximum of 24 mg daily is also used. Patients should be advised that drowsiness may occur with these drugs and affect their performance, e.g. in driving. Other rarer side-effects include hypotension, palpitations, arrhythmias, dizziness, extrapyramidal effects and sleep disturbances.
- Corticosteroids. See p. 584.
- Cysteinyl leukotriene receptor antagonists e.g. **montelukast** are used in aspirin-induced asthma.
- Monoclonal antibodies. Monoclonal antibodies against IgE, e.g. **omalizumab** SC injection, dose varies with IgE concentration and body weight. These inhibit the binding of IgE to basophils and mast cells, and are used in severe peanut allergy.
- Antigen-specific monotherapy (desensitization). Increasing sequential amounts of diluted antigen are given over prolonged periods in specialized centres. The exact mechanism of action is unknown. It is used in the prevention of insect venom anaphylaxis.
- Sublingual. For grass and tree pollen-induced conjunctivitis or rhinitis, a daily sublingual **grass pollen extract** is given four months before the start of the pollen season.
- Avoidance of allergen. If the allergen is known, an attempt should be made to avoid it with the help of dietitians.

Anaphylaxis

This life-threatening emergency is due to a systemic allergic reaction, which is rapid in onset. This reaction requires 'priming' by an antigen followed by re-exposure and the allergen must be systemically absorbed

---

Box 1.3 Acute anaphylaxis

Clinical features
- Bronchospasm
- Facial and laryngeal oedema
- Hypotension
- Nausea, vomiting and diarrhea
- For Management, see Fig. 20.3.

(ingestion or parenteral injection). Serum platelet-activating factor (PAF) levels have been found to correlate directly with the severity of anaphylaxis, whereas PAF acetylhydrolase (the enzyme that inactivates PAF) correlates inversely.

Causes
Allergens include:
- Foods: Nuts — peanuts (protein-arachis hypogaea Ara h 1–3), Brazil nuts, cashew nuts. Shellfish — shrimp (allergen Met e 1), lobster. Dairy products, egg and, more rarely, citrus fruits, mango, strawberry, tomato.
- Venoms: wasps, bees, yellow-jackets, hornets.
- Medications: antisera (tetanus, diphtheria), dextran, latex, some antibiotics and blood products.

Clinical features
The clinical features are shown in Box 1.3. Symptoms range from widespread urticaria and angio-oedema (laryngeal oedema, airway obstruction) to cardiovascular collapse, respiratory arrest and death. Initially there may only be tingling, warmth and itchiness. This is followed by a generalized flush, hypotension, bronchospasm, laryngeal oedema and cardiac arrhythmias; myocardial infarction can follow. Death can occur within minutes.

Emergency treatment
Treatment for **acute anaphylaxis** is shown in Emergencies in Medicine Fig. 20.3.

Non-emergency treatment
- Prevention by avoidance of triggering foods, particularly nuts and shellfish.
- Patient education in the self-administration of adrenaline (epinephrine); patients should always carry pre-loaded syringes.
- Desensitization, particularly if exposure is unavoidable or unpredictable, as in insect stings; this is carried out in specialist centres only.

Anxiety

Anxiety is common in the sick and hospitalized patient. Discussion of the cause of the anxiety with the patient, along with reassurance, is often sufficient to relieve the anxiety. Hyperventilation, which is a feature of anxiety, is described in Box 1.4

Benzodiazepines
These are used for the short-term relief of severe anxiety; their action is described on p. 22. Agents used are:

Kumar & Clark's Medical Management and Therapeutics

Box 1.4 The hyperventilation syndrome

Features
- Panic attacks — fear, terror and impending doom

Accompanied by some or all of the following:
- Dyspnoea (trouble getting a good breath in)
- Palpitations
- Chest pain or discomfort
- Suffocating sensation
- Dizziness
- Paraesthesia in hands and feet
- Peri-oral paraesthesiae
- Sweating
- Carpopedal spasms

Cause
- Overbreathing leading to a decrease in $Paco_2$ and a decrease in bicarbonate and therefore an increase in arterial pH (respiratory alkalosis), causing a decrease in ionised calcium and a relative hypocalcaemia

Diagnosis
- A provocation test — voluntary overbreathing for 2 mins — provokes similar symptoms
- Rebreathing from a large paper bag relieves them
- Blood gases to exclude severe asthma

Management
- Explanation and reassurance are given
- The patient is trained in relaxation techniques and slow controlled breathing
- The patient is asked to breathe into a closed paper bag

- Diazepam 2 mg 3 times daily, increased if necessary to 15–30 mg in divided doses per day
- Chlordiazepoxide 10 mg 3 times daily, increased if necessary to 100 mg in divided doses
- Oxazepam 15–30 mg (10–20 mg in the elderly) 3–4 times daily.
  The dose should be as small as possible to control symptoms.
- Side-effects (p. 23). Dependence and tolerance occur more frequently. Withdrawal symptoms are particularly severe after prolonged use and the drugs must be discontinued slowly. This period can range from 4 weeks to 1 year.

Beta-receptor adrenergic blockers

- Propranolol 20–40 mg 3 times daily is used to control the peripheral symptoms of anxiety such as palpitations, tremor and tachycardia. These drugs do not help control the underlying anxiety.

Management of the severely disturbed patient

Severely disturbed patients (see also p. 626) are usually seen in the accident and emergency department. The primary aims of management are the control of dangerous behaviour and establishment of a provisional

---

Box 1.5 Hallucination

A hallucination is defined as a perception in the absence of a stimulus. It is:
- a false perception and not a distortion
- perceived as inhabiting objective space
- perceived as having qualities of normal perception
- perceived alongside normal perceptions
- independent of the individual's will

---

diagnosis. The main causes are personality disorders, drug and alcohol abuse, and psychosis. For delirium tremens, see p. 627; hallucinations are desccribed in Box 1.5.

Three specific strategies are employed when dealing with the violent patient:

- **Reassurance and explanation.** Most disturbed patients are themselves frightened, as well as frightening, and may feel threatened by those around them. Staff should always explain the situation and their intentions.

- **Physical restraint.** Patients must be restrained from harming themselves and others. A sufficient number of trained staff must be available. At least one person per limb and two others are required if a sedating drug is to be given. Once brought under physical control, the patient should be held in the prone position to protect the airway and to allow an IM injection to be given. Care must be taken to ensure that neither the airway nor breathing is impeded, by having someone always present at the head of the patient. Patients should continue to be restrained until they have calmed down. If IM medications are given into the buttock, damage to the sciatic nerve is best avoided by injecting into the upper outer quadrant.

- **Medication.** Patients should be rapidly tranquillized if they have a psychosis.
  - A deep IM injection of **zuclopenthixol** in a dose ranging from 50 to 150 mg, together with **lorazepam** 0.5–1 mg, is the treatment of choice for rapid effect. Used in combination, they have a synergistic action.
  - Moderate doses of a neuroleptic, e.g. IM **chlorpromazine** 25–50 mg, 6-8-hourly, or a **benzodiazepine** can also be given at regular, comparatively short intervals (30–60 mins) IM.
  - An alternative regimen is IM **butyrophenone (haloperidol** 2–10 mg) in patients under 60 years old. This dose should be reduced in the elderly and those with known cardiac or hepatic disease. The patient should be observed for up to 1 hour before a further dose is administered.
  - In the case of continuing disturbance, it is preferable to administer an adjunctive IM benzodiazepine (**lorazepam** 2 mg) rather than a further dose of a neuroleptic.

Breathing, pulse rate and BP should be monitored for respiratory difficulty, arrhythmias and hypotension.

This procedure must be carefully documented and be within legal boundaries.

Kumar & Clark's Medical Management and Therapeutics

Falls

Falls are very common in older people, with about 15% resulting in serious injury. They are the commonest cause of fracture of the neck of femur in the elderly. Most hospitals have a 'falls' policy and patients are assessed for their risk of falling; this should be reviewed at regular intervals.

Assessment of risk

Assessment of the risk of falling should include: visual impairment, mobility (e.g. arthritis), impairment of activities of daily living, environment, nutrition, continence and cognitive status (confusion, agitation). The medication that patients are taking (particularly polypharmacy) should be reviewed (e.g. for any causing hypotension or sedation). Blackouts, muscle weakness, accidental trips and previous medical history should be ascertained.

Management

Investigations. Investigations to find an acute illness should include:

- FBC, U&E, LFTs, CRP, glucose, calcium
- CXR and urinary analysis for infection
- blood culture if pyrexial.

For chronic conditions:

- serum 25 hydroxy vitamin D
- cardiovascular assessment (ECG, e.g. for arrhythmias)
- neurological assessment (muscle weakness, gait disturbance, Parkinson's disease).

Prevention. This usually involves a multidisciplinary approach. Any abnormality detected should be addressed and reversed, if possible. For example, poor vision should be corrected, medication rationalized, and environmental hazards at home removed or modified. Medical treatment for conditions such as osteoporosis or cardiovascular disorders (common in the elderly, e.g. postural hypotension) may be required. Exercise and balance training can be very helpful in preventing falls. The nutritional status of the patient should be assessed and a proper healthy diet advised. Bone protectors (e.g. hip protector pads) are helpful in reducing the number of fractures of the neck of femur. Aids, such as walking sticks, tripods or Zimmer frames, might be suitable for some.

Insomnia

Insomnia is difficulty in sleeping; it can be due to mood disorders such as anxiety; drug use — both prescribed drugs such as steroids and drugs of abuse, or analgesics for pain — as well as excess alcohol consumption. The causes should be addressed prior to using a hypnotic.

Benzodiazepines

These are frequently used. They act at the benzodiazepine receptors, which are linked to the GABA receptors:

- Nitrazepam and flurazepam have a prolonged action. Dosages are nitrazepam 5–10 mg (dose halved in the elderly) and flurazepam 15–30 mg (15 mg in the elderly).
- Lorazepam, lormetazepam and diazepam have a shorter action and so have fewer hangover effects on the following day. Dosages are lorazepam 1–2 mg, lormetazepam 0.5–1.5 mg (500 mcg in the elderly) and diazepam 5–15 mg. These drugs should not be given for more than 4 weeks to avoid dependence.

- Side-effects include drowsiness, confusion and ataxia. Both tolerance and dependence can develop. An increase in aggression and anxiety is sometimes seen. All side-effects are more prevalent in the elderly. A withdrawal syndrome occurs on stopping any benzodiazepine, even a short-acting one which should always be done gradually. Symptoms include insomnia, anxiety, loss of appetite, tremor, confusion and a psychosis.

Non-benzodiazepines

- Zaleplon, zolpidem and zopiclone all act at the benzodiazepine receptor and are used for insomnia. Dosages are zaleplon 10 mg, zolpidem 10 mg (5 mg in the elderly) and zopiclone 3.75–7.5 mg at night. They should not be used in patients with severe hepatic or renal disease.
- Side-effects include headache, diarrhea, nausea, confusion and daytime drowsiness. Non-benzodiazepines do not cause any withdrawal symptoms but dependence has been reported.

The red eye

This is a common condition and can be a medical emergency. It can be associated with pain, a sticky, watery eye, reduced vision/visual loss and photophobia.

- A painful red eye with visual problems is due to glaucoma (see below), severe inflammation, acute anterior uveitis, infective endophthalmitis, or central corneal ulcers or abscesses.
- A painful eye without visual problems is due to early anterior uveitis, peripheral corneal ulcers or erosions, keratitis or anterior scleritis.
- Non-painful eyes may be associated with a purulent discharge (bacterial, viral, chlamydial, infective conjunctivitis); a sticky, watery discharge (hay fever, acute allergy, allergic conjunctivitis); grittiness (e.g. blepharitis, sicca syndrome); and photophobia (e.g. keratitis, herpes simplex, early iritis, corneal abrasion). Other causes, e.g. episcleritis, marginal ulcers, pterygium or rosacea keratitis, can produce a sector of redness.

Box 1.6 gives the red flags for a red eye. URGENT REFERRAL TO EYE CLINIC IS MANDATORY.

Kumar & Clark's Medical Management and Therapeutics

> **Box 1.6** Red flags for a red eye
>
> The following symptoms require urgent referral:
> - Severe pain
> - Photophobia
> - Reduced vision
> - Coloured haloes around point of light in a patient's vision
> - Proptosis
> - Smaller pupil in affected eye
>
> Plus, on medical assessment:
> - High intra-ocular pressure
> - Corneal epithelial disruption
> - Shallow anterior chamber depth
> - Ciliary flush

Conjunctivitis

This is the commonest cause of a red eye. There is inflammation causing soreness and a discharge but the visual acuity is usually, but not always, good. It can arise from a number of causes:

● Viral conjunctivitis (e.g. adenovirus) may be associated with a watery discharge and a cold or sore throat. It is commonly associated with chemosis, lid oedema and a palpable pre-auricular lymph node. Viral conjunctivitis can cause deterioration in visual acuity owing to corneal involvement (focal areas of inflammation). In 50% of patients the conjunctivitis is unilateral.

   • *Treatment* is usually self-limiting. Lubricants, together with a cold compress, can be soothing. Strict hygiene and keeping towels separate from the rest of the household reduce spread. Topical steroids are used in patients with corneal involvement or intense conjunctival inflammation.

● Bacterial conjunctivitis is uncommon (5%) and causes grittiness without visual problems. There is a mucopurulent discharge and conjunctivitis can be rapid in onset (e.g. gonococcus). Less acute inflammation can be due to *Haemophilus influenzae* and *Streptococcus pneumoniae*.

   • *Treatment* should be given promptly with oral and topical **penicillin** in gonococcal conjunctivitis to reduce the rate of corneal perforation. A Gram stain of the conjunctival swab can quickly confirm the presence of diplococci. Gonococcal conjunctivitis is a notifiable disease in the UK.

   • *Empirical treatment* for both subacute and chronic bacterial conjunctivitis involves a topical broad-spectrum antibiotic such as **chloramphenicol**. Swabs should be taken if these cases do not respond to this initial treatment.

● Allergic conjunctivitis causes an itchy, stringy discharge and can be due to various types viz. seasonal, perennial, vernal, atopic and giant papillary. Seasonal allergic conjunctivitis and perennial conjunctivitis affect 20% of the general population. The main symptoms include itching, redness, soreness, watering and a stringy discharge.

   • *Treatment* reduces the allergen load (e.g. dust) and antihistamine drops are given, e.g. **azelastine** and **emedastine**, along with topical mast cell-stabilizing agents such as **sodium cromoglicate** and **nedocromil**. **Olopatadine** has a dual action and is both an antihistamine and a mast cell stabilising agent. Corticosteroid drops should be avoided. Oral antihistamines help the itching.

Acute angle-closure glaucoma (AACG)

This is an ophthalmic emergency, presenting with an acute red, painful eye and blurred vision. The patient is unwell, with nausea, vomiting and headache. The eye is injected and tender; the cornea is hazy and the pupil is semi-dilated.

AACG usually occurs in the older person when there is a sudden rise in intra-ocular pressure (IOP) to levels greater than 50 mmHg.

● Treatment must be prompt to preserve the sight.

   • Give IV **acetazolamide** 500 mg (provided there are no contraindications) to reduce IOP. Instillation of **pilocarpine 4% drops** to constrict the pupil improves aqueous outflow and prevents iris adhesion to the trabecular meshwork.

- Other topical drops, such as β-blockers and prostaglandin analogues, can also be instilled if available, provided there are no contraindications.
- Give analgesia and antiemetics as required.
- Refer to an ophthalmologist immediately for reduction in IOP and monitoring. Other agents, e.g. oral glycerol or IV mannitol, can be administered to non-responding patients. Definitive treatment requires laser or surgery to make a hole in the periphery of the iris of both eyes.

Anterior uveitis (iritis)

The classical presentation is with a triad of redness, pain and photophobia. Vision is normal or blurred, depending on the degree of inflammation. Redness may be general or localized. On examination, keratic precipitates (KP) are seen on the corneal endothelium, with fibrin or hypopyon (pus), and the pupil may have adhered to the lens (posterior synechiae). The IOP may be normal or raised either due to cells clogging up the trabecular meshwork or because of posterior synechiae and reducing aqueous drainage.

● Treatment

- Reduce inflammation with topical steroids, e.g. dexamethasone 0.1% every 30–60 mins until the inflammation is controlled and then reduce to 4 times daily.
- Dilate the pupil with cyclopentolate 1% to prevent formation of posterior synechiae. Dilatation also allows fundoscopy to exclude posterior segment involvement.
- If the IOP is raised, treat with topical β-blockers, e.g. timolol 0.25%, prostaglandin analogues, e.g. latanoprost 50 mcg/mL once daily, or oral or IV acetazolamide 0.25 mg–1 g daily in divided doses.
- Refer to an ophthalmologist.

Pain management

Many patients complain of pain and require treatment, often without a precise diagnosis, e.g. non-specific headache. Before medication is prescribed, reassurance and explanation are often helpful.

Pain in palliative care is discussed on p. 292.

Analgesics, e.g. NSAIDs as used in rheumatic disorders, are discussed on p. 298. They (e.g. diclofenac 150 mg orally, IV, IM or rectally in 2–3 divided doses daily) are also useful in ureteric colic if renal function is normal and in post-operative musculoskeletal pain, for example.

Simple and compound analgesic agents

These include:

● Paracetamol (acetaminophen) 0.5–1 g orally, rectally or IV. Maximum dose 4 g per 24 hours. This has antipyretic and analgesic actions but is not an anti-inflammatory or antiplatelet drug, in contrast to aspirin. It does not produce gastric irritation. For post-operative pain, an IV infusion, 1 g every 4–6 hours, is given over 15 mins as a 10 mg/mL solution.

● Aspirin (non-selective COX-2 inhibitor) oral 200–900 mg, 4–6-hourly. Maximum dose 4 g daily. This has analgesic, antipyretic and anti-inflammatory actions, as well as an effect on platelets. Side-effects include gastrointestinal irritation. It is contraindicated in patients

Kumar & Clark's Medical Management and Therapeutics

under 16 years of age because of a risk of Reye's syndrome. Aspirin is rarely used in the UK for pain relief.

- Codeine (opioid) oral/IM 30–60 mg 4-hourly; maximum dose 240 mg per 24 hours. It has analgesic effects but is seldom given on its own for pain but rather used in combination with the above. Its main side-effect is constipation, and large doses over long periods can produce opiate addiction.

- Combinations of the drugs listed above are frequently used, e.g. **co-codamol**, 1–2 tablets 4-hourly (codeine and paracetamol; preparations with varying strengths of codeine are available); **co-dydramol**, 1–2 tablets 4–6-hourly (dihydrocodeine 10 mg and paracetamol 500 mg). Side-effects will be the same as those of paracetamol plus the opioids.

Severe pain

If simple analgesia or NSAIDs are ineffective, opioid analgesics are used.

- Tramadol 50–100 mg orally every 4 hours; 50–100 mg IV every 4–6 hours. Apart from its opioid action it enhances the serotonergic and adrenergic pathways. It has fewer typical opioid side-effects.

- Morphine is the opioid of choice. It is given by SC or IM injections, 10 mg (maximum 3 doses in 24 hours), titrated to response. It causes nausea and vomiting, and therefore an antiemetic, e.g. **metoclopramide** 10 mg, is usually given. Opioid side-effects include constipation, drowsiness and respiratory depression in high doses. IV morphine should be administered in an area of close observation because of the risk of respiratory depression.

   Diamorphine (heroin) is often used in place of morphine in the UK. It causes less nausea and hypotension than morphine. Please check dosages!

- Opioid reversal can be achieved with naloxone 0.4–2 mg IV. The dose (maximum 3 doses in 24 hours) can be incrementally increased by 100 mcg over 2 mins if there is an inadequate response. The half-life of naloxone is considerably shorter than that of morphine, so expect to administer the reversal agent on multiple occasions until opiates have been cleared.

Patient-controlled analgesia (PCA)

This consists of a pre-programmed pump allowing the patient to self-administer a pre-determined dose of a drug such as morphine. The dose (usually 1 mg initially) should be modified after taking into account the patient's age, weight and previous treatment with an opioid drug. Following a single dose the machine has a 'lockout' period (about 5 mins but this can be varied) when the patient cannot administer another dose until the first one has taken effect. Antiemetics may be required for the nausea.

Pressure ulcers (decubitus ulcers, bedsores)

Normal individuals feel the pain of continued pressure, and even during sleep, movement takes place to change position continually. However, ulcers can occur in the elderly and in immobile, unconscious or paralysed patients. They are due to skin ischaemia from sustained pressure over a bony prominence, usually the heel and sacrum. They can develop within 1–2 hours, particularly in patients on hard emergency room trolleys; 70% occur within 2 weeks of hospitalization. Once they develop, they are difficult to heal and are associated with an increased mortality. Pressure sores may be graded:

- Stage I: non-blanchable erythema of intact skin. This early stage can rapidly lead to ulcers if not dealt with urgently.
- Stage II: partial-thickness skin loss of epidermis/dermis (blister or shallow ulcer).
- Stage III: full-thickness skin loss involving subcutaneous tissue but not fascia.
- Stage IV: full-thickness skin loss with involvement of muscle/bone/tendon/joint capsule. Granulation will not occur over these tissues and formal surgical debridement and closure is indicated.

Prevention

Prevention is better than cure. Risk assessment is vital and is often provided by specialist 'tissue viability nurses'.

Several risk assessment tools have been devised, e.g. the **Norton scale** for pressure sores, the **Waterlow pressure sore risk assessment**. These enable staff to identify patients who are most at risk.

Skin care with daily inspection of the area is necessary, along with:

- pillows and fleeces to keep pressure off bony areas (e.g. sacrum and heels) and prevent friction
- special pressure-relieving mattresses and beds
- regular turning, but avoiding pressure on hips
- air-filled cushions for patients in wheelchairs
- adequate nutrition.

Treatment

- Non-irritant occlusive moist dressings (e.g. hydrocolloid).
- Adequate analgesia (opiates may be needed).
- Plastic surgery (debridement and grafting in selected cases).
- Treatment of underlying condition.

Further reading

General Medical Council: *Good Medical Practice*, London, 2006, GMC.
Kumar P, Clark M: *Kumar & Clark's Clinical Medicine*, ed 7, Edinburgh, 2009, Saunders.

Further information

www.mcpcil.org.uk/liverpool-care-pathway
Liverpool care of the dying pathway

Infectious disease 2

APPROACH TO THE PATIENT WITH A SUSPECTED INFECTION

Infectious diseases are the most common cause of illness in humans worldwide and can affect any organ. Fever is the cardinal symptom but not all infectious diseases will present with a fever. Fever can be defined as a temperature of $\geq 37.8°C$, although this may vary between 37.5°C and 38.0°C.

- **History** should include overseas travel; animal contact; exposure to sick individuals; tick, insect or animal bites; sexual activity with risk factors; IV drug users; leisure activity, e.g. freshwater-borne infections.
- **Examination** should include ears, eyes, mouth and throat, and all systems, including rectal, vaginal and penile examination for STIs. Rashes and lymphadenopathy are common in infectious diseases.
- **Investigations** may not be required, particularly in the primary healthcare setting if the patient is relatively well. In general, the following investigations should be conducted in anyone who is unwell and requires hospital attention:
  - FBC and ESR
  - blood cultures
  - serum save to microbiology
  - U&E, liver biochemistry, glucose and CRP
  - CXR
  - urinalysis and culture
  - if indicated by travel history — malaria — perform three blood smears if initial sample negative.
- **Management**
  - Take samples for cultures and tests above.
  - Give 'blind' antibiotics if the patient is unwell or if meningitis or septicaemia is likely. This 'blind' therapy should cover likely

Table 2.1 Causes of febrile illness in travellers returning from the Tropics and world-wide

Developing countries	Specific geographical areas (see text)
Malaria	Histoplasmosis
Schistosomiasis	Brucellosis
Dengue	**World-wide**
Tick typhus	Influenza
Typhoid	Pneumonia
Tuberculosis	Upper respiratory tract infection
Dysentery	Urinary tract infection
Hepatitis A	Traveller's diarrhea
Amoebiasis	Viral infection

pathogens with broad-spectrum antibiotics, e.g. IV cefotaxime 8-hourly is often used.
- The regimen should be changed when the organism (and sensitivities) are identified.

Returning travellers (Table 2.1)

There are number of common illnesses that occur only in certain areas. The history should cover all recent travel. Most tropical illnesses are uncommon in the countries in which they occur; upper respiratory tract infections, urinary tract infections and viral infections are still common worldwide. However, some illnesses, such as **malaria** or **dengue**, are common. WHO advises that fever occurring in a traveller 1 week or more after entering a malaria risk area and up to 3 months after departure is a medical emergency because of the mortality associated with *Plasmodium falciparum,* though there have been well-reported cases of *falciparum* infection occurring after 3 months. **Viral haemorrhagic fevers** are also seen in patients returning from endemic areas, though these are very rare infections. Websites are a useful source of up-to-date information on geographic medicine and epidemics (e.g. www.cdc.gov/travel/destinat.htm).

Fever of unknown origin (FUO)

One definition of a fever of unknown origin is 'a fever persisting for more than 2 weeks, with no clear diagnosis despite intelligent and intensive investigation'. The definition of FUO has also been refined to include classical FUO, nosocomial FUO, neutropenic FUO and HIV-related FUO.

The causes of FUO, when determined, are infections (20–40%), e.g. endocarditis, TB, Lyme disease; connective tissue disease, e.g. polymyalgia (15–20%); malignancy, e.g. lymphoma (10–30%); and miscellaneous (e.g. drugs).

Fever and rash

The presentation of fever and rash in an adult has many potential causes. These range from severe life-threatening infections, such as meningococcal sepsis or toxic shock syndrome, to the usually mild infections of parvovirus or enterovirus. Travel-related illnesses include dengue, typhus or typhoid. Illnesses such as syphilis or HIV seroconversion illness can also present with a fever and rash.

Investigations

Initial investigations should include the following:

- FBC, LFTs, CRP
- blood cultures (repeated)
- skin biopsy for microscopy (Gram stain), culture or PCR if appropriate
- appropriate imaging.

A low platelet count would tend to indicate either a viral infection or possibly malaria. A lymphopenia may also indicate a viral infection, whereas a neutrophilia occurs in a bacterial infection. Treatment may be delayed until a diagnosis is made or appears highly likely. However, if serious infection, such as meningococcal sepsis, is suspected, then antimicrobial therapy must be started immediately.

SYSTEMIC MULTI-SYSTEM INFECTIONS

Sepsis

Sepsis is a leading cause of death worldwide and is usually the result of an overwhelming bacterial infection. Most infections, whether bacterial, fungal or viral, initiate a systemic inflammatory response with the release of vasodilatory and pro-inflammatory substances, including cytokines, histamine and prostaglandins. This results in endothelial damage, capillary leak and vasodilatation, causing tissue hypoperfusion. Additionally, the coagulation pathway is activated by a number of cytokines, resulting in microthrombi and further tissue ischaemia. The mortality rate for severe sepsis remains about 30%.

Clinical features

Patients are pyrexial (occasionally hypothermic) and often hypotensive, and have rigors, warm peripheries and a bounding pulse. Hypotension may not be present, particularly in children and young adults. They can be hyperglycaemic or, in severe cases, hypoglycaemic.

A consensus definition (1991) of **sepsis immune response syndrome (SIRS)** for adults considers two or more of the following features to be present:

- heart rate > 90 beats per min
- body temperature < 36°C or > 38°C
- respiratory rate > 20 breaths per min or $Paco_2$ < 4.3 kPa
- white blood cell count < 4×10^9/L or > 12×10^9/L, or > 10% immature (band) forms on film.

Septicaemia is defined as SIRS plus the detection of a positive blood culture. **Bacteraemia** is the presence of bacteria in the bloodstream without SIRS or in an asymptomatic patient.

Severe sepsis is sepsis complicated by organ dysfunction or hypotension.

Septic shock is sepsis with hypotension in adults with a systolic BP < 90 mmHg, a mean arterial pressure < 60 mmHg, or a reduction of > 40 mmHg in the systolic BP from baseline.

Kumar & Clark's Medical Management and Therapeutics

Management

Sepsis and septic shock should be treated **urgently**, as should the bacterial cause of the infection.

● Patients should have close monitoring (intensive care) and be adequately supported with IV fluid volume replacement, inotropes and adequate oxygenation.

● Therapy to optimize the mixed venous oxygen saturation has been shown to improve survival from sepsis significantly.

● Adjunctive therapy of severe sepsis with **activated protein C (drotrecogin alfa activated)** may be of benefit. Evidence for other adjunctive therapies, such as the use of steroids, is disappointing. Tight glycaemic control is now not recommended (p. 539).

● Blood tests should include FBC, U&E, LFTs and CRP.

● Blood cultures × 2 (at least) should be taken from different sites prior to antibiotic therapy.

● Early IV **antibiotic therapy** should be given. The exact choice of antibiotic depends on the probable source of sepsis. If the source of sepsis is completely unknown, then choose antibacterial agents that treat a broad range of Gram-positive and Gram-negative bacteria (such as **co-amoxiclav** 1.2 g IV 3 times daily, **cefotaxime** 1 g twice daily IV to maximum of 8 g daily, plus **gentamicin** 5–7 mg/kg IV daily).

● **Neutropenic sepsis** may often be caused by *Pseudomonas aeruginosa* and these patients should be treated with an antipseudomonal β-lactam antibiotic (such as **piperacillin/tazobactam** 4.5 g 6-hourly IV infusion or **meropenem** 1 g 8-hourly) plus an aminoglycoside. If there is a permanent IV line in situ, then glycopeptides may need to be added. Failure of fever to resolve should indicate the need to investigate the possibility of a fungal or viral infection and/or to use a glycopeptide to treat resistant gram negative infections.

● **Asplenic patients** can develop sepsis from encapsulated organisms, e.g. *Streptococcus pneumoniae*, *Neisseria meningitidis* or *Haemophilus influenzae*. Give a third-generation cephalosporin (**ceftriaxone** IV infusion 2–4 g daily ± **vancomycin** 1–1.5 g IV infusion 12-hourly).

Meningococcal septicaemia

Neisseria meningitidis is found worldwide. There are five major serogroups. The organism carried asymptomatically in the nasopharynx of 5–20% of the general population. Invasion into the bloodstream (septicaemia-causing disease) depends on both host and bacterial factors.

Presentation is with the classic triad of headache, fever and neck stiffness, though this is not always the case (p. 54). Septicaemia causes septic shock with fever, myalgia and hypotension, and may be accompanied by a petechial or haemorrhagic rash. The case fatality rate is approximately 10%.

N.B. *If not treated immediately, patients can deteriorate rapidly, with shock, disseminated intravascular coagulation, multi-organ failure and death.*

Diagnosis

Diagnosis is frequently clinical with:

● presence of a rash (Fig. 2.1)

● Gram stain showing diplococci in CSF (not always necessary) or aspirate of petechiae

● culture of blood, CSF or aspirate

● PCR of above samples if necessary.

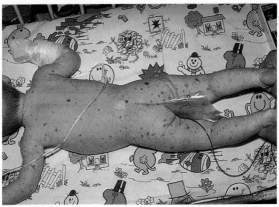

Fig. 2.1 Meningococcal septicaemia showing a purpuric rash.

Management (Box 2.1)

Start antibiotics *immediately*.

- cefotaxime 2 g 6-hourly IV for 7 days *or*
- benzyl penicillin 2.4 g 4-hourly by IV infusion.

Patient contacts in the household and 'kissing' contacts should be given prophylaxis with oral **rifampicin** 600 mg 6-hourly for 2 days or **ciprofloxacin** 500 mg single dose to eradicate bacteria from the nasopharynx. Group C disease contacts should be offered immunization.

> **Box 2.1** Meningococcal meningitis and meningococcaemia: emergency treatment
>
> Suspicion of meningococcal infection is a medical emergency requiring treatment immediately
>
> **Clinical features**
> - Petechial or non-specific blotchy red rash
> - Fever, headache, neck stiffness
>
> All these features may not be present — and meningococcal infection may sometimes begin like any apparently non-serious infection
>
> **Immediate treatment for suspected meningococcal meningitis at first contact before transfer to hospital or investigation**
> - Benzylpenicillin 1200 mg (adult dose) slow IV injection or intramuscularly
> - Alternative if penicillin allergy — cefotaxime 2 g IV ×4 daily
>
> In meningitis, minutes count; delay is unacceptable
>
> **On arrival in hospital**
> - Routine tests including blood cultures immediately
> - Watch out for septicaemic shock

Kumar & Clark's Medical Management and Therapeutics

Malaria

Malaria in humans is caused by *Plasmodium falciparum* (most severe form), *Plasmodium vivax*, *Plasmodium ovale*, *Plasmodium malariae* or rarely *Plasmodium knowlesi*, which are transmitted by the *Anopheles* mosquito. *P. vivax* and *P. malariae* may recur after many years, but *P. falciparum* and *P. malariae* do not recur, although individuals may be reinfected. *P. falciparum* causes a potentially fatal malaria that results in about 1–2 million deaths annually, most in children in sub-Saharan Africa. The other causes of malaria are very rarely fatal and may be regarded as the benign malarias.

Clinical features

Patients present with fever and other generalized features, such as malaise, headache, vomiting, diarrhoea and sweats, 10–21 days (occasionally months) after a mosquito bite. Symptoms can be mild or severe with complications (e.g. cerebral malaria) (see below). Repeated infections cause ill health, anaemia and hypersplenism with splenomegaly.

Diagnosis

- Peripheral blood film can detect asexual forms of the appropriate *Plasmodium*. This is usually done by microscopy. A single negative blood film examination does not exclude malaria and should be performed three times on three consecutive days. Speciation of malaria parasites should be performed by a skilled examiner if necessary. If there is any doubt as to the species or whether or not an infection is present, then the infection should be assumed to be *P. falciparum* until it can be proven otherwise.
- Antigen detection kits are available for *P. falciparum* and other malarias that rely on the detection of parasite histidine-rich protein 2 or lactate dehydrogenase.
- Real-time PCR for *P. falciparum* and some benign malarias is marginally more sensitive and specific than microscopy but is expensive, difficult to perform and not yet in routine clinical practice.

P. falciparum infection causes about 200 million infections worldwide annually. WHO advises that fever occuring in a traveller one week or more after entering a malaria risk area and up to three months after departure is a medical emergency because of the mortality associated with *P. falciparum*. Cases have been reported up to 5 years after leaving a malarial area. Three blood films should be performed. *Falciparum* malaria is divided into severe and uncomplicated forms.

Severe malaria can present differently in adults and children, but may be defined as the presence of the following features:
- Glasgow coma score ≤ 9/15
- hypoglycaemia (blood glucose ≤ 2.2 mmol/L)
- severe anaemia (Hb ≤ 5 g/dL)
- renal failure
- acidosis (pH < 7.25), hyperlactataemia (≥ 5 mmol/L)
- hyperparasitaemia (> 5%)
- Respiratory distress.

The case fatality rate of severe malaria remains between 15 and 30%, despite adequate antiparasitic treatment and good supportive management.

Management of uncomplicated *falciparum* malaria

The treatment of malaria varies, depending on the resistance patterns to antimalarial chemotherapy and will vary over time. Up-to-date advice

Table 2.2 Drug treatment of uncomplicated malaria in adults

Type of malaria	Drug treatment
Plasmodium vivax, P. ovale, P. malariae	**Chloroquine** 600 mg 300 mg 6 hours later 300 mg 24 hours later 300 mg 24 hours later
P. falciparum (almost all are resistant to chloroquine)	**Quinine** 600 mg 3 times daily for 7 days Plus **Doxycycline** 200 mg once daily for 7 days Or **Clindamycin** 450 mg 3 times daily for 7 days (**Fansidar** (SP) (pyrimethamine and sulfadoxine) 3 tablets as single dose with or following quinine) Or **Malarone** 4 tablets daily for 3 days Or **Riamet** (artemether with lumefantrine) 4 tablets 12-hourly for 3 days
	Alternative therapy **Artesunate-mefloquine** 12/25 mg/kg daily for 3 days Or **Dihydroartemisinin/piperaquine** 6.3 mg/kg daily for 3 days

should be sought if there are doubts as to the appropriate therapy. There is very little chloroquine-sensitive *falciparum* malaria. Treatments for uncomplicated *falciparum* malaria are shown in Table 2.2.

Management of severe *falciparum* malaria (Box 2.2)

- In non-endemic countries, all cases of *falciparum* malaria should be admitted to hospital for at least 1–2 days to ensure there is no immediate deterioration. It can be a medical emergency and require intensive care therapy.
- Artesunate 2.4 mg/kg single bolus by IV injection can be given if available, then at 12 and 24 hours, thereafter daily until oral medication can be tolerated. It does not cause hypoglycaemia. A recent trial found a lower death rate in patients with severe malaria treated with artesunate compared to quinine-treated patients. Artemisinin resistance has been reported in Cambodia. Artesunate is also available as rectal suppositories. However, if artesunate is difficult to obtain then quinine therapy should not be delayed.
- Quinine salts is an alternative. 20 mg/kg IV loading dose (max. 1.2 g) given over 4 hours, followed by 10 mg/kg IV over 4 hours 3 times daily should be used to treat severe malaria. IV administration may induce

> **Box 2.2** Drug treatment of severe chloroquine-resistant *P. falciparum* malaria in adults
>
> **Full hospital facilities**
> - **Artesunate** 2.4 mg/kg by IV injection, then 1.2 mg/kg over 4 hours every 8 hours
>
> *or*
> - **Quinine salt** 20 mg/kg IV infused over 4 hours, followed by 10 mg/kg
>
> **No infusion available**
> - **Quinine dihydrochloride** (diluted 1:1 in water) given by divided IM injection (regimen as for IV) — half into each thigh
>
> **No injection available**
> - **Artemisinin** rectal suppositories (limited availability)
> - Rectal **quinimax** or **quinine**

hypoglycaemia, and any patient receiving IV quinine should have a glucose infusion and regular (4-hourly) blood glucose monitoring. Quinine may be given orally as soon as the patient is able to tolerate oral medication (600 mg 3 times daily) to complete a week of therapy.

- Exchange transfusion is of unproven benefit in the treatment of severe malaria; it has a number of complications and should only be used in adults with a parasitaemia of > 10% after specialist advice has been sought.

Management of non-*falciparum* malaria

Non-*falciparum* malarias can be treated with oral **chloroquine** 600 mg, then 300 mg after 8 hours, then 300 mg daily for 2 days. There is some reported chloroquine-resistant malaria in Papua New Guinea and treatment can be with **riamet** or **malarone** (dosages in Table 2.2). *P. vivax* and *P. ovale* have hypnozoites that may persist and cause a recurrence of infection many years later. Patients with *vivax* or *ovale* infection should receive **primaquine** 15 mg daily for 2–3 weeks following successful treatment, to eradicate hepatic hypnozoites and prevent relapse. Anyone who is about to receive primaquine should have their glucose-6-phosphate dehydrogenase (G6PD) status checked, as primaquine use is associated with haemolysis in patients with G6PD deficiency (p. 216). WHO guidelines www.who.int/topics/malaria/en.

Prevention of malaria

- Avoidance of mosquito bites with mosquito repellants and permethrin-impregnated bed-nets can reduce transmission of malaria by similar amounts to chemoprophylaxis. The advice given to travellers to the tropics about the risks of malaria at their destinations and the need for malaria chemoprophylaxis should be up to date, as it changes over time.
- Currently available alternatives for chemoprophylaxis in adults are **atovaquone/proguanil** (**malarone** 1 tablet daily), **mefloquine** 250 mg weekly and **doxycycline** 100 mg daily.
- Chloroquine-resistant *P. falciparum* is so common that there are very few places where **chloroquine** 300 mg weekly/**proguanil** 200 mg daily prophylaxis can currently be recommended.

- **Prophylaxis** should usually be started a week (malarone — only 1 day) before travel and continued for 4 weeks after return. It should also be stressed in advice to patients that malaria chemoprophylaxis is not 100% effective; should they become febrile after return from a malarial area, they should still suspect malaria.

Dengue

Dengue is caused by a flavivirus that is carried by the daytime-biting *Aedes* mosquito. It is found throughout most of the tropics and is particularly common in South-East Asia and the Caribbean. The incubation period is about 5–7 days.

Clinical features

An acute febrile illness with very severe musculoskeletal pain, severe headache with retro-orbital pain, severe malaise, lymphadenopathy and sometimes a maculo-papular rash occur. The fever subsides after 3–4 days and then returns.

Dengue haemorrhagic fever (DHF) may occur as a result of a second or subsequent infection with a different dengue serotype and may be caused by an abnormal immune response to dengue infection. It presents with severe bleeding (haematemesis and melaena), a severe capillary leak and hypotension.

Investigations

Investigations show a low platelet count, normal white cell count and sometimes mildly abnormal liver biochemistry. See Figure 2.2 for the course and timing of diagnosis.

Treatment

There are no specific antiviral therapies currently available for the treatment of dengue fever but adequate fluid replacement in DHF is essential; blood transfusion is given if necessary. Corticosteroids are of no proven benefit. Convalescence is slow.

Leptospirosis

Leptospirosis is a zoonosis caused by a number of species of the genus *Leptospira*. Leptospirosis is found worldwide, but is particularly common

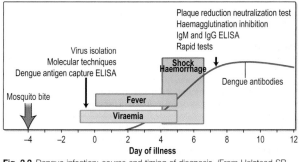

Fig. 2.2 Dengue infection: course and timing of diagnosis. (From Halstead SB 2007, with permission.)

in South-East Asia. A chronic renal infection in the animal reservoir (usually rodents) is the usual source of infection in humans, disease in humans being acquired through contact with water contaminated with rodent urine. Around 90% of infections are thought to result in a self-limiting febrile illness, but some result in a severe and potentially fatal illness. The incubation period is 5–14 days.

Clinical features

The main features of severe leptospirosis are fever, anorexia, jaundice, myalgia, conjunctival suffusion, and hepatic and renal failure. The case fatality rate of severe leptospirosis is about 5–40%.

Diagnosis

Diagnosis of leptospirosis is by culture or serological tests. There should be early liaison with the laboratory, as specialized culture techniques improve diagnosis.

Treatment

Treatment of severe disease is with **benzyl penicillin** 1.2 g IV 4 times daily or **ceftriaxone** 1 g IV daily. **Doxycycline** 100 mg twice daily may be used in mild disease. Jarisch–Herxheimer reactions have been reported after treatment.

Plague

Sporadic cases (as well as occasional epidemics) of plague occur world-wide, the majority in sub-Saharan Africa, although disease is occasionally seen in the southern states of the USA. Plague is caused by a Gram-negative bacillus, *Yersinia pestis*. The main reservoirs are rodents. The usual vector is the rat flea.

Clinical features

Clinical manifestations of plague are bubonic, septicaemic, pneumonic, pharyngeal and meningitis.

Diagnosis

Diagnosis is by clinical suspicion and culture of *Y. pestis* from blood, sputum or aspirate of a bubo. A rapid immunodermatographic dipstick test is also available, and has high sensitivity and specificity.

Treatment

The treatment of choice is **streptomycin** 15 mg/kg IM twice daily for at least 7 days or **gentamicin** 5 mg/kg IV daily for 10 days. Oral **tetracycline**, **quinolones** and **chloramphenicol** are also effective. Post-exposure prophylaxis is with **doxycycline** or **ciprofloxacin**.

Brucellosis

Brucellosis is a zoonosis and nearly all human infections result from direct or indirect exposure to animals. Farmers, veterinarians and abattoir workers are particularly at risk. Spread is following direct contact with infected animals or by the consumption of unpasteurized dairy products from cows, goats or sheep. The pathogens are members of the genus *Brucella*: in humans usually *B. abortus*, *B. melitensis* and *B. canis*. Brucellosis has a worldwide distribution, although it has been eliminated from the UK. It is especially common in the Mediterranean, India and the Arabian Peninsula.

Clinical features

The onset is insidious, with an incubation period about 2–4 weeks. Symptoms are initially non-specific, although specific ones include an 'undulant' fever, malodorous sweat and a peculiar taste in the mouth. Brucellosis can affect nearly any organ of the body and includes lymphadenopathy, hepatosplenomegaly, sacro-iliitis, arthritis, osteomyelitis and meningoencephalitis. Chronic brucellosis can last over a year. Symptoms may also recur over long periods.

Investigations

- White cell count is normal/low. CRP and ESR are variable.
- Blood and bone marrow cultures (which have a higher yield) should be performed. *Brucella* may also be cultured from CSF, lymph nodes or liver biopsies. There should be liaison with the laboratory, as a prolonged incubation is required and laboratory transmission of *Brucella* should be prevented.
- Serological tests with rising antibody titres on ELISA may aid diagnosis if culture results remain negative.

Treatment

- WHO recommends treatment for 6 weeks with **doxycycline** 200 mg daily and **rifampicin** 600–900 mg daily, but relapses occur.
- **Doxycycline** 200 mg daily for 6 weeks and **streptomycin** 1 g IM daily for 2–3 weeks or **gentamicin** are also used.

Listeriosis

Listeria monocytogenes causes an infection of many animal species. It is also widespread in the environment in soil and decayed matter. The organism can grow at low temperatures and may be transmitted in foods such as unpasteurized cheeses and pâtés.

Clinical features

- In healthy adults, *Listeria* causes a self-limiting febrile gastroenteritis, the incidence of which is unknown. A brainstem encephalitis can occur in healthy adults; CSF examination may be normal, although these patients are often bacteraemic and MRI may be useful.
- In pregnant women, neonates, and elderly or immunosuppressed patients, *Listeria* can cause serious problems.
  - *In pregnancy* bacteraemia usually occurs in the last trimester and presents as a flu-like illness, but infection of the fetus can lead to septic abortion, premature labour and stillbirth. Early treatment may prevent fetal loss but the rate remains about 50%.
  - *In neonates Listeria* may manifest as an early-onset sepsis in the premature infant, acquired in utero. A second, late-onset form occurs about 2 weeks after birth and usually presents as a meningitis.
  - *In the elderly and the immunocompromised Listeria* usually causes meningitis or bacteraemia; a variety of other focal infections have been described.

Investigations

Listeriosis is established by culture of blood, CSF or other body fluids.

Treatment

The treatment of choice for adult listeriosis is **ampicillin** plus **gentamicin**. **Co-trimoxazole** is also effective.

Q fever

Infection with the obligate intracellular pathogen *Coxiella burnetii*, which is widespread in many animals, is the cause of Q fever. Transmission to

Kumar & Clark's Medical Management and Therapeutics

humans is usually via dust, aerosol and unpasteurized milk; spore formation means that the infection can remain in the environment for long periods.

The incubation period is 2–4 weeks. Onset is insidious, with fever, myalgia and headache, but pneumonia and hepatitis may occur. Occasionally, endocarditis or other focal infections may cause chronic illness.

- Diagnosis is made serologically or by nested PCR (low sensitivity).
- Treatment is with **doxycycline** 200 mg daily for 14 days. The addition of chloroquinine is used in chronic infection.

Lyme disease

Lyme disease is found in North America, Europe and Asia, and is caused by infection with the spirochaete *Borrelia burgdorferi*, of which there are several genomic species. It is a zoonosis transmitted to man by ixodid ticks, the main animal reservoir being deer or occasionally other mammals. Infections usually occur after visiting woodland.

There are three stages of Lyme infection:

- Stage 1 disease is a localized infection, presenting about a week after the tick bite with erythema migrans (a macular rash), lymphadenopathy, and associated fever and headache.
- Stage 2 disease occurs several days to weeks after the appearance of erythema migrans. Some patients may develop a more widespread rash, and after several weeks or months around 15% of untreated cases develop neurological complications such as meningitis, encephalitis, cranial or peripheral neuritis, or radiculopathies. About 5% of patients develop cardiac involvement. Myalgia and arthritis may also occur at this stage.
- Stage 3 disease commonly causes a chronic arthritis (usually of the knees), but may also cause chronic encephalomyelitis and other neurological disorders or acrodermatitis chronica atrophicans. The evidence for persistent infection at this stage is lacking.

Diagnosis

This may occasionally be established by finding spirochaetes in CSF or skin samples. Serodiagnosis is usually performed to confirm the diagnosis, with an IgM response detectable in the first month. Some care should be taken in interpreting results, as false positives may occur.

Treatment

- Amoxicillin 500 mg 3 times daily for 14–21 days or **doxycycline** 100 mg twice daily for 14–21 days can be used to treat early infection or isolated facial palsies. The duration of amoxicillin or doxycycline treatment should be increased to 30–60 days for stage 2 disease.
- Ceftriaxone 2 g IV daily for 14–28 days should be used if there is neurological involvement or cardiac involvement, e.g. second- or third-degree atrioventricular block.
- Prevention is necessary in tick-infested areas with repellants and protective clothing. Ticks must be removed promptly.

Visceral leishmaniasis

Visceral leishmaniasis (kala-azar) is caused by *Leishmania donovani*, *L. infantum* or *L. chagasi*, and is present in India, Asia, Africa, the Mediterranean and South America. In central India, humans are the main host and the disease occurs in epidemics. In most other areas, it is a zoonosis; the main animal reservoirs are dogs and foxes, although in Africa it is carried by rodents. Visceral leishmaniasis is a common opportunistic infection of advanced HIV disease in Mediterranean coastal regions.

Clinical features

The incubation period is usually 1–2 months but may be much longer. Fever and splenomegaly are common features, pancytopenia and hepatomegaly are often present, and lymphadenopathy is common in Africa. If the infection is untreated, death usually occurs within a year with worsening pancytopenia and weight loss.

Diagnosis

This is confirmed by finding the parasite in aspirates of bone marrow, liver, lymph node or spleen, though in inexperienced hands these can occasionally be mistaken for histoplasmosis.

● Nucleic acid amplification and specialized culture techniques are available from specialist centres.
● Serology can be useful.

Treatment

● The drug of choice is IV **amphotericin B** (preferably given in the liposomal form), but this is expensive and is not widely available in many areas where the disease is prevalent.
● **Miltefosine** may be an oral alternative to amphotericin B.
● In areas where resources are limited, **pentavalent antimony salts** are used, but these are toxic drugs and should be given after specialist advice.

Rickettsial diseases

Rickettsia and the closely related species, *Orientia*, are small intracellular bacteria that are spread by arthropods (ticks, lice, mites). The reservoir of infection is usually mammalian (often rodent) but may be human. The incubation period is 4–21 days and rickettsial illnesses are characterized by fever, rash and headache. A black spot or *eschar* may be present at the site of the tick bite, which is painless. Renal failure and haematological, neurological or cardiovascular abnormalities may complicate the illness, but these are rare.

Diagnosis

This can be confirmed serologically.

Treatment

● **Doxycycline** 100 mg twice daily for 5–7 days and **rifampicin** 600 mg daily are also effective if tetracyclines cannot be used.
● Prophylaxis for scrub typhus is with weekly oral **doxycycline** 200 mg, but only in highly endemic areas.

Epstein–Barr virus (EBV)

This herpes virus commonly causes infections, mainly in adolescents and young adults worldwide. It is probably transmitted in saliva and by aerosol.

Clinical features

● Infectious mononucleosis (sometimes referred to as glandular fever) produces a fever, headache, malaise, lymphadenopathy and sore throat. A transient macular rash is common if amoxicillin is given. Mild hepatitis and splenomegaly are common. **Severe complications**, such as meningoencephalitis, myocarditis and splenic rupture, are rare.

- A post-viral syndrome may occasionally occur after the acute infection, with patients feeling lethargic for a number of months. Like other herpes viruses, EBV remains latent for life but reactivation in the immunocompetent is controversial.

EBV is implicated in the aetiology of a number of malignancies, including Burkitt's lymphoma, nasopharyngeal carcinoma and post-transplant lymphoma, and in HIV disease with primary cerebral lymphoma, Hodgkin's lymphoma and oral leucoplakia.

Investigations
- Specific IgG and IgM EBV antibodies detect the infection.
- PCR is available for the detection of EBV DNA in CSF and other body fluids; this may be particularly useful in the diagnosis of meningoencephalitis or primary cerebral lymphoma in HIV infection.

Treatment
Most cases of EBV infection require no specific treatment. The efficacy of antiviral treatment of EBV-associated tumours or EBV in immunosuppressed patients remains unproven; steroids may be of use in some complications, such as thrombocytopenia or haemolysis.

SKIN AND SOFT-TISSUE INFECTIONS

Skin infections result in a number of different conditions. The most common organisms causing skin infections are group A streptococci and *Staphylococcus aureus*.

- Impetigo — weeping exudative area, often on the face, with a honey-coloured crust on the surface due to *Staph. aureus* or group A streptococci.
- Cellulitis — confluent erythema of the skin, often tender. Cellulitis affects the lower leg or sometimes the face, and is associated with a high temperature. It is commonly caused by a streptococcus, or less frequently a staphylococcus.
- Folliculitis — inflammation of hair follicles, presenting as tender papules and pustules. Folliculitis is very commonly caused by *Staph. aureus*.
- Boils — deep-seated inflammation of the skin, causing painful red swellings, sometimes with pus. Boils are usually caused by staphylococci.

Treatment
Treatment should be started empirically and should cover both *Staph. aureus* and streptococcal infections. If oral therapy is appropriate, then **flucloxacillin** 500 mg 4 times daily and **amoxicillin** 500 mg 3 times daily are reasonable choices; the duration of therapy depends on response, but is usually around a week. **Clindamycin** 300–450 mg 4 times daily, **clarithromycin** 500 mg orally 2 times daily for 7 days or another macrolide is used in penicillin-allergic patients.

In severe or extensive infections, high-dose IV **benzyl penicillin** 1.2–1.8 g IV 4-hourly and **flucloxacillin** 1–2 g IV 6-hourly will be required. High-dose IV **clindamycin** or a **macrolide** is used in penicillin-allergic patients. Collections of pus may need to be drained, and in cellulitis elevation of the affected limb speeds recovery.

Meticillin-resistant *Staph. aureus* (MRSA)

The *mec-A* gene in *Staph. aureus* makes it resistant to meticillin, oxacillin, flucloxacillin and nearly all other β-lactam antibiotics. The incidence of MRSA has increased over the last 25 years and in some hospitals more than 50% of *Staph. aureus* are MRSA; the prevalence of community-acquired MRSA is increasing.

Like meticillin-sensitive *Staph. aureus (MSSA)*, MRSA is usually a harmless skin colonizer, particularly in hospital inpatients. However, both can cause a variety of invasive infections, e.g. soft-tissues infections, bacteraemias, pneumonias and line infections. The case fatality rate of invasive MRSA infections is greater than that of MSSA. Eradication of MRSA carriage is possible, though sometimes difficult. Isolation of patients, strict hand washing, good IV catheter care and other infection control procedures should be observed. Control of the use of antibiotics in hospitals and good infection control policies are vital to prevent spread.

Community-acquired MRSA (CA-MRSA) may have different resistance profiles to hospital strains (often retaining sensitivities) as regards tetracycline, clindamycin and co-trimoxazole. It often produces the exotoxin Panton–Valentine leucocidin and is an increasingly common cause of soft-tissue infections, particularly in the USA (USA300 strain).

Treatment

Treatment of MRSA infection depends on the source of the infection and the sensitivity of the MRSA.

Antibiotics active against MRSA include the glycopeptides (vancomycin and teicoplanin), rifampicin, the tetracyclines and fusidic acid.

- Serious invasive MRSA infections should, in general, be treated with a glycopeptide (e.g. **vancomycin** 1 g IV twice daily), and often a second agent is added, such as **rifampicin** for MRSA pneumonia, **fusidic acid** for MRSA osteomyelitis, or **gentamicin** or **rifampicin** for MRSA endocarditis.
- MRSA bacteraemia should be treated for at least 2 weeks but, for example, MRSA endocarditis or osteomyelitis must be treated for longer.
- Less serious infections, such as mild cellulitis, can be treated with two oral agents, such as a **tetracycline**, co-trimoxazole or a combination of fusidic acid and **rifampicin**.
- Newer agents include **linezolid**, **quinupristin/dalfopristin**, **daptomycin** and **tigecycline**. **Linezolid** may have advantages over vancomycin; linezolid has better penetration into lung tissue and skin, but the clinical benefit is yet to be confirmed. These new drugs should not yet be used as first-line treatment for MRSA infections.

Glycopeptide-intermediate *Staph. aureus* (GISA) and vancomycin-resistance in *Staph. aureus* (VRSA)

- GISA develops because of changes in cell wall synthesis.
- VRSA, which has acquired the *van A* gene from vancomycin-resistant enterococci, has also been reported but is rare.

Staphylococcal toxic shock syndrome (TSS)

TSS is an acute febrile illness characterized by a generalized erythematous rash that nearly always starts within the first 24 hours of illness, desquamating after about 1 week. The most common symptoms include fever

(>40° C), hypotension, and diffuse rash with desquamation. TSS ranges in severity from a mild disease to a severe life-threatening illness. It is due to toxin production by *Staph. aureus*. TSS toxin-1 (**TSST**-1) acts as a superantigen that stimulates non-specific T-cell proliferation. For streptococcal toxic shock syndrome, see below.

In the early 1980s, most cases of TSS were in menstruating females and associated with retained tampons. Recently, TSS has been less often associated with menstruation.

- Treatment is by removal of the source of the staphylococcal infection and treatment with **flucloxacillin** 1–2 g IV 4 times daily.

Post-streptococcal syndromes

Strep. pyogenes infections usually cause localized throat or skin infections. However, there are a number of immune-associated, generalized complications of *Strep. pyogenes*.

Rheumatic fever

This is a multi-system inflammatory disorder, occurring in children and young adults as a result of a pharyngeal infection with a group A streptococcus. It is due to molecular mimicry between cell wall M proteins of some group A streptococcus strains, and cardiac laminin and myosin and synovial membrane. Rheumatic fever is much less common in Western Europe and the USA than in other parts of the world; this may be due in part to the treatment of streptococcal infections, e.g. sore throats. The diagnosis of rheumatic fever is made according to the revised Duckett–Jones criteria. The major criteria are carditis, polyarthritis, chorea, erythema marginatum and subcutaneous nodules, while the minor criteria include fever and arthralgia.

- Diagnosis. This is made on the basis of two or more major criteria, or one major criterion plus two or more minor criteria, with evidence of recent streptococcal infection, e.g. positive throat cultures or raised antistreptolysin O titre.
- Treatment
  - **Aspirin/NSAIDs** produce a dramatic response.
  - **Bed rest** is advised. **Steroids** are used if carditis is present but their efficacy remains unproven.
  - Streptococcal infections should be eradicated with oral **phenoxymethylpenicillin** 500 mg 4 times daily for 10 days.
- Prophylaxis. Oral **phenoxymethylpenicillin** 250 mg twice daily, until the age of 20 years or for 5 years after the latest attack, is used for prophylaxis against further episodes of rheumatic fever. This is most common after an episode of carditis. **Erythromycin** is used if the patient is allergic to penicillin.
- Complications. Chronic rheumatic valvular disease develops in just over half of those who have acute rheumatic fever complicated by carditis (after 10–20 years). The mitral and aortic valves are mainly affected.

Other post-streptococcal syndromes

- Scarlet fever is a diffuse, erythematous, 1–2 mm, 'sandpaper'-like rash that results from the production of pyrogenic exotoxin (erythrogenic toxin, types A, B and C) produced by group A streptococcus, usually after a pharyngeal infection. The rash usually starts on the head and then proceeds downwards, but sparing the palms and soles. The rash often exhibits a linear character in the axillary folds (Pastia's lines). Scarlet fever is diagnosed clinically and with a culture-positive throat swab.

- Streptococcal toxic shock syndrome (STSS) is a febrile illness associated with a streptococcal infection. It is similar to staphylococcal TSS and results from the production of superantigens produced by streptococcal infections.
- Glomerulonephritis — see p. 343.

Cat scratch fever

This is caused by *Bartonella henselae*. Regional lymphadenopathy occurs 1–2 weeks after infection. This resolves after weeks or months and is not accompanied by systemic symptoms. **Doxycycline** can be used.

Herpes simplex (HSV)

HSV1 is spread by direct contact and droplet infection. The primary illness produces a fever with painful blisters on the face or a painful gingivostomatitis. Recrudescence of HSV blisters appears as cold sores.

- Treatment is with topical aciclovir; if infection is severe, use oral **aciclovir** 200 mg 5 times daily for 5 days.

Myositis

Pyomyositis is an acute bacterial infection of skeletal muscle that is usually caused by *Staph. aureus* and occasionally by streptococci or other organisms.

- Treatment is with prompt surgical debridement with **benzyl penicillin** 1.2 g IV 4 times daily and **flucloxacillin** 500 mg 4 times daily.

Gas gangrene

Gas gangrene is caused by infection with *Clostridium perfringens* or occasionally with other species of *Clostridia*. It is characterized by the absence of pus and the presence of gas in the tissues. It may be difficult to distinguish from necrotising fasciitis, except during surgery, though the presence of gas on X-ray and crepitation in the tissues is useful.

- Treatment is with prompt surgical debridement and high-dose **benzyl penicillin** 2.4 g IV 6 times daily and **clindamycin** 1.2 g IV 4 times daily. Hyperbaric oxygen therapy is also advised, although there is no RCT to support the use of this therapy.

Necrotising skin and soft-tissue infections

These are defined as soft-tissue infections spreading along the fascial planes with or without an overlying cellulitis. They are serious infections with mortality as high as 40%. Clinically, these patients are very unwell and pain is a prominent symptom, out of proportion to the skin findings. The causative organism is usually group A streptococcus, though other organisms can cause this syndrome; if the infection follows abdominal surgery or a testicular infection (Fournier's gangrene), then mixed infections with anaerobic and aerobic organisms (synergistic gangrene) occur. *Vibrio vulnificans* infection may be contracted from sea water.

- Diagnosis is made clinically and these patients should be rapidly assessed by a specialist surgeon. High white cell count and high CRP are usually present. US/CT may be helpful but should not delay early surgery.

- **Treatment** is with wide and aggressive surgical debridement, which may need to be repeated on a number of occasions.
  - Antibiotic therapy for group A streptococcus is with high-dose **benzyl penicillin** 2.4 g IV 6 times daily and **clindamycin** 1.2 g IV 4 times daily.
  - If a synergistic infection is suspected, then treatment should cover anaerobes and Gram-negative organisms; suitable drugs could include **ampicillin**, **gentamicin** and **metronidazole**; **ampicillin**, **gentamicin** and **clindamycin**; or **co-amoxiclav**, **gentamicin** and **metronidazole**.

Bite wounds

The major problem resulting from bite wounds is infection, but this will depend on the site, extent and cause.

- Dog bites. These are the commonest type of bite (80%) but only a few become infected. The oral flora of dogs contains streptococci, staphylococci, *Pasteurella multocida* and *Capnocytophaga canimorsus*.
  - *Treatment.* If the bite is infected, give **co-amoxiclav** 500 mg 8-hourly for 7 days. This can also be used as prophylaxis for 3–5 days.
- Cat bites. Most of these become infected and prophylaxis with co-amoxiclav should always be given.
  - *Treatment.* If the bite is infected, give **co-amoxiclav** or **doxycycline** 100 mg daily. Increase the duration to 2 weeks for cellulitis and longer for osteomyelitis.
- Wild animal bites. The danger here is rabies and vaccination must be given (p. 56). **Co-amoxiclav** is a reasonable choice for prophylaxis.

General measures for bite wounds

- Investigations include culture of swabs from wounds.
- Foreign bodies should be removed and the wound irrigated.
- Do not suture unless the bite is on the face.
- Elevate if possible.
- Give antibiotics as above.
- If there is a fracture, X-ray the relevant area. Vaccinate against rabies (p. 57).

Varicella zoster virus (VZV) infection

Primary infection with VZV is in childhood in Europe and the Americas. In some countries (e.g. in South Asia) transmission is different, with more infections in adults.

The primary infection with VZV causes **chickenpox**, which almost never occurs again in the same person. Chickenpox is infectious from 2 days before the start of the rash until all the vesicles have crusted. The incubation period of chickenpox is 14–21 days. There is a brief 'flu-like prodromal illness, which may be absent in the young. A rash then develops, with macules rapidly progressing to vesicles, mainly on the head and trunk. The rash occurs in 'crops', with skin lesions in all stages typically present on the body. Eventually, the vesicles crust and heal without scarring. Chickenpox is highly infectious and is spread from infected lesions and by the respiratory route. After recovery, VZV remains latent for life in spinal nerve roots. The illness tends to be more severe in adults, particularly pregnant women, smokers and the immunosuppressed. **Complications** of chickenpox include pneumonia, bacterial superinfection of skin lesions and meningo-encephalitis. VZV can cross the placenta and infection in pregnancy leads to fetal damage in about 2% of cases, mostly in infections before 20 weeks' gestation.

Shingles is a secondary reactivation of latent VZV infection in the distribution of one or sometimes two dermatomes. The vesicles of shingles are identical to those in chickenpox. Shingles mainly affects the elderly but can occur at any age. Post-herpetic neuralgia may occur after herpes infection and causes severe debilitating pain. Shingles involving the ophthalmic division of the trigeminal nerve has a high rate of complications. Disseminated shingles infection can occur in the immunosuppressed patients (particularly in late HIV infection), when the rash is seen over many dermatomes and appears similar to chickenpox. Shingles lesions may transmit infection to non-immune individuals.

Diagnosis

Diagnosis is clinical but, if necessary, can be confirmed with immunofluorescence, electron microscopy or viral culture of vesicle fluid.

Treatment

- Healthy children with chickenpox usually require no treatment and infection results in lifelong immunity.
- Adults with chickenpox should be given antiviral treatment, if they present within 72 hours of onset, with **aciclovir** (800 mg oral 5 times daily for 7 days) or oral **valaciclovir** or **famciclovir**.
- Severe VZV infection, particularly in the immunosuppressed or pregnant women, should be treated with **IV aciclovir** (10 mg/kg IV 3 times daily).
- Zoster immune immunoglobulin (ZIG) can be used as post-exposure prophylaxis in the immunocompromised or pregnant, with no past infection with chickenpox who has been exposed to VZV.
- An effective varicella vaccine is available but is not recommended as routine in all countries.
- Shingles is also treated with **aciclovir** (800 mg orally 5 times daily for 7 days), as early treatment reduces the duration of symptoms and the occurrence of neuralgia.
- Prophylactic therapy with **aciclovir** can be used to prevent HSV and VZV in immunocompromised patients. In the USA **varicella zoster vaccine** is recommended for all people over 65 years.

Leprosy (Hansen's disease)

Leprosy is caused by *Mycobacterium leprae*, an acid-fast bacillus. The majority of cases are in India and Brazil. The prevalence of leprosy has decreased since a successful WHO treatment campaign.

The incubation period is very variable but is usually 2–6 years. The signs of leprosy are usually skin lesions, usually anaesthetic and thickened peripheral nerves. Leprosy is classified between two polar extremes of tuberculoid (high degree of cell-mediated immunity (CMI)) and lepromatous (impaired CMI), depending on the host's immune reaction to the infection (Ridley–Jopling system).

Diagnosis and treatment

It is not possible to culture *M. leprae* but diagnosis is made clinically and on microscopic examination of tissue. The type of treatment and its duration depend on the type of leprosy. **Rifampicin**, **clofazimine** and **dapsone** are the main drugs used (p. 87).

RESPIRATORY INFECTIONS

Upper respiratory tract infections

Pharyngitis

Most throat infections are caused by viruses and do not need antimicrobial therapy, but it is difficult to differentiate between viral and bacterial causes in all patients. Patients with three of the following are more likely to have bacterial rather than viral infection: fever, purulent tonsils, cervical lymphadenopathy and absence of cough. *Strep. pyogenes* (Lancefield group A β-haemolytic streptococcus) is the major bacterial cause of pharyngitis and is commoner in the age group 5–15. A history of contact with a patient with proven *Strep. pyogenes* infection is helpful in diagnosis.

- **Investigations.** Rapid antigen detection tests may be helpful but, like throat cultures, will also be positive in those who have throat colonization with *Strep. pyogenes*.
- **Treatment.** If antibacterial treatment is given, the first choice should be oral **phenoxymethylpenicillin** 500 mg 4 times daily for 10 days. **Amoxicillin** and **ampicillin** should not be given unless infection with EBV can be ruled out. For penicillin-allergic patients, a macrolide (e.g. **erythromycin** 250 mg 4 times daily or 500 mg twice daily) or an oral **cephalosporin** can be given for 10 days. Rarer bacterial causes of pharyngitis include *Arcanobacterium haemolyticum*, which can be treated with erythromycin.

Diphtheria

See p. 49.

Acute laryngo-tracheobronchitis (croup)

This causes paroxysms of cough with breathlessness and stridor. It is caused initially by viral infections, e.g. parainfluenza, complicated by bacterial infection. The voice is hoarse with a barking cough (croup) and audible laryngeal stridor.

- **Treatment.** Oral **corticosteroids** and **nebulized adrenaline (epinephrine)** are helpful. Oxygen with adequate rehydration is necessary.

Epiglottitis

This presents with a sudden onset of fever, sore throat and stridor, which may rapidly progress to complete airway obstruction. In children, the bacterial causes of epiglottitis include group A streptococcus, *Strep. pneumoniae* and *Staph. aureus*. Capsulated strains of *H. influenzae*, e.g. type b, are now rare in countries that immunize against this pathogen (Hib vaccine). A swab from the epiglottis may reveal the causative organism, but this could potentially provoke airway obstruction and should only be carried out if facilities for intubation are present. Blood cultures should also be taken.

- **Treatment. Cefotaxime** 50 mg/kg IV 4 times daily or **ceftriaxone** 50 mg/kg IV daily is the first-choice agent. For patients who are allergic to cephalosporins, **chloramphenicol** 25 mg/kg IV 4 times daily is used. Epiglottitis is rare in adults but the spectrum of bacteria is similar to that seen in children and cefotaxime, ceftriaxone or chloramphenicol can be used at adult doses.

Coryza

Coryza (the common cold) is caused by viruses. There are currently no effective antimicrobial treatments.

Sinusitis

Most episodes of sinusitis are viral and will resolve without antimicrobial therapy. The symptoms of bacterial infection are maxillary/facial pain, and purulent discharge after 7–10 days. The likely organisms are *Strep. pneumoniae, H. influenzae, Moraxella catarrhalis,* group A streptococcus, *Staph. aureus* and anaerobes in chronic infection.

- Treatment. Appropriate antibacterials include **amoxicillin** 500 mg 3 times daily for 7 days, oral **doxycycline** 200 mg, followed by 100 mg daily for 7 days or **erythromycin** 250 mg 4 times daily or 500 mg twice daily for 7 days. If there is a failure to respond or the patient has recently received antibacterial treatment, **co-amoxiclav** 625 mg 3 times daily for 7 days or **ciprofloxacin** 500 mg twice daily for 7 days, combined with **metronidazole** 400 mg twice daily for 7 days, can be used. Chronic infection usually requires surgery.

Otitis media

This is predominantly an infection of children. Most episodes are viral and will resolve without antimicrobial treatment. Although bacterial infection may occur with *Strep. pneumoniae, H. influenzae,* group A streptococcus and *Staph. aureus,* use of antibacterials is of questionable value, as most cases get better without treatment.

- Treatment. If the child remains unwell for more than 3 days, antibacterials can be used, including **amoxicillin** (< 2 years, 125 mg 3 times daily; 2–10 years, 250 mg 3 times daily; > 10 years, 500 mg 3 times daily, all for 5 days). If the patient is allergic to penicillin, **erythromycin** (< 2 years, 125 mg 4 times daily; 2–8 years, 250 mg 4 times daily; > 8 years, 250–500 mg 4 times daily) can be given for 5 days or **azithromycin** (15–25 kg, 200 mg daily; 26–35 kg 300 mg; 36–45 kg 400 mg daily) for 3 days.

Diphtheria

Diphtheria is caused by pharyngeal or cutaneous infection with **toxigenic** strains of *Corynebacterium diphtheriae* and, rarely, toxigenic strains of *C. ulcerans.* Classical diphtheria presents with a membranous pharyngitis, cervical lymphadenopathy and oedema of the surrounding soft tissues. The membrane, which is not always present, is typically grey, thick and adherent. Laryngeal involvement also occurs, and causes hoarseness and stridor. **Nasal diphtheria** may present as a bloody nasal discharge. **Cutaneous diphtheria** is commoner in tropical countries and usually affects the legs. The lesions start as vesicles and progress to form ulcers.

- Diagnosis. Diagnosis relies on a combination of clinical and laboratory findings, with the demonstration of a toxigenic isolate of *C. diphtheriae* from throat, nose or skin swabs.
- Treatment. A combination of antitoxin to neutralize the toxin and antibacterials to eradicate the organism is needed, though the benefit of antitoxin in cutaneous infection is uncertain. Appropriate antibacterials include **IV erythromycin** 40 mg/kg a day, until the patient can swallow, when oral **erythromycin** 500 mg 4 times daily or oral **phenoxymethylpenicillin** 250 mg 4 times daily can be given. Antibacterials should be given for 14 days and a throat swab taken to check for elimination of the organism. If the culture is still positive, a further 10 days' treatment is needed. Cases should also be **immunized** in the convalescent stage. **Close contacts** require antibacterial prophylaxis with **erythromycin** 500 mg 4 times daily for 7 days. If cultures are positive from close contacts, a further 10 days' treatment is needed. Those contacts who

Kumar & Clark's Medical Management and Therapeutics

have not been immunized in the preceding 12 months require vaccine. Non-toxigenic strains of *C. diphtheriae* may cause severe pharyngitis, which can be treated with **oral erythromycin** 500 mg 4 times daily for 7 days or **phenoxymethylpenicillin** 250 mg 4 times daily for 7 days.

Measles

This is a vaccine-preventable viral infection and no specific antiviral treatment is available. The incubation period ranges from 7 to 18 days. There is a prodromal illness with fever, conjunctivitis, cough and often diarrhoea. This is followed, usually 2 or 3 days later, with a rash that starts on the face and spreads to the trunk, lasting for 4–7 days. Measles is a self-limiting illness but complications are relatively frequent. **Diagnosis** is by demonstration of viral antigen on PCR in nasopharyngeal aspirates or urine, or by demonstration of IgM antibody in blood or saliva. Otitis media and pneumonia may follow and antibacterials can be used for these complications. **Inosine pranobex** has been used to treat the rare complication, subacute sclerosing panencephalitis, but there is little evidence of any benefit.

Mumps

This is a vaccine-preventable viral infection and no specific antiviral treatment is available. The incubation ranges from 18 to 21 days. Mumps is a febrile illness characterized by inflammation of the salivary glands, particularly the parotids, which are swollen and tender. It is a self-limiting illness and complications are rare. Aseptic meningitis, orchitis and oophoritis and pancreatitis may occur. **Diagnosis** is usually by demonstration of IgM antibody in blood or saliva.

Rubella (German measles)

Rubella is a worldwide viral disease spread by droplets. The incubation is 14–21 days; the rash begins 7 days after the onset of malaise, fever, conjunctivitis and lymphadenopathy. The rash is pinkish red, macular and discrete. Treatment is supportive and complications are rare. Congenital rubella syndrome affects fetuses in ~80% of women who contract the disease in the first trimester.

Prevention is with the MMR vaccine.

Lower respiratory tract infections

Influenza

Influenza A and influenza B viruses are a cause. The incubation period is from 1 to 4 days, and patients present with fever, headache, malaise, generalized aches, cough and sore throat. Secondary bacterial infection is common and secondary pneumonia caused by *Staph. aureus* has a mortality of 20%. Rapid diagnosis can be made by antigen detection or the nucleic acid amplification test (NAAT) from nasopharyngeal aspirate or throat washings, and acute and convalescent serology. Prevention by immunization is necessary in people over 65 years of age, those who are immunosuppressed, those with chronic respiratory, cardiac, renal and liver disease, and those with diabetes mellitus.

- **Treatment.** The neuraminidase inhibitors, **oseltamivir** 75 mg twice daily for 5 days and **zanamivir** 10 mg by inhalation twice daily for 5 days, can shorten duration of illness and may reduce complications if started as soon as possible after symptoms start (no more than 48 hours after onset).

- **Prophylaxis.** Oseltamivir 75 mg orally once daily for 7 days following exposure, or for up to 6 weeks during an epidemic, is used if current vaccine does not cover the circulating strain of the virus. **Amantadine** and **rimantadine** may also be used for treatment and prophylaxis, although adverse effects are common.

- **H1N1.** A variant H1N1 virus, originally seen only in pigs, caused an influenza in humans initially in 2009, with mostly mild symptoms. However, deaths have occurred and many countries have been affected. This virus is susceptible to oseltamivir, although resistance is found.
- **Avian flu.** In 1997 and again in 2004 and 2005, the avian H5N1 strain of influenza A was found in humans, initially transmitted from poultry but also spreading from human to human. The illness is similar to but more severe than that caused by other influenza viruses.

Pertussis (whooping cough)

Whooping cough is a vaccine-preventable acute bacterial infection caused by *Bordetella pertussis*. The incubation period ranges from 7 to 13 days. **Clinically**, three stages of illness are recognized: a catarrhal stage, a paroxysmal stage and a convalescent stage. In infants, adolescents and adults, these stages may not be so obvious. In adults, a chronic cough may the only symptom. **Complications** of infection include bronchopneumonia and seizures, which are more likely in infants.

- **Diagnosis.** This can be confirmed by culture of *B. pertussis* from a pernasal swab or by PCR from the same specimen. Cultures and PCR are more likely to be positive in the early stages of infection. Serology can also be useful for diagnosis later in the infection.
- **Treatment.** Treatment should be confined to those who are diagnosed within 21 days of onset of symptoms. Antibacterials have little effect on resolution of symptoms but can reduce infectivity of the case. **Erythromycin** (< 2 years, 125 mg 4 times daily; 2–8 years, 250 mg 4 times daily; others, 500 mg 4 times daily, all for 7 days) is given. Cases are likely to be no longer infectious after 5 days of treatment. Patients should complete their immunization schedule for pertussis. Unimmunized or partly immunized contacts of infectious cases can be given prophylaxis with **erythromycin** (< 2 years, 125 mg 4 times daily; 2–8 years, 250 mg 4 times daily; others, 500 mg 4 times daily, all for 7 days). **Azithromycin** (15–25 kg, 200 mg daily; 26–35 kg, 300 mg daily; 36–45 kg, 400 mg daily; adults, 500 mg daily, for 5 days) can also be used. **Contacts** should also be immunized unless it is certain that they have completed a full schedule previously.

Pneumonia

See p. 505.

Tuberculosis

See p. 512.

Lung abscess

The pathogenesis of lung abscess is variable. It may follow **pneumonia** (especially aspiration pneumonia), bacteraemic spread (e.g. IV drug users), foreign body, or bronchial obstruction with a tumour. Bacteria include anaerobes, enteric Gram-negative bacilli, *Strep. milleri*, *Strep. pneumoniae* and *Staphylococcus aureus*, especially in right-sided endocarditis. Lung abscess presents with fever, night sweats, breathlessness, and a cough with foul-smelling sputum.

- **Investigations.**
  - CXR — cavity formation
  - Blood and sputum culture

- **Treatment.** Treatment will be led by culture results but suitable agents include **clindamycin** 450 mg 4 times daily or 600 mg IV 4 times daily, or **cefotaxime** 1 g IV 3 times daily and **metronidazole** 500 mg IV 3 times daily, or **co-amoxiclav** 1.2 g IV 4 times daily. If *Staph. aureus* is isolated, **flucloxacillin** 500 mg IV 4 times daily and **oral sodium fusidate** 500 mg 3 times daily are used. The duration of treatment will depend on response and many patients will need surgical drainage or broncho-scopic relief of obstruction.

CARDIOLOGICAL INFECTIONS

Infective endocarditis (IE)

IE is a severe life-threatening infection that still has a high mortality despite advances in cardiac surgery and antibacterial therapy. It predominantly affects individuals with structural abnormalities of the cardiac valves, which may be congenital or acquired. IE occurs following a bacteraemic spread to the valve. **Bacteraemia** may follow dental or other surgical procedures or as a result of infection at another site. IV drug users are also at risk. Endocarditis may also result from infected intravascular devices in hospital patients. The commonest bacterial causes of IE are α-haemolytic streptococci, enterococci and *Staph. aureus*; in prosthetic valve IE, coagulase-negative staphylococci are most common.

Clinical features

Symptoms include fever, malaise and weight loss. Embolic phenomena and vasculitic lesions may also be evident. A new valvular murmur may be heard. The duration of symptoms often reflects the bacterial aetiology. IE caused by *Staph. aureus* usually has an acute presentation, often with neurological complications, e.g. cerebrovascular events. IE caused by α-haemolytic streptococci has a more indolent presentation over weeks or months. Patients with right-sided endocarditis may present with a lung abscess.

Diagnosis

The Duke Criteria are the established way of making the diagnosis clinically.

- **Blood cultures** are the key diagnostic investigation. At least three sets of samples should be taken and there should be liaison with the micro-biology department.
- **Trans-thoracic echocardiogram** is a rapid, non-invasive investigation and has a high specificity for visualizing vegetations, although sensitiv-ity is 60–75%.
- **Trans-oesophageal echocardiography (TOE)** has a higher sensitivity and specificity for abscess formation because of the physical proximity of the transducer to the aortic root. A negative echo does not exclude the diagnosis in a patient with a fever but it does lower the probability.
- **Inflammatory markers**, e.g. ESR and CRP, are raised and liver biochem-istry is usually mildly deranged.
- **Microscopic haematuria** is almost always present.

Treatment

High concentrations of IV antibiotics are required for prolonged periods to achieve successful treatment, as IE still carries a substantial morbidity and mortality. Empirical antibiotic treatment is started only after cultures are taken and is then adjusted according to the culture results. The treatment should continue for 4–6 weeks.

- Clinical endocarditis culture results awaited with no suspicion of staphylococci: **benzyl penicillin** 1.2 g 4-hourly, **gentamicin** 80 mg every 12 hours.
  - *If suspected staphylococcal endocarditis:* **vancomycin** 1 g 12-hourly, **gentamicin** 80 mg 8-hourly.
  - *If cardiac prosthesis, penicillin allergy or MRSA:* vancomycin and rifampicin.
- When culture is confirmed:
  - *Streptococcal endocarditis:* penicillin-sensitive: treatment as above.
  - *Enterococcal endocarditis:* **amoxicillin** 2 g 4-hourly, **gentamicin** 80 mg 12-hourly.
  - *Staphylococcal endocarditis:* **vancomycin** 1 g 12-hourly, or **flucloxacillin** 2 g 4-hourly or **benzyl penicillin** 1.2 g 4-hourly plus **gentamicin** 80–120 mg 8-hourly. **Vancomycin** and **gentamicin** levels must be monitored. Choice will depend on sensitivities. Liaise with an infectious diseases expert.
- Prophylactic therapy prior to invasive procedure: not necessary unless there is an infection at the site of the proposed intervention (see national guidelines).

Pericarditis

Pericarditis is inflammation of the pericardium, giving rise to chest pain and a pericardial friction rub, with concave upward elevation of the ST segment in all leads on the ECG. **Acute infective pericarditis** is caused by viruses, e.g. Coxsackie B and echovirus, and by a variety of bacteria, including *Strep. pneumoniae* (following pneumonia), *Staph. aureus,* group A streptococcus and *N. meningitidis.* In acute bacterial pericarditis, fever and signs of heart failure due to tamponade occur. TB presents less acutely! Diagnosis of bacterial pericarditis including TB can be confirmed by culture of pericardial fluid. Pericardial biopsy may be needed to diagnose TB.

- Treatment will be guided by culture findings but empirical therapy with **cefotaxime** 1 g IV 3 times daily is suitable. If *Staph. aureus* is suspected, **flucloxacillin** 2 g IV 4 times daily should be added.

Non-infective pericarditis occurs following a myocardial infarct (p. 445), in malignant disease (lung cancer, lymphoma), in uraemia and after surgery.

Chronic pericarditis
See p. 460.

Myocarditis

Acute inflammation of the myocardium is commonly due to viruses, e.g. Coxsackie, adenoviruses or influenza viruses. It can also be caused by rickettsial, fungal, bacterial or parasitic infections, drug hypersensitivity, autoimmunity and other factors. Presentation is with palpitations, chest pain, breathlessness and fatigue.

- Investigations: CXR, ECG, viral antibodies, PCR, echo and nasopharyngeal swab. A myocardial biopsy may be helpful.
- Treatment: depends on the cause. Antiviral agents are not usually helpful.

RHEUMATOLOGICAL INFECTIONS

Infective arthritis

See p. 321.

Osteomyelitis

See p. 323.

NEUROLOGICAL INFECTIONS

Meningitis

Meningitis is inflammation of the meninges; it is usually caused by infection, although rarely it results from a non-infectious cause. Infectious causes of meningitis include bacterial (including TB), viral and fungal (e.g. cryptococcal). Acute bacterial meningitis is a medical emergency and should be considered in any patient with fever and neurological symptoms, especially if there is a history of other infections or head trauma.

Clinical features

- Meningitis usually presents with headache, neck stiffness, photophobia and fever. Vomiting, myalgia, impaired consciousness and rash are often present, particularly in bacterial meningitis. In acute bacterial infection there is usually intense malaise, fever, rigors, severe headache, photophobia and vomiting.
- Signs of meningitis include fever, rash, a positive Kernig's sign, neck stiffness and head jolt; of these signs, the head jolt is one of the more reliable.

Investigations

In bacterial meningitis there is usually a **neutrophilia** and a **raised CRP**.

- CT should be performed immediately if raised intracranial pressure (ICP) is suspected (e.g. loss of consciousness).
- CSF examination by lumbar puncture (LP) is carried out in the absence of contraindications (e.g. signs of raised ICP, papilloedema or impaired consciousness). **N.B.** *If a petechial rash is present, indicating meningococcal infection, IV penicillin or cefotaxime must be given IMMEDIATELY* and an LP is not necessary. In cases without a meningococcal rash, CSF examination confirms the diagnosis and gives information about cause, prognosis and antibiotic sensitivities. An LP is still useful even if antibiotics are given beforehand, or if the LP is deferred until the patient is stabilized.
- PCR of blood for *N. meningitidis* is helpful if LP is not possible or the CSF is culture-negative.
- Viral stool and throat cultures, as well as **viral PCR of CSF**, will often detect the viral cause of meningitis.

Treatment

Treatment is with antimicrobial therapy and supportive measures, including maintenance of airways and electrolyte balance. **Dexamethasone** 0.15 mg/kg 4 times daily for 4 days is given, especially if *Strep. pneumoniae* meningitis is suspected, although corticosteroids should be avoided if septic shock is a factor.

- Initial therapy with 'unknown cause' should be with **cefotaxime** 2 g IV 4 times daily or **ceftriaxone** 2 g IV twice daily. Alternative antibiotics (if the patient is allergic) include **benzyl penicillin** 2.4–4.8 g daily IV in 4 divided doses and **chloramphenicol** oral or IV infusion 50 mg/kg in 4 divided doses for β-lactam allergy.

- *N. meningitidis* (see also p. 33 and Box 2.1) is treated with IV **benzyl penicillin**. Alternatively, high-dose **cefotaxime** 2 g IV 4 times daily or **ceftriaxone** 2 g IV twice daily for about 7 days (at least 5 days after the patient is febrile) is given. For close contacts, prophylaxis and eradication, see p. 33.
- *Strep. pneumoniae* is treated with **cefotaxime** 2 g IV 4 times daily for 10–14 days or **benzyl penicillin** (see above). **Vancomycin** 1 g IV twice daily, though CSF penetration may be poor, and **rifampicin** can be given if there is known or suspected resistance. **Dexamethasone** 0.15 mg/kg 4 times daily for 4 days should also be given.
- *L. monocytogenes* (suspect in patients > 55 years old or the immuno-suppressed) is treated with **ampicillin** 2 g IV 4 times daily or with **gentamicin** slow IV infusion 3–5 mg/kg/day in 2 divided doses for 3–4 weeks. Listeria is resistant to cephalosporins.

Other forms of meningitis

- Tuberculous meningitis presents with vague headaches, lassitude, ano-rexia and vomiting. Evidence of meningism takes weeks to develop. LP shows high protein and low glucose levels.
  - *Treatment* with anti-TB drugs (p. 87) is often on a presumptive basis. A glucocorticoid should also be given (adults, equivalent to pred-nisolone 20–40 mg if on rifampicin; otherwise 10–20 mg).
- Viral meningitis This presents with fever, headache, photophobia and meningism similar to bacterial meningitis but often less severe. Viral meningitis is usually a self-limiting condition lasting 4–10 days, although a headache may persist for some time. The CSF usually con-tains lymphocytes.
  - *Treatment* is symptomatic.

Encephalitis

Encephalitis is inflammation of the brain that usually results in fever, impaired consciousness, confusion and occasionally convulsions. The cause is usually viral; the most common causes of encephalitis in Europe are HSV, enterovirus, mumps, EBV, VZV and influenza. Often, viral aetiol-ogy is presumed but never confirmed. Bacterial causes of encephalitis include listeria, syphilis, mycoplasma, and Lyme disease. There are a number of causes of encephalitis that occur in certain specific areas, which include **Japanese B encephalitis** and **enterovirus** in South-East Asia, Ross River fever in Australia, rabies in many countries, and West Nile encepha-litis in Egypt and Sudan. Outbreaks of encephalitis occur, such as a West Nile virus outbreak in the USA.

Investigations

- CT or MRI may show areas of oedema, particularly temporal lobe changes in HSV encephalitis.
- EEG usually shows typical slow waves.
- CSF shows a raised lymphocytic count.
- CSF PCR may be diagnostic.
- Viral serology (blood and CSF) is helpful.
- Brain biopsy is occasionally performed.

Treatment

Herpes simplex encephalitis has a high case fatality rate and high-dose **aciclovir** 10 mg/kg IV 3 times daily, infused over 1 hour, should be given for 2–3 weeks if it is suspected. Seizures are treated with anticonvulsants.

Prophylaxis

Vaccines are available against Japanese encephalitis for travellers to endemic areas in Asia. Tick-borne encephalitis vaccine is also available.

Brain abscess

Brain abscesses present with fever, headache and features of raised ICP and a space-occupying lesion. Abscesses usually develop over weeks but can develop more quickly (particularly cerebellar abscesses). Brain abscesses arise by local spread from the paranasal sinuses and teeth (streptococci and anaerobes), and are occasionally caused by *Pseudomonas* infection from otitis externa or staphylococcal infection from penetrating trauma. Haematological spread of bacteria causes brain abscesses, usually from endocarditis. Brain abscesses are often the result of infections with mixed organisms. Immunosuppressed patients develop abscesses with unusual organisms such as *Toxoplasma* or *Nocardia*.

Investigations

● Neutrophilia and raised CRP are usual, though not invariable.
● MRI or CT with contrast will identify brain abscesses as ring enhancing lesions. These scans will also identify focal collections in the skull or sinuses.

Treatment

Expert advice should be sought from neurosurgeons on the need for surgical drainage and there should be close liaison with the laboratory for appropriate antibiotic advice. The site of the infection and likely infecting agents will guide empiric therapy, e.g. **cefuroxime** 2 g IV 6 hourly plus **metronidazole** 500 mg IV 8 hourly (add **flucloxacillin** if staphyloccus suspected).

Cerebral malaria

See p. 34.

Rabies

Rabies is a Lyssavirus, which causes an infection that is nearly always fatal in humans. Rabies is found in most countries, though it is absent from a number including the UK, Australia and New Zealand. Nearly any mammal may carry rabies and bites should be considered as potential sources of infection. The incubation period ranges from a few weeks to several years; in general, it is inversely related to the distance from the bite to the brain. Rabies may present as either **paralytic rabies**, which takes the form of an ascending paralysis (similar to **Guillain–Barré syndrome**) or furious rabies. **Furious rabies** initially presents with tingling at the site of the bite, along with fever and headache. About 2 weeks later, there is an encephalitic illness marked by hyperexcitability, precipitated by sounds or visual stimuli. Pharyngeal spasms (hydrophobia) when trying to drink or eat occur in about half the cases of furious rabies. On **examination** there is hyperreflexia and evidence of sympathetic over-activity. The patient goes on to develop convulsions, respiratory paralysis and cardiac arrhythmias. Death usually occurs about 10–14 days later.

- **Diagnosis.** This is clinical but can be confirmed by detecting the virus in blood, saliva or CSF by PCR, viral culture or immunofluorescence. Skin biopsies can show histological, **immunofluorescence** or PCR evidence of rabies.
- **Treatment.** There is no known treatment for rabies once the disease is established and therapy should be to keep the patient comfortable.
- **Prophylaxis.** Both pre- and post-exposure prophylaxis are available. **Human diploid cell vaccine** (HDCV) is relatively safe (though expensive) and may be given if there is any doubt of an exposure to rabies. HDCV given at 0 and 1 month provides protection against rabies, with booster doses given at 1 year and then every 1–3 years. For post-exposure prophylaxis the wound should be cleaned carefully and left open. **Human rabies immunoglobulin** should be given immediately if the patient had not been previously immunized (20 U/kg half infiltrated around the wound and half IM). HDCV 1 mL IM on days 0, 3, 7, 14 and 28 should then be given.

Neurocysticercosis

This is acquired by ingestion of tapeworm eggs from contaminated food or water. It is a major global health challenge. Infection is endemic in Latin America, Africa, India and much of South-East Asia. Neurocysticercosis presents with epilepsy; other neurological patterns include brainstem dysfunction, cerebellar ataxia, hydrocephalus and rarely dementia, arachnoiditis and vasculitis. Most infected people remain symptomless.

Investigations
- Brain CT and MRI are helpful but sometimes not diagnostic.
- Serological tests indicate infection but not activity.

Management
- Management consists primarily of the control of seizures with **anticonvulsants**. **Praziquantel** and **albendazole** are used but surgery is sometimes needed for giant brain cysts or hydrocephalus.

Tetanus

Clostridium tetani is found in soil and disease results from a contaminated wound. Neonatal tetanus can result from contamination of the umbilical stump. Following an incubation of a few days to several weeks, there is malaise and spasm of the masseter muscle (lockjaw) and of the facial muscles, giving a grinning expression (risus sardonicus). Painful reflex spasms occur, with arching of the neck and back (opisthotonus), respiratory impairment and autonomic dysfunction (tachycardia, labile BP, sweating and cardiac arrhythmias). Death is from aspiration, hypoxia, respiratory failure, cardiac arrest or exhaustion.

Diagnosis
- Diagnosis is clinical.
- Rarely, *C. tetani* is isolated from wounds.

Management
- Suspected tetanus
  - Clean/debride the wound.
  - Give human tetanus immunoglobulin (HTIG) 250–500 U.
  - Give an IM injection of tetanus toxoid.

Kumar & Clark's Medical Management and Therapeutics

Established tetanus

- Give supportive medical and nursing care.
- Nurse in a quiet, isolated, well-ventilated, darkened room.
- Give benzodiazepines to control spasm and sedate the patient.
- Intubation and mechanical ventilation may be required.
- A magnesium sulphate infusion decreases the need for antispasmodics.
- Antibiotics: give IV **metronidazole** 500 mg daily. Penicillin and cephalosporins are also effective.
- Anti-toxin: give HTIG sodium. If this is unavailable, give immune equine tetanus Ig 10 000 U IM but expect a high incidence of allergic reaction.
- When the patient recovers, give active immunization, as immunity is incomplete following tetanus.

GASTROINTESTINAL INFECTIONS

Gastroenteritis (see also p. 135)

Diarrhoea as a result of infectious intestinal disease is common and is caused by a wide variety of viruses, bacteria and protozoa. The majority of infections worldwide are **viral** and these are responsible for high infant mortality rates in the developing world. Viruses include rotavirus, adenoviruses, astrovirus and calicivirus (norovirus and sapoviruses).

- Diagnosis. This is usually clinical but, if necessary, electron microscopy, antigen detection tests or PCR on stools can be used. Protozoa can be identified by microscopy of stool specimens.
- Treatment. There are no specific antiviral treatments available but rehydration therapy is often necessary (see below).

Common **bacterial** causes include non-typhoidal *Salmonellae, Campylobacter* spp., and strains of *Escherichia coli*, which have been classified according to their pathogenic mechanisms, e.g. enterotoxigenic *E. coli* (ETEC), enteropathogenic *E. coli* (EPEC), enteroinvasive *E. coli* (EIEC), enteroaggregative *E. coli* (EaggEC) and enterohaemorrhagic *E. coli*, which produce verocytoxin (VTEC). **Cholera** caused by *Vibrio cholerae* is still common in many parts of the world. *Shigella* spp. cause bacillary dysentery with bloody stools.

- Treatment. The major risks with bacterial infections are dehydration and, in some cases, malnutrition. **Rehydration** can be accomplished by use of an oral rehydration solution (ORS) (Table 2.3). There is overwhelming evidence that this is life-saving; IV fluids are required only in severe cases or when there is excessive vomiting.
- Antibiotics. In most cases, symptoms will resolve without antibiotics. If symptoms are severe, e.g. ≥ 6 unformed stools per day and/or fever, tenesmus or blood, antibacterials are given (Table 2.4).
  - *Shigella infections* are treated with **co-trimoxazole** 960 mg twice daily for 3 days or **ciprofloxacin** 500 mg twice daily for 3 days.
  - *ETEC, EPEC and EIEC infection* can be treated with the same antibiotics, but they should not be used for infection with **VTEC strains** such as *E. coli* O157, as there is evidence that antibacterials increase the risk of complications such as haemolytic uraemic syndrome.
  - Campylobacter *infection* can be treated effectively with oral **erythromycin** 500 mg twice daily for 5 days, but increasing resistance with quinolones means that **ciprofloxacin** will be less helpful.

Table 2.3 Oral rehydration solutions (ORS) and IV solutions used in moderate and severe diarrhoea

Type of solution	Salts (mmol/L)			Glucose	Substance added (per L water)
	Na+	K+	Cl-		
Oral WHO new reduced osmolality formulation	75	20	65	75	2.6 g NaCl 2.9 g Na citrate 1.5 g KCl 13.5 g glucose
Cereal-based	85	–	80	–	80 g cooked rice 5 g salt (NaCl)
Household	85	–	80	111	20 g glucose 5 g salt (NaCl)
UK/Europe	35–60	20	37	90–200	Pre-prepared solutions
IV Ringer's lactate	131	4	109	0	Pre-prepared solution

- *Non-typhoidal* Salmonella does not usually need treatment unless the symptoms are severe or there are the following risk factors: patient < 6 or > 50 years, prosthesis present, valvular heart disease, severe atherosclerosis, immune suppression or malignancy. **Ciprofloxacin** 500 mg twice daily for 5–7 days or **ceftriaxone** 60 mg/kg IV daily dose can then be used.
- *Cholera* usually responds to **doxycycline** 300 mg single dose, tetracycline 500 mg 4 times daily for 3 days and **co-trimoxazole** 960 mg twice daily, or a single dose of a quinolone, e.g. **oral ciprofloxacin** 1 g or **azithromycin** 1 g, which help to shorten duration of diarrhoea and also reduce the infectivity of the patient.
- *Giardia intestinalis diarrhoea* is treated with **metronidazole** 2 g daily for 3 days or **tinidazole** 2 g as a single dose.
- *Entamoeba histolytica infection* is treated with oral **metronidazole** 800 mg 3 times daily for 5 days or **tinidazole** 2 g daily for 2–3 days, followed by **diloxanide furoate** 500 mg 3 times daily for 10 days to eradicate cysts.
- *Cyclospora cayetanensis infection* is treated with **co-trimoxazole** 960 mg twice daily for 7 days.
- *Cryptosporidium hominis infection* lacks effective treatments.

Clostridium difficile-associated diarrhoea

C. difficile-associated diarrhoea (CDAD) occurs most frequently after exposure to cephalosporins, quinolones and clindamycin, but most antibiotics have been causal. Elderly hospitalized patients are often affected. Hospital-acquired infections remain frequent. Severity ranges from mild diarrhoea to severe pseudomembranous colitis with development of a

Table 2.4 Antibiotics in adult acute bacterial gastroenteritis

Condition	Indications	Drug of choice	Other drugs	Benefits
Dysentery	Most patients	Ciprofloxacin 500 mg twice daily	Nalidixic acid 1 g 4 times daily Ampicillin 500 mg 4 times daily Co-trimoxazole 960 mg twice daily	Relieve symptoms Shorten illness Decrease transmission
Cholera	All patients	Ciprofloxacin	Tetracycline 250 mg 4 times daily Azithromycin Nalidixic acid Co-trimoxazole	Relieve symptoms Shorten illness Decrease transmission
Empirical therapy of watery diarrhoea	Severe symptoms Prolonged illness Elderly patients Immunosuppressed	Ciprofloxacin	Azithromycin 500 mg once daily Co-trimoxazole	Relieve symptoms Shorten illness May decrease complications
Travellers' diarrhoea	Rarely used	Ciprofloxacin	Co-trimoxazole	Relieve symptoms Shorten illness
Treatment of confirmed *Salmonella, Shigella, Campylobacter*	Symptoms not improving (rarely needed)	Ciprofloxacin Azithromycin	Erythromycin Co-trimoxazole	May shorten illness
Clostridium difficile	Most cases (unless symptoms resolved)	Metronidazole 400 mg three times daily	Vancomycin 125 mg 4 times daily	Relieve symptoms Shorten illness

toxic megacolon and bowel perforation. Diarrhoea may be the only symptom, whereas in severe disease there is fever as well. Severe disease may be defined as including the following features:

- white cell count > 15×10^9/L
- acute rising creatinine (> 50% of baseline)
- fever > 38.5°C
- evidence of severe colitis.
- Diagnosis. Diagnosis of CDAD can be made by detection of *C. difficile* toxins in the stool on ELISA or cell culture. **Pseudomembranous colitis** is seen at sigmoidoscopy.
- Treatment. Fluid loss can be severe, requiring IV rehydration (p. 611). Some patients will improve when the offending precipitating antibacterial is stopped. For non-severe disease, oral **metronidazole** 400 mg 3 times daily for 7–10 days is the treatment of choice. An alternative is oral **vancomycin** 125 mg 4 times daily for 7–10 days. In severe disease oral vancomycin is recommended 125–500 mg oral 4 times daily for 10–14 days. If the patient cannot take oral medication, **metronidazole** may be given by the IV route, 500 mg 3 times daily for 7–10 days. Relapse of diarrhoea after treatment is common. IVIG may be considered in severe disease. Some patients may respond simply to repeat treatment but many do not. Pulsed tapering courses of metronidazole or vancomycin have been used. Toxic megacolon may require colectomy.
- Prevention. Prevention requires isolation of infected patients and good hygiene, including hand washing with soap and water by patients and healthcare workers. Reduction in the hospital use of cephalosporins reduces the risk.

Enteric fever (typhoid and paratyphoid fever)

Typhoid fever is a systemic bacterial infection caused by *Salmonella typhi*. The incubation period ranges from 1 to 3 weeks. Presentation is variable and the severity of symptoms can range from mild to severe toxaemia. Common symptoms are fever, headache, malaise, nausea and a dry cough, with constipation or diarrhoea.

Diagnosis

Blood culture is usually positive in the first 2 weeks. *S. typhi* may also be isolated from bone marrow. Culture of faeces and urine can also be performed, although it should be noted that these cultures may also be positive in chronic carriers. Several rapid antibody detection tests have been developed with good sensitivity, though relatively poor specificity.

The symptoms of paratyphoid fever are similar but usually less severe. Paratyphoid fever is caused by *Salmonella paratyphi A*, *S. paratyphi B* and *S. paratyphi C*.

Treatment

Treatment is governed by the severity of illness and the susceptibility of the organism. Quinolones are the most effective antibacterial treatment for both adults and children when the organism is susceptible. In many parts of the world, patients will not be admitted to hospital and for mild illness **ciprofloxacin** 15 mg/kg daily for 5–7 days is commonly used. Quinolones are not licensed for use in children but the benefit in this situation outweighs the risk. For severe illness requiring hospital admission,

ciprofloxacin 15 mg/kg daily for 10–14 days is recommended. In the case of reduced quinolone susceptibility (demonstrated by nalidixic acid resistance), alternatives for mild disease include **azithromycin** 8–10 mg/kg daily for 7 days and **cefixime** 20 mg/kg daily for 7–14 days. For severe disease with nalidixic acid-resistant isolates, **cefotaxime** 80 mg/kg IV daily or **ceftriaxone** 60 mg/kg IV daily for 10–14 days is given.

Gastrointestinal tuberculosis

TB can affect the intestine as well as the peritoneum. Intestinal TB is due to reactivation of primary disease caused by *Mycobacterium tuberculosis*. Bovine TB occurs in areas where milk is unpasteurized and is rare in Western countries.

Clinical features

These are abdominal pain, weight loss, anaemia, fever with night sweats, obstruction, right iliac fossa pain or a palpable mass. The ileocaecal area is most commonly affected, but the colon and, rarely, other parts of the gastrointestinal tract can be involved.

Diagnosis

- **Small bowel follow-through** will show transverse ulceration and diffuse narrowing of the bowel, with shortening of the caecal pole.
- **US or CT** shows additional mesenteric thickening and lymph node enlargement.
- **Histology and culture** of tissue is desirable but not always possible. Specimens can be obtained by colonoscopy or laparoscopy, but laparotomy is required in some cases.

Treatment

Drug treatment is similar to that of pulmonary TB: rifampicin, isoniazid, ethambutol and pyrazinamide (p. 87). In gastrointestinal TB treatment should last 1 year.

Peritonitis

Spontaneous bacterial peritonitis (SBP)

The yearly risk of developing spontaneous bacterial peritonitis (SBP) for patients with ascites and cirrhosis has been estimated to be as high as 29%. See Chapter 6 (p. 189) for Diagnosis and Treatment.

Peritonitis secondary to large bowel perforation, ruptured appendix or ruptured diverticulum

This is caused by organisms that are part of the normal bowel flora, namely enteric Gram-negative bacilli, anaerobes and enterococci.

- **Treatment.** An antibacterial combination such as **amoxicillin** 1 g IV 4 times daily, **metronidazole** 500 mg IV 3 times daily and **gentamicin** 5 mg/kg IV daily is suitable, as is monotherapy with **meropenem** 1 g IV 3 times daily, **co-amoxiclav** 1.2 g IV 3 times daily or **piperacillin/ tazobactam** 4.5 g IV 3 times daily. A combination of a cephalosporin, e.g. **cefotaxime** 2 g IV 3 times daily, and **metronidazole** 500 mg IV 3 times daily can also be used, but cephalosporins have no activity against enterococci. Antibacterials alone are often insufficient therapy and appropriate surgical drainage or peritoneal washouts must be performed.

Peritonitis with continuous peritoneal dialysis (CAPD)

Peritonitis is also a risk for patients undergoing CAPD. Infection usually occurs as a result of bacteria entering the peritoneum via the dialysis catheter or following an exit site infection. The common bacterial causes are coagulase-negative staphylococci, *Staph. aureus* and Gram-negative bacilli, including *P. aeruginosa*. Fungal infection with *Candida* spp. also occurs. Patients usually present with a 'cloudy bag', often without other symptoms.

- **Diagnosis.** Peritoneal fluid should be sent for cell count, Gram stain and culture. Infection has been defined as > 100 white blood cells per microlitre, with > 50% neutrophils seen on microscopy. Culture is improved if large volumes of peritoneal dialysate are concentrated by centrifugation. Around 20% of cultures are sterile despite raised cell counts.
- **Treatment.** Empiric treatment is usually intraperitoneal and includes **vancomycin** (< 60 kg body weight 1.5 g; > 60g body weight 2 g, and left in bag for 6 hours) and an aminoglycoside, e.g. **gentamicin** 0.6 mg/kg and left in bag for 6 hours, or **vancomycin** and oral **ciprofloxacin** 500 mg orally twice daily for 4 days. Once a pathogen is identified, treatment can be more specific. Infection with coagulase-negative staphylococci is usually treatable, but an exit site infection with *Staph. aureus* and Candida peritonitis usually requires removal of the dialysis catheter. Cultures yielding enteric Gram-negative bacilli are suggestive of peritonitis following bowel perforation and urgent surgical intervention will be required.

Tuberculous peritonitis

This is the second most common form of abdominal TB.

- In the **wet type**, ascitic fluid should be examined for protein concentration (> 20 g/L) and tubercle bacilli (rarely found).
- In the **dry form**, patients present with subacute intestinal obstruction, which is due to tuberculous small bowel adhesions.
- In the **fibrous form**, patients present with abdominal pain, distension and ill-defined irregular tender abdominal masses.
- **Diagnosis.** The diagnosis of peritoneal TB can be supported by findings on US or CT screening (mesenteric thickening and lymph node enlargement). A histological diagnosis is not always required before instituting treatment.
- **Treatment.** Drug treatment is similar to that of pulmonary TB (p. 87).

HEPATOBILIARY AND PANCREATIC INFECTIONS

Pancreatitis

See p. 170.

Hepatitis

See p. 179.

Cholecystitis

See p. 172.

Cholangitis

See p. 173.

Kumar & Clark's Medical Management and Therapeutics

Liver abscess (see also p. 194)

A liver abscess may occur following intestinal sepsis, e.g. appendicitis, biliary sepsis or, more rarely, bacteraemic spread from a more distant focus. The bacteria most frequently involved are enteric Gram-negative bacilli, *Streptococcus milleri*, enterococci and anaerobes. Blood cultures may yield the organism.

Treatment

- *Percutaneous or surgical drainage* is sometimes required.
- *Suitable antibacterials* are a combination of **amoxicillin** 1 g IV 4 times daily, **metronidazole** 500 mg IV 3 times daily and **gentamicin** 5 mg/kg IV daily, or monotherapy with **meropenem** 1 g 3 times daily, **co-amoxiclav** 1.2 g 3 times daily or **piperacillin/tazobactam** 4.5 g IV 3 times daily.
- *Entamoeba histolytica* liver abscess can be diagnosed serologically. Treatment is with **metronidazole** 400 mg or 500 mg IV 3 times daily for 5–10 days. **Tinidazole** 1.5–2 g daily for 3–6 days is an alternative.
- *Aspiration* of an amoebic abscess is indicated if rupture is suspected or there is failure to improve after 72 hours of metronidazole. Aspiration can improve penetration of metronidazole and may need to be repeated.
- *Diloxanide furoate* 500 mg orally 3 times daily for 10 days should be given after metronidazole or tinidazole to eradicate intestinal cysts.

GENITOURINARY INFECTIONS

Lower urinary tract infection (LUTI)

LUTI is common in women, in whom it usually occurs in a normal urinary tract. In contrast, LUTI is rare in men and children, and these patients should be investigated for anatomical urinary tract abnormalities. LUTI may occasionally result in a potentially life-threatening Gram-negative bacteraemia. LUTI is characterized by dysuria, urgency, fever, polyuria, suprapubic tenderness or frequency.

Diagnosis

Urinary dipsticks for both white cells and nitrites together are highly sensitive and provides a quick, simple confirmation of a LUTI. Bacteriuria and pyuria correlate well with the presence of infection. Quantitative culture often yields more than 10^8 bacteria/L, but lower counts may indicate infection in the presence of pyuria or acute dysuria.

Treatment

The most common causative organism of LUTI is *E. coli*; the next most common are *Proteus mirabilis*, *Klebsiella aerogenes*, *Staphylococcus saprophyticus* and *Enterococcus*. The sensitivities of these organisms vary greatly across the world. In particular, sensitivities to amoxicillin and trimethoprim vary greatly and the empirical treatment of LUTI must be based on local antibiotic sensitivities. In the UK, the empirical treatment of uncomplicated LUTI may be with **trimethoprim** 200 mg twice daily for 3–7 days, **nitrofurantoin** 50 mg 4 times daily for 7 days or an oral cephalosporin for 7 days. A urine culture should be obtained and antibiotic changes based on culture results.

In pregnancy, asymptomatic bacteriuria requires treatment. Women should have their urine routinely dipstick-tested in the first trimester;

with a positive result, urine should be sent for microscopy and culture, and appropriate antibiotics that are safe in pregnancy should be started e.g. **cefadroxil** 500 mg × 2 for 7 days.

Upper urinary tract infections (UUTI)

UUTI presents with fever, flank pain and LUTI symptoms. These infections are severe and often require hospital admission.

Diagnosis

Urine specimens are similar to those in LUTI, showing significant bacteriuria and pyuria. Blood cultures are also frequently positive. Causative agents are similar to those of LUTI. Non-invasive studies, such as US or CTKUB, should be performed to rule out intrarenal abscess, anatomical abnormalities or renal stones.

Treatment

Patients with mild to moderate illness who are able to take oral medication can be safely treated as outpatients with quinolones, e.g. **ciprofloxacin** 250–500 mg twice daily for 10–14 days. Patients with a more severe or systemic illness and those unable to tolerate oral treatment should be initially given parenteral therapy, with an appropriate empirical therapy based on local antibiotic sensitivities. The choice would include co-amoxiclav, third-generation cephalosporins, fluoroquinolones or aminoglycosides. As with LUTI, changes to antibiotic therapy should be guided by the results of a urine culture if there is no response to the initial empirical therapy. In pregnant women give cefuroxime 750 mg–1.5 g IV 3 times daily for 48 h, switching to oral amoxicillin 500 mg 8 hourly.

Urinary catheter-related infections

Urinary tract infection is one of the most common causes of healthcare-associated infections and indwelling urinary catheters are linked with a greatly increased risk of a urinary tract infection. Urinary catheters are commonly colonized with bacteria, and the presence of bacteria in a urine sample from a catheterized patient does not necessarily imply that treatment should be given. If there are symptoms of a urinary tract infection, then treatment should be prescribed, the choice of the most appropriate antibiotic varying according to local antibiotic sensitivities. If the catheter can be removed, then this should be done. There is no agreement as to whether an aminoglycoside antibiotic should be given during a urinary tract infection to 'cover' a catheter change.

Epididymitis

Epididymitis is usually caused by *Neisseria gonorrhoeae* or *Chlamydia trachomatis* in sexually active men, or by enteric organisms or TB in older men. Diagnosis and therapy should be directed accordingly.

Prostatitis

Acute prostatitis presents as fever, dysuria, and an extremely tender prostate on examination. Chronic prostatitis is usually asymptomatic, but occasionally lower back pain, testicular discomfort and dysuria are noted. Quantitative urine cultures performed both before and after prostatic massage and NAAT on urine or swab are performed for diagnosis.

Prostatitis is usually the result of Gram-negative infection. Treatment is with quinolones, e.g. **ciprofloxacin** 500 mg twice daily for 28 days.

SYSTEMIC FUNGAL INFECTIONS

Candidiasis

This is the most common fungal infection in humans. *Candida albicans* is the major pathogen. This and other species that are pathogenic to humans are commensals in the oropharynx and gastrointestinal tract.

- **Clinical features.** Vaginal infection (p. 72) and oral thrush are common. They are seen in the very young and the elderly, and in patients who have had antibiotic therapy. Any organ in the body can be invaded in the immunosuppressed. Candidal oesophagitis presents with painful dysphagia. Cutaneous candidiasis typically occurs in intertriginous areas. It is also a cause of paronychia. **Chronic mucocutaneous candidiasis** is a rare manifestation, usually occurring in children, and is associated with a T-cell defect.
- **Diagnosis.** Scrapings from infected lesions, tissue secretions or blood cultures (in invasive disease) can demonstrate the fungus.

Treatment

- *Oral lesions* respond to **nystatin** 500 000 U every 6 hours, oral **amphotericin B** 10 mg lozenge dissolved in the mouth 4 times daily for up to 2 weeks, or **fluconazole** 50 mg daily for 2 weeks.
- *Systemic infections* require parenteral therapy; possible treatment includes **fluconazole** 400 mg daily, or **caspofungin** 70 mg on the first day then 50 mg daily. In neutropenic patients liposomal amphotericin 3–5 mg/kg/day or caspofungin or voriconazole are recommended.

Histoplasmosis

Histoplasma capsulatum infection occurs worldwide but the disease is commonly seen in Ohio and the Mississippi river valley, where over 80% of the population have been subclinically exposed. Transmission is mainly by inhalation of the spores, which can survive in moist soil for years.

Clinical features

- *Primary pulmonary histoplasmosis* is usually asymptomatic, with radiological features similar to those seen with the Ghon primary complex of TB (p. 512). Calcification in the lungs, spleen and liver occurs in patients from areas of high endemicity. When symptomatic, primary pulmonary histoplasmosis generally presents as a mild 'flu-like illness, with fever, chills, myalgia and cough. The systemic symptoms are pronounced in severe disease.
- *Chronic pulmonary histoplasmosis* produces pulmonary cavities, infiltrates and characteristic fibrous streaking from the periphery towards the hilum on X-ray.
- *Disseminated histoplasmosis* resembles disseminated TB clinically. Fever, lymphadenopathy, hepatosplenomegaly, weight loss, leucopenia and thrombocytopenia are common.
- **Diagnosis.** Diagnosis is made by culturing the fungi or by demonstrating them on histological sections. The histoplasmin skin test is only of diagnostic value when it converts from a negative to a positive result.

- **Management.** Only symptomatic patients require therapy. **Itraconazole** or **ketoconazole** is indicated for moderate disease. Severe infection is treated with **IV amphotericin B** for 1–2 weeks, followed by oral **itraconazole** 200 mg twice daily for 6 months

Aspergillosis

This is caused by *Aspergillus fumigatus* (the most common), *A. flavus* and *A. niger*. These fungi are ubiquitous in the environment and are often found on decaying leaves and trees. Humans are infected by inhalation of the spores. Three major forms of the disease are recognized:

- **Allergic bronchopulmonary aspergillosis (rare)** is an exaggerated immune response to aspergillus which leads to proximal bronchiectasis. Eosinophilic pneumonia occurs, particularly in late autumn and winter, with a wheeze, cough, fever and malaise. Peripheral blood eosinophil count is usually raised. Total levels of IgE are usually extremely high (both that specific to *Aspergillus* and also the non-specific type). Skin-prick testing to protein allergens from *A. fumigatus* gives rise to positive immediate skin tests. Sputum may show eosinophils and mycelia, and precipitating antibodies are usually, but not always, found in the serum.
  - *Treatment.* **Prednisolone** 30 mg daily produces rapid clearing of the pulmonary infiltrates; intermittent long-term treatment with prednisolone 10–15 mg daily is usually required. **Itraconazole** 200 mg daily is also used and improves pulmonary function.
- **Aspergilloma and invasive aspergillosis.** *A. fumigatus* grows within previously damaged lung tissue, forming a ball of mycelium within lung cavities (called an **aspergilloma**). A round lesion, with an air 'halo' above it, is seen on CXR. With continuing antigenic stimulation, large quantities of precipitating antibody are seen in the serum. Massive haemoptysis may occur and requires resection of the area of damaged lung containing the aspergilloma. Antifungal agents are not helpful. **Invasive aspergillosis** is seen with immunosuppression and requires aggressive antifungal **Voriconazole** 6 mg/kg × 2 for 24 hours then 4 mg/kg IV or orally is the treatment of choice. **Caspofungin** and **amphotericin B** is used liposomal 3–5 mg/kg day (p. 89).

Cryptococcosis

Cryptococcus neoformans has a worldwide distribution and is spread via the droppings of birds, especially pigeons. Transmission is by inhalation of the spores into the lungs, which produces a granulomatous reaction; pulmonary symptoms are uncommon. Pulmonary lesions include lung cavitation, hilar lymphadenopathy and pleural effusions. Meningitis usually occurs in immunocompromised patients with AIDS or lymphoma and often develops subacutely.

- **Diagnosis.** A positive Indian ink stain or latex cryptococcal antigen test performed on the CSF is diagnostic. Tissue biopsies may demonstrate characteristic encapsulated yeasts.
- **Treatment.** **Amphotericin B** 0.7–1.0 mg/kg daily IV, alone or in combination with **flucytosine** 100–200 mg/kg daily for 2 weeks, is followed by **fluconazole** 400 mg daily. Therapy should be continued for 8 weeks with meningitis. **Fluconazole** has greater CSF penetration and is used when toxicity is encountered with **amphotericin B** and **flucytosine**, and as maintenance therapy in immunocompromised patients, especially those with HIV (p. 114).

Coccidioidomycosis

Coccidioides immitis, a soil saprophyte, is found in the southern USA, Central America and parts of South America. Transmission is by inhalation of spores.

- **Clinical features.** The majority of patients are asymptomatic. Acute pulmonary coccidioidomycosis presents with fever, malaise and cough, after an incubation period of about 10 days. Erythema nodosum, erythema multiforme, phlyctenular conjunctivitis and, less commonly, pleural effusions may occur. Complete recovery is usual.
- **Diagnosis.** The organism can be identified in respiratory secretions or tissue samples by histopathology. Cultures are not usually performed. Tests include the highly specific latex agglutination and precipitin tests (IgM), which are positive within 2 weeks of infection and decline thereafter. Other tests include complement fixation, ELISA and radioimmunoassay. A complement-fixation test (IgG) performed on the CSF is diagnostic of coccidioidomycosis meningitis; it becomes positive within 4–6 weeks and remains so for many years.
- **Treatment.** Mild pulmonary infections are self-limiting and require no treatment, but progressive and disseminated disease require urgent therapy. **Itraconazole** 200 mg for 6 months or **fluconazole** 400–600 mg for 6 months is the treatment of choice for primary pulmonary disease, with more prolonged courses for cavitating or fibronodular disease. Fluconazole in high dose (600–1000 mg daily) is given for meningitis.

Blastomycosis

Blastomycosis is caused by *Blastomyces dermatitidis* and is found in North America.

- **Clinical features.** Blastomycosis primarily involves the skin, presenting as non-itchy papular lesions that later develop into ulcers with red verrucous margins. Pulmonary solitary lesions are found and are radiologically similar to the Ghon focus of TB. Fever, malaise and cough occur, and bone lesions are common.
- **Diagnosis.** The organism is found in histological sections or by culture from lesions; results can be negative in up to 50% of patients. ELISA may be helpful in the diagnosis but there is some cross-reactivity between *Blastomyces* and *Histoplasma* antibodies.
- **Treatment.** **Itraconazole** 200–400 mg is used for mild to moderate disease for up to 6 months. Fluconazole is also used. In severe or unresponsive disease and in the immunocompromised, **amphotericin B** 0.7–1.0 mg/kg/day (max. 2.5 g) or liposomal amphotericin for several weeks followed by oral azole therapy is recommended.

Pneumocystis jiroveci infection

This is seen in adults associated with immunodeficiency states, particularly AIDS, and is discussed on page 112.

HELMINTHIC INFECTIONS

Worm infections are very common in developing countries. Multiple infections with different helminths are common in endemic areas. Mass treatment programmes are carried out, usually annually, to keep the total worm load down (see Table 2.5). Treatment of trematodes and intestinal nematodes is shown in Tables 2.6 and 2.7 respectively.

Table 2.5 Drugs used in mass treatment programmes for helminth infections (alone or in combination)

Drug	Infection
Diethylcarbamazine (DEC)	Loiasis
	Filariasis
Ivermectin	Loiasis
	Filariasis
	Onchocerciasis
	Strongyloidiasis
Albendazole	Filariasis (with DEC)
	Intestinal helminths
Praziquantel	Schistosomiasis

Table 2.6 Treatment of trematode infections

Parasite	Drug and dose
Schistosoma mansoni	Praziquantel 40 mg/kg single dose*
S. haematobium	Praziquantel 40 mg/kg single dose*
S. japonicum	Praziquantel 60 mg/kg single dose*
Paragonimus spp.	Praziquantel 25 mg/kg 8-hourly for 3 days
Chlonorchis sinensis	Praziquantel 25 mg/kg 8-hourly for 2 days
Opisthorcis spp.	Praziquantel 25 mg/kg 8-hourly for 1 day
Fasciolopsis buski	Praziquantel 25 mg/kg 8-hourly for 1 day
Fasciola hepatica	Triclabendazole 10 mg/kg single dose†

*May be split to minimize nausea.
†Repeated if necessary.

Table 2.7 Drugs used for treating human intestinal nematodes (single dose unless otherwise stated)

Drug	Dosage	Ascaris	Hookworm	Enterobius	Trichuris	Strongyloides
Piperazine	75 mg/kg	++	+	++	–	–
Pyrantel pamoate	10 mg/kg	++	+	++	–	–
Oxantel pamoate	10 mg/kg	++	+	n/a	++	–
Albendazole	400 mg*	++	++	++	+	+
Mebendazole	500 mg†	++	++	++	+	+
Tiabendazole	25 mg/kg*	n/a	n/a	n/a	n/a	++
Levamisole	5 mg/kg	++	+	n/a	n/a	–
Ivermectin	200 mcg/kg‡	n/a	n/a	n/a	n/a	++

++, Highly effective; +, moderately effective; –, ineffective; n/a, drug not used for this indication/no data available.

*Twice daily for 3 days in strongyloidiasis.

†WHO recommended dose for developing countries; in UK commonly given as 100 mg single dose for threadworm, or 100 mg twice daily for 3 days for whipworm.

‡Once daily for 2 days.

SEXUALLY TRANSMITTED INFECTIONS

Sexually transmitted infections (STIs) are very common worldwide.

Risk factors for most STIs are similar and therefore multiple infections frequently coexist, some of which may be asymptomatic. Because of this, all patients presenting with a possible STI should be screened for syphilis, chlamydia, gonorrhoea and trichomoniasis, and should be offered HIV testing.

People seeking advice for STIs are usually anxious and concerned about confidentiality, and are sometimes embarrassed. The clinic setting should ensure privacy and adhere to strict confidentiality. STIs should ideally be treated in a genitourinary clinic.

In addition to a history of both genital and generalized symptoms, a travel and drug history will aid diagnosis and allow contact tracing to be carried out. Treatment of sexual partners is an essential part of the control of STIs.

Investigations

In general, send urethral, vaginal, urine, and sometimes oral and rectal swabs for culture and NAAT, along with appropriate serological tests for diagnosis. Investigations should also include screening for hepatitis (A, C and B), and HIV screening should be offered.

Herpes simplex virus (HSV)

Genital herpes is caused by the human herpes simplex virus (usually type 2). It is characterized by painful genital vesicles and ulceration. Like other human herpes viruses, herpes simplex virus remains dormant but can reactivate with recurrences. The diagnosis of genital herpes is made clinically but should be confirmed by viral culture or immunofluorescence. As herpes infection is so common, all genital ulcers should be cultured for herpes virus. Antiviral therapy is effective if begun within 5 days of the start of the infection, whilst there are new lesions.

Treatment

Treatment should be with **aciclovir** 200 mg 5 times a day, **famciclovir** 250 mg 3 times daily or **valaciclovir** 500 mg twice daily for 5 days; IV therapy is necessary to treat complications if the patient is unable to tolerate oral therapy. HIV-positive patients need to be treated for 10 days. Suppressive therapy with **aciclovir** 400 mg twice daily for recurrent confirmed genital herpes infections is used for severe or frequent recurrences.

Syphilis

Treponema pallidum infection causes syphilis. The natural history of syphilis is divided into the following entities:

- **Primary syphilis** develops within several weeks of exposure and involves a chancre (painless, indurated, superficial ulceration).
- **Secondary syphilis** is characterized by multi-system involvement within the first 2 years following infection: generalized polymorphic, (usually) non-itchy rash, often affecting the palms and soles, mucocutaneous lesions and generalized lymphadenopathy. Less commonly, other complications such as meningitis occur.
- **Tertiary syphilis** includes cardiovascular, gummatous and neurological disease (tabes dorsalis, meningovascular syphilis or general paresis), which occurs after a period of latency (early or late).

Kumar & Clark's Medical Management and Therapeutics

Investigations

Microscopic diagnosis of primary syphilis is made by dark-field microscopy of exudates from a chancre. **Serology** is the mainstay of the diagnosis of syphilis. A cardiolipin (non-treponemal) serological test, such as the rapid plasma reagin (**RPR**) test or the Venereal Disease Research Laboratory (**VDRL**) test, detects non-specific treponemal antigens and becomes positive a few weeks into the infection; it then becomes negative again after several months. Specific treponemal serological tests, such as the fluorescent treponemal antibody absorption test (**FTA**), the *Treponema pallidum* haemagglutination test (TPHA) and the *Treponema pallidum* particle agglutination assay (**TPPA**), become positive after several months and remain positive for life. The treponemal enzyme immunoassay (**EIA**) (IgG and IgM) is also available; the IgM becomes positive after about 2 weeks and the IgG after 5 weeks. Screening with an EIA (IgG and IgM) or both a non-specific (RPR/VDRL) and a specific test (FTA/TPPA) is recommended. The serology cannot differentiate between syphilis and other treponemal diseases such as yaws and pinta. CSF serology is necessary to diagnose neurosyphilis.

Treatment

- **Early syphilis** is treated with **procaine penicillin** G 750 mg IM daily for 10 days. **Doxycycline** 100 mg twice daily for 14 days, **erythromycin** 500 mg 4 times orally daily for 14 days or **azithromycin** 500 mg daily for 10 days is also used in cases of penicillin allergy.
- **Late latent syphilis** is treated with **procaine penicillin** 750 mg IM daily for 17 days or **doxycycline** 200 mg twice daily for 28 days.
- **Neurosyphilis** is treated with **procaine penicillin** 2 g IM daily for 17 days plus probenecid 500 mg 4 times daily for 17 days, or in case of penicillin allergy **doxycycline** 200 mg twice daily for 28 days. Patients with neurological syphilis should be given **prednisolone** at the start of the therapy to avoid the Jarisch–Herxheimer reaction), although the evidence for its efficacy is poor.

Chancroid

Chancroid is caused by *Haemophilus ducreyi*. It is relatively uncommon in Europe and North America, but a common cause of ulcerative genital lesions in Africa and Asia. Chancroid presents as painful, non-indurated genital ulcers with tender inguinal lymphadenopathy that suppurates.

- **Diagnosis.** Diagnosis of chancroid requires culture and microscopy of *H. ducreyi* from a genital lesion or lymph node aspirate.
- **Treatment.** Treatment regimens are **ceftriaxone** 250 mg IM single dose, **azithromycin** 1 g daily single dose, **ciprofloxacin** 500 mg twice daily for 3 days or **erythromycin** 500 mg 4 times daily for 7 days.

Trichomoniasis

Trichomonas vaginalis is a flagellated protozoan that causes a vaginitis. Clinical symptoms include a foul-smelling frothy vaginal discharge, dysuria and genital inflammation (cervical petechiae), though many infections are asymptomatic. Men are usually asymptomatic but may present with discharge or dysuria.

- **Diagnosis.** Microscopy of vaginal fluid shows motile trichomonads on a saline wet mount of discharge.

- Treatment. **Metronidazole** 2.0 g single dose or metronidazole 400–500 mg twice daily for 5–7 days is used. Metronidazole is contraindicated in pregnancy so intravaginal **clotrimazole** 100 mg (suppositories) daily for 7 days may be used for symptomatic relief, although definitive treatment later is usually required.

Candidiasis

Vulvovaginal candidiasis is a common cause of an itchy vaginitis caused by *Candida* spp. and is not sexually transmitted. It presents with a thick, white vaginal discharge and intense vulvar inflammation, pruritus and occasionally dysuria. In men, candidiasis is often asymptomatic but can cause a balanitis.

- **Diagnosis** is usually made clinically, but is supported by microscopy and culture.
- Treatment with **topical clotrimazole** (cream or suppository) or **fluconazole** 150 mg oral single dose is usually effective, but infections are often recurrent.

Bacterial vaginosis

Bacterial vaginosis (BV) is the most frequent cause of vaginal discharge in women of childbearing age. It is characterized by a replacement of vaginal lactobacilli leading to overgrowth of predominantly anaerobic organisms (*Gardnerella vaginalis*, *Prevotella* and *Mobiluncus* spp.) and a rise in vaginal pH; it is not, strictly speaking, an STI. BV presents as a homogeneous, thin, vaginal discharge that smoothly coats the vaginal walls. There is minimal genital inflammation. Clue cells are found on microscopy; the pH of vaginal fluid is > 4.5 and there is a fishy odour on adding 10% KOH.

- Treatment is with **metronidazole** 400–500 mg twice daily for 5–7 days, metronidazole 2 g single dose, **clindamycin** (2% cream) 4 times daily for 7 days or clindamycin 300 mg twice daily for 7 days. Recurrence is common.

Human papilloma virus

Anogenital warts are caused by the human papilloma virus (HPV), of which over 100 genotypes have been identified. Warts may be single or multiple, and are usually easy to diagnose on naked eye examination, but if in doubt diagnosis may be confirmed histologically. There may be occult lesions and HPV (not all types) is associated with carcinoma.

- Treatment is with cryotherapy, chemical applications such as **podophyllin**, **podophyllotoxin**, **imiquimod** and **interferon**, or surgical removal. No single therapy is always effective and recurrences are common. An effective vaccine is now available and should be given to females aged 12–13 years.

Gonorrhoea

Gonorrhoea is caused by infection with *Neisseria gonorrhoeae*, a Gram-negative diplococcus. Men usually present with urethral discharge and/or dysuria but infection may be asymptomatic. Rectal infection may cause anal discharge or pain but pharyngeal infection is usually asymptomatic. In women gonorrhoea is often asymptomatic but vaginal discharge and lower abdominal pain occur.

On examination men usually have a purulent urethral discharge, and rarely, epididymal tenderness or balanitis is seen. In women examination is often normal, but there may be a mucopurulent cervical discharge and cervical contact bleeding, and rarely, lower abdominal tenderness.

- **Diagnosis.** Diagnosis is by NAAT (PCR-based) on urine or microscopy and culture of urethral and cervical samples.
- **Treatment.** There is increasing resistance of *N. gonorrhoeae* to commonly used antibiotics, especially in South-East Asia. The antibiotic treatment of gonorrhoea should reflect local resistance patterns. **Cefix-ime** 400 mg as a single dose or **ciprofloxacin** 500 mg as a single dose are common first-line therapies; **ofloxacin** 400 mg as a single dose is an alternative. **Quinolone** resistance is becoming increasingly common. Patients should return 72 hours after completing treatment for a test of cure.

Chlamydia

Genital infection with *Chlamydia trachomatis* is very common. Approximately 40% of non-gonococcal urethritis is caused by *C. trachomatis*. This infection is maintained at such high rates because it may be symptomless in both men and women. Most infections are asymptomatic but in men may present as dysuria or urethral discharge. In women chlamydia presents as vaginal discharge, intermenstrual bleeding or lower abdominal pain. Rectal infection may occasionally cause proctitis.

- **Diagnosis** is often made on clinical suspicion (after excluding other diagnoses), as tests are not completely sensitive. Diagnosis may be made by culture, immunofluorescence or NAAT.
- **Treatment** is with **doxycycline** 100 mg twice daily for 7 days, **azithro-mycin** 1 g orally as a single dose. Erythromycin 500 mg 4 times daily for 14 days is an alternative although test of cure at 28 days is recommended as there is a significant rate of treatment failure.

ANTIMICROBIAL DRUGS

These drugs are categorized as antibacterials, antivirals, antifungals, antiprotozoals and antihelminthics.

Mode of action

Antimicrobials have many and varied mechanisms of action, e.g. inhibition of an organism's cell wall or inhibition of protein or nucleic acid synthesis. The essential property is **selective toxicity** to the microbe rather than the host. In the case of bacteria, the result is either death of the bacterium (**bactericidal**) or inhibition of the bacterium's growth (**bacteriostatic**). Though the terms bacteriostatic and bactericidal are defined in vitro, their applicability to treatment has been questioned.

General principles of use

Antimicrobials are widely used for treatment or for prophylaxis, but are also widely misused. Overuse can lead to resistance. The following general principles should be followed to guide the use of these agents:

- **Necessity for treatment** should be decided on the clinical evidence of infection, the availability of other more appropriate therapy (e.g. surgical drainage of an abscess) and an evaluation of whether the benefits of treatment outweigh the risks (e.g. side-effects).
- **Cultures of appropriate sites and sensitivities** must be obtained prior to commencing antibiotics, except in certain circumstances (e.g. meningococcal disease).

- **Choice** of antimicrobial will depend on sensitivity to the causative bacterium and whether the agent will reach the site of infection. More than one drug may be required but any contraindications and possible drug reactions should be checked.
- **Dose** will vary with the patient's age and weight, the presence or absence of renal and liver dysfunction, and the site and severity of infection.
- **Route of administration** depends on the absorption kinetics.
  - *Oral therapy* is cost-effective and non-invasive but depends on good gastrointestinal absorption.
  - *Intramuscular injections* are painful and may be contraindicated in bleeding disorders.
  - *Intravenous therapy* is used in severe infections, particularly when high concentrations in the blood are required quickly.
  - *Switch from IV to oral therapy.* This should be as soon as possible when the signs and symptoms of infection have improved and the patient is haemodynamically stable and able to take oral fluids. N.B. Remember IV therapy is extremely expensive e.g. IV **metronidazole** is approximately 15 times the oral cost.
  - *Topical antibiotics* can be used for skin, eye or ear infections.
  - *Rectal (suppositories or foam) antibiotics* are usually cheaper but are not always appropriate.
- **Duration of therapy** depends on the nature of the infection and the clinical response. The optimum duration of therapy is not known for many infections. Good evidence exists for treatment of TB, bacterial pharyngitis, urinary tract infection and endocarditis.

Antimicrobial prophylaxis

Prophylaxis is the use of a drug to prevent infection. The antimicrobial used should be given at the appropriate time, by the appropriate route and for the appropriate duration. The choice of antibacterial agent is also dictated by the likely sensitivity of the organisms expected to be encountered.

Situations in which prophylaxis is needed include the following:

- before a surgical procedure with a risk of infection, e.g. bowel or gynae-cological surgery or implantation of surgical prostheses
- after an individual has been exposed to an infectious agent, e.g. *N. meningitidis*
- before an individual has been exposed to an infectious agent *but is not yet ill*, e.g. antimalarial prophylaxis for *P. falciparum* infection
- when post-splenectomy chemoprophylaxis is required (see Box 7.1, p. 205).

Chemoprophylaxis to prevent endocarditis after procedures in patients with high-risk heart lesions is controversial. Procedures can introduce a bacterium but there is no evidence that this leads to endocarditis. The UK is unusual in that it has issued guidance that chemoprophylaxis is never required; most other countries recommend chemoprophylaxis in high-risk cases.

Adverse effects

- **Toxicity.** Antimicrobials may be harmful to the patient. Minor side-effects, such as nausea, are common. Antimicrobials may be ototoxic, nephrotoxic, hepatotoxic or neurotoxic. Some are contraindicated in pregnancy because of potential teratogenicity, and in breast feeding because the agent is present in the milk. **N.B.** *Always check the dose and route of administration.*

● Interactions. Antimicrobials may interact with a wide range of other drugs, e.g. rifampicin, warfarin or the oral contraceptive pill (p. 11).

Failure of antimicrobial therapy

Antimicrobials may fail for a variety of reasons and this does not always indicate **resistance** or necessitate a change in antimicrobial therapy. The common reasons for failure of antimicrobial therapy are:
● poor compliance
● wrong diagnosis, wrong choice of drug, failure of drug to reach the site of infection
● inadequate dose, duration or route of administration
● bacterium has become resistant, superinfection with resistant organism
● antimicrobial started too late
● antimicrobial is inactivated by another drug, or metabolized or excreted more quickly than normal
● other treatment such as surgery is required, e.g. drainage of an abscess, removal of an infected intravascular device.

Antimicrobial resistance

Resistance may be due to there being no active site for the antimicrobial agent, cell wall impermeability or the destruction or modification of the antimicrobial itself. Reduced drug uptake and increased drug excretion (efflux) can also play a part.

Not all organisms are sensitive to all antimicrobial agents; some are intrinsically resistant. Antimicrobial resistance may also develop (acquired resistance) in organisms that were previously sensitive, as a result either of mutation or of horizontal transferral of resistance genes by conjugation, transfer of plasmids or other mobile genetic elements.

Antimicrobials are commonly prescribed drugs and resistance can easily develop with overuse. It is imperative that they should be prescribed rationally and only when necessary. A number of resistant organisms already exist, e.g. meticillin-resistant staphylococci, ESKAPE organisms (*Enterococcus faecium, Staphylococcus aureus, Klebsiella pneumoniae, Acinetobacter baumanni, Pseudomonas aeruginosa,* and *Enterobacter* species). A recent resistance in Klebsiella *pneumoniae* contains NDm-1 (New Delhi metallo-beta-lactamase-1), a transmissable genetic element encoding multiple resistant genes. The worrying factor is that it can spread across many bacterial genes.

Antimicrobial policies/guidelines

Most hospitals operate an antibacterial policy to reduce the development of resistance, to achieve economy and to reduce the frequency of hospital-acquired infections. The latter has been achieved by the reduction in use of broad-spectrum antibiotics.

Antibacterial drugs

These drugs may be classified according to their chemical structure (e.g. β-lactam agents, aminoglycosides, quinolones), their mode of action (e.g. inhibitors of cell wall synthesis, inhibitors of protein synthesis) or their spectrum of activity (e.g. antituberculous agents, antistaphylococcal agents).

Below is a brief description of the commonly used antibacterial agents listed according to chemical structure; some are listed by mode of action and some by spectrum of activity.

β-lactams

These antibiotics contain a β-lactam ring structure; they interfere with bacterial cell wall synthesis and are bactericidal. They include the penicillins, cephalosporins, carbapenems and monobactams.

Penicillins

Patients should always be asked if they are sensitive to penicillin prior to its administration. In general, patients with a history of atopy (asthma, eczema and hay fever) have a higher risk of anaphylactic reactions to penicillins.

Penicillin is active against streptococci, including most pneumococci, meningococci, *Corynebacterium diphtheriae* and treponemes. Most strains of *Staphylococcus aureus* and *Neisseria gonorrhoeae* are now resistant because of the production of β-lactamase. IM preparations, e.g. benzyl penicillin, procaine penicillin and the derivatives of benzyl penicillin, such as benthamine penicillin or benzathine penicillin, are less frequently used but are still useful in the treatment of syphilis (p. 72).

- *Benzyl penicillin (penicillin G).* Dose 2.4–4.8 g daily in 4 divided doses IM or by slow IV infection or infusion.
- *Phenoxymethylpenicillin (penicillin V).* This is poorly absorbed enterally and oral bioavailability is low. It is mainly used for streptococcal sore throats and prophylaxis against recurrent rheumatic fever (250 mg twice daily).
- *Broader-spectrum penicillins.* **Ampicillin** 250 mg to 1 g 6-hourly orally or 500 mg 4–6-hourly IV and **amoxicillin** 250–500 mg 8-hourly orally or 0.5–1 g 6–8-hourly IV. The spectrum of activity includes that of basic penicillins but also covers enterococci and some Gram-negative bacteria, e.g. *Haemophilus influenzae*, some Enterobacteriaceae. However, these antibiotics are hydrolysed by β-lactamase enzymes, e.g. those found in *Staph. aureus*, *N. gonorrhoeae* and some *H. influenzae*. Thus almost all staphylococci, 20% of *H. influenzae* and 60% of *Escherichia coli* are resistant.
- *Penicillinase-resistant penicillins.* The first semisynthetic β-**lactamase**-stable compound to be used was **meticillin,** which has been replaced by the isoxazolyl penicillins. These are β-lactamase-stable penicillins that are active against *Staph. aureus*, e.g. **flucloxacillin** orally 500 mg 6-hourly or IM or IV infusion 0.5–1 g 6-hourly. Meticillin-resistant *Staph. aureus* (MRSA — see p. 43) is also resistant to this agent. Strains of *Staph. aureus* that remain sensitive to isoxazolyl penicillins are often referred to as MSSA (meticillin-sensitive *Staph. aureus*). **Nafcillin** has a spectrum of activity similar to the isoxazolyl penicillins and is used mostly in North America (2 g IV 4–6-hourly). **Temocillin** 1–2 g 12-hourly IM or IV infusion is active against Gram-negative bacteria and is stable to many β-lactamases. It is best reserved for treating β-lactamase-producing Gram-negative bacteria, those isolates resistant cephalosporins such as cefotaxime and ceftazidime.
- *Antipseudomonal penicillins.* These are semi-synthetic derivatives that have an expanded spectrum of activity against Gram-negative bacteria, including *Pseudomonas aeruginosa*. Examples include the **ureidopenicillins** such as **piperacillin** (combined with tazobactam 4.5 g 8-hourly IV), and the **carboxypenicillins** such as **ticarcillin** (combined with clavulanic acid 3.2 g 6–8-hourly IV). These agents are

often used as empirical therapy in neutropenic sepsis. They are usually used in combination with a β-lactamase inhibitor, as the latter broadens the spectrum of activity.

- *β-lactam/β-lactamase inhibitor combinations.* These include **co-amoxiclav** 500 mg 8-hourly orally, a combination of **amoxicillin** and the β-lactamase inhibitor **clavulanic acid**; **piperacillin** and the inhibitor **tazobactam**; **ampicillin** and the inhibitor **sulbactam**; **ticarcillin** and **clavulanic acid**. The spectrum of activity is that of the β-lactams plus expanded activity against Gram-negatives, including *Pseudomonas*, MSSA and also most anaerobic organisms.
- *Mecillinams.* **Pivmecillinam** 200–400 mg 8-hourly orally is active against Gram-negative bacteria, including *Klebsiella*, *Enterobacter*, *Salmonella* and *E. coli*, but not *Pseudomonas*.

Cephalosporins

These β-lactams have an advantage over penicillins in that they are more resistant to hydrolysis by β-lactamases but are still inactive against MRSA and enterococci. Cephalosporins are often classified by 'generations', with succeeding generations having a wider Gram-negative spectrum. This classification is not always helpful, as not all cephalosporins of the same generation have the same activity. For example, some have less activity against Gram-positive organisms, particularly staphylococci. Cephalosporins also produce adequate CSF concentrations in the presence of meningeal inflammation.

Oral cephalosporins are used frequently for treatment of urinary tract infections, but because of extremely poor oral bioavailability most are usually used parenterally.

The IV agents are commonly used for empirical treatment of septicaemia and neutropenic sepsis. They are often used in combination with an **aminoglycoside** and **metronidazole**, in abdominal sepsis. In severe community-acquired pneumonia they are usually combined with a macrolide. These drugs are also widely misused when an antimicrobial with a narrower spectrum may be better. Patients on these broad-spectrum agents are prone to the development of *Clostridium difficile*-associated diarrhoea.

- *First generation.* These oral agents are active against staphylococcal and streptococcal infections. They include **cefalexin** 250 mg 4 times daily increasing to 1–1.5 g 6–8-hourly for severe infections, and **cefadroxil** 0.5–1 g twice daily for skin and soft-tissue infections and 1 g daily for urinary tract infections.
- *Second generation.* These are more effective than first-generation agents against *E coli*, *Klebsiella* spp. and *Proteus mirabilis*, but less effective against Gram-positive organisms. They include **cefuroxime** 250 mg orally twice daily for mild upper respiratory tract infections, or 750 mg 3 times daily IM or IV, rising to 1.5 g 6–8-hourly for severe infections. For meningitis, use 3 g IV 8-hourly. This drug is also useful for community-acquired pneumonia, urinary tract infections, and soft-tissue and skin infections. **Cefaclor** 250 mg oral 8-hourly, or 500 mg 8-hourly for severe infections, is used for sensitive Gram-positive and Gram-negative bacteria.
- *Third generation.* These penetrate the CSF better than the second-generation drugs. They are broad-spectrum and more potent against anaerobic Gram-negative bacteria. They are useful in severe septicaemia and can also be used for urinary tract infections, pneumonia and

intra-abdominal infections, usually combined with metronidazole. They include **cefotaxime** 1 g twice daily IM or IV, increased in severe infections, e.g. meningitis, to 2 g 6-hourly. It has greater activity against many Gram-negatives and also retains some anti-Gram-positive activity, e.g. for streptococci. **Ceftriaxone** IV 1 g daily over 2–4 mins or by IV infusion, rising to 2–4 g in severe infections, has similar activity to cefotaxime but a longer half-life, allowing once-a-day dosing. **Ceftazidime** 1 g 3 times daily IV, 2 g IM 8-hourly for broad-spectrum cover in meningitis, is a parenteral third-generation agent with a spectrum of activity extended to include *P. aeruginosa*. **Cefoperazone** 2–4 g IV 12-hourly has similar activity to ceftazidime. **Cefixime** 200 mg twice daily and **cefpodoxime** 200 mg twice daily are the only orally available third-generation drugs and are used for upper and lower respiratory and urinary tract infections.

- *Fourth generation.* **Cefepime** 0.5–2 g IV 8–12-hourly has good activity against Gram-negatives, including *P. aeruginosa*. It has better activity against Gram-positive bacteria such as MSSA than the third-generation agents, and is used in febrile neutropenic infections.
- *Fifth generation.* **Ceftobiprole** (IV and oral) and **Ceftaroline** have a similar broad spectrum action but also include MRSA, pseudomonas and enterococcei.

Carbapenems

These agents are stable to many β-lactamases, including extended spectrum β-lactamases (ESBLs) and AmpC-producing organisms. Currently available carbapenems are not active against MRSA. The Gram-negative organism, *Stenotrophomonas maltophilia*, which may cause sepsis in immunocompromised patients, is also resistant by virtue of the production of **metallo-β-lactamase** enzyme. Such enzymes have also been found in some other Gram-negatives, including some isolates of *P. aeruginosa*. Examples of carbapenems include:

- *Imipenem* 0.5 mg 4 times daily IV infusion has a broad spectrum of activity, including aerobic and anaerobic Gram-positive and Gram-negative bacteria. It is used in combination with a specific enzyme inhibitor, cilastatin, which blocks its renal inactivation. It is slightly more active against enterococci compared to the others in this group. **Imipenem** and **meropenem** are used in the empirical treatment of sepsis, including neutropenic sepsis, and polymicrobial infections, e.g. abdominal sepsis, or when ESBL-producing organisms are suspected, or in infections with multi-resistant *Acinetobacter*, when they are sensitive. Imipenem should not be used for the treatment of CNS infection or in people prone to fitting, as it is neurotoxic in high doses or in patients with chronic kidney disease.
- *Meropenem* 500 mg 8-hourly IV infusion is similar to imipenem but, as it is stable to the renal enzyme, it does not require cilastatin. It is the preferred antibiotic in this class for CNS infections.
- *Ertapenem* 1 g once daily IV infusion has a longer half-life but has no activity against *P. aeruginosa*. It is used for community-acquired pneumonia.
- *Doripenem* 500 g 4 times daily IV infusion is used for hospital-acquired pneumonia and complicated urinary tract and abdominal sepsis.

Kumar & Clark's Medical Management and Therapeutics

- Monobactams. **Aztreonam** 2 g twice daily IV infusion, a parenteral drug, is the only member of this class of drug that has been used widely. Monobactams are active against a wide range of Gram-negative organisms but not active against Gram-positive or anaerobic organisms, meaning that aztreonam should not be used on its own empirically.
- Toxicity of β-lactams. Generally β-lactams are very safe. Hypersensitivity reaction occurs in 1–10% of patients, causing rashes, urticaria and anaphylaxis (< 0.05%). Hypersensitivity is to the basic penicillin structure and therefore occurs with all penicillins and all β-lactam antibiotics. Rarely, an encephalopathy occurs. Intrathecal injections should *not* be given, as they can cause a fatal encephalopathy. Ampicillin produces a rash in 90% of patients with infective mononucleosis who receive the drug. Co-amoxiclav causes a cholestatic jaundice six times more frequently than amoxicillin itself; this is commoner in patients over 65 years. Flucloxacillin rarely causes a cholestatic jaundice, which can occur several weeks after the drug is stopped.

Aminoglycosides

Aminoglycosides bind to the 30S subunit of the bacterial ribosome and interfere with protein synthesis. They are bactericidal. This group includes **gentamicin**, **netilmicin**, **amikacin**, **tobramycin** and **streptomycin**. These agents are poorly absorbed from the gut and must be given parenterally. They are active predominantly against Gram-negative bacteria, including *P. aeruginosa*. Many strains of *Staph. aureus* are sensitive to aminoglycosides. There are differences in the activity of the different agents, with bacteria resistant to some of the aminoglycosides as a result of the production of aminoglycoside-modifying enzymes. The substrate range of these enzymes varies so, for example, an organism that is resistant to **gentamicin** may still be sensitive to **amikacin**. These drugs are rarely used as monotherapy and are usually given in combination with a β-lactam. Streptococci and enterococci are resistant to aminoglycosides, but when used in combination with a β-lactam, synergy occurs. Thus many regimens for treatment of infective endocarditis include an aminoglycoside. Gentamicin and amikacin are now commonly given as a single daily dose.

- Gentamicin is given by slow IV injection over 3 mins, or by slow IV infusion, either 5 mg/kg as a single daily dose or 3–5 mg/kg/day in divided doses 8-hourly.
- Amikacin is used in serious Gram-negative infections resistant to gentamicin. It is given by slow IV injection or infusion 15 mg/kg as a single daily dose or in 2 divided doses. For severe infections use a maximum of 22.5 mg/kg/day in 3 divided doses. Amikacin is also used occasionally for the treatment of TB or infections caused by non-tuberculous mycobacteria.
- Streptomycin IM 0.5–1 g daily is mainly used for treatment of TB when other drugs cannot be used, e.g. because of resistance.
- Tobramycin 1 mg/kg daily every 8 hours by slow IV injection or infusion, increasing to 5 mg/kg daily for severe infections has similar activity to gentamicin. It can also be used by inhaler for treatment of *P. aeruginosa* in cystic fibrosis (can cause bronchospasm).
- Netilmicin 4–6 mg/kg daily in 2 or 3 divided doses has a similar spectrum of activity to gentamicin.

Side-effects: aminoglycosides are nephrotoxic and therapeutic drug monitoring is essential (p. 365). Nephrotoxicity is reversible if detected early but permanent damage can occur. Use cautiously in liver disease. Ototoxicity can be vestibular or due to cochlear damage. Aminoglycosides should not be used along with ototoxic diuretics, e.g. furosemide.

- Neomycin is used as a topical agent for the treatment of eye and ear infections.

Macrolides

Macrolides and ketolides inhibit protein synthesis by binding to the 50S subunit of the bacterial ribosome and interfere with protein synthesis. They are bacteriostatic.

- Erythromycin has a similar range of activity to penicillin and thus is often used to treat infections where β-lactams are contraindicated because of allergy, e.g. those caused by streptococci and *Staph. aureus*. However, resistance in these organisms is becoming commoner. Some isolates of MRSA remain sensitive. Erythromycin is commonly used to treat community-acquired pneumonia, as it is active against *Mycoplasma pneumoniae* and *Legionella pneumophila*. Erythromycin can be given orally 250–500 mg 6-hourly, rising to 4 g daily in severe infections. It can also be given by IV infusion in severe infections, 50 mg/kg daily in divided doses 6-hourly.
- Clarithromycin, e.g. 250–500 mg twice daily orally, is an erythromycin derivative that has a similar spectrum to erythromycin but greater activity. Tissue concentrations are higher. It is used for respiratory tract infections and otitis media. It is also given in combination with other drugs (e.g. amoxicillin and omeprazole) for the eradication of *Helicobacter pylori*.
- Azithromycin, e.g. 500 mg once daily for 3 days orally, has better activity than erythromycin against some Gram-negative organisms such as *H. influenzae* but less activity against Gram-positive bacteria. It is also used for the treatment of upper and lower respiratory tract infections and otitis media. Macrolides have good intracellular penetration and azithromycin is useful for the treatment of *Salmonella typhi* and *S. paratyphi* infections (500 mg once daily for 7 days). It is also useful for genital *Chlamydia* infections and non-gonococcal urethritis (1 g single dose). It is used in the WHO SAFE approach (p. 93) for trachoma (20 mg/kg as a single dose) and also in the treatment and prophylaxis of *Mycobacterium avium intracellulare* in patients with HIV infection (p. 117).
- Telithromycin is a ketolide derivative of erythromycin with a similar spectrum of activity to the other macrolides. It is used in the treatment of respiratory tract infections (800 mg daily for 5 days).

Nausea, vomiting and diarrhoea are common gastrointestinal **side-effects**, which are less frequent with clarithromycin and azithromycin. Rashes and abnormal liver biochemistry occur, as does prolongation of the QT interval.

Glycopeptides

Glycopeptides interfere with bacterial cell wall synthesis and are bactericidal.

- Vancomycin is active only against Gram-positive organisms. Absorption from the gut is poor so it is only used parenterally, except when it is given orally to treat *C. difficile*-associated diarrhoea (125 mg 6-hourly). Vancomycin IV infusion 1 g 12-hourly is reserved for situations when other agents cannot be used, e.g. against MRSA. It is also used for the treatment of neutropenic sepsis and also IV line-associated infections. Some strains of enterococci are now resistant to glycopeptides, so-called glycopeptide-resistant enterococci (GRE), and reduced susceptibility has also developed in some strains of MRSA, which are termed glycopeptide-intermediate *Staphylococcus aureus* (GISA).

- Teicoplanin is used once daily 200–400 mg by IV infusion.

Side-effects: vancomycin is nephrotoxic and therapeutic drug monitoring is needed. Trough levels are most useful, aiming for 5–10 mg/L. With normal renal function the level should be measured before the fourth dose, but if there are renal problems wait for the result before giving the next dose. Vancomycin causes histamine release, leading to the red man syndrome if given rapidly. Teicoplanin is less nephrotoxic but still requires monitoring in patients with poor renal function or to check that therapeutic concentrations have been achieved.

Tetracyclines

Tetracyclines bind to the 30S subunit of the bacterial ribosome; they interfere with protein synthesis and are bacteriostatic. Tetracyclines are natural microbial products or semisynthetic derivatives. They are broad-spectrum agents with activity against many commonly encountered Gram-positive and Gram-negative organisms, as well as *Chlamydia* spp., *M. pneumoniae*, rickettsia, *Coxiella burnetii* (Q fever), and the agents of Lyme disease and syphilis. The majority of preparations are for oral administration. In terms of microbiological activity there is little to choose between the various tetracyclines. Use of these agents for the treatment of common bacterial infection has been limited due to the development of resistance, but they are still commonly employed in the treatment of infections caused by chlamydiae, i.e. urethritis, cervicitis and lymphogranuloma venereum. Minocycline, in particular, has also found a role in the treatment of acne and rosacea. In combination with other drugs, tetracyclines can be used for brucellosis. Tetracyclines can also be used to treat syphilis, and in the treatment and prophylaxis of malaria.

- Tetracycline 250–500 mg 4 times daily is also used in some *H. pylori* eradication regimens if other treatments have failed. Its absorption can be inhibited by chelation with cations in milk, milk products, iron, aluminium, magnesium and zinc.
- Doxycycline is given as 200 mg 1st day, then 100 mg daily orally.
- Minocycline 100 mg twice daily can occasionally cause irreversible pigmentation.
- Demeclocycline hydrochloride is given as 150 mg 6-hourly or 300 mg 12-hourly.
- Lymecycline is given as 408 mg 12-hourly (for at least 8 weeks in acne). Higher doses are used for severe infections.
- Oxytetracycline is given as 250–500 mg 6-hourly.
- Tigecycline 50 mg IV infusion 12-hourly is a glycylcycline agent, structurally related to the tetracyclines. It is a derivative of minocycline. It has a similar mechanism of action to the tetracyclines but remains active against some organisms that are resistant to tetracycline, as well as having activity against MRSA and GRE. It is currently reserved for complicated abdominal and soft-tissue infections caused by multiple antibacterial-resistant organisms.

Side-effects: nausea and photosensitivity are common. Tetracyclines should not be given to children and breast feeding mothers because of deposition in growing bone and teeth, causing yellowing and enamel defects. Demeclocycline can cause reversible nephrogenic diabetes insipidus and acute kidney injury. Hypersensitivity is common.

Quinolones

Quinolones affect bacterial DNA synthesis by inhibiting the action of bacterial topoisomerases. They are bactericidal and are active against Gram-positive and Gram-negative bacteria. Oral and IV preparations are available for most of these agents. MRSA is commonly resistant to the quinolones and there is increasing resistance to many bacteria, as the agents are widely used.

- Ciprofloxacin 250–750 mg twice daily oral, IV infusion 200–400 mg twice daily over 30–60 mins (for severe infections) is active mostly against Gram-negatives and useful for complicated urinary tract infections, gastrointestinal infections and gonorrhoea. It does have some activity against Gram-positive organisms but is not adequate for the treatment of pneumococcal infections. Ciprofloxacin can be used as prophylaxis for close contacts of meningococcal infection and following exposure to *Bacillus anthracis*.
- Norfloxacin 400 mg twice daily has a similar spectrum of activity but its use has been confined mainly to the treatment of urinary tract infections. For prophylaxis to prevent recurrent urinary infections norfloxacin may be given for up to 12 weeks.
- Ofloxacin 200–400 mg daily is used for urinary tract infections and for gonorrhoea, genital chlamydia and pelvic inflammatory disease. It is also available as a topical agent for the treatment of eye and ear infections.
- Moxifloxacin 400 mg once daily for 5–10 days is used for the treatment of pneumonia caused by β-lactam-resistant pneumococci, sinusitis and chronic bronchitis, and is also playing an increasing role in the treatment of TB, especially multi-drug-resistant TB.
- Levofloxacin 250–750 mg daily for 7–10 days; infusion 50 mg once to twice daily given over 60 mins is active against Gram-positive and Gram-negative organisms, and is used as second-line therapy in community-acquired pneumonia.
- Nalidixic acid 900 mg 6-hourly for 7 days was the first quinolone and is used in urinary tract infections only.

Gastrointestinal **side-effects** include nausea, vomiting, abdominal pain and diarrhoea; skin problems include rash, pruritus and, rarely, toxic epidermal necrolysis; neurological disturbances include headaches, drowsiness and dizziness, particularly in the elderly and confused. Prolongation of the QT interval occurs, particularly with moxifloxacin and levofloxacin, and these should not be used in patients taking class I or III antiarrhythmics. Nalidixic acid should not be used in porphyria. There is an age-related tendon inflammation/rupture and those with tendonitis or taking corticosteroids should not be given the drug. The young and pregnant/breast feeding women can develop an arthropathy. Patients on these agents are also prone to the development of *C. difficile*-associated diarrhoea. There are many drug interactions.

Sulphonamides and trimethoprim

- Sulphonamides are bacteriostatic by competitive inhibition of folate synthesis; they have a broad range of activity. However, because of resistance they are now rarely used for treatment of bacterial infections, other than for urinary tract infections in many parts of the world.

Sulfadiazine and sulfadoxine are combined with **pyrimethamine** and used as treatment for the protozoal infections, toxoplasmosis and malaria (p. 35) *respectively*. **Sulfamethoxazole** is combined with **trimethoprim** as **co-trimoxazole**. **Sulfasalazine** is a combination of **5-aminosalicylic acid** and **sulfapyridine** and is used in inflammatory bowel disease (p. 157)

- **Trimethoprim** is a synthetic diaminopyrimidine drug with a broad range of bactericidal activity against Gram-positive and Gram-negative bacteria, but not anaerobes. It exerts its action by inhibiting bacterial dihydrofolate reductase, an enzyme required for folate synthesis. It is mostly used for the treatment of urinary tract infections and respiratory tract infections (200 mg 12-hourly).

- **Co-trimoxazole** is a combination of **trimethoprim** and **sulfamethoxazole**, and is bactericidal. It is available orally 960 mg 12-hourly. It can also be given by IV infusion 980 mg, rising to 1.44 g 12-hourly in severe infections. It penetrates the tissues well, including the CNS, bone and prostate. Its use for bacterial infections should be limited to treatment of nocardiosis, Whipple's disease, some atypical mycobacterial infections, and infections with *Stenotrophomonas maltophilia*. Co-trimoxazole has a major role in the treatment and prophylaxis of *Pneumocystis* pneumonia in HIV infection (p. 112). However, since HAART therapy, its use has declined. **Side-effects** include nausea, vomiting, headache and a variety of rashes. Prolonged use causes folate deficiency and megaloblastic anaemia. Stevens–Johnson syndrome, toxic epidermolysis and blood dyscrasias (e.g. thrombocytopenia) preclude its common usage. Avoid in elderly patients, as deaths have been reported.

Nitroimidazoles

- **Metronidazole** 500 mg 3 times daily orally or by IV infusion is active against anaerobic bacteria and some protozoa. Its antibacterial effect works by breaking or causing destabilization of DNA. Metronidazole has no activity against aerobic bacteria and is used for the treatment of suspected or proven anaerobic infections, e.g. abdominal or dental infections and brain abscesses. It is also used for *C. difficile*-associated diarrhoea, bacterial vaginosis and tetanus, and in combination with other drugs for the eradication of *H. pylori*. It has a major use as prophylaxis for abdominal surgery, and is also used for the treatment of protozoal infections, e.g. amoebiasis (p. 136) and *Giardia* (p. 136). A topical formulation is useful for reducing the odour caused by anaerobic infection of ulcers.

- **Tinidazole** 500 mg twice daily has a longer half-life than metronidazole but is used similarly.

Side-effects are vomiting, a metallic taste in the mouth and a peripheral neuropathy after prolonged use. There is also a disulfiram-like reaction with alcohol. Both drugs enhance the anticoagulant effect of warfarin.

Chloramphenicol

Chloramphenicol orally or by IV infusion 50 mg/kg in 4 divided doses inhibits protein synthesis by binding to the 50S subunit. It is well absorbed and used for life-threatening infections. It has a broad spectrum of activity against many Gram-positive and Gram-negative bacteria, including anaerobes. It is now rarely given systemically but is still used occasionally for the treatment of brain abscesses, typhoid and some complicated respiratory tract infections or meningitis, when other agents are not suitable. A topical preparation is very useful for the treatment of eye and ear infections.

Side-effects can be serious and include irreversible aplastic anaemia, limiting its use. Gastrointestinal (nausea, vomiting, diarrhoea) and neurological (peripheral neuropathy, optic neuritis, headaches, depression) side-effects occur.

Fusidic acid

Sodium fusidate 500 mg 3 times daily orally or IV inhibits bacterial protein synthesis and is bacteriostatic. It is active predominantly against Gram-positive organisms, and *Staph. aureus* in particular. If used as a single agent resistance can develop and therefore it should always be combined with another drug when treating serious staphylococcal infection such as osteomyelitis or infective endocarditis. The oral preparation, sodium fusidate, is well absorbed and is less likely to cause disturbance of liver function than the IV fusidic acid. The oral suspension of fusidic acid is less well absorbed and therefore higher doses are required. Topical preparations can also be used for skin infections and eye infections, although there are concerns over the development of resistance.

Side-effects include occasional hepatic toxicity.

Oxazolidinone

Linezolid oral 600 mg 12-hourly for 10–14 days or IV infusion over 30–120 mins is one of the newest antibacterial agents. It inhibits protein synthesis by binding to the bacterial 50S ribosomal subunit at its interface with the 30S subunit. It is bacteriostatic. It is active against Gram-positive infections only. Its use should be reserved for multi-resistant Gram-positive infections, such as those caused by MRSA or GRE. Oral and IV preparations are available.

Side-effects: diarrhoea, nausea, vomiting, taste disturbances and tongue discoloration occur. Linezolid is a reversible non-selective monoamine oxidase inhibitor and thus has many potential drug interactions. Patients treated for over 28 days are also at risk of developing thrombocytopenia, anaemia, leucopenia and severe optic neuropathy (patients should report eye symptoms immediately).

Polymyxins

These are cyclic peptides that are active against Gram-negative bacteria only. They disrupt bacterial cell membranes and are bactericidal. **Polymyxin B** and **colistin (polymyxin E)** are the two agents in use. Neither is absorbable as an oral drug. Polymyxin B is mainly used topically for ear infections. Colistin is also used topically for ear infections but is also available as an IV preparation (slow IV infusion 1–2 million U 8-hourly). Because of toxicity, this is reserved for infections when other agents cannot be used, e.g. multiple-resistant *Acinetobacter*. Nebulized colistin is also used for treatment of cystic fibrosis infections. **Colistin** can be given orally 1.5–3 million U 8-hourly, in combination with other drugs, for gastrointestinal decontamination in neutropenic patients and in some patients on the ICU.

Side-effects are dose-related neuro- and nephrotoxicity and polymyxins should not be given with aminoglycosides or other nephrotoxic agents.

Other antibiotics

- Clindamycin is given as 150 mg 6-hourly up to 450 mg 6-hourly in severe infections; IV infusion 0.6–2.7 g daily in 2–4 divided doses. The mode of action is similar to that of the macrolides. Clindamycin is active against Gram-positive bacteria, in particular *Staph. aureus* and streptococci, as well as having good activity against anaerobes. It is used mainly in the treatment of bone and joint infections, serious *Streptococcus pyogenes* infections and mixed infections where anaerobes are suspected. Topical clindamycin can be used for the treatment of bacterial vaginosis. The major **side-effect** is *C. difficile* diarrhoea, which limits its usage. It also causes rashes, nausea, vomiting and abnormal liver biochemistry.

- Streptogrammins inhibit protein synthesis as a result of binding to the 50S subunit of the bacterial ribosome and interfering with transfer RNA function. They are bacteriostatic. **Quinupristin** and **dalfopristin** are given together and are active mostly against Gram-positive organisms, with the exception of *Enterococcus faecalis*. Use is limited to treatment of infections caused by MRSA or vancomycin-resistant enterococci (VRE) (not *E. faecalis*). They do not cross the blood–brain barrier. The combined drugs (7.5 mg/kg IV 8-hourly) must be given by IV infusion via a central line. **Virginiamycin** and **pristinamycin** are other drugs in this class. **Side-effects** include nausea, diarrhoea, myalgia and arthralgia.

- Rifamycins include **rifampicin** (p. 87), which has a wide spectrum of activity against Gram-positive and Gram-negative bacteria, and even some protozoa and viruses. However, its main role is as an antituberculous agent. This drug is sometimes used in combination with others for the treatment of brucellosis and also serious infections caused by *Staph. aureus*, including MRSA. It is also used as prophylaxis in close contacts of meningococcal and invasive *H. influenzae* type b infections.

- Daptomycin 4 mg/kg IV infusion daily is a lipopeptide with activity against Gram-positive bacteria similar to vancomycin. It is bactericidal as a result of disrupting the bacterial cell membrane potential. It is used for complicated skin and soft-tissue infections, and for infections caused by multiple-resistant bacteria such as MRSA and VRE. **Side-effects** are gastrointestinal disturbances (nausea, vomiting, diarrhoea and occasionally abdominal pain and constipation), and hepatic and renal impairment. Myalgia, muscle weakness and myositis are uncommon but the creatine phosphokinase should be monitored. Daptomycin interferes with the assay for the prothrombin time.

- Nitrofurans include **nitrofurantoin** 50 mg 3 times daily, the only commonly used antibacterial of this group. It has activity against a wide variety of bacteria but is used almost exclusively as an oral preparation for the treatment and prevention of urinary tract infections. *Proteus* spp. and *P. aeruginosa* are resistant. **Side-effects** include nausea, brown urine and, rarely, pulmonary complications (e.g. pneumonitis and fibrosis) and peripheral neuropathy.

- Methenamine 1 g 12-hourly orally for 3 weeks at a time is converted to formaldehyde in acidic urine in the bladder and is used for lower urinary tract infections. **Side-effects** include dysuria and haematuria; the drug is contraindicated in glaucoma and renal impairment.

Antituberculosis drugs

These agents are always used in combination to prevent development of resistance. Four drugs for 2 months (after which the sensitivities are available) and two drugs for a further 4 months is the standard regimen for unsupervised treatment. Formulations comprising combinations of these drugs are available. See p. 87 for details of all treatments for TB and infections with non-tuberculous mycobacteria.

- Rifampicin 600 mg oral daily plays a major role in the initial and continuation phases of treatment of TB. It is well absorbed orally, though IV preparations are also available. Hepatotoxicity can be a problem and LFTs must be monitored. Patients should be warned that their body secretions stain orange–red and therefore contact lenses should not be worn.

- Rifabutin 150–450 mg daily single dose has a similar spectrum of activity but also includes activity against some non-tuberculous mycobacteria such as *Mycobacterium avium intracellulare* (p. 117). **Side-effects** include gastrointestinal disturbance, hepatotoxicity (liver biochemistry should be monitored) and interstitial nephritis. Patients should be warned that their body secretions stain orange–red and therefore contact lenses should not be worn.

- Isoniazid (INH) 300 mg oral daily is also used in the initial and continuation phases of TB treatment in combination with other drugs. It has potent activity against replicating *M. tuberculosis*. It is well absorbed orally but parenteral preparations are also available. **Side-effects** include hepatotoxicity (20% have raised liver enzymes), which is commoner in patients who are slow acetylators. Isoniazid can be used a single agent for prophylaxis against TB infection. A peripheral neuropathy can develop, as isoniazid disrupts the tryptophan pathway and therefore pyridoxine 10 mg daily is given prophylactically.

- Ethambutol 15 mg/kg daily for 2 months is active against not only *M. tuberculosis* but also many non-tuberculous mycobacteria. It is used mostly in the initial phase of TB treatment in combination with other drugs. Peak and trough levels should be measured. It is also has a role in the treatment of non-tuberculous mycobacteria such as *M. avium intracellulare* and is well absorbed orally. The major **side-effect** is optic neuritis and patients must be monitored for this. Visual acuity should be checked prior to treatment and patients told to stop the drug immediately if any eye symptoms develop. There is decreased red–green colour perception.

- Pyrazinamide 2 g daily oral is active against *M. tuberculosis* only; it kills mycobacteria replicating in macrophages. It is used mostly in the initial phase of TB treatment in combination with other drugs. *Mycobacterium bovis* is always resistant. The major **side-effect** is hepatotoxicity with high doses and a rising bilirubin requires cessation of therapy.

- Streptomycin is an aminoglycoside that is normally used in drug-resistant cases only. It is given by IM injection 15 mg/kg (max. 1 g). **Side-effects** are ototoxicity and nephrotoxicity; therapeutic monitoring must be performed in patients with renal disease.

- Other agents used mainly for multi-drug-resistant (MDR)-TB (resistant to isoniazid and rifampicin) and extensive drug-resistant (XDR)-TB (also resistant to any quinolone and at least one of kanamycin, capreomycin and amikacin), which are increasingly common problems in some parts of the world. Many other agents can be used. These include the macrolide **clarithromycin**, the aminoglycoside **amikacin** and the quinolones, e.g. **moxifloxacin**, as well as agents from several unrelated groups of antimicrobials. Other drugs include **capreomycin, cycloserine**, **ethionamide** (and the related drug prothionamide) and

Kumar & Clark's Medical Management and Therapeutics

para-aminosalicylic acid (PAS). Treatment of non-tuberculous myco-bacteria is complex and expert advice should be sought.

Antileprotic drugs

- Treatment is normally with **rifampicin** 600 mg once monthly super-vised, combined with one or two agents for 12 months, usually dapsone and clofazimine depending on the type of disease (p. 47).
- **Clofazimine** (for leprosy 300 mg once monthly supervised *and* 50 mg daily self-administered) has good activity against several species of mycobacteria, as well as some anti-inflammatory properties. It is well absorbed orally.
- **Dapsone** (for leprosy 100 mg daily *or* 1–2 mg/kg daily self-administration for those less than 35 kg) is active against many myco-bacteria and some protozoa. It is well absorbed orally. **Side-effects** include haemolysis, methaemoglobinaemia, neuropathy, headaches and vomiting.
- Many other drugs, including **clarithromycin**, **minocycline** and **ofloxacin**, have good activity against *Mycobacterium leprae*. However, the activity of rifampicin is superior and these other drugs should only be used as reserve agents.

Antifungal agents

Polyenes

Polyenes bind to and disrupt the fungal cell membrane. Nystatin and amphotericin have a wide spectrum of activity against many fungi. They are not absorbed orally.

- **Nystatin** is used for the treatment of intestinal candidiasis.
- **Amphotericin** can be used topically for the same indications as nystatin but is also available for IV administration. It is used for treatment of systemic fungal infections, e.g. cryptococcosis and histoplasmosis, and also infections in immunocompromised patients, including aspergillosis and candidaemia. Lipid formulations of amphotericin are less toxic, so that higher doses can be given. These preparations are expensive. Different preparations of IV amphotericin vary and brand names should be specified to avoid mistakes. **Side-effects** of amphotericin include nephrotoxicity, which is dose-related. Anaphylactic reactions occur and an initial test dose should be given before the first infusion. Anorexia, nausea, vomiting and diarrhoea occur, and occasionally muscle and joint pain.

Azoles

The azoles block the action of the fungal enzyme 14-α-demethylase and thus inhibit the formation of ergosterol, a molecule that is a constituent of the fungal cell membrane.

Imidazoles

This group of agents has a broad range of antifungal activity.

- *Clotrimazole, sulconazole, econazole, ketoconazole, miconazole and tioconazole* are mainly used as topical agents to treat candidal and dermatophyte infections, as they are poorly absorbed from the gastrointestinal tract.
- *Ketoconazole* is better absorbed and can be given orally, but hepa-totoxicity is a problem and therefore its use is limited and it has been largely replaced by the newer triazoles.

Triazoles

- *Fluconazole* 100–400 g daily is active against most species of *Candida* and also against *Cryptococcus neoformans*. It is well absorbed orally and penetrates the CSF well. It can also be given intravenously. It is used for the treatment of mucosal and invasive candidal infections and also for cryptococcal infection, usually to prevent relapse following primary treatment with other agents. It also has a role as prophylaxis in immunocompromised patients.
- *Itraconazole* 100–400 mg daily is also used for the treatment of mucosal *Candida* infections. It may be active against some fluconazole-resistant isolates. It also has a role in the treatment of invasive aspergillosis. Oral absorption can be a problem in patients with neutropenia and AIDS, and heart failure may occur following prolonged use.
- *Voriconazole* 400 mg twice daily has a broader range of activity and is used in the treatment of resistant candidal infections such as *Candida krusei*, invasive aspergillosis and some mould infections that may be seen in immunocompromised patients. It also has good activity against *Histoplasma capsulatum*.
- *Posaconazole* 400 mg twice daily is used for invasive aspergillosis not responding to other antifungals.

Gastrointestinal **side-effects** of nausea and diarrhoea, and rashes are common. Liver biochemistry should be checked weekly, as hepatitis is a serious but rare complication. Heart failure can occur with prolonged use of itraconazole. It should not be given intravenously in patients with heart failure. Renal failure (eGFR < 30 mL/min) causes the accumulation of hydroxy-β-cyclodextrin (**the vehicle for itraconazole and voriconazole**) and the usage of these drugs should be avoided. Voriconazole also commonly causes visual disturbances.

Echinocandins

The echinocandins inhibit the synthesis of glucan, a constituent of the fungal cell wall.

- Caspofungin has cidal activity against *Candida* spp. It is also active against *Aspergillus*. Its is usually reserved for treatment of infections in immunocompromised patients by IV infusion 50 mg daily. This IV drug usually retains activity against *Candida* spp. that are resistant to azoles and triazoles and to *Aspergillus terreus*, which is usually resistant to amphotericin. It has no activity against *C. neoformans*. Data on this drug's activity against other fungi are limited, although it is known to be poorly active against *Fusarium* spp. and *Rhizopus* spp.
- Anidulafungin 100 g daily IV after loading dose of 200 mg is also used in invasive candidiasis.
- Micafungin 100 mg daily IV for 14 days is used for invasive candidiasis.

Other antifungals

- Flucytosine is activated by deamination within the fungus to form 5-fluorouracil, which acts as an antimetabolite. This agent is given by IV infusion over 30 mins, 50 mg 4 times daily, and is active against *Candida* spp. and *C. neoformans*. If used as a single agent, resistance develops, so flucytosine is used in combination with **amphotericin** when treating invasive candidal infections and cryptococcosis. It has good penetration into the CSF. Therapeutic drug monitoring is needed, especially if renal function is poor — optimal levels are 25–50 mg/L (200–400 µmol/L), toxic levels > 80 mg/L (620 µmol/L). **Side-effects** are nausea, vomiting, diarrhoea, liver toxicity (monitor liver biochemistry), thrombocytopenia, leucopenia and anaemia.

- Griseofulvin 500 mg daily is deposited in keratin. It inhibits fungal mitosis. This oral agent has activity against dermatophytes and is used when topical therapy has failed or is not indicated, e.g. in nail infections. In adults other newer agents are now preferred, but griseofulvin is still used for scalp dermatophyte infections in children.

- Allylamines include **terbinafine**, which inhibits the fungal enzyme, squalene epoxidase, involved in the biosynthesis of ergosterol, a constituent of the fungal cell membrane. This is the preferred agent for the treatment of dermatophyte infections in adults. Oral preparations are available for the treatment of nail infections (250 mg daily for 6–12 weeks) and topical agents for ringworm.

Antiviral agents

Drugs used for herpes virus infections

- Aciclovir belongs to a group of agents that are activated by phosphorylation by viral thymidine kinase to become competitive inhibitors of viral DNA polymerase and hence viral DNA synthesis. It is active against herpes simplex viruses (HSV) types 1 and 2, and varicella zoster virus (VZV). It has little inhibitory activity against Epstein–Barr virus (EBV) and even less against cytomegalovirus (CMV). Aciclovir is available as topical, oral and IV preparations. It is used topically for the treatment of eye and lip infections with HSV in immunocompetent patients. For HSV infections in immunocompromised patients and in neonates, HSV encephalitis and HSV genital infections, systemic treatment must be used. Systemic aciclovir is also used for the treatment of chickenpox and shingles, which are caused by VZV.

- Valaciclovir is a prodrug of aciclovir. It is used orally for HSV infections of the skin and mucous membranes (including genital infections) and for shingles, and prophylactically against CMV infection following renal transplantation and for suppression of recurrent genital herpes.

Side-effects of aciclovir and valaciclovir include gastrointestinal effects of nausea, vomiting, abdominal pain and diarrhoea, rash, fatigue, headaches and photosensitivity. Neurological effects (more common with valaciclovir) of confusion, hallucination and convulsions are rare. Very rarely, hepatitis and acute kidney injury occur. High doses of valaciclovir in the immunosuppressed can also cause bone marrow depression, haemolytic uraemic syndrome and thrombotic thrombocytopenic purpura.

- Penciclovir has a similar mechanism of action and range of antiviral activity to aciclovir. It is used as a topical agent to treat herpes labialis.

- Famciclovir 750 mg daily is a prodrug of penciclovir and is given orally to treat shingles and for the treatment and suppression of genital herpes. **Side-effects** include headache, nausea and diarrhoea.

- Idoxuridine is an inhibitor of DNA synthesis and is active against HSV-1, HSV-2 and VZV. It is too toxic to be given systemically and has been used as a **topical agent** for the treatment of HSV keratitis, herpes labialis, genital herpes and shingles. It has been mostly superseded by aciclovir.

- Ganciclovir is closely related to aciclovir. It is activated by virus-dependent phosphorylation and is active against herpes viruses. It is 10–50 times more active against CMV than aciclovir and is used for the treatment of severe CMV infection, including retinitis, in immunocompromised patients.

- Valganciclovir is an orally administered prodrug of ganciclovir. It is used for the induction and maintenance treatment of CMV retinitis and also as prophylaxis against CMV in solid organ transplantation. **Side-effects**: myelosuppression can be a major problem.

- Cidofovir inhibits viral **DNA synthesis** following non-viral dependent phosphorylation. It is active against human herpes viruses, including CMV and EBV. Because activation of this drug is not dependent on viral thymidine kinase, it maintains activity against mutants resistant to aciclovir. It also has activity against many other viruses, such as adenoviruses, polyoma viruses, papilloma viruses and pox viruses. **Side-effects**: cidofovir is nephrotoxic and causes iritis and uveitis responsive to topical corticosteroids. It is given by IV infusion 5 mg/kg over 1 hour weekly for 2 weeks, then every 2 weeks. It is preceded by 1 L of 0.9% saline over 1 hour and oral **probenecid** 2 g 3 hours before. Probenecid is repeated 1 g at 2 hours and 8 hours after cidofovir infusion. Cidofovir is confined to the treatment of CMV retinitis in AIDS patients, in whom other drugs cannot be used.

- Foscarnet is an inhibitor of HSV DNA polymerase. It is a toxic drug and its use is limited to the treatment of CMV infections in immunocompromised patients when ganciclovir cannot be used, e.g. because of resistance. It can also be used for HSV infections resistant to aciclovir. It is given by IV infusion 60 mg/kg 3 times daily for 2 weeks, then maintenance 60 mg/kg daily. Nephrotoxicity is its main **side-effect** and patients should be given 1 L of 0.9% saline before and during the infusion.

Drugs used for viral hepatitis
See p. 183.

Drugs used for HIV infection
See p. 100.

Drugs used for influenza

- Neuraminidase inhibitors. **Oseltamivir** 75 mg 12-hourly and **zanamivir** 10 mg inhaled as powder twice daily for 5 days inhibit viral **neuraminidase** and thus prevent new viruses emerging from the host cell. They are active against both influenza A and influenza B viruses. Oseltamivir is given orally, whereas zanamivir is given by the inhalational route. Both can be used for treatment and prophylaxis (75 mg for 7 days after exposure or up to 6 weeks during an epidemic). Treatment should start within 48 hours of the onset of symptoms if possible. Resistance has recently been described with some H1N1 subtypes. **Side-effects** include gastrointestinal symptoms, fatigue, headache, insomnia and epistaxis. Hypersensitivity reactions, hepatitis and Stevens–Johnson syndrome are very rare. Zanamivir can very rarely cause bronchospasm and urticaria.

- Adamantanes. **Amantadine** is active against influenza A virus only and exerts its antiviral action by interfering with a viral protein, M2, which is an ion channel necessary for fusion of the viral envelope with the endosome of the host cell. It can be used for treatment and prophylaxis but has been superseded for the treatment of influenza by the neuraminidase inhibitors. Resistance can occur.

Drugs used for respiratory syncytial virus (RSV)

- Ribavirin can be used by the inhalational route to treat bronchiolitis in infants. Care must be taken that pregnant women are not exposed to the aerosol.
- Palivizumab IM 15 mg/kg once a month is a monoclonal antibody against RSV. It is used for prophylaxis in infants and children at risk of severe disease, i.e. those born before 35 weeks' gestation, those with bronchopulmonary dysplasia and those with heart disease. It is given at the start of and during the RSV season.

Side-effects: for ribavirin, see p. 186. Palivizumab can cause injection site reactions, fever, rash, nervousness and gastrointestinal problems.

Other antivirals

- Inosine pranobex is a nucleoside that has been used for the treatment of mucocutaneous HSV infection, genital warts (human papilloma virus infection) and subacute sclerosing panencephalitis (SSPV) caused by measles virus. There is little evidence of beneficial effect in any of these conditions.
- Pleconaril is an oral agent that inhibits replication of picorna viruses by preventing viral attachment to host cells. It has been used to treat severe enteroviral infections, such as those seen in patients with agammaglobulinaemia and in neonates. Trials for use in treatment of the common cold have also taken place.

Antiprotozoal agents

Drugs from several families, including antibacterials, are used in the treatment of protozoal infections. The main groups of drug are described below.

Antimalarial agents (p. 35)

- Quinolines. This group contains **quinine**, **quinidine**, **chloroquine**, **amodiaquine**, **mefloquine** and **primaquine**. These agents are used primarily for prophylaxis and/or treatment of malaria. Quinine remains one of the treatments of choice for severe malaria, though it does cause hypoglycaemia and blood glucose need to be closely monitored. Chloroquine was an excellent antimalarial agent but resistance is now widespread; it is no longer useful against *falciparum* malaria but remains the treatment of choice in most non-*falciparum* types. **Mefloquine** remains an effective prophylactic agent but its use has been somewhat limited by concerns about neuropsychiatric adverse events.
- Artemisinins. This class includes the drugs **artemisinin**, **artesunate**, **artemether** and **dihydroartemisinin**. They are available for IV, IM, rectal and oral administration. Artemisinins are rapidly active against parasites in the peripheral blood. Unlike quinine, they are not associated with hypoglycaemia. Recent studies have shown promise for IV artesunate in the treatment of severe malaria, though IV artesunate produced to Good Manufacturing Processes standards is still unavailable. Artemisinins should always be used in **combination** with other agents for the treatment of uncomplicated malaria.
- Sulphonamides. Sulphonamides, pyrimethamine, dapsone and **proguanil** all act against *falciparum* malaria by inhibiting folate metabolism. These agents have been widely used in the treatment of non-severe

falciparum malaria, particularly sulfadoxine/pyrimethamine (**Fansidar**), though its use is now being limited by increasing resistance.

- Other antimalarials. **Atovaquone** in combination with the antifolate **proguanil** is effective prophylaxis and treatment for uncomplicated malaria. The antibiotic, doxycycline, has been used for chemoprophylaxis, and **clindamycin** has been used in combination with **quinine** for the treatment of *falciparum* malaria.

Other antiprotozoal agents

- Organometals. The pentavalent antimonial **sodium stibogluconate** 20 mg of antimony/kg for 21 days or **meglamine antimonite** (in India) is used in the treatment of visceral leishmaniasis.
- Antibacterials and antifungals used in the treatment of protozoal infections. **Metronidazole** and **tinidazole** are used for the treatment of amoebiasis and of *Giardia*, *Blastocystis hominis* and *Trichomonas vaginalis* infection. **Co-trimoxazole** can be used for *Cyclospora cayetanensis* and *Isospora belli*. **Sulfadiazine** (in combination with pyrimethamine) and the macrolides **spiramycin** and **azithromycin** are used for toxoplasmosis. The aminoglycoside **paromomycin** can be used for the treatment of intestinal protozoa. **Amphotericin** can be used for visceral leishmaniasis.
- Others. **Pyrimethamine**, a folate antagonist, is used for the treatment of malaria, usually in combination with sulfadoxine. **Pentamidine** is used for antimonial-resistant leishmaniasis. Mepacrine can be used for malaria and also for *Giardia* infection. **Diloxanide furoate** is used for the treatment of asymptomatic intestinal amoebiasis, as it eradicates the cysts.

Antihelminthic agents

Helminths include **cestodes** (tapeworms), **trematodes** (flukes) and **nematodes** (roundworms). The agents used come from several groups.

- Benzimidazoles are synthetic compounds with a broad range of activity against intestinal nematodes. The three main drugs, **albendazole**, **mebendazole** and **tiabendazole** (thiabendazole), have good activity against threadworms (*Enterobius vermicularis*), roundworms (*Ascaris lumbricoides*), whipworms (*Trichuris trichiura*) and hookworms (*Ancylostoma duodenale*, *Necator americanus*), and the encysted larvae of *Trichinella spiralis*. Tiabendazole and albendazole have good activity against *Strongyloides stercoralis* and the canine and feline hookworm larvae that cause cutaneous larva migrans. Albendazole is used in conjunction with surgery for the treatment of hydatid disease caused by the cestodes *Echinococcus granulosus* and *E. multilocularis*. Albendazole is also used in the treatment of cysticercosis.
- Piperazine is a synthetic agent used for the treatment of threadworm and roundworms.
- Levamisole 120–150 mg as a single dose is highly active against the roundworm *A. lumbricoides* and hookworms.
- Niclosamide 2 g as a single dose is active against the cestodes *Taenia saginata* (beef tapeworm), *Taenia solium* (pork tapeworm), *Diphyllobothrium latum* (fish tapeworm) and *Hymenolepis nana* (dwarf tapeworm).
- Diethylcarbamazine is a derivative of piperazine. It is active against the adults and microfilaria of *Loa loa*. It kills the microfilaria of *Brugia malayi* and *Wuchereria bancrofti*, and slowly kills the adults of these species. It

is active against the microfilaria, but not the adults, of *Onchocerca volvulus*.

- **Praziquantel** is active against a wide range of cestodes, including *Taenia saginata* (beef tapeworm), *Taenia solium* (pork tapeworm), *Diphyllobothrium latum* (fish tapeworm) (single dose 5–10 mg/kg) and *Hymenolepis nana* (dwarf tapeworm) (single dose 25 mg/kg), and against trematodes, including all the human **schistosomes**, *Fasciolopsis buski*, *Clonorchis sinensis*, *Metagonimus yokogawai*, *Heterophyes heterophyes*, *Opisthorchis viverrini* and *Paragonimus westermani* (Table 2.6).
- **Ivermectin** has broad antihelminthic activity. It is used in the treatment of *Onchocerca volvulus*, cutaneous larva migrans and strongyloidiasis (150–200 mcg/kg dose).

Further reading

Halstead SB: Dengue, *Lancet* 370:1644–1652, 2007.

Nathanson E, Nunn P, Uplekar M, et al: MDR tuberculosis — critical steps for prevention and control, *New Engl J Med* 363:1050–1058, 2010.

Van de Beek D, Drake JM, Tunkel AR: Nosocomial bacterial meningitis, *New Engl J Med* 362:146–154, 2010.

Further information

http://BNF.org
British National Formulary

www.brit-thoracic.org.uk
British Thoracic Society

www.hpa.org.uk/infections/topics_az/antimicrobial_resistance/guidance.htm
Health Protection Agency

www.idsociety.org
Infectious Disease Society of America

www.nice.org.uk
NICE guidelines

www.ncbi.nlm.nih.gov/entrez/query.fcgi
Online Microbiology textbook (Medical Microbiology, Baron S, ed 4)

www.sanfordguide.com/
Sanford Guide

Human immune deficiency virus and AIDS

3

CHAPTER CONTENTS

INTRODUCTION

- Over 33 million people worldwide have human immune deficiency virus (HIV) infection.
- The human, societal and economical costs are huge.
- HIV1 is a human retrovirus. It infects CD4 lymphocytes.
- Acquired immuno-deficiency syndrome (AIDS) is characterized by infection with opportunistic organisms and malignancy. The onset of development of AIDS following HIV infection can range from months to years (the median incubation period is 10 years).
- Effective therapy has reduced the mortality and morbidity.
- Routes of acquisition. HIV can be isolated from many body fluids and tissues but the majority of infections are transmitted via semen, cervical secretions and blood.
  - *Sexual intercourse (vaginal and anal).* Heterosexual intercourse accounts for most infections; circumcision reduces infection rates.
  - *Mother to child (transplacental, perinatal, breast feeding).* Without intervention, between 15% and 40% of babies born to HIV-infected mothers in Africa become infected.
  - *Contaminated blood, blood products and organ donations.*
  - *Contaminated needles.* These are involved in IV drug use, infections and needle-stick injuries.

PATHOGENESIS

- HIV enters through the wet mucous membranes of the genital tract and infects CD4-bearing dendritic cells and macrophages, which transport the virus to the regional lymph nodes.
- CCR5 and CKCR4 facilitate binding of virus particles to the CD4 T-lymphocytes.
- Once in the draining lymph node, HIV particles are exposed to other cell types, including CD4-bearing T-helper cells.
- Viral replication occurs at an astonishing rate and can be detectable by a rising viral load.
- The adaptive immune system responds by the proliferation and activation of HIV-specific lymphocytes. HIV has a preference for infecting activated CD4 T-cells, which become depleted.

- HIV spreads beyond the lymph nodes, and is capable of infecting memory CD4 T-cells in the bowel; ~60–80% of memory CD4 T-cells are destroyed within the first 17 days of infection in the bowel. Immunosuppression allows opportunistic infections.

There is a progressive loss of CD4 T-cells during the course of infection, increasing the immunosuppression level. In a minority of patients the CD4 T-cell counts are maintained at levels that are not immunosuppressive (long-term non-progressors), possibly related to viral and host genetic factors.

DISEASE MANIFESTATIONS OF HIV INFECTION

These can be due to HIV itself, to the treatment of HIV and lastly to immunosuppression, which leads to opportunistic infections (p. 111) and cancer (p. 117).

HIV infection

Acute seroconversion

Symptoms and signs may be detected from 1 to 4 weeks after exposure to HIV. Often no symptoms are recalled at all. Common mild symptoms include fever, lethargy, myalgia, arthralgia, sore throat and lymphadenopathy. Frequently, a maculopapular skin rash is seen, and nervous system involvement with headache and photophobia is not uncommon. Rarely, myelopathy, peripheral neuropathy, facial palsy, Guillain–Barré syndrome and radiculopathy can be seen. As the adaptive immune response develops, many of these features regress with the fall in viral load.

- Treatment is predominantly symptomatic.

HIV-associated nephropathy (HIVAN)

This presents with renal insufficiency and gross proteinuria late in the course of HIV infection and predominantly in patients of African origin. Without treatment, patients progress rapidly to end-stage kidney disease. Biopsy shows focal segmental glomerulosclerosis.

- Initial management is as for presentation of acute kidney injury. Other reversible causes should be excluded. Co-infection with hepatitis viruses should be ruled out, as this can cause differing glomerular nephritides. Biopsy may be necessary to confirm the diagnosis.
- Treatment is with anti-retroviral medication, which usually produces a dramatic response; ACE inhibitors are also beneficial. Necessary supportive therapy, including dialysis, should be given whilst the response to the primary treatments is being assessed. Prednisolone appears to be beneficial in some patients.

HIV-associated dementia

HIV enters the CNS early after the acute infection, affecting oligodendrocytes, microglia and astrocytes. However, symptoms are only seen in patients who have been HIV-infected for a number of years; they include changes in personality, intellect and coordination.

- Diagnosis is usually one of exclusion.
- Treatment with highly active anti-retroviral therapy (HAART) is associated with an improvement in symptoms in over half the patients treated. Whether CNS penetration is essential for this effect is not clear. AZT has the most evidence of efficacy. Other anti-retrovirals that have good CNS penetration include abacavir and the non-nucleoside reverse transcriptase inhibitor (NNRTI) class of drugs (p. 94).

Manifestations due to treatment of HIV

Mitochondrial toxicity and lactic acidosis

- Mitochondria have their own genome, which utilizes the enzyme, γ-DNA polymerase, for replication. Unfortunately, γ-DNA polymerase, like viral reverse transcriptase, recognizes nucleotide reverse transcriptase inhibitors (NRTIs) as nucleosides, leading to chain termination and interruption of the mitochondrial life cycle.
- Organ damage occurs when sufficient mitochondria within a tissue are affected for normal function not to be maintained.
- Different NRTIs affect different organ systems preferentially. Mitochondrial toxicity can be seen affecting the peripheral nerves, pancreas, liver, muscle and bone marrow. Pancreatitis should be treated, but with medication stopped. Myopathy and peripheral neuropathy can improve with a change of medication.
- Liver toxicity can lead to the potentially fatal problem of lactic acidosis. Symptoms and signs of this are non-specific and include nausea, malaise, weight loss and abdominal pain. Investigations may show abnormal liver enzymes. A blood lactate measurement with ABG should be done. Specialist advice should be sought in any patient on NRTIs with an acidotic pH and a raised blood lactate.

Lipodystrophy and metabolic syndrome

This is likely to be a heterogenous condition of overlapping syndromes, with differing aetiologies. The syndrome is associated with treatment with protease inhibitors (PIs) and some NRTIs. However, aspects of this condition can occur in patients never exposed to these medications.

The main components of the syndrome are dyslipidaemia, insulin resistance and diabetes (metabolic syndrome), visceral/breast fat accumulation and diminution of subcutaneous fat mass. The changes in appearance can lead to problems with adherence to medication. Lipodystrophy is associated with an increased cardiovascular risk, partly due to dyslipidaemia and diabetes.

Current recommendations include avoiding the use of **stavudine**, and of zidovudine if possible. Exercise and diet have been associated with mild improvements.

Severe dyslipidaemia requires treatment with statins or fibrates. Dyslipidaemia and lipoatrophy require a switch of therapy. Bioadsorbable and permanent substances have been injected to correct subcutaneous lipoatrophy.

Immune reconstitution inflammatory syndrome (IRIS)

This occurs in severely immunosuppressed people on HAART, when their immune system starts to recover. They mount an inflammatory response with an exacerbation of symptoms.

APPROACH TO THE PATIENT

Initial diagnosis

The routine tests for screening are ELISA techniques confirmed with Western blot assay. However, antibodies may not appear until 3 months.

Simple, rapid HIV antibody screening assays are available using blood, urine and saliva. These tests are very sensitive and may give false positive results. Confirmatory tests are necessary using highly sensitive ELISAs that can detect HIV antibodies at 6–8 weeks after infection.

In patients with undetermined/negative HIV serology, the diagnosis of an acute infection is by demonstrating a high viral load or a positive p. 24 antigen (which disappears after 8 weeks of infection).

Investigations and monitoring

Initial assessment

All clinicians should be of the competence necessary to obtain consent for an HIV test. The British HIV Association provides a list of associated presenting conditions for which an HIV test may be indicated (http://www.bhiva.org/cms1222621.asp). Many patients are diagnosed when they present themselves to a sexual health clinic.

Following diagnosis:

- Take a history with details of route of transmission, probable length of time infected and any symptoms of seroconversion.
- Carry out baseline investigations (Box 3.1) to assess current immune function.
- Take a medication history, noting any reactions.
- Seek evidence of co-infection with hepatitis.

Box 3.1 Baseline investigations in a newly diagnosed asymptomatic patient with HIV infection

Haematology
- FBC, differential count and film

Biochemistry
- Serum, liver and renal function
- Fasting serum lipid profile
- Fasting blood glucose

Immunology
- Lymphocyte subsets
- HLA-B*5701 status

Virology
- HIV antibody (confirmatory)
- HIV viral load (copies per mL)
- HIV genotype
- Hepatitis serology (A, B and C)
- Cytomegalovirus antibody

Microbiology
- Toxoplasmosis serology
- Syphilis serology
- Screen for other STIs

Other
- Cervical cytology
- CXR if indicated
- Human T-cell lymphotropic virus (HTLV)-1 serology in patients of African origin
- Glucose-6-phosphate-dehydrogenase (G6PD) status

(Based on British HIV Association guidelines 2008)

A full examination, including fundoscopy, neurological examination and palpation of all lymph node groups, is carried out.

The acutely unwell patient with HIV infection may be suffering from multiple opportunistic infections, and all symptoms and signs should not be attributed to HIV itself.

CD4 count

(Normal range 400–1200 mm^3.)

- Helper T-cells bearing the marker CD4 are infected with HIV. The absolute concentration of CD4 T-cells within blood has proven correlations with disease stage and risk of disease progression.
- Primary prophylaxis is indicated at CD4 counts below 200 to protect against *Pneumocystis jiroveci*, and below 100 to prevent toxoplasmosis.
- A good response to HAART correlates with a rise in the CD4 count, which is a good indication of the patient's immune status.
- CD4 counts are performed every 3 months in asymptomatic patients (Box 3.1), but more frequently if unexpected changes are seen in either the clinical state or the viral load of the patient.

The viral load

Transitory changes in the viral load occur with intercurrent infection and vaccination. Thus treatment decisions should never be made on a one-off aberrant viral load reading without other clinical or laboratory evidence to support its validity.

A number of assays are available, the commonest being the reverse transcription polymerase chain reaction (RT-PCR). The most sensitive test is able to detect 20 copies of viral RNA/mL.

- The viral load is an independent indicator of disease progression, i.e. the higher the viral load, the more likely the patient is going to progress to severe immunosuppression and AIDS.
- It can also be used as a marker of treatment success. HIV can only develop resistance if it is allowed to replicate actively whilst in the presence of the drug. Successful treatment is dependent on the prevention of resistant strains emerging. An aim of treatment is to reduce the viral load to below the level of detection within 3 months. Persistently detectable viral loads indicate ongoing viral replication and correlate with the development of resistance and treatment failure; they would usually warrant a change in the management of the patient. Thus, the viral load is used to assess:
  - the rate of immune decline in those patients 'off' treatment
  - treatment success in those patients on treatment. Measurements should be done every 3 months in asymptomatic patients, but more frequently if unexpected changes are seen in the clinical state or CD4 count.

Genotyping

- Genotype variations within HIV exist between viral subtypes and also point mutations associated with retroviral drug usage.
- Phenotype variations give an indication of possible drug resistance, although they do not detect low levels of resistant viruses (< 20% of viral populations).
- In the absence of medication, the dominant viral species will revert back to wild type relatively quickly.
- Delay in resistance testing once medication is stopped can lead to missing resistant mutants in a patient failing a drug regimen.

- Transmission of the drug-resistant virus can occur, accounting for poor response to first-line therapy.

Thus all newly diagnosed patients should be tested for resistance, and lack of a significant fall in the viral load by 4–8 weeks requires further testing to look for minority viral species not evident at the time of initiation of therapy.

Phenotyping

This is also used to detect resistance. HIV replication in vitro in the presence of anti-retrovirals (ARVs) is tested. However, assays are complex and not widely available.

HIGHLY ACTIVE ANTI-RETROVIRAL THERAPY (HAART)

In order to be successful, anti-retroviral treatment has to prevent the emergence of resistant strains of virus within the patient. Because of the error-prone nature of viral reverse transcriptase, mutations arise with the ongoing viral life cycle. Reduction of this viral proliferation rate to as low as possible prevents the development of these mutations. Treatment with one or two anti-retroviral medications in the majority of patients is insufficient to reduce this rate to levels that would prevent the emergence of resistance. It is only with the use of at least three agents that the rate of viral cycling is reduced to preventative levels. Alongside viral suppression, immune reconstitution can occur, which can be monitored by rising CD4 count.

Available anti-retroviral medications, along with their side-effects, are shown in Table 3.1.

Available drugs

Nucleoside reverse transcriptase inhibitors (NRTIs)

- Zidovudine (AZT), when used as monotherapy, leads to resistant mutations appearing within the reverse transcriptase gene in months. A combined formulation with **lamivudine (3TC)**, i.e. **Combivir (AZT/3TC)** has proven popular due to the decreased pill burden. Cross-resistance with other drugs in this class is a problem. Switching AZT to abacavir can reduce the rate of fat loss. The drug should not be used with D4T, as they antagonize each other's effects. Bone marrow toxic effects can be increased by probenecid, ganciclovir, doxorubicin, co-trimoxazole, pyrimethamine and sulfadiazine.
- Stavudine (D4T) is a thymidine analogue like zidovudine. Its major problems with lipodystrophy and peripheral neuropathy have led to it becoming obsolete but it is still used in some countries. Specific mutations in the reverse transcriptase gene can confer cross-resistance between this drug and lamivudine (3TC), **emtricitabine** (FTC) and abacavir (ABC). Antagonistic interactions between AZT and D4T occur. Co-prescribing with other medications that are particularly neurotoxic is not advised.
- Abacavir (ABC) is a guanosine analogue that has a good side-effect profile in the majority of patients and crosses the blood–brain barrier. It is available in two combination pills: one as a triple combination with AZT and 3TC, and one as a combination with 3TC. It can be used once daily with 3TC. The triple nucleotide regime alone is now not recommended, as studies have called into doubt its effectiveness when

compared with other NNRTI- or PI-based regimes. Hypersensitivity reactions are a major problem. If two differing hypersensitivity symptoms occur, stop the medication. In most cases, **once stopped, the medication must *never* be restarted**. In patients whose prescription for abacavir has been stopped for another reason, restarting the medication should be done with regular monitoring. Viral resistance to ABC occurs in a stepwise fashion, and the appearance of mutants with low-level resistance does not impede the drug's efficacy. However, with the appearance of large numbers of AZT-associated mutations in the reverse transcriptase gene, the drug significantly loses potency.

- Lamivudine (3TC) is a popular cytosine analogue that is effective when used as part of an NNRTI- or PI-based combination regime. It can be given once daily. In general, the drug is well tolerated. Resistance to this medication develops rapidly, the commonest reverse transcriptase mutation occurring at codon 184 (M184V/I). This drug, as well as FTC, is effective in the treatment of hepatitis B.

- Didanosine (DDI) is effective as part of a combination regime in the treatment of HIV, and is available in once-daily or twice-daily formulations. Strict dietary restrictions (it must be taken 2 hours before or after food on an empty stomach) in its administration have clouded its common use (Table 3.1). The enteric-coated form is taken once daily but still has to be taken at least 2 hours before or 2 hours after any oral intake other than water. Given the number of other HIV medications that are recommended to be taken with food, this complicates the dosing regimen. The formulation contains calcium and magnesium antacids. There is evidence of cross-resistance with other NRTIs. It interacts with tenofovir, causing decreased levels of both.

- Emtricitabine (FTC) is a cytosine analogue that is active against both hepatitis B and HIV, though it is not currently recommended for the treatment of hepatitis B. It is available in a once-daily formulation and in a combination formulation with tenofovir. FTC has been compared with D4T and 3TC, and shows equivalence or improvement over the more established therapies. No studies have looked at possible interactions between FTC and other cytosine analogues (DDC and 3TC). However, with the evidence of competition between D4T and AZT, it is not recommended that they be co-prescribed. The mutation at codon 184 (M184V/I) of the reverse transcriptase gene that confers resistance to 3TC also confers resistance to FTC. The virus strains carrying this mutation are more susceptible to AZT.

Nucleotide reverse transcriptase inhibitors

- Tenofovir (TFV). Nucleoside analogues have to be intracellularly phosphorylated to become the active form of the drug — a nucleotide. Tenofovir is already in the phosphorylated form and is equivalent to other NRTIs. Tenofovir can be used as a switch medication for those patients experiencing lipid abnormalities with stavudine (D4T). It should not be used with DDI, as a fall in CD4 count can occur. Tenofovir has activity against hepatitis B and is first-line therapy in co-infected (HIV and HBV) patients, alongside 3TC. Renal dysfunction, most commonly a proximal renal tubular defect seen with the Fanconi syndrome, requires monitoring. Mutation at codon 64 of the reverse transcriptase gene (also seen with ABC) can confer resistance. The M184V/I mutation, as with AZT, can confer some increased susceptibility to this medication.

Table 3.1 Anti-retroviral drugs available in the UK

Drug name (alphabetical order)	Dose/regimen	Metabolism	Recognized side-effects
Nucleoside/nucleotide* reverse transcriptase inhibitors (NRTIs)			
Abacavir (ABC)	600 mg (one 600 mg tablet or two 300 mg tablets) once daily	No food restrictions	Hypersensitivity reaction, linked with HLA-B*5701, potentially fatal. Fever, rash, GI effects, headaches, puffy throat and face
Didanosine (DDI)	400 mg once daily (> 60 kg), 250 mg once daily (< 60 kg), one capsule/day	30–60 mins before food	Nausea, diarrhoea, polyneuropathy, pancreatitis. Association with mitochondrial dysfunction and lactic acidosis. Lipodystrophy
Emtricitabine (FTC)	200 mg (one capsule) once daily	No food effects. Renal excretion	Headache, nausea, diarrhoea and skin pigmentation. Modify dose if creatinine clearance is < 50 mL/min, lactic acidosis and liver disease
Lamivudine (3TC)	One 300 mg or two 150 mg tablets once daily	No food effects. Well absorbed with high bioavailability	Nausea, headache, rash, peripheral neuropathy, myelosuppression. Association with mitochondrial dysfunction and lactic acidosis
Stavudine (D4T) (seldom used)	40 mg (one tablet) twice daily. Reduce to 30 mg twice daily < 60 kg	High bioavailability. Competes with zidovudine for intracellular activation by phosphorylation so do not use together	Polyneuropathy, lipoatrophy, GI effects, megaloblastic changes. Mitochondrial dysfunction and lactic acidosis (fatal)
Tenofovir (TFV)	One 245 mg tablet once daily	After food	Hypophosphataemia, renal toxicity

Zidovudine (AZT)	250–300 mg (one capsule) twice daily	Well absorbed with good bioavailability. No food effects	Nausea, headache, insomnia, skin and nail pigmentation, myelosuppression, megaloblastic changes. Liver abnormality, lipoatrophy. Association with mitochondrial dysfunction and lactic acidosis
Non-nucleoside reverse transcriptase inhibitors (NNRTIs)			
Efavirenz (EFV)	600 mg (one tablet) once daily, ideally at night	Metabolized by cytochrome p. 450 3A (mixed inducer and inhibitor)	Contraindicated in pregnancy. Rash, toxic epidermal necrolysis, CNS effects (vivid dreams, agitation, hallucinations, depression)
Nevirapine (NEV)	200 mg (one tablet) once daily for first 14 days, then 200 mg (one tablet) twice daily	High bioavailability, long half-life, wide tissue distribution. Induces its own metabolism, hence dose escalation. No food effects	Nausea, fatigue, headache and GI symptoms, Muscle pains. Rash, toxic epidermal necrolysis, hepatic toxicity
Etravirine (TMC125)	200 mg (two 100 mg tablets) twice daily	After food. Substrate and inducer of CYP3A4, substrate and inhibitor of CYP2C9 and CYP2C19	Hypersensitivity reaction, erythema multiforme, nausea
Protease inhibitors (PIs) (all given with ritonavir)			
Atazanavir (ATZ)	300 mg once daily (two 150 mg capsules) + ritonavir 100 mg once daily	Cytochrome p. 450 3A4 inhibitor and substrate. Take with food; no concomitant antacids	Hyperbilirubinaemia. Haematuria. Fewer lipid abnormalities than some other PIs
Darunavir	600 mg (two 300 mg tablets) + ritonavir 100 mg twice daily	Take with food. Cytochrome p. 450 3A4 inhibitor and substrate	Rash, toxic epidermal necrolysis, erythema multiforme, hyperlipidaemia. Diarrhoea, nausea, headache, lipodystrophy

Table 3.1 Continued

Drug name (alphabetical order)	Dose/regimen	Metabolism	Recognized side-effects
Fosprenavir Amprenavir (AMP)	700 mg (one tablet) + ritonavir 100 mg twice daily 600 mg + ritonavir 100 mg twice daily	With food. Cytochrome p. 450 3A4 inhibitor, inducer and substrate	Rash, diarrhoea, nausea, vomiting. Peri-oral tingling. Hyperlipidaemia, lipodystrophy, liver dysfunction, toxic epidermal necrolysis
Indinavir (IND)	800 mg (two 400 mg tablets) + ritonavir 100 mg twice daily	1 hour before or 2 hours after food. Cytochrome p. 450 3A4 inhibitor	Nausea, headache, fatigue, vomiting, rash, dry skin, worsening thrombocytopenia and anaemia. Nephrolithiasis, hyperbilirubinaemia, alopecia, hyperlipidemia, lipodystrophy
Lopinavir/ ritonavir (LPV/ RIT)	400 mg + ritonavir 100 mg (two tablets) twice daily	With food. Cytochrome p. 450 3A4 inhibitor and substrate	GI intolerance, nausea, vomiting and diarrhoea. Hyperlipidemia, lipodystrophy. Rare — kidney stones, liver dysfunction, pancreatitis
Ritonavir (RIT) (seldom used alone)	600 mg (six 100 mg capsules) twice daily	With food. Cytochrome p. 450 3A4 — powerful inhibitor	GI intolerance, nausea, vomiting, diarrhoea, peri-oral paraesthesia, hyperlipidemia, lipodystrophy, metallic taste. Renal failure
Saquinavir (SAQ)	1000 mg (two 500 mg tablets) + ritonavir 100 mg twice daily	Take with food. Cytochrome p. 450 inhibitor and substrate. Avoid garlic	GI intolerance, nausea, diarrhoea, headache, hyperlipidaemia, lipodystrophy
Tipranavir (TPR)	500 mg (two 250 mg capsules) + ritonavir 200 mg twice daily	With food	GI side-effects. Rare cases of intracranial bleeding, rash, hyperlipidemia, lipodystrophy. Liver toxicity — monitor

Integrase inhibitors			
Raltegravir	400 mg (one tablet) twice daily	Take with or without food. Metabolism via UGT1A1 glucuronidation	Diarrhoea, nausea, headache, myopathy and rhabdomyolysis
Fusion inhibitors			
Enfuvitide, T-20	90 mg (1 mL) twice daily by SC injection		Reaction at injection site. Hypersensitivity
Co-receptor blockers			
Maraviroc	300 mg twice daily	Blocks the CCR5 chemokine co-receptor. Take with or without food. Cytochrome p. 450 substrate	Hepatotoxicity, pyrexia, rash, hypotension
Fixed-dose combinations			

Combivir AZT 300 mg/3TC 150 mg
Kivexa Abacavir 600 mg/3TC 300 mg
Truvada Tenofovir 245 mg/FTC 200 mg
Trizivir Abacavir 300 mg/AZT 300 mg/3TC 150 mg
Atripla Tenofovir 300 mg/FTC 200 mg/efavirenz 600 mg
Kaletra Lopinavir 200 mg/ritonavir 50 mg — 2 tablets per day

N.B. Check all doses and side-effects in local formularies, e.g. *British National Formulary.*

Cross-resistance can occur between tenofovir and AZT or D4T. Despite this, the risk of cross-resistance with other NRTIs is relatively low. Interactions also occur between tenofovir and atazanavir or lopinavir. There is no evidence of interactions with methadone, anti-TB medication, 3TC, efavirenz and the oral contraceptive pill.

Non-nucleoside/nucleotide reverse transcriptase inhibitors (NNRTIs)

- Efavirenz (EFV) has proven efficacy as a first-line agent when combined with two NRTIs (not used in pregnancy). A previous psychiatric history should be taken into account in view of the dysphoria that can occur with this drug. Most side-effects will present themselves shortly after treatment is started. Liver dysfunction occurs and is more common in patients co-infected with hepatitis viruses, as efavirenz is an inducer of liver cytochrome p. 450 3A4 enzyme. Rash is common but rarely severe. Efavirenz is currently not recommended for use in women considering pregnancy. Both efavirenz and nevirapine have long half-lives.

- Nevirapine (NEV) can be as effective as PIs when combined with two NRTIs. Nevirapine, alongside AZT, has the best CNS penetration of the currently used medications. Nevirapine is taken as two tablets, which can be taken together or as a split dose. It has a low genetic barrier to resistance, and mutations at codons 103, 181, 190 and 188 of the viral reverse transcriptase gene are associated with resistance to both efavirenz and nevirapine. Like efavirenz, it has a long half-life. The **common side-effects** include a rash that can vary from mild and self-limiting (for 2–4 weeks) to more severe, requiring the medication to be stopped. Starting the medication at a low dose and then gradually increasing it reduces the incidence of the milder rash. Abacavir and nevirapine should not be started at the same time, as distinguishing the cause of a hypersensitivity reaction can be difficult. Liver toxicity is a serious side-effect associated with nevirapine, and has both genetic and environmental risk factors. Nevirapine is not recommended in men with CD4 counts > 400, women with CD4 counts > 250, or in patients with hepatitis virus co-infection. It is a potent inducer of the cytochrome p. 450 3A4 enzyme, and hence has many drug interactions.

- Etravirine is a drug that has recently become available; it has activity against virus resistant to other NNRTIs. It has a unique molecular flexibility, thought to account for its greater barrier to the development of resistant virus. Severe rashes have been reported as a side-effect.

Protease inhibitors (PIs)

PIs block the action of the viral protease, which cleaves large viral polypeptide chains into functioning proteins. The functioning viral protease, integrase, and reverse transcriptase enzymes are all products of protease activity. Viral protease has a fold in its quaternary structure that the inhibitors fit into, altering the protease's catalytic activity. Mutations in the amino acids that make up the fold can impair the association of the drug with the fold and consequently lead to resistance. New virus particles can be assembled in the presence of PI medication, but these are non-infectious and hence the viral life cycle is interrupted.

- Ritonavir (RIT) is often prescribed specifically for its ability to boost the levels of another co-administered PI. It is a liver and gut enzyme inhibitor and can therefore increase the levels of other PIs and their half-life. By doing this, it can improve the side-effect profiles and dosing requirements of other PIs. It does not cross the blood–brain barrier. It can only be stored for 1 month at room temperature; thus the patient has to keep stocks refrigerated. The **side-effects** are one of the chief reasons why this drug is now rarely prescribed as the sole PI, but are less of a problem with the low-dose boosting regimen. As with the other PIs, there is cross-resistance of varying degrees across the whole class. In cases of ritonavir resistance the virus is almost always resistant to indinavir, and to a lesser extent nelfinavir and saquinavir. Ritonavir is a potent liver enzyme inhibitor and thus interacts with a number of other medications, potentially raising their levels dangerously.

- Lopinavir (LPV), combined with appropriate NRTIs, is the first-line PI agent of choice. Its use in naïve (previously untreated with lopinavir) patients enables individuals to have fully suppressed viral loads at 6 years after the initiation of therapy. Lopinavir is co-formulated with **ritonavir**, another PI. Ritonavir is a potent inhibitor of the liver enzyme that metabolizes lopinavir, and thus potentiates its action. Lopinavir can be effective in patients who have previously been given PIs, even in the presence of small numbers of PI resistance-conferring mutations. As with other members of this class, body fat changes associated with blood dyslipidaemia can occur. Mutations in the viral protease gene can confer resistance to all drugs in this class. Lopinavir has a high genetic barrier to resistance and a number of these mutations appear to be necessary before phenotypic resistance emerges.

- Fosamprenavir/amprenavir (AMP) is inferior to other PIs in treatment-naïve patients and is not recommended for use in this group of patients. This may be due to poor adherence secondary to a large and difficult pill burden (eight very large tablets a day) and side-effects. Ritonavir-boosted amprenavir is effective in patients who have resistance to nelfinavir, indinavir, ritonavir and saquinavir, and consequently it has a role in patients who have virologically failed therapy. Fosamprenavir is a prodrug of amprenavir, which in trial data has demonstrated equivalence with other PIs in treatment naïve patients. It has been put forward as an alternative to lopinavir in treatment-naïve patients because of the low incidence of PI cross-resistance in patients who fail fosamprenavir treatment; this allows other PIs to be held for effective second-line therapy. It is a sulphonamide and therefore a history of previous allergic reactions to sulphonamides makes them at risk of further reaction.

- Indinavir (IND) in combination is able to sustain a reduction in the viral load below the level of detection. Indinavir by itself requires relatively strict dietary requirements and three times a day dosing. For these reasons, together with the implications for adherence, indinavir is now usually prescribed as part of a ritonavir-boosted regimen. Resistance can occur rapidly if dosing is suboptimal. The appearance of four or more mutations in the susceptible codons of the protease gene can confer high-level resistance. Indinavir is metabolized by the liver and thus interacts with other liver enzyme inhibitors and inducers.

- Atazanavir (ATZ) is only recommended for use in treatment-experienced patients. It is as effective in first-line therapy as efavirenz and nelfinavir in some studies. It is the only PI currently available that is suitable for once-daily dosing. Haematuria has been reported in patients taking this drug. It appears that atazanavir-treated patients have less harmful lipid changes than those treated with other PIs such as efavirenz. There is also evidence of an improvement in lipodystrophy upon switching from another regimen. Like other PIs, atazanavir is a p. 450 3A4 inhibitor and consequently has a wide range of interactions. Atazanavir resistance emerges with increasing numbers of mutations in the viral protease gene. An interesting mutation at codon 150 of the viral protease gene confers resistance to atazanavir but increases sensitivity to other PIs. Hyperbilirubinaemia is a frequent side-effect but is not associated with liver enzyme changes and rarely causes cessation of treatment.

- Saquinavir (SAQ) has a long record of effectiveness in the treatment of HIV. Hard gel saquinavir is nearly always prescribed as a combination with ritonavir. To prevent problems with adherence, medicines that symptomatically treat these **side-effects** can be given prior to the prescription. As with other drugs of this class, treatment is associated with lipodystrophy. Resistance is associated with mutations at codons 48 and 90 of the protease gene. Saquinavir inhibits not only cytochrome p. 450 3A4, but also P-glycoprotein, and consequently interacts with a number of other drugs.

- Tipranavir (TPR) is a non-peptidic PI, which inhibits the protease enzyme. Due to its different chemical structure, viral strains resistant to other PIs are sensitive to tipranavir. It is used in treatment-experienced patients, with favourable results. In combination with the fusion inhibitor, T20, results are even more promising. No data are available yet on this drug's use in treatment-naïve patients. Rash is potentially worse with the oral contraceptive pill. Tipranavir was developed with a view to treating patients with cross-class resistance to PIs. For resistance to develop, a number of mutations must occur in the protease gene. The codons at which these occur differ from the ones that confer cross-class resistance.

- Darunavir is a boosted PI that received approval for use in treatment-experienced patients in 2008 and approval for use in treatment-naïve patients in 2009. Studies have shown favourable results compared to lopinavir. Mild to moderate rash is seen in some patients; other **side-effects** reported include diarrhoea, headache, vomiting, abdominal pain and constipation. Reported drug interactions include atorvastatin, pravastatin, rifabutin, saquinavir, lopinavir and maraviroc.

Integrase inhibitors

- Raltegravir is a selective inhibitor of HIV integrase, which blocks viral replication by preventing the insertion of HIV DNA into the human DNA genome. It is only used in patients who are resistant to many anti-retrovirals.

Fusion inhibitors

Two glycoproteins on the surface of HIV (gp120 and gp41) are used to engage and bind to the host T-cells. Engagement of gp120 with CD4 exposes the hydrophobic tip of gp41, which dives straight to the nearest hydrophobic environment, the host T-cell's bilipid membrane.

- Enfuvirtide works by binding to gp41 and preventing the fusion of HIV's viral envelope with the host T-cell. Its use is in patients who have failed a number of other regimens. It is the only HIV drug that has to be taken subcutaneously and injections have to be prepared daily. A needle-free method of delivery has been developed using a carbon dioxide-powered jet, with fewer incidences of injection site reactions. Injection site reactions are currently the most common **side-effects** (95%). These vary between an itchy rash, red, swollen or puffy skin, hardened skin or injection site cysts or nodules. Other reported effects include bacterial pneumonia, headache, insomnia, neuropathy and eosinophilia. No interactions between T-20 and other drugs have been noted so far. Resistance mutations to T-20 can occur rapidly, in the gene encoding viral gp41. However, there is good evidence that resistance to other classes of drugs does not leave patients resistant to T-20.

Co-receptor blockers

● Maraviroc, a chemokine receptor antagonist, blocks the cellular CCR5 receptor entry by CCR5 trophic strains of HIV. It is used with other anti-retrovirals in patients previously treated. Its use is hampered by the need for a phenotypic test of viral tropism prior to use.

Indications for anti-retroviral therapy

Symptomatic HIV infection

● In individuals with evidence of a disease related to immunosuppression, treatment should be initiated irrespective of the CD4 count and viral load.
● TB, though being an AIDS-defining illness, is not strictly an opportunistic infection, as immunocompetent patients can have the disease. Hence there is debate as to whether pulmonary TB infection in the context of HIV is an absolute indication for the initiation of therapy in the absence of evidence of other immunosuppression.

Asymptomatic HIV infection

● *CD4 count < 200 at diagnosis.* Start treatment immediately. This is the level often used in countries with poor resources and inadequate HAART supplies.
● *CD4 counts < 350.* Start treatment when the patient is ready, and certainly no later than CD4 < 200.
● *Asymptomatic patients with CD4 counts > 500 with a low CD4 percentage, hepatitis B/C or cardiovascular risk.* Special consideration is necessary and treatment may be indicated.

Currently, there is little evidence that treatment during *primary infection* of HIV alters the natural course of the disease. However, there is evidence that treatment during primary infection can preserve anti-HIV-specific CD4 responses, which are usually lost early in the disease. It is therefore recommended that patients be offered entry into a clinical trial of treatment.

Starting therapy

There is a wide range of drugs available for the treatment of HIV. Standard therapy is two NRTIs, e.g. **tenofovir** and **emtricitabine**, combined with either a **ritonavir**-boosted PI, e.g. **lopinavir**, or an NNRTI, e.g. **efavirenz**, except in women wishing to become pregnant. The choice between the two is debatable. The lower resistance of NNRTIs to mutation is used as an argument for their use as first-line therapy, in that they are less likely to be successful when used as a second-line agent.

Other options include boosted **saquinavir**- and boosted **fosamprenavir**-based regimens. Evidence is not sufficient for the use of boosted **atazanavir** in naïve patients.

● Changing therapy because of virologic failure. Patients should be considered for a change in therapy if their viral load rises to > 400 copies/mL on two separate occasions at least 1 month apart. A resistance test should be carried out, and assessment made of potential causes such as poor adherence, drug interactions and side-effects. The new regimen should contain at least three drugs that resistance testing and past history suggest would have antiviral activity in vivo. In patients with evidence of multiple multi-class drug resistance, the aim of treatment shifts from maintaining an undetectable viral load to one of preserving immunological function. In patients with stable CD4 counts (50–100), delaying new combinations containing just one new drug to a time when more drugs may become available is also advised.

● Structured treatment interruptions. These were tried but recent data suggest that patients do less well than on conventional therapy.

Adherence

For treatment to be effective the patient must adhere to the required dosing schedules and dietary requirements for anti-retroviral medication. Levels of adherence below 95% have been associated with poor responses and the emergence of resistant virus. Greater understanding of factors that can improve adherence is required.

● Patient factors include:
  • An understanding of living with HIV, and optimizing motivation and commitment to maintain this.
  • Social and behavioural factors that may impact upon an individual's adherence to difficult medication regimes.
  • Mental health illness, which needs to be treated effectively.
● Regime factors include:
  • Noting individual patient preferences for regimen characteristics, such as pill burden, pill size, dosing frequency and dietary requirements.
  • Informing patients of likely toxicities and encouraging them to report these to the clinician.
  • Noting potential drug interactions and making necessary dose adjustments.

The clinician should be aware of the full range of support services that can help with these factors.

Adherence should be monitored regularly in the clinic and recorded in the notes. The management of any failing therapy must include a comprehensive review to assess whether poor adherence has led to the problem, and ways in which this can be avoided in the future.

Choice of drugs (Table 3.1)

The drug regimen used for starting therapy must be individualized to suit each patient's needs.

● Nucleoside reverse transcription inhibitor (NRTI). The combination of two NRTIs to form a backbone to the treatment is increasingly influenced by both efficacy and ease of administration. The availability of the once-daily, one-tablet, fixed-dose combinations, Truvada (TFV/FTC) and Kivexa (ABC/3TC), has led to the majority of patients who are naïve to medication being prescribed one of these as their 2NRTI backbone. Combivir (AZT/3TC), with a twice-daily dosing schedule and poorer toxicity profile, is less frequently prescribed.

● Non-nucleoside reverse transcriptase inhibitor (NNRTI). The decision about use of an NNRTI or a boosted PI will depend on the particular circumstances of each patient but, following clinical trial data, an

NNRTI-based regimen is most commonly prescribed to treatment-naïve patients.

- **Efavirenz** is frequently used, having demonstrated good durability over time, and potency at low CD4 counts and in high viral loads. It has the advantage of once-daily dosing but is associated with CNS side-effects (Table 3.1) and is contraindicated in pregnancy. A fixed-dose preparation of efavirenz co-formulated with Truvada (**Atripla**) allows for a 'one pill once a day' regimen.
- **Nevirapine** is of equivalent potency to efavirenz but has a higher incidence of hepatotoxicity and rash and is taken twice daily. Toxicity is greater in women and in those with higher CD4 counts. It is contraindicated in women with CD4 counts > 250 cells and in men with counts > 400. However, it is a useful alternative to efavirenz if CNS side-effects are troublesome and in women with lower CD4 counts who wish to conceive.
- **Etravirine** is a second-generation NNRTI, active against drug-resistant strains and useful in treatment-experienced patients.
- **Protease inhibitor (PI).** This class of drugs has demonstrated excellent efficacy in clinical practice. A PI combined with a low dose of ritonavir (a boosting PI) provides a pharmacokinetic advantage and is now most commonly used in naïve patients. When this approach is used, the half-life of the active drug is increased, allowing greater drug exposure, fewer pills with enhanced potency and minimized risk of resistance. The disadvantage is a possible risk of greater lipid abnormalities, particularly raised fasting triglycerides. **Darunavir/ritonavir**, **lopinavir/ritonavir** and **fosamprenavir/ritonavir** (all taken twice daily) are recommended for first-line therapy, with **saquinavir/ritonavir** as an alternative. All three regimens commonly cause gastrointestinal disturbance and lipid abnormalities. **Atazanavir/ritonavir** is a once-daily regimen.

Currently, treatment-naïve patients should be treated with two NRTIs, with either an NNRTI or a PI. Despite interest in the use of PI monotherapy in some situations, the current data do not support its use in treatment-naïve patients.

OPPORTUNISTIC INFECTION IN THE HAART ERA

Fungal infection

Candidiasis

Candidiasis is caused by infection with various *Candida* species, the commonest being *C. albicans*. Genital infection is frequently seen in the immunocompetent population, but in immunosuppressed individuals, **oral candidiasis** appears, with removable white plaques or even erythematous patches. Oesophageal disease produces pain and difficulty with swallowing, and indicates severe immunosuppression. Cerebral and pulmonary disease also occurs.

- Diagnosis is confirmed by tissue samples, but often is retrospective following a good response to a trial of treatment.

Treatment

- *Skin infection* can be treated with creams such as **clotrimazole**.
- *Oral disease* can be treated with **nystatin** pastilles or **fluconazole** oral solution. In more severe oral and oesophageal disease, systemic

treatment is warranted with **fluconazole** 50–200 mg daily for 7 days or **itraconazole** 200–400 mg for 7–14 days.

- *Systemic infections* can be treated with **liposomal amphotericin B** when very severe.

Cryptococcosis

Cryptococcosis is caused by infection with the yeast-like fungus, *Cryptococcus neoformans*. Patients are at risk when their CD4 counts fall < 100. Cryptococcosis presents with meningism, neurological dysfunction and sometimes pulmonary symptoms.

- **Diagnosis** is confirmed by the presence of organisms seen with India ink stain or the detection of the cryptococcal antigen within blood or CSF. Patients can develop extremely high CSF pressures, and may need repeated lumbar puncture or even insertion of a ventro-peritoneal shunt.
- **Treatment** is divided into 'induction' and 'maintenance' phases.
  - *Induction* is usually with **liposomal amphotericin B** 3 mg/kg IV daily. There is some evidence that the addition of **flucytosine** 100 mg/kg/day in 4 divided doses can be helpful in resistant cases.
  - *Maintenance* is with oral **fluconazole** 400 mg daily, which can be stopped if a sustained immune recovery is seen following the initiation of HAART.

Aspergillosis

Infection occurs with a neutropenia, CD4 count < 50 mm^3, use of steroids and previous *Pneumocystis* infection. It presents with fever, dry cough and breathlessness. Extrapulmonary disease can occur in skin, brain, spleen, liver, heart and pancreas. *Aspergillus* species can often be found asymptomatically in the lung, and diagnosis is by demonstration of invasive infiltration within the lung or by detection of the organism in an atypical site.

- **Treatment** is with voriconazole 400 mg twice daily for 2 doses, followed by 200 mg twice daily. Amphotericin is an alternative.

Histoplasmosis

Histoplasmosis is usually caused by *Histoplasma capsulatum*, and leads to fever, weight loss, shortness of breath and skin lesions. Hepatosplenomegaly, neurological dysfunction, lymphadenopathy and bone marrow suppression occur.

- **Diagnosis** can be confirmed by growing samples from affected sites. A urine antigen test is available.
- **Treatment** is initially with an induction phase of **amphotericin B** 1–3 mg/kg daily IV or **itraconazole** 200 mg twice daily for 2 days, then 200 mg daily for a maximum of 12 days, followed by a maintenance phase also using **itraconazole** 200 mg daily.

Pneumocystis infection

Infection is caused by *P. jiroveci*, an atypical fungus. It is found in patients with CD4 counts < 200. Patients complain of shortness of breath on exertion, fever, dry cough, weight loss, malaise and chest pain or tightness. Oxygen desaturation can be demonstrated on exercise. All patients need ABG measurement. Treatment can be started presumptively in patients with risk factors.

- **Diagnosis** should then be confirmed by demonstration of the organism, obtained from either induced sputum or bronchoalveolar lavage. A CT scan shows a bilateral ground-glass appearance in the lung fields, indicating an alveolitis.

- **Primary prophylaxis** has a proven role for the prevention of this condition in patients with CD4 counts < 200. Oral **co-trimoxazole** 960 mg daily oral or 960 mg oral 3 times weekly is usually used. If this is not tolerated, **aerosoled pentamidine** 300 mg nebulized every 3–4 weeks, **dapsone** 50–100 mg daily oral or **atovaquone** 750 mg oral twice daily may be used. Primary or secondary prophylaxis can be stopped if a CD4 count > 250 is achieved with HAART and then maintained.
- **Treatment for primary infection** is with **co-trimoxazole** 120 mg/kg IV or oral in 2–4 divided doses for 14–21 days. Other options include **pentamidine** 4 mg/kg IV infusion for 14 days or (for mild disease) 600 mg inhaled for 3 weeks, **atovaquone** 750 mg twice daily oral, and **dapsone** and trimethoprim (**dapsone 100 mg once daily oral; trimethoprim 20 mg/kg oral**) in divided doses, both for 14–21 days. **Atovaquone** should not be used for severe cases.

Patients with severe disease (defined by a PaO_2 < 8 kPa) should also be treated with a steroid (e.g. **methyl prednisolone 40 mg** for the first 5 days) to prevent ARDS.

Protozoal infection

Toxoplasmosis

Toxoplasmosis is caused by *Toxoplasma gondii* infection and is transmitted by ingesting undercooked meat. Disease is usually caused by reactivation of dormant tissue cysts within the brain, when a previously infected patient becomes immunocompromised. Reactivation presents with symptoms such as fever, confusion and headache with focal signs due to multiple mass lesions within the cranium. A brain imaging study often reveals typical multiple ring-enhancing lesions.

- **Diagnosis** is usually confirmed retrospectively by response to treatment. A brain biopsy is occasionally indicated.
- **Treatment** with oral **sulfadiazine** 2 g 4 times daily for up to 6 weeks and oral **pyrimethamine** 75 mg once daily has proven efficacy. Less common treatments include oral **clindamycin** 600 mg 4 times daily with **pyrimethamine** in patients with sulphonamide allergy. **Atovaquone** and **fansidar** have also been used successfully. Repeat brain scan 2 weeks after initiation of therapy should show radiological improvement, the absence of which may indicate another diagnosis. Treatment is continued for 6 weeks, followed by maintenance therapy with lower doses of **sulfadiazine** 500 mg 4 times daily and **pyrimethamine** 25 mg daily, **clindamycin** and **pyrimethamine** or **atovaquone**. Maintenance treatment can be stopped if a sustained immune recovery is seen with HAART.
- **Prophylaxis.** All newly diagnosed HIV-positive patients should have *Toxoplasma* serology carried out. Patients who are negative for *Toxoplasma* should be advised to avoid handling and eating undercooked meat. Serology-negative patients should also avoid handling cats. Prophylaxis is given in patients with CD4 counts < 200 until immunity is restored with HAART. **Co-trimoxazole**, prescribed for prevention of *Pneumocystis*, is an effective option for prophylaxis, as is the combination of **dapsone** and **pyrimethamine**. Nebulized pentamidine does not provide effective prophylaxis for this protozoal infection.

Cryptosporidiosis

Cryptosporidiosis is caused by infection with *Cryptosporidium parvum* and leads to chronic diarrhoea and/or sclerosing cholangitis. Diarrhoea can be large-volume and intermittent, or small-volume and frequent, depending on the site of infection. Sclerosing cholangitis presents with deranged liver biochemistry with or without jaundice. Diagnosis is with stool samples (up to six samples may be required) or bowel biopsy. No specific treatments have been proven to be effective in the treatment of cryptosporidiosis; however, patients who successfully immune-reconstitute with HAART will eventually eradicate the organism.

Viral infection

Cytomegalovirus (CMV)

Cytomegalovirus is a member of the herpes virus family. In immunocompetent individuals primary infection leads to a mild, self-limiting, flu-like illness. Fifty percent of the general population have been exposed. Previous CMV exposure can be detected by CMV serology. **Reactivation** occurs with severe immunosuppression (usually CD4 counts < 50), and can lead to retinitis, encephalitis, adrenalitis, oesophagitis, colitis and pneumonitis. Regular screening for CMV retinitis should be carried out in all patients with CD4 counts < 50, as symptoms are often non-specific. Fundoscopy in active disease reveals white exudates with haemorrhages. Other presentations depend on the organ system involved. The histological hallmark of CMV disease is the presence of owl's eye inclusion bodies on biopsy specimens.

- Diagnosis of retinitis is clinical. The presence of blood or CSF PCR positivity is an indication to commence treatment, as this is a marker of current or imminent disease.
- Treatment is with **ganciclovir** 5 mg/kg IV twice daily for 14–21 days, **foscarnet** 90 mg/kg twice daily IV for 14–21 days or **cidofovir**. The drugs are usually prescribed to be given by the IV route. However, intravitreal injections of **ganciclovir** and **foscarnet** can be used for active retinitis. Oral **valganciclovir** 900 mg daily is also an effective treatment for acute CMV retinitis. Systemic treatment with these agents is associated with **side-effects** that can be limiting. The patient needs to remain on lifelong treatment, unless significant immune reconstitution is seen.

Herpes simplex virus (HSV)

Exposure to the herpes simplex viruses is common and causes cold sores, genital disease and even encephalitis in immunocompetent individuals. In HIV infection, all these presentations are possible and, in addition, oesophagus, colon, liver, eye and lung can all be affected. Skin and genital disease is often more common, greater in severity and longer in duration.

- Diagnosis is usually by PCR-based assays of lesional samples.
- Treatment is with **aciclovir** (mild: 200–400 mg oral five times daily for 5 days, severe: 5 mg/kg IV 8 hourly, encephalitis 10 mg/kg IV 3 times daily for 7-14 days), **valaciclovir, famciclovir, foscarnet and cidofovir** all having activity against this virus.

JC virus

The JC virus is a papova virus that can lead to progressive multifocal leucoencephalopathy (PML). It is seen in patients with CD4 counts < 100.

Presentation is with cognitive impairment and confusion, but focal neurological signs are detectable in most patients on presentation. White matter disease, with non-enhancing high-signal lesions seen on T_2-weighted MRI, is the classical radiological finding. JC virus can be detected in CSF by PCR techniques. Brain biopsy is the only definitive diagnostic procedure. The only specific treatment available is **cidofovir**, but data are inconclusive on its efficacy. Immune reconstitution is associated with improved survival but, despite this, PML remains a life-threatening condition with a poor prognosis.

Hepatitis B virus (HBV)

HBV shares common routes of transmission with HIV. At diagnosis all patients with HIV should be screened for co-infection. Hepatitis B infection does not hasten HIV disease progression in co-infected individuals. However, HIV infection accelerates the liver disease, and increasing risks of cirrhosis and hepatocellular carcinoma occur with co-infection. Hepatitis B vaccination should be given to all HIV patients who are HBsAg negative.

- **Diagnosis** is by hepatitis serology, with measurement of HBV DNA (p. 181).
- **Treatment** of patients with co-infection of HIV and HBV is with a combination of **tenofovir** with **emtricitabine** or **lamivudine**, along with other anti-retrovirals. If patients only require HBV treatment, they should receive antivirals not active against HIV, e.g. **PEG interferon**.
- **Other management** consists of informing patients of the dangers of alcohol, offering vaccination to contacts (Box 3.2), and giving specific anti-HBV treatments (p. 183).

Hepatitis C virus (HCV)

HCV and HIV share some common routes of infection, e.g., via blood products, although sexual and vertical transmission of HCV is rare. All patients should be screened for co-infection at presentation. HIV infection appears to hasten the process of liver damage to which chronic HCV infection can lead. There are conflicting data on whether hepatitis C infection hastens HIV disease progression.

- **Diagnosis** is usually via serology. PCR tests of HCV RNA are useful to quantify viral load.
- **Treatment** should include advice on alcohol avoidance, prevention of further transmission, vaccination against HBV if negative, and consideration for specific HCV antiviral therapy (p. 186).

Bacterial infection

Respiratory infection

Patients with HIV have impaired B-cell function due to the lack of appropriate T-cell 'help'. Consequently, HIV-infected patients are at increased risk of infection from a wide range of bacteria, including *Streptococcus*, *Haemophilus*, *Pseudomonas* and *Klebsiella* species. Patients should be vaccinated with both pneumococcal and *Haemophilus* vaccines.

Mycobacterium TB

Patients who are infected with HIV are likely to reactivate latent TB disease and have higher rates of extrapulmonary disease. There is also evidence that recent exposure to the tubercle bacillus causes a significant number of new presentations and that active TB can increase the rate of progression of HIV.

> **Box 3.2** Use of vaccines in HIV-infected adults
>
> **Vaccines that can be used in all HIV-infected adults (all inactivated)**
> - Anthrax
> - Cholera — WC/rBS
> - Hepatitis A
> - Hepatitis B
> - *Haemophilus influenzae* b (Hib)
> - Influenza — parenteral
> - Japanese encephalitis
> - *Meningococcus* — MenC
> - *Meningococcus* — ACWY
> - *Pneumococcus* — PPV23
> - Poliomyelitis — parenteral (IPV)
> - Rabies
> - Tetanus-diphtheria (Td)
> - Tick-borne encephalitis
> - Typhoid — ViCPS
>
> **Vaccines that are contraindicated in all HIV-infected adults**
> - Cholera — CVD103-HgR (live)
> - Influenza — intranasal (live)
> - Poliomyelitis — oral (OPV) (live)
> - Typhoid — Ty21a (live)
> - Tuberculosis (BCG) (live)
> - Smallpox (vaccinia) (live)
>
> **Vaccines that can be used only in asymptomatic HIV-infected adults with a current CD4 count > 200 cells/mm³**
> - Measles, mumps, rubella (MMR)
> - Varicella
> - Yellow fever

- Clinical features of TB comprise night sweats, weight loss, hepato-splenomegaly and lymphadenopathy. Pulmonary TB presents with symptoms of chest pain, chronic productive cough and haemoptysis. Virtually any extrapulmonary site can be involved, including CNS, gastrointestinal tract, genitourinary tract and joints.
- Treatment is increasingly problematic due to the emergence of drug-resistant TB. Multiple drug resistance (MDR) occurs worldwide in about 20% of cases, with 2% having extensive drug resistance (XDR, p. 514). Nosocomial transmission of XDR is an increasing problem. To establish the presence of resistance rapidly, samples must be sent to the reference laboratory for molecular detection of species and resistance. Early morning sputum samples, pleural aspiration and biopsy if effusion is present, along with bronchial washings, may all be necessary to diagnose pulmonary disease. For extrapulmonary disease, tissue samples should not all be placed in formalin and sent to histopathology; some should be sent in a dry sterile container for microbiological culture. As large a volume of CSF should be sent to be tested for suspected CNS disease. Bone marrow and liver biopsy may be necessary for suspected

miliary disease. It is essential that treatment be carried out with at least four separate drugs to which the organism is sensitive (p. 86).

Mycobacterium avium intracellulare (MAI)

Most MAI infections occur in patients with CD4 counts < 50. Infections are caused by *M. avium* and *M. intracellulare*. Presentation is usually with fever, fatigue, anorexia, weight loss and diarrhoea. Signs include lymphadenopathy, hepatosplenomegaly and jaundice. A raised serum alkaline phosphatase is often seen on investigation.

- Diagnosis is confirmed by isolation of the organisms, usually via blood culture into a specialized *Mycobacterium* culture flask. Two sets are sufficient to make the diagnosis in most cases.
- Treatment is with **ethambutol**, one **macrolide antibiotic** and **rifabutin**. Treatment was previously continued for life. However, there is evidence that it can be stopped once a sustained immunological response is seen with HAART.

Prevention of opportunistic infection

The key strategies are:
- avoidance of infection
- chemoprophylaxis when appropriate
- immunization (Box 3.2)
- HAART.

HIV-RELATED MALIGNANCIES

Non-Hodgkin's lymphoma (NHL)

Patients at all ranges of CD4 count are at risk of NHL but the incidence increases with falling CD4 count. Epstein–Barr virus (EBV) is isolated from a large number of HIV NHLs.

Primary CNS lymphoma

NHL involving the CNS with no peripheral involvement is termed primary CNS lymphoma. EBV is involved in nearly 100% of HIV primary CNS lymphomas. Presentation is with neurological dysfunction.

- Diagnosis is confirmed by CNS imaging; the presence of EBV DNA in the CSF has a specificity of over 90%. Biopsy is sometimes necessary to confirm the diagnosis or exclude other conditions.
- Treatment is usually with radiotherapy but the prognosis for this condition, even in the HAART era, is extremely poor.

Primary effusion lymphoma

This rare entity is associated with human herpes virus 8 (HHV8), the virus that causes Kaposi's sarcoma. Fluid accumulations in the serous cavities (pericardium, pleura and peritoneum) contain lymphomatous cells. Solid tissue disease may be present. Patients present late and the prognosis is poor.

Kaposi's sarcoma (KS)

In HIV infection KS is associated with HHV8 infection. The majority of initial presentations comprise skin involvement, ranging from macular pigmented lesions to larger truncal plaques, which may be associated with painful localized oedema on the trunk. KS has been found to affect every organ system in the body, apart from the brain. In treatment of patients with minor skin lesions anti-retroviral therapy alone may be adequate. Intralesional injections can help patients with more severe limited cutaneous disease. Patients with more severe or visceral involvement often

Kumar & Clark's Medical Management and Therapeutics

warrant radiotherapy or chemotherapy. HAART may cause regression of the lesions and prevent new ones emerging.

Cervical/anal cancer

These cancers are associated with infection by the human papilloma virus. Cervical cancer is an AIDS-defining illness. The pre-malignant lesion of cervical cancer can be detected on screening, which should occur yearly. Anoscopic cytology has been used as a screening tool for anal cancer. Therapeutic options include surgical excision and laser ablation for small lesions. The treatment for established cancers is the same as for non-HIV-infected individuals.

Further reading

Barnett T, Whiteside A: *AIDS in the Twenty-First Century, Disease and Globalisation*, ed 2, London, 2006, Palgrave.

Chadwick DR, Geretti AM: Immunization of the HIV infected traveler, *AIDS* 21:787–794, 2007.

Dolin R: A new class of anti-HIV therapy, *New Engl J Med* 359:1509–1511, 2008.

Palella FJ Jr, Baker RK, Moorman AC, et al: Mortality in the highly active antiretroviral therapy era: changing causes of death and disease in the HIV outpatient study, *J Acquir Immune Defic Syndr* 43(1):27–34, 2006.

Simoni JM, Pearson CR, Pantalone DW, et al: Efficacy of interventions in improving highly active antiretroviral therapy adherence and HIV-1 RNA viral load. A meta-analytic review of randomized controlled trials, *J Acquir Immune Defic Syndr* 43(Suppl 1):S23–S35, 2006.

Taylor BS, Carr JK, Salminen MO, et al: The challenge of HIV-1 subtype diversity, *New Engl J Med* 358:1590–1603, 2008.

Young T, Arens F, Kennedy G, et al: Antiretroviral post-exposure prophylaxis (PEP) for occupational HIV exposure. *Cochrane Database Syst Rev* 21(1):CD002835 2007(1), 2007.

Further information

http://bashh.org
British Association for Sexual Health and HIV

www.bhiva.org
British HIV Association (BHIVA)

www.i-base.info/
HIV i-Base. HIV treatment information

www.aidsmap.com/
National AIDS Manual. Aidsmap information on HIV and AIDS

www.hiv-druginteractions.org/
University of Liverpool. HIV drug interactions

http://hivdb.stanford.edu/
University of Stanford. HIV Drug Resistance Database

http://www.aidsinfo.nih.gov/guidelines/
US Department of Health and Human Services. Clinical Guidelines Portal

Nutrition 4

DIETARY REQUIREMENTS

Energy

Food is necessary to provide the body with energy. The SI unit of energy is the joule (J), and 1 kJ = 0.239 kcal. The conversion factor of 4.2 kJ, equivalent to 1 kcal, is used in clinical nutrition.

Energy expenditure gives a reasonably accurate estimate of dietary requirements. Daily energy expenditure is the sum of:

- the basal metabolic rate (BMR)
- the thermic effect of food eaten
- occupational activities
- non-occupational activities.

- BMR. This is usually taken from standardized tables that require knowledge of the subject's age, weight and sex.
- Physical activity. The physical activity ratio (PAR) is expressed as multiples of the BMR for both occupational and non-occupational activities of varying intensities.
- Total daily energy expenditure:

$$BMR \times [\text{Time in bed} + (\text{Time at work} \times PAR) + (\text{Non-occupational time} \times PAR)]$$

The estimated 'average' daily requirement is:

- for a 55-year-old female: 8100 kJ (1940 kcal)
- for a 55-year-old male: 10 600 kJ (2550 kcal).

This figure is at present made up of 50% carbohydrate, 35% fat and 15% protein plus or minus 5% alcohol. In developing countries, however, carbohydrate may constitute more than 75% of the total energy input, and fat less than 15% of the total energy input.

Energy requirements increase during the growing period, with pregnancy and lactation, and sometimes following infection or trauma. In general, the increased BMR associated with inflammatory or traumatic conditions is counteracted or more than counteracted by a decrease in physical activity, so that total energy requirements are not increased.

In the basal state, energy demands for resting muscle are 20% of the total energy required, abdominal viscera 35–40%, brain 20% and heart 10%. There can be more than a 50-fold increase in muscle energy demands during exercise.

Protein

In the UK the adult daily reference nutrient intake (RNI) for protein is 0.75 g/kg, with protein representing at least 10% of the total energy intake. Most affluent people eat more than this, consuming 80–100 g of protein per day. The total amount of nitrogen excreted in the urine represents the balance between protein breakdown and synthesis. In order to maintain nitrogen balance, at least 40–50 g of protein are needed. The amount of protein oxidized can be calculated from the amount of nitrogen excreted in the urine over 24 hours using the following equation (most proteins contain about 16% of nitrogen):

Grams of protein required = Urinary nitrogen $\times 6.25$

In practice, urinary urea is more easily measured and forms 80–90% of the total urinary nitrogen (N). In healthy individuals urinary N excretion reflects protein intake. However, urinary N excretion does not match intake either in catabolic conditions (negative N balance), or during growth or repletion following an illness (positive N balance).

Protein contains many amino acids.

- **Indispensable (essential) amino acids.** These are tryptophan, histidine, methionine, threonine, isoleucine, valine, phenylalanine, lysine and leucine. They cannot be synthesized and must be provided in the diet.
- **Dispensable (non-essential) amino acids.** These can be synthesized in the body, but some may still be needed if there are insufficient precursors in the diet.

Animal proteins, such as those in milk, meat and eggs, are of high nutritional value, as they contain all indispensable amino acids. Conversely, many proteins from vegetables are deficient in at least one indispensable amino acid.

In **developing countries**, adequate protein intake is achieved mainly from vegetable proteins. By combining foodstuffs with different low concentrations of indispensable amino acids (e.g. maize with legumes), protein intake can be adequate, provided enough vegetables are available.

Amino acids may be utilized to synthesize products other than protein or urea. For example, haem requires glycine.

Fat

Dietary fat is chiefly in the form of triglycerides, which are esters of glycerol and free fatty acids. Fatty acids vary in chain length and in saturation. Unsaturated fatty acids are monounsaturated or polyunsaturated. The hydrogen molecules related to these double bonds can be in the *cis* or the *trans* position; in most natural fatty acids in food, they are in the *cis* position.

The **essential fatty acids** (EFAs) are linoleic and α-linolenic acids, both of which are precursors of prostaglandins. Eicosapentaenoic and docosahexaenoic acids are also necessary, but can be made to a limited extent in the tissues from linoleic and linolenic; thus a dietary supply is not essential.

Synthesis of triglycerides, sterols and **phospholipids** is very efficient, and even with low-fat diets, subcutaneous fat stores can be normal.

Dietary fat provides 37 kJ (9 kcal) of energy per gram. A high fat intake has been implicated in the causation of cardiovascular disease, cancer (e.g. breast, colon and prostate), obesity and type 2 diabetes. It is suggested that the consumption of saturated fatty acids should be reduced, accompanied by an increase in monounsaturated fatty acids, e.g. oleic acids (the 'Mediterranean diet'), or polyunsaturated fatty acids, e.g. linoleic acid. Any increase in polyunsaturated fats should not, however, exceed 10% of the total food energy, particularly as this requires a big dietary change.

Increased consumption of partially hydrogenated vegetable and fish oils in margarines has led to a higher *trans* fatty acid consumption, and their intake should not be above more than the current estimated average of 5 g per day or 2% of the dietary energy. This is because **trans fatty acids** (also called *trans* fats) behave as if they were saturated fatty acids, with an increase in the risk of cardiovascular disease. A total ban of trans fats is in place in many countries.

The **current recommendations for fat intake** for the UK are as follows:

- Total fat intake should be no more than 35% of the total dietary energy, and restriction to 30% is desirable.
- Saturated fatty acids should provide ~10% of the dietary energy.
- *cis*-Monounsaturated acids (mainly oleic acid) should continue to provide approximately 12% of the dietary energy.
- *cis*-Polyunsaturated acids should provide 6% of dietary energy, and are derived from n-6 and n-3 polyunsaturated fatty acids, which should provide approximately 0.5% of total energy intake.

Cholesterol is found in all animal products. Eggs are particularly rich in cholesterol, which is virtually absent from plants. The average daily intake in the UK is 300–500 mg. Cholesterol is also synthesized, and only very high or low dietary intakes will significantly affect blood levels.

Essential fatty acid deficiency may accompany protein–energy malnutrition (PEM), but it has been clearly defined as a clinical entity only in patients on long-term parenteral nutrition who are given glucose, protein and no fat. Alopecia, thrombocytopenia, anaemia and a dermatitis occur within weeks, with an increased ratio of triene (n-9) to tetraene (n-6) in plasma fatty acids.

Carbohydrate

Carbohydrates are readily available in the diet, providing 17 kJ (4 kcal) per gram of energy (15.7 kJ (3.75 kcal) per gram monosaccharide equivalent).

Carbohydrate intake comprises the polysaccharide (starch), the disaccharides (mainly sucrose) and the monosaccharides (glucose and fructose). Carbohydrate is cheap compared with other foodstuffs; a great deal is therefore eaten, usually more than required.

PROTEIN–ENERGY MALNUTRITION

Starvation uncomplicated by disease is relatively uncommon in developed countries, although some degree of undernourishment is seen in very poor areas. Most nutritional problems occurring in the population at large are due to eating wrong combinations of foodstuffs, such as an excess of refined carbohydrate or a diet low in fresh vegetables. Undernourishment associated with disease is common in hospitals and nursing homes. Surgical complications, with sepsis, are a common cause.

The majority of the weight loss, leading to malnutrition, is **due to poor intake secondary to the anorexia associated with the underlying condition**. Disease may also contribute by causing malabsorption and increased catabolism, which is mediated by complex changes in cytokines, hormones, side-effects of drugs and immobility. The elderly are particularly at risk of malnutrition because they often suffer from diseases and psychosocial problems such as social isolation or bereavement.

- In the fed state, insulin/glucagon ratios are high. Insulin promotes synthesis of glycogen, protein and fat, and inhibits lipolysis and gluconeogenesis.
- In the fasted state, insulin/glucagon ratios are low. Glucagon acts mainly on the liver and has no action on muscle. It increases glycogenolysis and gluconeogenesis, as well as increasing ketone body production from fatty acids. It also stimulates lipolysis in adipose tissue. Catecholamines have a similar action to glucagon but also affect muscle metabolism. These agents both act via cyclic adenosine monophosphate (cAMP) to stimulate lipolysis, producing free fatty acids that can then act as a major source of energy.
- During weight loss, uncomplicated by disease, the proportion of lean to fat tissue loss (or proportion of energy derived from protein metabolism) is greater in thin than in overweight/obese individuals.

Clinical features

Patients are sometimes seen who have loss of weight or malnutrition as the primary symptom (failure to thrive in children). Mostly, however, malnourishment is only seen as an accompaniment of some other disease process, such as malignancy. Severe malnutrition is seen mainly with advanced organic disease or after surgical procedures followed by complications. Three key features that help in the detection of chronic PEM in adults are described below. These features are also used in the Malnutrition Universal Screening Tool (see Fig. 4.1):

- The body mass index (BMI): calculated as weight/height^2 (kg/m^2):
  - probable risk of chronic PEM: < 18.5 kg/m^2
  - possible risk of chronic PEM: 18.5–20 kg/m^2
  - little or no risk of chronic PEM: > 20 kg/m^2.

  In patients with oedema or dehydration the BMI may be somewhat misleading.
- Weight loss in the previous 3–6 months:
  - $> 10\%$, high risk
  - 5–10%, possible risk
  - $< 5\%$, low/no risk of developing PEM.
- Acute disease effect: Diseases that have resulted or are likely to result in no dietary intake for more than 5 days are associated with a high risk of malnutrition (e.g. prolonged unconsciousness, persistent swallowing problems after a stroke, or prolonged ileus after abdominal surgery).
- Other factors:
  - History of decreased food intake/loss of appetite.
  - Clothes becoming loose-fitting (weight loss) and a general appearance indicating obvious wasting.
  - Physical and psychosocial disturbances likely to have contributed to the weight loss.

PEM leads to a depression of the immunological defence mechanism, resulting in a decreased resistance to infection. It also detrimentally affects muscle strength, and produces fatigue, poor wound healing and decreased psychological function (e.g. depression, anxiety, hypochondriasis, loss of libido).

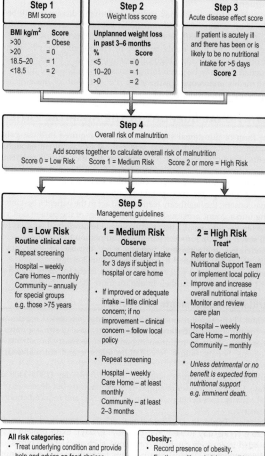

Step 1
BMI score

BMI kg/m^2	Score
>30	= Obese
>20	= 0
18.5–20	= 1
<18.5	= 2

Step 2
Weight loss score

Unplanned weight loss
in past 3–6 months

%	Score
<5	= 0
10–20	= 1
>0	= 2

Step 3
Acute disease effect score

If patient is acutely ill
and there has been or is
likely to be no nutritional
intake for >5 days
Score 2

Step 4
Overall risk of malnutrition

Add scores together to calculate overall risk of malnutrition
Score 0 = Low Risk   Score 1 = Medium Risk   Score 2 or more = High Risk

Step 5
Management guidelines

0 = Low Risk
Routine clinical care

• Repeat screening

Hospital – weekly
Care Homes – monthly
Community – annually
for special groups
e.g. those >75 years

1 = Medium Risk
Observe

• Document dietary intake
for 3 days if subject in
hospital or care home

• If improved or adequate
intake – little clinical
concern; if no
improvement – clinical
concern – follow local
policy

• Repeat screening

Hospital – weekly
Care Home – at least
monthly
Community – at least
2–3 months

2 = High Risk
Treat*

• Refer to dietician,
Nutritional Support Team
or implement local policy
• Improve and increase
overall nutritional intake
• Monitor and review
care plan

Hospital – weekly
Care Home – monthly
Community – monthly

* Unless detrimental or no
benefit is expected from
nutritional support
e.g. imminent death.*

All risk categories:
• Treat underlying condition and provide
help and advice on food choices,
eating and drinking when necessary.
• Record malnutritional risk category.
• Record need for special diets and
follow local policy.

Obesity:
• Record presence of obesity.
For those with underlying conditions,
these are generally controlled before
the treatment of obesity.

Fig. 4.1 Malnutrition Universal Screening Tool (MUST). Reproduced with
permission from the British Association for Parenteral and Enteral Nutrition
(BAPEN): http://www.bapen.org.uk.

Treatment

When malnutrition is obvious and the underlying disease cannot be corrected at once, some form of nutritional support is necessary. Nutrition should be given enterally if the gastrointestinal tract is functioning adequately. This can most easily be done by encouraging the patient to eat more often and by giving a high-calorie supplement. If this is not possible, a liquefied diet may be given intragastrically via a fine-bore tube or by a percutaneous endoscopic gastrostomy (PEG). If both of these measures fail, parenteral nutrition is given.

NUTRITIONAL SUPPORT IN THE HOSPITAL PATIENT

Some form of nutritional supplementation is required in those patients who cannot eat, should not eat, will not eat or cannot eat enough. All patients should be screened on admission for their nutritional requirements and a care plan drawn up by a trained multidisciplinary team. Plans are discussed with patients and consent is taken for any invasive procedure (e.g. naso-gastric tube, parenteral nutrition). If the patient is unable to give consent, the healthcare team should act in the patient's best interest, taking into account previously expressed wishes of the patient and views of the family. It is usually necessary to provide nutritional support for:

- all severely malnourished patients on admission to hospital
- moderately malnourished patients who, because of their physical illness, are not expected to eat for more than 3–5 days
- normally nourished patients expected not to eat for more than 5 days or to eat less than half their intake for more than 8–10 days.

Nutritional requirements for adults

- **Water.** Typical requirements are ~2–3 L/day. Increased requirements occur in patients with large-output fistulae, naso-gastric aspirates and diarrhoea. Reduced requirements are often necessary in patients with oedema, hepatic failure, renal failure (oliguric and not dialysed) and brain oedema.
- **Energy.** Typical requirements are ~7.5–10.0 MJ/day (1800–2400 kcal/day). Disease increases resting energy expenditure but decreases physical activity. Extra energy is given for repletion and reduced energy for obesity.
- **Protein.** Typically 10–15 g N/day (62–95 g protein/day) or 0.15–0.25 g N/kg/day (0.94–1.56 g protein/kg/day). Extra protein may be needed in severely catabolic conditions, such as extensive burns.
- **Major minerals.** Typical requirements for sodium and potassium are 70–100 mmol/day. Increased requirements occur in patients with gastrointestinal effluents (see Table 11.2). The excretion of these minerals in various effluents can provide an indication of the additional requirements. Low requirements may be necessary in those with fluid overload (or patients with hypernatraemia and hyperkalaemia). The requirements of calcium and magnesium are higher for enteral than for parenteral nutrition because only a proportion of these minerals is absorbed by the gut.
- **Trace elements.** The requirements for enteral and parenteral nutrition are similar for trace elements such as iodide, fluoride and selenium that are well absorbed. For other trace elements, such as iron, zinc, manganese and chromium, the requirements for parenteral nutrition are

substantially lower than for enteral nutrition. Daily requirements are shown in Table 4.1.

● Vitamins. Many vitamins are given in greater quantities in patients receiving parenteral nutrition than in those receiving enteral nutrition. This is because patients on parenteral nutrition may have increased requirements, partly because of severe disease, partly because they may already have depleted pools of vitamins, and partly because some vitamins degrade during storage. Vitamin K is usually absent from parenteral nutrition regimens and therefore it may need to be administered separately. Daily vitamin requirements are shown in Table 4.2.

Table 4.1 Daily dietary electrolyte and trace element requirements

Electrolyte/trace element	Daily requirement
Na^+	70–220 mmol
K^+	60–120 mmol
Mg^{2+}	5–20 mmol
Ca^{2+}	15–20 mmol
Zn^{2+}	50–100 µmol
Mn^{2+}	120 µmol
Fe^{2+}	70 µmol
Cu^{2+}	20 µmol
Cl^-	70–220 µmol
PO^{-3}	15–25 µmol
F^-	50 µmol
I^-	1 µmol

Table 4.2 Daily requirements of fat-soluble and water-soluble vitamins

Vitamin	Daily requirement
Fat-soluble A (retinol)	700 mcg
D (cholecalciferol)	No dietary intake required (if fully ambulant)
K	1 mcg/kg body weight
E (α-tocopherol)	10 mg
Water-soluble B_1 (thiamin)	0.4 mg per 1000 kcal
B_2 (riboflavin)	1.3 mg
Niacin	6.6 mg per 1000 kcal
B_6 (pyridoxine)	15 mcg per g of dietary protein
B_{12} (cobalamin)	1.5 mcg
Folate	200 mcg
C (ascorbic acid)	40 mg

Enteral nutrition (EN)

Feeds can be given by various routes:

- By mouth. Food can be supplemented with solid or liquid supplements. These can be given by using blenderized food or milk-based drinks. Various formulae are available. Advice should be obtained from a dietitian.
- By fine-bore nasogastric tube (Box 4.1).
- By PEG. PEG is useful for patients who need enteral nutrition for a prolonged period (e.g. more than 30 days), such as those with swallowing problems following a head injury, or elderly people after a stroke. A catheter is placed percutaneously into the stomach under endoscopic control.
- By needle catheter jejunostomy. A fine catheter is inserted into the jejunum at laparotomy and brought out through the abdominal wall.

Diet formulation

A polymeric diet with whole protein and fat can be used (Box 4.2), except in patients with severely impaired gastrointestinal function who may require a predigested (i.e. elemental) diet. In these patients, the nitrogen source is purified low-molecular-weight peptides or amino acid mixtures, with the fat sometimes being given partly as medium-chain triglycerides. Appropriate diets can be used for patients with, for example, chronic kidney disease (low protein) or anorexia (e.g. high-nitrogen or high-calorie diets).

Management

Daily amounts of enteral diet vary between 2 and 2.5 L, and the full amount can be started immediately.

Box 4.1 Enteral feeding via nasogastric tube

The procedure should be explained to the patient and consent taken.

Procedure
- Insert a fine-bore tube intranasally with a wire stylet
- Confirm the position of the tube in the stomach by aspiration of gastric contents and auscultation of the epigastrium
- Check by X-ray if aspiration or auscultation is unsuccessful

Problems
- No satisfactory way of keeping nasogastric tubes in place (up to 60% come out)

Main complications
- Regurgitation and aspiration into bronchus
- Erosive tissue damage in the nose or pharynx
- Blockage of the naso-gastric tube. Regular flushing of the tube is necessary
- Gastrointestinal side-effects, the most common being diarrhoea (worse with antibiotic therapy)
- Metabolic complications, including hyperglycaemia and hypokalaemia, as well as low levels of magnesium, calcium and phosphate

---

Box 4.2 Standard enteric diet, providing 8.4 MJ per day (= 2000 kcal)

Energy
- Carbohydrate as glucose polymers (49–53% of total energy)
- Fat as triglycerides (30–35% of total energy)

Nitrogen
- Whole protein (10–14 g of nitrogen/day)

Additional
- Electrolytes, vitamins and trace elements

Features
- Ratio of energy to nitrogen kJ : g = 620 : 1 (kcal : g = 150 : 1)
- Osmolality = 285–300 mOsm/kg

Hypercatabolic patients require a high supply of nitrogen (15 g daily) and often will not achieve positive N balance until the primary injury is resolved.

The success of enteral feeding depends on careful supervision of the patient, as there are frequent mechanical complications (e.g. tube occlusion) and often the full daily amount given is less than prescribed. Monitoring of weight, biochemistry and diet charts should be performed daily, as hypokalaemia, hyponatraemia, hypophosphataemia and hyperglycaemia (requiring insulin therapy) often occur.

Parenteral nutrition

Peripheral parenteral nutrition

Specially formulated mixtures for peripheral use are available, with a low osmolality and containing lipid emulsions. Heparin and corticosteroids can be added to the infusion and local application of glyceryl trinitrate patches reduces the occurrence of thrombophlebitis and prolongs catheter life. Peripheral cannulae can be inserted into a mid-arm vein (20 cm) and can last up to 5 days. A longer (60 cm) peripherally inserted central catheter (PICC) inserted into an antecubital fossa vein has its distal end lying in a central vein; here there is less risk of thrombophlebitis and hyperosmolar solutions can be given. With careful management, these catheters can last for up to a month. Peripheral parenteral nutrition is often preferred initially, allowing time to consider the necessity for inserting a central venous catheter.

Total parenteral nutrition via a central venous catheter (TPN)

A silicone catheter is placed into a central vein, usually using the infraclavicular approach to the subclavian vein (Box 4.3). The skin-entry site should be dressed carefully and not disturbed unless there is a suggestion of catheter-related sepsis.

- **Complications** following catheter placement include central vein thrombosis, pneumothorax and embolism, but the major problem is catheter-related sepsis. Organisms, mainly staphylococci, enter along the side of the catheter, leading to septicaemia. Sepsis can be prevented by careful and sterile placement of the catheter, by not removing the dressing over the catheter entry site, and by not giving other substances

> ### Box 4.3 Central catheter placement for parenteral nutrition
>
> This should be performed only by experienced clinicians under aseptic conditions in an operating theatre.
>
> Give an explanation and obtain consent from the patient.
>
> - The patient is placed supine with 5° of head-down tilt to avoid air embolism
> - The skin below the midpoint of the right clavicle is infiltrated with 1–2% lidocaine and a 1 cm skin incision is made
> - A 20-gauge needle on a syringe is inserted beneath the clavicle and first rib, and angled towards the tip of a finger held in the suprasternal notch
> - When blood is aspirated freely, the needle is used as a guide to insert the cannula through the skin incision and into the subclavian vein
> - The catheter is advanced so that its tip lies in the distal part of the superior vena cava
> - A skin tunnel is created under local anaesthetic using an introducer inserted through a point about 10 cm below and medial to the incision and passed upwards to the incision
> - The proximal end of the catheter (with hub removed) is passed backwards through the introducer to emerge 10 cm below the clavicle, where it is sutured to the chest wall
> - The original infraclavicular entry incision is now sutured
> - Complications during insertion include arterial puncture, pneumothorax and brachial plexus injury

(e.g. blood products, antibiotics) via the central vein catheter. Sepsis should be suspected if the patient develops fever and leucocytosis. In two-thirds of cases, organisms can be grown from the catheter tip after removal. Treatment involves removal of the catheter and appropriate systemic antibiotics.

Nutrients

With TPN it is possible to provide sufficient nitrogen for protein synthesis and calories to meet energy requirements. Electrolytes, vitamins and trace elements are also necessary. All of these substances are infused simultaneously.

Nitrogen source

Most patients receive at least 11–15g N per day, in the form of synthetic L-amino acids.

Energy source

This is provided by glucose, with additional calories provided by a fat emulsion. Fat infusions provide a greater number of calories in a smaller volume than can be provided by carbohydrate. Fat infusions are not hypertonic and they also prevent EFA deficiency.

EFA deficiency has been reported in long-term parenteral nutritional regimens without fat emulsions. It causes a scaly skin, hair loss and delay in healing.

Electrolytes, vitamins and trace elements

Initially, the electrolyte status should be monitored on a daily basis and electrolyte solutions given as appropriate (see Tables 4.1 and 4.2).

Water-soluble vitamins can be given daily but **fat-soluble vitamins** should be given weekly, as overdose can occur. A **trace-metal** solution is available for patients on long-term parenteral nutrition, but if the patient requires blood transfusions trace-metal supplements are not needed.

Administration and monitoring

- Peripheral parenteral nutrition is administered via 3 L bags over 24 hours, with the constituents being premixed under sterile conditions. Table 4.3 shows the composition, which provides 9 g of nitrogen and 1700 calories in 24 hours.
- Central venous TPN regimens are based on premixed 3 L bags in most hospitals. A standard parenteral nutrition regimen, which provides 14 g of nitrogen and 2250 calories over 24 hours, is also given in Table 4.3. Monitoring includes:
- Blood tests. Daily plasma electrolytes and glucose. Twice-weekly FBC, liver biochemistry and function, calcium, phosphate. Magnesium and zinc weekly.
- Nutritional status. Weekly weight and skin-fold thickness.
- Nitrogen balance (p. 120) assessment. This requires complete collections of urine.

Table 4.3 Examples of parenteral nutrition regimens

	Constituent	Amount
Peripheral: all mixed in 3 L bags and infused over 24 hours		
Nitrogen	L-amino acids 9 g/L	1 L
Energy	Glucose 20%	1 L
	Lipid 20%	0.5 L
	+ Trace elements, electrolytes, water-soluble and fat-soluble vitamins, heparin 1000 U/L and hydrocortisone 100 mg; insulin is added if required. Nitrogen 9 g, non-protein calories 7206 kJ (1700 kcal)	
Central: all mixed in 3 L bags and infused over 24 hours		
Nitrogen	L-amino acids 14 g/L	1 L
Energy	Glucose 50%	0.5 L
	Glucose 20%	0.5 L
	+ Lipid 10%	0.5 L Fractionated soya oil 100 g/L, soya oil 50 g, medium-chain triglycerides 50 g/L
	+ Electrolytes, water-soluble and fat-soluble vitamins, trace elements, heparin and insulin may be added if required. Nitrogen 14 g, non-protein calories 9305 kJ (2250 kcal)	

Complications

- Catheter-related: (see above).
- Metabolic (e.g. hyperglycaemia — insulin therapy is usually necessary).
- Fluid and electrolyte disturbances.
- Hypercalcaemia.
- Liver dysfunction: steatosis, cholestasis, fibrosis and cirrhosis, usually after 3–4 months of TPN. Transient abnormal liver biochemistry is common in the early stages of TPN and usually resolves spontaneously.
- Metabolic bone disease: after 3 months of TPN, osteopenia and osteomalacia occur.

NUTRITIONAL SUPPORT IN THE HOME PATIENT

In both high- and low-income countries there is considerably more undernutrition in the community than in hospital. However, the principles are very similar: detection of malnutrition and the underlying risk factors; treatment of underlying disease processes and disabilities; correction of specific nutrient deficiencies and provision of appropriate nutritional support. A systematic review of the use of nutritional supplements in the community came to the following conclusions:

- Acceptability and compliance are likely to be better when a choice of supplements (differing in type, flavour and consistency) and the schedule are decided in conjunction with the patient and/or carer.
- Supplements are generally of value in patients with a BMI < 20 kg/m^2.

Enteral tube feeding

This is often given at home. The commonest reason for starting home tube feeding is for swallowing difficulties in patients with stroke, motor neurone disease, multiple sclerosis and Parkinson's disease.

- A PEG is used rather than a nasogastric tube in most patients, as long-term feeding is necessary.
- The swallowing capabilities of patients should be assessed regularly in order to avoid unnecessary tube feeding.

Home parenteral nutrition

This is practised much less frequently, usually for patients with intestinal resection and the short bowel syndrome. The potential value of intestinal transplantation in patients with long-term intestinal failure is still being assessed.

REFEEDING SYNDROME

The refeeding syndrome can occur within hours of refeeding by the oral, enteral or parenteral route. It is under-recognised and can be fatal. It involves a shift from the use of body fat as an energy source during starvation to the use of carbohydrate as an energy source during refeeding. This augments insulin release and there is rapid intracellular transport of phosphate, magnesium and potassium, resulting in hypophosphataemia, hypomagnesaemia and hypokalaemia.

- Phosphate concentration. Phosphate concentration in the serum can fall within hours to < 0.4 mm/L (1 mg/dL), which results in widespread organ dysfunction (muscle weakness, parathesiae, cardiac failure, immune suppression, coma, hallucinations and fits).

- **Fluid overload.** Fluid overload leading to cardiac failure and pulmonary oedema occurs due to poor cardiac function from malnutrition.
- **Glucose intolerance.** Refeeding with carbohydrate can lead to severe hyperglycaemia, as insulin levels are low and there is increased insulin resistance. Thiamin deficiency can be precipitated, leading to the Wernicke–Korsakoff syndrome. Intravenous thiamine should be given before refeeding in those at risk.
- **Cardiac arrhythmias.** Prolonged QT with ventricular tachyarrhythmias occurs, leading to sudden death.

Management

All malnourished patients must be monitored frequently, both clinically (with physical examination and daily weighing) and biochemically, and starting before initial feeding.

Initially, refeeding over the first 3–7 days is limited to 800 mL/day plus insensible losses of fluid. Changes in body weight are a general indication of fluid requirements. Daily calorie intake should be 15–20 kcal/kg with approximately 100 g carbohydrates and 1.5 g protein per kg body weight. Sodium should be to 60 mmol/day (1.5 g).

Adjustments to the initial regimen depends on clinical response but should always be increased slowly.

Further reading

National Institute for Health and Clinical Excellence: *Guidelines for nutrition support in adults. Clinical guidelines 32*. London, 2008, NICE.
Ziegler TR: Parenteral nutrition in the critically ill patient, *New Engl J Med* 361:1088–1097, 2009.

Further information

http://www.who.int/nutgrowthdb/
World Health Organisation site provides information on worldwide nutrition issues, resources and research

http://www.bapen.org.uk
British Association for Parenteral and Enteral Nutrition

Kumar & Clark's Medical Management and Therapeutics

Gastrointestinal disease 5

CHAPTER CONTENTS

SYMPTOMS

Dyspepsia and indigestion

The term dyspepsia is used to describe a variety of upper abdominal symptoms, including nausea, heartburn, acidity, pain or discomfort, wind, fullness or belching. The term indigestion is used by patients to describe any symptom that is food-related. Indigestion is common and most people will have experienced it at some time.

History
This should elicit any 'alarm' features (Box 5.1).

Investigations
See p. 144.

Treatment
Treatment is with antacid therapy (Table 5.1).

Nausea and vomiting

Many gastrointestinal conditions are associated with vomiting, but nausea and vomiting without abdominal pain are frequently non-gastrointestinal in origin, e.g. acute infections, CNS disease and drug ingestion.

- Early-morning vomiting is seen in pregnancy, alcohol dependence and in some metabolic disorders (e.g. uraemia).
- Large volumes of vomit suggest intestinal obstruction; faeculent vomit suggests low intestinal obstruction or the presence of a gastrocolic fistula, while projectile vomiting is due to gastric outflow obstruction.
- Chronic nausea and vomiting with no other abdominal symptoms usually have a psychological cause.

Treatment
Many patients require no therapy. Food is usually withheld and fluids only are allowed. With more persistent vomiting, IV fluids, e.g. 0.9% saline (p. 369), are given for dehydration and correction of electrolyte abnormalities. A naso-gastric tube is inserted if there is bowel obstruction.

> ### Box 5.1 Alarm symptoms
>
> - Persistent vomiting
> - Dysphagia
> - Weight loss
> - Anorexia
> - Haematemesis or melaena

Table 5.1 Antacid therapy

Class of drug	Drug	Dose
H_2-receptor antagonists	Cimetidine	400 mg twice daily
	Famotidine	40 mg daily
	Nizatidine	300 mg daily
	Ranitidine	300 mg daily
Proton pump inhibitors	Esomeprazole	20 mg daily
	Lansoprazole	30 mg daily
	Omeprazole	20 mg daily
	Pantoprazole	40 mg daily
	Rabeprazole	20 mg daily
Antacids	Aluminium hydroxide	10–20 mL 3 times daily
	Magnesium carbonate	10 mL 3 times daily
	Magnesium trisilicate	10–20 mL 3 times daily
	Aluminium and magnesium complexes	10 mL between meals and at bedtime
Others	Alginates and antacids	2 tablets twice daily
	Chelates and complexes, e.g. tripotassium, dicitratobismuthate, sucralfate	2 tablets twice daily

- Hyoscine 300 mcg is the most effective drug for motion sickness.
- Antihistamines, e.g. **cyclizine** 50 mg oral/IM/IV 3 times daily, oral **cinnarizine** 15 mg and oral **promethazine** 25–75 mg, are also used for motion sickness and in nausea and vomiting with vertigo. Drowsiness and antimuscarinic side-effects, such as urinary retention, dry mouth, photophobia (dilatation of the pupil), confusion and constipation (p. 137), occur.
- Dopamine receptor antagonists
  - *Phenothiazines*, e.g. **prochlorperazine** 10 mg oral 3 times daily, **perphenazine** 4 mg 3 times daily oral, **trifluoperazine** 2–4 mg oral in divided doses and **chlorpromazine** 10–25 mg orally 4–6-hourly, are useful for vomiting produced by drugs or surgery and in nausea

associated with vertigo. Drowsiness, acute dystonic reactions and other extrapyramidal **side-effects** occur.

- *Metoclopramide* is given 10 mg 3 times daily orally or intravenously for all causes of vomiting, with high doses often given by intravenous infusion for cytotoxic drug-induced vomiting. It is a pro-kinetic agent with additional central effects.
- *Domperidone* 10 mg 3 times daily oral is predominantly used for cytotoxic drug-induced vomiting. It has few central effects, as it does not cross the blood–brain barrier easily. **Side-effects of metoclopramide and domperidone** include sedation and acute dystonia, although dystonia is less with domperidone. Both drugs should be avoided in pregnancy.
- *Serotonin (5HT₃) antagonists* are mainly used for cytotoxic drug-induced vomiting and post-operatively. **Granisetron** 1–2 mg is given 1 hour before cytotoxic treatment, then 2 mg daily. **Ondansetron** is given as 8 mg 1–2 hours before treatment, then 8 mg every 12 hours. **Side-effects** include constipation, headache and rash.
- *Synthetic cannabinoid* (nabilone 1 mg twice daily) is used for cytotoxic-induced vomiting refractory to other treatments. **Side-effects** include drowsiness, ataxia (these two can persist for 72 hours) and visual disturbance. Avoid in patients with a history of psychiatric disorder and in the elderly.
- *Neurokinin receptor antagonist* (**aprepitant** 125 mg 1 hour before chemotherapy, then 80 mg daily for 2 days) is used as an adjunct to dexamethasone and 5HT₃ treatment. **Side-effects** include gastrointestinal problems, headaches and dizziness. Do not use when the patient is breast-feeding.

Diarrhoea

Acute diarrhoea

Acute diarrhoea is very common and is usually due to dietary indiscretion, infectious agents, toxins or drugs, e.g. antibiotics, magnesium-containing antacids, or laxatives. It is usually self-limiting and ceases in 24–48 hours with no treatment.

- *Watery diarrhoea.* Viral infections with rotavirus, enteric adenovirus and norovirus are common and usually cause acute watery diarrhoea. *Salmonella, Campylobacter* and non-invasive *Escherichia coli* and *Clostridium difficile* may also cause watery diarrhoea.
- *Bloody diarrhoea (dysentery).* This can occur due to *Shigella, Campylobacter, Salmonella,* invasive *E. coli* subtypes and *C. difficile.*
- Investigations
  - *Stool culture.* *Salmonella, Shigella, Campylobacter* and *E. coli* can all be detected on culture. Detection of viral particles requires electron microscopy, which is not performed routinely.
  - *Ova, cysts and parasites.* Amoebiasis and giardiasis should be considered in returning travellers with diarrhoea.
  - *C. difficile toxin.* *C. difficile* infection is associated with the use of broad-spectrum antibiotics and is a common cause of diarrhoea in hospitalized patients. It is diagnosed by the presence of toxin in stools.
  - *Flexible sigmoidoscopy.* This may be useful in protracted cases to allow mucosal assessment and biopsy.

- Treatment
  - *Oral rehydration solutions* (p. 59) containing glucose and electrolytes are useful to prevent dehydration. IV rehydration is generally required only in severe cases or in the very young and very old.
  - *Antidiarrhoeal drugs* may impair clearance of the pathogen but can be given for symptomatic relief.
  - *Loperamide* 2–4 mg 4 times daily is a non-absorbed opioid that stimulates receptors in the enteric nervous system to reduce peristalsis and fluid secretion. It has the advantage of being non-euphoria-inducing, has no antimuscarinic side-effects and dependence does not occur. Adverse effects include nausea.
  - *Codeine* 30–60 mg oral 4 times daily acts in a similar way to loperamide but is systemically absorbed; opioid side-effects occur.
  - *Co-phenotrope* 2 tablets 4 times daily contains an opioid (diphenoxylate) and an antimuscarinic agent (atropine) which reduces colonic motility. It has antimuscarinic side-effects (p. 134).

All produce constipation if given frequently.

- Specific therapy
  - *Antibiotic therapy.* Most bacterial causes of diarrhoea are self-limiting (lasting only days) and antibiotics are not necessary. Quinolones (e.g. **ciprofloxacin** 500 mg twice daily) may decrease the severity and duration of symptoms.
  - **C. difficile.** A course of 10–14 days of oral **metronidazole** 400 mg 3 times daily. Oral **vancomycin** 125 mg 4 times daily is used for resistant cases. Oral **vancomycin** and IV **metronidazole** are used in patients not responding to **vancomycin** and with life-threatening infections.
  - *Amoebiasis.* Diagnosis is confirmed by the presence of trophozoites or cysts of *Entamoeba histolytica* in the stool, or by serum antibody tests. Treatment is with oral **metronidazole** 800 mg 3 times daily for 5–10 days or **tinidazole** oral 2 g daily for 2–3 days. Oral **paromomycin** 500 mg 3 times daily for 7 days or oral **diloxanide furoate** 500 mg 8-hourly for 10 days should be given to clear parasites from the bowel.
  - *Giardiasis.* Diagnosis is clinical. Trophozoites of *Giardia intestinalis* in stool or duodenal aspirate are not usually found. Therapy consists of oral **metronidazole** 2 g a day for 3 consecutive days or **tinidazole** 2 g orally single dose.

Diarrhoea in patients with HIV infection

Chronic diarrhoea is a common symptom in patients with HIV infection (p. 96). *Cryptosporidium* is the commonest pathogen isolated. Other infective causes include cytomegalovirus, *Mycobacterium avium* and *Giardia intestinalis*. Stool culture with examination for ova, cysts and parasites should be performed, together with flexible sigmoidoscopy/colonoscopy and biopsy.

- **Treatment** should be directed at individual causes. Some suggest empiric therapy with **metronidazole** for *Giardia*. Non-infective causes of diarrhoea associated with HIV disease include a specific enteropathy, lymphoma and Kaposi's sarcoma. All these conditions are less common with highly active anti-retroviral treatment (HAART).

Chronic diarrhoea

Chronic diarrhoea refers to diarrhoea of more than 4 weeks' duration. It can be due to a variety of causes (usually non-infective) including inflammation (inflammatory bowel disease), drugs (metformin, statins), functional factors, malabsorption or cancer (change in bowel habit), the treatments for which are described elsewhere.

● Clinical features
  ● *Steatorrhoea* suggests excessive fat in the stool and is due to malabsorption and pancreatic disease.
  ● *Bloody diarrhoea* suggests active colonic inflammation and is most commonly due to inflammatory bowel disease.
  ● *Watery diarrhoea* is the most common presentation and encompasses the broadest range of diagnoses. When standard investigations have proved unhelpful, a 72-hour assessment of stool weights may be helpful. The stool weights per day are not normally performed but in general: < 250 g is normal (frequency of defecation is often interpreted as diarrhoea by patients with, for example, irritable bowel syndrome); between 300 and ~800–900 g is probably organic (Crohn's disease); > 1000 g may be due to laxative abuse or a neuroendocrine tumour, e.g. VIPoma, causing profuse watery diarrhoea.
● Investigations. These include rectal examination, sigmoidoscopy, stool culture and ova, cysts and parasites, followed by a colonoscopy or barium follow-through, depending on type of diarrhoea. Small bowel MRI is replacing barium follow-throughs.
● Treatment. Treatment is usually directed at the cause, but symptomatic treatment as above is appropriate whilst investigations are ongoing or when specific therapy has failed to provide relief.

Constipation

This term is used for the infrequent passage of stool (< 2 per week), straining > 25% of the time or passage of hard stools and incomplete evacuation. Headache, malaise, halitosis, abdominal bloating and discomfort are often attributed to constipation without any factual evidence.

Constipation can come on acutely and, in the older patient, may indicate an organic disorder. Chronic constipation lasting years is usually functional.

Local anal diseases, e.g. fissures or haemorrhoids, are associated with constipation, as are some drugs, e.g. opiates, antimuscarinics, calcium channel blockers (such as verapamil), antidepressants and iron, and systemic disorders, e.g. hypothyroidism, hypercalcaemia and diabetes mellitus.

Rectal examination, flexible sigmoidoscopy/colonoscopy or CT pneumocolon (barium enema is being used less) may be necessary to rule out structural diseases in recent-onset constipation.

Treatment

● Lifestyle changes. Lifestyle changes, including a high fluid intake and regular exercise, help. Dietary fibre is mainly non-starch polysaccharides (NSP), which are soluble or insoluble. **Soluble fibre** (e.g. psyllium, ispaghula, calcium polycarbophil — found in the flesh of fruits, vegetables and grains) is broken down and fermented by colonic bacteria, increasing stool bulk. **Insoluble fibre** (wheat bran, corn) also increases the bulk of stools but can sometimes make symptoms worse, e.g. wind. Dietary fibre should be increased to up to 30 g a day. This is achieved by increasing consumption of bread, potatoes, fruit and vegetables and reducing sugar intake in order to avoid an increase in total calories. Unprocessed bran added to food increases fibre but many find

Kumar & Clark's Medical Management and Therapeutics

> **Box 5.2** Laxatives and enemas
>
> **Bulk-forming laxatives**
> - Dietary fibre
> - Wheat bran
> - Methylcellulose
> - Mucilaginous gums — sterculia
> - Mucilaginous seeds and seed coats, e.g. ispaghula husk
>
> **Stimulant laxatives (stimulate motility and intestinal secretion)**
> - Phenolphthalein
> - Bisacodyl
> - Anthraquinones — senna, dantron (only for the terminally ill)
> - Docusate sodium
> - Methyl naltrexone (for opiate-induced constipation)
> - Lubiprostone
>
> **Osmotic laxatives**
> - Magnesium sulphate
> - Lactulose
> - Macrogols
>
> **Suppositories**
> - Bisacodyl
> - Glycerol
>
> **Enemas**
> - Arachis oil
> - Docusate sodium
> - Hypertonic phosphate
> - Sodium citrate

it unpalatable. **Bulk-forming laxatives** increase faecal mass, which stimulates peristalsis, and are of use in those individuals with small hard stools where dietary fibre cannot be sufficiently increased. **Ispaghula husk** 3.5 g twice daily or **methylcellulose** 1.5–3 g twice daily is used.

- Laxatives (Box 5.2)
  - *Osmotic laxatives* are non-absorbable salts or carbohydrates that increase the amount of water retained in the large bowel and should be used as first-line drugs. **Lactulose** 15 mL twice daily is a semi-synthetic non-absorbed disaccharide. As a side-effect it can cause cramps and flatulence. **Macrogols**, inert polymers of ethylene glycol (1–3 sachets daily), are not fermented so gas is not formed and distension does not occur. **Magnesium salts** 5–10 g daily are dissolved in a glass of hot water before breakfast; they work in 2–4 hours.
  - *Stimulant laxatives* increase intestinal motility and can consequently cause abdominal cramps. They are contraindicated in intestinal obstruction. Benign pigmentation of the colon (melanosis coli), colonic atony due to smooth muscle atrophy and damage to the myenteric plexus occur and so these drugs should not be used long-term. **Bisacodyl** 5–10 mg at night (tablets or suppositories), or dantron –**co-danthrusate** 1–2 capsules at night is indicated only in terminally

ill patients (because of evidence of carcinogenicity in animal studies). **Senna** is given as 15–30 mg at night and increasing gradually.

- *Lubiprostone* is a bicyclic fatty acid, which opens chloride channels, increasing intestinal water secretion. It is used in the irritable bowel syndrome with constipation.
- *Methylnaltrexone* is an opioid antagonist and is effective in opioid-induced constipation without reducing the analgesic effect. It is given subcutaneously.
- *Faecal softeners* (e.g. liquid paraffin) can be given and arachis oil per rectum helps to soften impacted faeces.
- *Bowel-cleansing solutions* are used as pre-operative or pre-procedural regimens to empty the bowel. They should not be used routinely as laxatives. They are used in combination with a low-residue diet for the 48 hours prior to the procedure. They include **sodium picosulphate** 10 mg sachets; 2 sachets on the day before the procedure; a mixture of **macrogols**, **sodium sulphate** and **bicarbonate** 4 L 4–6 hours before the procedure; and **magnesium carbonate mixture** 2 sachets on the day before the procedure. Very elderly patients must be observed to avoid dehydration.
- *Prucalopride* is now used for resistant constipation.

● Biofeedback. For some patients chronic constipation is due to a failure of coordination of the process of defecation. Biofeedback has been shown to be of benefit in these patients and is used in some specialized centres.

GASTRO-OESOPHAGEAL REFLUX DISEASE

Reflux is extremely common in the general population, causing mild indigestion and heartburn.

Heartburn is the major feature and is mainly due to direct stimulation of the hypersensitive oesophageal mucosa, but also partly caused by spasm of the distal oesophageal muscle. It is aggravated by bending, stooping or lying down and may be relieved by antacids. The patient may complain of a burning pain on drinking hot liquids or alcohol.

Regurgitation of food and 'acid' into the mouth occurs, particularly when the patient is bending or lying flat. Aspiration into the lungs, producing pneumonia, is unusual without an accompanying stricture, but cough and nocturnal asthma from regurgitation and aspiration can occur. The differential diagnosis of the retrosternal pain from angina can be difficult; 20% of cases admitted to a coronary care unit have gastro-oesophageal reflux disease (GORD).

Investigations

Under the age of 45 years, all patients should be treated initially without investigations, unless there are alarm symptoms (Box 5.1).

● Fibre-optic oesophagoscopy is used to confirm the presence of oesophagitis, i.e. a red friable mucosa with ulceration in severe cases (erosive oesophagitis). For non-erosive reflux disease (NERD), see below.

● 24-hour ambulatory pH monitoring is used in patients with atypical symptoms and for assessment prior to surgery.

● Impedance uses a catheter to measure the resistance to flow of 'alternating current' of the contents of the oesophagus. Combined with pH monitoring, both acid and alkaline reflux can be detected.

Treatment

- **General measures.** Many patients with reflux symptoms (~50%) can be treated successfully with simple antacids, loss of weight, and raising the end of the bed at night. Precipitating factors should be avoided, with a reduction in alcohol and chocolate consumption and cessation of smoking. These measures are simple to say yet difficult to carry out, but are useful in mild cases. Medication that potentiates reflux, e.g. antimuscarinics, calcium channel blockers and bisphosphonates, should be stopped if possible.

- Medical treatment (Table 5.1)
  - *Simple antacids* include **magnesium trisilicate** and **aluminium hydroxide**, which are readily available over the counter. The former tends to cause diarrhoea whilst the latter causes constipation. Many antacids contain sodium, which may exacerbate fluid retention; aluminium hydroxide has less sodium than magnesium trisilicate. **Alginate-containing antacids** 10 mL 3 times daily form a gel or 'foam raft' with gastric contents and thereby reduce reflux. They are available over the counter in the UK.

  - *H_2-receptor antagonists* (e.g. **cimetidine** 400 mg twice daily, **ranitidine** 150 mg daily, **famotidine** 20 mg twice daily and **nizatadine** 150 mg twice daily) are used for acid suppression if the above measures fail, and can be obtained over the counter. These drugs are well tolerated. **Side-effects** include diarrhoea, abnormal liver biochemistry, headaches, dizziness, rashes, and rarely, cardiac arrhythmias, confusion and hallucinations in the elderly. Gynaecomastia and impotence are occasionally seen with cimetidine.

  - *Proton pump inhibitors (PPIs)* (e.g. **omeprazole** 20–40 mg daily, **rabeprazole** 20 mg daily, **lansoprazole** 30 mg daily, **pantoprazole** 40 mg daily, **esomeprazole** 40 mg daily) inhibit gastric hydrogen-potassium ATPase. Dispersible tablets to put on the tongue are available for lansoprazole and omeprazole. PPIs produce almost complete reduction of gastric acid secretion and are the drugs of choice for all but mild cases. Patients with ongoing symptoms need prolonged treatment, often for years. Sometimes a lower dose, e.g. omeprazole 10 mg, is sufficient for maintenance. **Side-effects** include gastrointestinal problems of nausea, vomiting, abdominal pain and diarrhoea. Other uncommon side-effects include fatigue, dizziness and sleep disturbances. Serious side-effects are rare.

  - *Prokinetic agents* metoclopramide 10 mg 3 times daily and **domperidone** 10 mg 3 times daily are dopamine antagonists (for side-effects, see p. 644). They are occasionally helpful, as they enhance peristalsis and speed gastric emptying. Cisapride has been withdrawn because it increases the Q–T_c interval and the risk of arrhythmias.

- **Surgery.** Surgery should never be performed for a hiatus hernia alone. The properly selected case with severe reflux symptoms confirmed by pH monitoring and with oesophagitis on oesophagoscopy responds well to surgery. Repair of the hernia and additional antireflux surgery (e.g. a modified Nissen fundoplication) is performed laparoscopically. Results show an improvement in symptoms in up to 80% of cases. The indications for surgery are not always clear, as medical therapy with PPIs is so effective; a young patient requiring years of drug treatment is one common indication. Patients with oesophageal dysmotility unrelated to acid reflux do less well than those with proven reflux.

Non-erosive reflux disease (NERD)

These cases include patients with reflux symptoms. They often do not respond to a PPI. Patients are usually female and often the symptoms are functional (p. 167).

Complications

- Peptic stricture usually occurs in patients over the age of 60. The symptoms are those of dysphagia over a long period preceded by severe heartburn. Treatment is by dilatation of the stricture and a PPI is given to achieve anacidity. Occasionally, surgery for continued reflux is required. Intermittent dysphagia is more classical of a Schatzki ring than a peptic stricture.

- Barrett's oesophagus. This occurs as a result of longstanding reflux (Fig. 5.1). It consists of columnar epithelium with intestinal metaplasia extending upwards into the lower oesophagus and replacing normal squamous epithelium. Barrett's oesophagus (even short segment < 3 cm) is pre-malignant for **adenocarcinoma**. Risk factors for progression are male sex, age > 45 years, length of segment > 8 cm, early age of onset and duration of symptoms of GORD, the presence of ulceration and stricture and a family history. Dysplasia is patchy and biopsies from all four quadrants (every 2 cm) of the Barrett's segment must be performed. There is some evidence that anti-reflux surgery leads to Barrett's regression. Patients without dysplasia do not require **surveillance**. Low-grade dysplasia requires regular endoscopic surveillance. High-grade dysplasia is now treated by radiofrequency ablation using the HALO system or local endomucosal resection. Endoscopic ablation therapy with photodynamic therapy or laser is also used.

- Adenocarcinoma. Patients with weekly reflux symptoms were nearly 8 times more likely to develop adenocarcinoma than those without symptoms in one study. The greater the frequency, severity and the duration of reflux symptoms, the greater the risk.

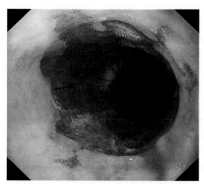

Fig. 5.1 Barrett's oesophagus. Endoscopic view showing a segment of columnar-lined oesophagus (arrowed)

Kumar & Clark's Medical Management and Therapeutics

OTHER OESOPHAGEAL DISORDERS

Achalasia

Achalasia is characterized by aperistalsis in the body of the oesophagus and failure of relaxation of the lower oesophageal sphincter (LOS) on initiation of swallowing.

The disease presents at any age with a long history of intermittent dysphagia for both liquids and solids, and regurgitation of food from the dilated oesophagus. Aspiration pneumonia may result. Severe retrosternal chest pain due to vigorous non-peristaltic contraction of the oesophagus occurs, particularly in younger patients.

- Barium swallow will show dilatation of the oesophagus, lack of peristalsis and often synchronous contractions. The lower end gradually narrows like a bird's beak.
- Manometry shows aperistalsis of the oesophagus, as well as failure of relaxation of the LOS.
- Oesophagoscopy is necessary to exclude a small carcinoma at the lower end of the oesophagus.

Treatment

- **Endoscopic balloon dilatation** is performed to produce a sustained reduction of the LOS by disrupting the circular muscle with balloon dilatation under fluoroscopic guidance. Greater diameters of dilatation are used (30–40 mm) than for dilatation of peptic strictures. The risk of perforation is therefore higher and occurs in 3–5% cases. An effective symptom response occurs in 80% of patients; most patients require 2–3 dilatations over a 5-year period. Younger patients tend to have a shorter duration of response.
- **Botulinum toxin** acts to prevent the release of acetylcholine from peripheral nerves, thus inducing muscle paralysis. Although controversial, it can be injected quadrantically in 25 U aliquots at the squamocolumnar junction. Studies have shown reasonable response rates but the duration of response ranges between 7 and 11 months. This therapeutic option is attractive for elderly patients, as it is low-risk and easy to administer repeatedly.
- **Heller's surgical myotomy** is a well-established surgical procedure and can now be performed with a minimally invasive laparoscopic approach. The duration of response is excellent, with 85–90% of patients describing a good symptomatic response at 5 years. Consequently, the surgical approach is often preferred in younger patients. The associated mortality is in the region of 1%. To prevent reflux, some surgeons combine this laparoscopic operation with a partial fundoplication (see below).
- **Pharmacological therapy** with smooth muscle relaxants such as calcium channel blockers (nifedipine) and nitrates can be given preprandially. They are less effective than other measures.

GORD is a common complication, with all successful treatments necessitating PPI therapy in most patients.

Diffuse oesophageal spasm

This disorder causes chest pain and dysphagia, is diagnosed by oesophageal manometry and is characterized by simultaneous non-peristaltic oesophageal contractions occurring after 20% or more swallows. Barium swallow may show a corkscrew appearance. Nutcracker oesophagus is a variant of diffuse oesophageal spasm characterized by very high-amplitude peristalsis (> 200 mmHg).

- Treatment. Sublingual nifedipine 10 mg 3 times daily should be tried initially. When the spasm is associated with GORD, acid suppression is given.

Rings and webs

A number of rings and webs have been described throughout the oesophagus that may cause dysphagia (difficulty in swallowing). They can usually be treated at endoscopy by dilatation.

Eosinophilic oesophagitis

This usually occurs in young white male patients who have a long history of dysphagia, food impaction, heartburn and oesophageal pain. Endoscopically there is mucosal furrowing, loss of vascular pattern and prominent circular folds. Histologically there is a characteristic infiltration with eosinophils (the oesophagus is usually devoid of eosinophils). The cause is unknown but there may be a personal or family history of allergic diseases. Food allergy may be a causative factor.

- Treatment is with a PPI, swallowing inhaled steroid preparations, e.g. **fluticasone** or **oral steroids**. Liquid budesonide is used.

Oesophageal infections

Infection is a cause of painful swallowing (odynophagia) and is seen particularly in the immunosuppressed, the debilitated, patients on antibiotics and those with AIDS. Oral lesions may make the diagnosis obvious, e.g. thrush, but endoscopy with cytology and biopsy is often necessary. *Candida* is treated with oral **nystatin** 400–600 000 U 4 times daily. **Fluconazole** 100 mg daily for 2 weeks is used for more severe cases and IV **amphotericin** B 0.3–0.5 mg/kg/day for systemic infection. Herpes simplex is treated with oral **aciclovir** 400 mg 5 times daily for 7 days but may require IV therapy 5 mg/kg 8-hourly for 5 days. Cytomegalovirus is treated with **ganciclovir** IV infusion 5 mg/kg 12-hourly. Prophylactic treatment with nystatin or amphotericin is required for all patients on large doses of immunosuppressive therapy.

Chemical oesophagitis

- Drugs, such as bisphosphonates, potassium, NSAIDs, aspirin and iron, can cause a variety of oesophageal disorders, e.g. oesophagitis, ulcers, erosions and strictures, presenting as odynophagia or dysphagia. An oesophagoscopy should be performed. Treatment depends on the lesion and stopping the offending drug if possible.
- Ingestion of household products (e.g. intentional or accidental in young children), such as bleach, toiletries and disinfectants, can cause corrosion of the mouth and of the pharyngeal and oesophageal mucosa. Gastric aspiration, lavage or dilution or neutralization of alkali is contraindicated. Careful upper gastrointestinal endoscopy is required to assess damage. Strictures occur in the long term. If there is life-threatening pharyngeal or laryngeal oedema, endotracheal intubation is necessary.

Oesophageal perforation or rupture

The commonest cause is endoscopic dilatation, usually of malignant strictures. Small lesions heal spontaneously (with nil by mouth and broad-spectrum antibiotics), but many require insertion of an oesophageal stent. Rupture can also occur after forceful vomiting, when it presents with severe chest pain and collapse. Treatment is surgical.

PEPTIC ULCER DISEASE

Peptic ulcers are mainly due to *Helicobacter pylori* infection or non-steroidal anti-inflammatory drugs (NSAIDs), including aspirin.

Helicobacter pylori

This is a spiral-shaped, Gram-negative, urease-producing bacterium. It is found in the gastric antrum and in areas of gastric metaplasia in the duodenum, in 95% of patients with a duodenal ulcer and 75% of patients with a gastric ulcer. *H. pylori* is also present in people with no ulcer disease and in up to 80% in people from developing countries. It can be identified by the following methods:

● Non-invasive:
  ● *^{13}C urea breath test.* The measurement of $^{13}CO_2$ in the breath, after ingestion of ^{13}C urea, is very sensitive (98%) and specific (95%) for the presence of *H. pylori*.
  ● *Serological tests.* These detect IgG antibodies to *H. pylori* and are 80% sensitive and specific. They are used in diagnosis and in epidemiological studies. IgG titres may take up to 1 year to fall by 50% after eradication therapy and therefore are not useful for confirming eradication or the presence of a current infection.
  ● *Stool immunoassay.* The overall sensitivity is about 90% with a specificity of 95% for the presence of *H. pylori*.
● Invasive (endoscopy): Gastric biopsies are added to urea in a gel containing phenol red (CLO test). If *H. pylori* is present, the urease enzyme splits the urea to release ammonia, which raises the pH of the solution and causes a rapid colour change. Biopsies can also be cultured and sensitivities to antibiotics can be ascertained. *H. pylori* can be detected histologically.

Eradication therapy for *H. pylori*

Treatment is based on a PPI (**omeprazole** or **lansoprazole**) plus two antibiotics (from **clarithromycin**, **amoxicillin**, **tetracycline** and **metronidazole**) for 1 week. Because of metronidazole resistance in 20–50% and no resistance to amoxicillin, the preferred regimen was **omeprazole 20 mg, amoxicillin 1 g and clarithromycin 500 mg**, all twice daily for 1 week.

With the increase in clarithromycin resistance many are now using quadruple therapy with omeprazole 20 mg × 2 daily, tripotassium dicitrate bismuthate 120 mg × 4 daily, tetracycline 500 mg × 4 daily and metronidazole 500 mg × 3 daily for 2 weeks. These should be taken 30 mins before a meal, antacids and milk avoided for half an hour before or after; patients should be warned that bismuth may blacken their tongue.

Reinfection after successful eradication occurs in < 1%. In developing countries, where compliance is often poor and antibiotic resistance high, failure of eradication is common.

Tinidazole or tetracycline is occasionally used in some regimens with antisecretory drugs and other antibiotics.

Treatment failures (< 10% with good compliance) are treated with bismuth plus a PPI plus two antibiotics for 2 weeks.

Aspirin and other NSAIDs

These drugs cause gastric mucosal damage in 50% of patients taking them regularly and ~30% will have ulcers on endoscopy. Only 5% have symptoms and only 1–2% have a major problem, i.e. gastrointestinal bleed. In patients who develop problems, NSAIDs should be stopped and for established ulcers, a PPI should be prescribed. *H. pylori* eradication is unhelpful. When stopping NSAIDs is *not* possible, use an NSAID with low gastrointestinal side-effects at the lowest possible dose, e.g. ibuprofen 1–2 g daily, and prophylactic cytoprotective therapy, e.g. a PPI (**omeprazole** 20 mg daily) or **misoprostol**, which is a synthetic analogue of prostaglandin E1 and is given as 200 mcg 4 times per day. The main side-effects of this latter agent are diarrhoea and abdominal pain, and so it is not often used.

Prophylactic therapy

This is necessary for all high-risk patients, i.e. those over 65 years, those with a peptic ulcer history, particularly with complications, and patients on therapy with corticosteroids or anticoagulants. An alternative is to give a COX-2 NSAID, which causes less mucosal damage (p. 298), but long-term cardiovascular risk is a problem.

General measures for peptic ulcer disease

Stopping smoking helps ulcers heal. Eradication of *H. pylori* is judged on the relief of symptoms, except in patients with complications of peptic ulcer disease in whom eradication should be checked by a ^{13}C urea breath test or stool immunoassay. A patient with a gastric ulcer should be re-endoscoped at 6 weeks to check healing and to exclude a malignant ulcer. **Antacids** are of no value for ulcer healing but may help pain relief. The choice depends on the formulation, side-effects and buffering capacity. For example, a compound alginate 15 mg 4 times a day may be given.

Complications of peptic ulcer

These include haemorrhage (p. 151).

● **Perforation** is becoming increasingly uncommon because of better medical therapy. Duodenal ulcers perforate more commonly than gastric ulcers, usually into the peritoneal cavity. Treatment is surgical and *H. pylori* should be eradicated.

● **Gastric outlet obstruction** is now uncommon but can occur due to duodenal ulcer oedema or subsequent scarring. There is projectile vomiting and a succussion splash may be demonstrated clinically. Metabolic alkalosis can occur due to loss of acid. Those with duodenal oedema may settle but the majority are treated with dilatation, stenting or surgery.

GASTROINTESTINAL HAEMORRHAGE

Acute upper gastrointestinal bleeding

Haematemesis is the vomiting of blood from a lesion proximal to the distal duodenum. **Melaena** is the passage of black tarry stools; the black colour is due to altered blood — 50 mL or more is required to produce this. Melaena can occur with bleeding from any lesion in areas proximal to and including the caecum.

Unaltered or 'maroon blood' passed per rectum can be due to an upper gastrointestinal bleed if the bleed is massive.

Clinical approach to the patient

All cases with a recent (i.e. within 48 hours) significant gastrointestinal bleed should be seen in hospital. In many, no immediate treatment is required, as often there has been only a small amount of blood lost and the patient's cardiovascular system can compensate for this. Approximately 85% of patients stop bleeding spontaneously within 48 hours.

Immediate management (Box 5.3)

This involves taking a rapid history to determine the likely aetiology of the bleeding and carrying out an examination. Note the age of the patient and make a rapid assessment of the haemodynamic state. Look for pallor, cold nose, tachycardia and low BP, i.e. 'shock', and also for evidence of co-morbidity, i.e. cardiac failure, ischaemic heart disease, renal and malignant disease or signs of chronic liver disease. Co-morbidity adversely effects outcome. Give oxygen to shocked patients. Take blood for Hb, U&E, LFTs, coagulation studies, and grouping and cross-matching.

- Blood volume. The major principle is to restore the blood volume rapidly to normal. This can best be achieved by transfusion of blood via one or more large-bore 14–18 IV cannulae. A central venous catheter is useful in the severely shocked and elderly. It may be necessary to give

---

> **Box 5.3** Management of acute gastrointestinal bleeding
> (see also Fig. 20.4)
>
> - History and examination. Note co-morbidity
> - Monitor pulse and BP half-hourly
> - Take blood for haemoglobin, urea, electrolytes, liver biochemistry, coagulation screen, group and cross-matching (2 U initially)
> - Establish IV access — 2 large-bore IV cannulae; central line if brisk bleed or if patient is elderly or has co-morbidities
> - Give blood transfusion/colloid if necessary. Indications for blood transfusion are:
>   - Shock (pallor, cold nose, systolic BP < 100 mmHg, pulse > 100 bpm)
>   - Hb < 10 g/dL in patients with recent or active bleeding
> - Oxygen therapy if hypoxic
> - Urgent endoscopy in shocked patients/liver disease
> - Continue to monitor pulse and BP
> - Re-endoscope for continued bleeding/hypovolaemia
> - Angiography if bleeding continues
> - Surgery if bleeding persists

a colloid, e.g. **gelofusine**, initially to a severely shocked patient whilst blood products are awaited. Occasionally, with a massive bleed, O negative blood can be given.

- *Rate of blood transfusion* must be monitored; the pulse rate and venous pressure are good guides to transfusion requirements.
- *Anaemia* does not develop immediately after a bleed as haemodilution has not taken place, and therefore the Hb level is a poor indicator of the need to transfuse. If, however, the Hb level is low (< 10 g/dL) and the patient has either bled recently or is actively bleeding, transfusion is usually necessary.

● **Correction of coagulopathy.** All anticoagulants, antiplatelet agents and NSAIDs should be stopped if possible. Significant coagulopathy should be corrected with **fresh frozen plasma** (FFP) (15 mL/kg) and cryoprecipitate (about 20 mL). **IV vitamin K** (10 mg) should be given if the coagulopathy is due to warfarin or liver disease, but as its action is delayed for up to 24 hours FFP is also usually required. Platelet infusion is indicated if the platelet count is $< 50 \times 10^9/L$.

● **Naso-gastric tube insertion.** Insertion of naso-gastric tube is not normally required. It is occasionally useful in confirming the diagnosis and ensuring an empty stomach prior to oesophagogastroduodenoscopy (OGD).

● **Timing of upper gastrointestinal endoscopy.** Whenever possible, OGD should be performed within 24 hours, as it allows diagnosis, risk stratification (Table 5.2) and early discharge. However, as the majority of upper gastrointestinal bleeds stop spontaneously, most patients can wait to have an OGD performed within normal working hours. **Emergency endoscopy** should be reserved for patients with a high likelihood of either persistent bleeding or recurrent bleeding. Rockall et al (Table 5.3) found the likelihood of rebleeding and mortality could be predicted on the basis of five factors and devised a simple scoring system to allow risk assessment. Although the full scoring system requires endoscopy, the first three factors can be used in isolation to provide an initial assessment to determine the need for emergency endoscopy. There should be a lower threshold for emergency endoscopy in patients with known or likely oesophageal varices (e.g., minor coffee ground vomit).

Table 5.2 Risk of recurrent bleeding in peptic ulceration

Endoscopic appearance	Risk
Active bleeding	55%
Visible vessel	45%
Adherent clot	20%
Flat spot	10%
Clean base	5%

Kumar & Clark's Medical Management and Therapeutics

Table 5.3 Rockall risk assessment score in non-variceal upper gastro-oesophageal haemorrhage

a) Rockall risk assessment score

Variable	0	1	2	3
Age	< 60	60–70	> 70	–
Shock	None	Pulse > 100 bpm Systolic BP < 100 mmHg	Pulse > 100 bpm Systolic BP < 100 mmHg	–
Co-morbidity	None		Cardiac disease or any major co-morbidity	Chronic kidney disease, liver failure, disseminated malignancy
Diagnosis	Mallory–Weiss tear or no lesion	All other diagnoses	Malignancy of upper gastrointestinal tract	–
Stigmata (endoscopy)	None or dark spot		Blood in upper gastrointestinal tract, adherent clot, visible or spurting vessel	–

Score: < 3 Excellent prognosis; > 8 High risk of death.
(BSG Endoscopy Committee 2002, with permission)

b) Rebleed and mortality risk according to Rockall score

Risk score	Predicted rebleed (%)	Predicted mortality (%)
0	5	0
1	3	0
2	5	0
3	11	3
4	14	5
5	24	11
6	33	17
7	44	27
8+	42	41

Management of specific acute upper gastrointestinal disorders

Mallory–Weiss tears (5% of diagnoses found on endoscopy for acute UGI haemorrhage)

These appear as linear mucosal tears at the gastro-oesophageal junction. They are often no longer visible by the time endoscopy is performed. Most patients stop bleeding spontaneously and early discharge within 24 hours is usually possible.

Oesophagitis (10%)

As described on p. 140, this should be treated with high-dose oral PPI therapy, e.g. omeprazole 40 mg daily.

Oesophageal varices (10%)

Oesophageal varices are portosystemic collaterals, which occur due to portal hypertension usually secondary to cirrhosis of the liver. In the upper gastrointestinal tract they occur most commonly at the gastro-oesophageal junction and the fundus of the stomach, although duodenal varices also occur occasionally.

Oesophageal varices are easily seen at endoscopy as blue/purple vascular swellings that form columns running the length of the oesophagus. They can be graded according to their number and size, with longer, larger columns being more likely to bleed. Microtelangiectasia on the surface of the varix, usually described as a cherry red spot, are also associated with an increased risk of bleeding. In contrast to upper gastrointestinal bleeds, in general, only 40% of variceal bleeds stop spontaneously and therefore urgent endoscopic intervention is required. Even in patients with cirrhosis, upper gastrointestinal bleeding can still be caused by peptic ulcers rather than varices.

- **General management.** Patients with variceal bleeding are often unstable and require admission to an ICU or HDU. CVP monitoring is frequently required, and endotracheal intubation for airway protection should be performed if there is agitation or a decreased conscious level.
- Pharmacotherapy
  - *Terlipressin* 1–2 mg IV 4-hourly for 48 hours is an analogue of vasopressin and causes selective vasoconstriction of the splanchnic vasculature. This leads to a reduction in portal pressure and has been shown to reduce mortality from variceal bleeds. **Side-effects** include coronary ischaemia and myocardial infarction. Terlipressin should not be used in those with ischaemic heart disease.
  - *Octreotide* 50–100 mcg bolus, then 25–50 mcg/hour for 3–5 days, a somatostatin analogue, has a similar effect to glypressin but does not have the same ischaemic side-effects.
  - *Antibiotics* are needed for bacterial infections, which occur in one-third to two-thirds of patients with variceal bleeds. Patients with untreated bacterial infections have a higher risk of continued bleeding and recurrent bleeding. All patients with variceal bleeding should receive a broad-spectrum antibiotic (e.g. **ciprofloxacin** 500 mg twice daily or third-generation cephalosporin).
  - *Lactulose and phosphate enemas* may be needed. Due to the increased production of ammonia caused by the digestion of blood, patients with cirrhosis frequently develop encephalopathy subsequent to a variceal bleed. Enemas with **lactulose** 10 mL 4 times daily and **phosphate** 1 twice daily are therefore commenced early in treatment.
- Endoscopic therapy
  - *Oesophageal banding.* This is the first-line endoscopic treatment for oesophageal varices, both acutely and as secondary prophylaxis. A rubber band is placed via an endoscope over the varix, leading to its strangulation and necrosis. Bands are placed on each varix just above the oesophago-gastric junction (OGJ) and 5–8 bands can be applied before the endoscope must be removed in order to reload. Variceal banding has a higher success rate (85–95%) than injection sclerotherapy (80%) for the control of acute variceal bleeding and the rates of complications are lower. The procedure should be repeated every 2 weeks after the initial bleed until the varices are obliterated.

Kumar & Clark's Medical Management and Therapeutics

- *Injection sclerotherapy.* Injection of the sclerosant causes coagulation necrosis, followed by thrombosis with inflammation and scarring of the surrounding tissue, leading to variceal obliteration. The most commonly used sclerosant is **ethanolamine** (5%). Between 1 and 3 mL of sclerosant is injected into each varix just above the oesophago-gastric junction (OGJ). Necrotic ulcers are present in 90% of patients the day after injection and rates of complication with stricture formation and perforation are high (up to 20%).
- *Balloon tamponade.* A Sengstaken–Blakemore tube can be used as a temporizing measure for a maximum of 24 hours, when other interventions have failed or are not available. It consists of a tube with an oesophageal and a gastric balloon, which is placed either under direct vision or endoscopically via the mouth into the stomach. The gastric balloon is then inflated with either 500 mL air or 200–300 mL of water and 50 mL of radio-opaque water-soluble contrast depending on manufacturer's recommendation. An X-ray is essential to check tube position. Gentle traction is applied to pull the gastric balloon against the gastro-oesophageal junction, compressing the bleeding vessels. Inflation of the oesophageal balloon above 35 mmHg is associated with a high incidence of oesophageal perforation and therefore is rarely done. It should only be used in ICU with sedation, and endotracheal intubation is required.
- *Transjugular intrahepatic portosystemic shunt (TIPS).* In this radiological procedure a guidewire is passed from the jugular vein into the liver; an expandable metal stent is then passed over the guidewire into the liver to form a channel between the systemic and portal circulations. This decompresses the portal system and is an effective treatment for uncontrolled or recurrent variceal bleeding. The principal **side-effect** is worsening encephalopathy.
- Surgery (used when all the forms of therapy described above have failed):
  - *Oesophageal transection* — can be performed as an emergency procedure for uncontrolled bleeding.
  - *Shunt surgery* — portocaval or distal splenorenal shunts can be performed as an elective procedure in those with recurrent variceal bleeding when other measures have failed.

Gastric varices

Gastric varices should be treated pharmacologically with **terlipressin** and **antibiotics**; endoscopic therapy with banding or sclerosants is usually ineffective. Endoscopic injection with tissue adhesive agents such as **N-butyl cyanoacrylate** (histoacryl) has been reported as being effective in up to 90% of cases. This liquid forms a hard polymer on contact with blood, which plugs the bleeding varix. TIPS should be considered early and surgery may be necessary.

- **Prevention of recurrent variceal bleeding.** The risk of recurrence is 60–70% over a 2-year period. Long-term measures to prevent this are:
  - *Oral propranolol.* Give an adjusted dose to reduce the resting pulse rate by 25%. This will also prevent bleeding from portal gastropathy.
  - *Endoscopic treatment.* Banding at 2-weekly intervals leads to obliteration of varices but follow-up is necessary as varices return (30–40% per year).

Patients with cirrhosis and varices who have not bled should be given propranolol.

Peptic ulcers (50%)

Gastric and duodenal ulcers are the commonest cause of significant upper gastrointestinal bleeding. The risk of continued bleeding and rebleeding can be predicted on the basis of the endoscopic appearance of the ulcer (Box 5.3). This in turn determines the required medical and endoscopic therapy.

Larger ulcers (> 2 cm) and those located on the lesser curve of the stomach and the posterio-inferior wall of the duodenal bulb also have a higher risk of rebleeding.

- Management
  - *Medical therapy.* Stability of clot is favoured by a high gastric pH, with clot lysis occurring at a pH < 6. **PPI therapy** is more effective than H_2-antagonists in preventing recurrent bleeding. In ulcers with active bleeding, visible vessels or adherent clot, **IV omeprazole** 80 mg IV bolus followed by 8 mg/hour infusion reduces the rebleed rate to 7% compared to 23% with placebo. Most rebleeds occur within 72 hours and therefore the infusion should be continued for this period of time. For ulcers with a clean base or flat spot, an oral PPI is sufficient. **H. pylori eradication therapy** should be commenced immediately if a CLO test is positive (p. 144).
  - *Endoscopic therapy.* Endoscopic therapy is not required for ulcers with a clean base or flat spot but should be attempted for those with active bleeding or a visible vessel. Adherent clot should be removed to expose any visible vessels. It is now agreed that bimodal therapy should be employed. Any two of the following should be used:
    a) **adrenaline (epinephrine) injection** — **1:10000 adrenaline** injected quadrantically around the bleeding point (2–3 mL per injection)
    b) **thermal coagulation** —with either heater probe or bipolar electrocoagulation
    c) **mechanical devices** — endoscopically placed clips that can apply tamponade to the bleeding point.
    When an initial attempt at endoscopic therapy fails, it is common to undertake a second procedure. However, the case should be discussed with surgical colleagues and preparations made for surgery should the patient rebleed.
  - *Therapeutic angiography.* Options at angiography include selective intra-arterial vasopressin infusion or embolotherapy with micro-coils, gelatin or polyvinyl alcohol particles. Technical success rates of 50–90% have been reported. Therapeutic angiography is used when endoscopy fails to control the bleeding.
  - *Surgery.* Due to improvements in endoscopic and medical therapy, the requirement for surgery for the treatment of bleeding peptic ulcers has declined dramatically over the last few decades. However, it is still occasionally required when other interventions have failed. Ligation of the bleeding vessel is performed.

Erosive gastritis and duodenitis (10–20%)

This should be treated with oral PPI therapy and *H. pylori* eradication if the CLO test is positive.

Kumar & Clark's Medical Management and Therapeutics

Oesophageal and gastric cancer (<4%)

Bleeding points on the tumour can be treated with similar endoscopic therapy to that employed for gastric and duodenal ulcers. Endoscopic therapy with argon plasma coagulation (APC) or NAG laser therapy may also be useful.

Prognosis

The mortality from gastrointestinal haemorrhage has shown little change from 5–12% over the years, despite many changes in management, mainly because of a demographic shift to more elderly patients with co-morbidity. The lowest mortality rates are achieved in dedicated medical/surgical gastrointestinal units. Early therapeutic endoscopy has not so far lowered mortality, although rebleeding episodes are reduced.

GI haemorrhage in specific circumstances

Bleeding after percutaneous coronary intervention (PCI)

This occurs in approximately 2% of patients undergoing PCI (who are on antiplatelet therapy), and has a high mortality of 5–10%. Urgent endoscopy should be performed with appropriate therapy, for example, for an ulcer. A PPI should be given intravenously. Management is difficult, as cessation of antiplatelet therapy has a high risk of acute stent thrombosis and also an associated high mortality. Using a risk assessment score (e.g. Rockall, p. 148), a reasonable approach is to stop all antiplatelet therapy in high-risk patients but to continue in low-risk ones. These patients should be under the combined care of a cardiologist and a gastroenterologist.

Acute lower gastrointestinal bleeding

Massive bleeding from the lower gastrointestinal tract is rare. Conversely, small bleeds from haemorrhoids occur very commonly. Massive bleeding is usually due to diverticular disease or ischaemic colitis (p. 166).

Initial management

Initial management is similar to that of upper gastrointestinal bleeding (p. 146). Additional immediate investigations are rectal examination, proctoscopy and sigmoidoscopy.

- **Colonoscopy** performed within 24 hours of presentation gives the best chance of making a diagnosis. A rapid bowel cleanser should be given first, either orally or via an naso-gastric tube, to ensure good visibility.
- **Mesenteric angiography** is useful both diagnostically and therapeutically. The mesenteric vessels are selectively cannulated and contrast is injected to look for extravasation into the gastrointestinal lumen. The minimum bleed rate required is 0.5 mL/min. Embolization of the bleeding vessel can be performed but carries the risk of bowel infarction. Intra-arterial infusions of vasopressin can also be given.

The majority of lower gastrointestinal bleeds settle with supportive management. However, surgical removal of the affected part of bowel is occasionally required.

Management of specific acute lower gastrointestinal disorders

Angiodysplasia

This refers to abnormal blood vessels most commonly found in the caecum and proximal ascending colon. They are also associated with

Hereditary haemorrhagic telangiectasia (HHT), renal disease, von Wille-brand's disease and aortic stenosis. Treatment is usually endoscopic, with thermal modalities and argon plasma coagulopathy (APC). In HHT, hor-monal therapy with oestrogen–progesterones (oestradiol 0.035–0.05 mg; norethisterone 1 mg twice daily) has also been tried but evidence for efficacy is conflicting. **Side-effects** include gynaecomastia and erectile dysfunction.

Meckel's diverticulum

This is a congenital abnormality in the ileum, approximately 60 cm from the ileocaecal valve. It is usually symptomless but can ulcerate and bleed. Treatment is surgical removal.

Radiation proctitis

Radiation damage causing superficial vascular abnormalities can occur months to years after exposure to radiation therapy. In the rectum it causes proctitis and rectal bleeding. It is refractory to most treatments, although endoscopic APC therapy may be effective. Sucralfate enemas and also formalin swabs, inserted into the rectum for 2 mins, have also been tried.

Occult/chronic gastrointestinal bleeding

All men and post-menopausal women with iron deficiency anaemia should be investigated for possible blood loss from the gastrointestinal tract. The history and examination may indicate the most likely site of bleeding, but if no clue is available, it is usual to investigate both the upper and lower gastrointestinal tract endoscopically at the same session ('top and tail').

Initial investigations

- **Upper gastrointestinal endoscopy with duodenal biopsy** – to exclude an upper gastrointestinal malignancy and coeliac disease.
- **Colonoscopy** – to exclude a colonic neoplasm.

If these investigations are normal, the patient can be treated with oral iron replacement therapy (p. 202) and only investigated further should anaemia recur.

Further investigations

- **Small bowel follow-through** is often the next investigation but diagnos-tic yield is low and many advocate proceeding straight to capsule endoscopy.
- **Wireless capsule endoscopy** involves swallowing a tiny video camera which is moved by peristalsis though the bowel and transmits images to a recorder carried on a belt.
- **New enteroscopy techniques** with a single and double balloon show a similar diagnostic yield to the wireless capsule.
- **Radio-labelled red cell scan** involves red blood cells labelled with ^{99}-technetium, which are given intravenously to the patient and passed into the gut at the point of bleeding. This is detected as a pool of tracer by a gamma camera but a minimum bleed rate of approximately 0.1 mL/min is required. If positive, this technique can localize the bleeding source in 80% of cases.
- **Mesenteric angiography**.

Treatment

Individual diagnoses are treated as appropriate.

MALABSORPTION

Coeliac disease

Coeliac disease (CD) is a chronic inflammatory response to the gliadin component of gluten in patients who are mainly DQ2/DQ8-positive. Gluten is contained in cereals, wheat, rye and barley. There is a loss of villi (villus atrophy) with crypt hyperplasia in the mucosa of the proximal small bowel and an increase in intra-epithelial lymphocytes. Coeliac disease can present at any age. Patients can be asymptomatic or present with non-specific tiredness and malaise or gross malnutrition. Routine blood tests showing anaemia, with a combination of iron, B12 or folate deficiency, is now a common presentation. Common gastrointestinal symptoms range from diarrhoea, steatorrhoea, abdominal bloating, mouth ulcers and angular stomatitis.

Investigations

These include:

- **Anti-tissue tranglutaminase IgA antibodies.** This cheap, quick ELISA technique has high sensitivity (85–100%) and specificity (97–100%). Levels return towards normal within 1–2 months of starting a gluten-free diet. The test is therefore useful in monitoring compliance.
- **Anti-endomysial IgA antibodies.** This immunofluorescence technique uses umbilical cord tissue and has high sensitivity (84–100%) and specificity (94–100%).
- **IgA deficiency.** IgA-deficient patients are 10–20 times more likely to develop coeliac disease and have false-negative serological tests.
- **HLA DQ2/DQ8.** A positive test demonstrates a high risk of having coeliac disease.
- **Duodenal biopsies.** Gastroscopy with four distal duodenal biopsies still represents the gold standard for diagnosis.

Management

All patients with coeliac disease should be referred to a dietitian for a gluten-free diet (GFD). The avoidance of gluten should be emphasized even in the asymptomatic patient because of the increased risk of osteoporosis and malignancy (which is reduced by a strict diet). Folate deficiency is present in 50% of patients and iron deficiency is common; initial replacement therapy is given. Most patients respond to a GFD; a few require corticosteroids or azathioprine. All patients diagnosed with coeliac disease should undergo a bone densitometry scan (dual energy X-ray absorptiometry, DEXA) to assess for osteoporosis, which should be treated with bisphosphonates (p. 324), and monitored yearly. **Pneumococcal vaccination** is necessary due to the occurrence of splenic atrophy.

Dermatitis herpetiformis is a gluten-sensitive enteropathy with a sub-epidermal, blistering rash, mainly on the extensor surfaces. It is treated with **dapsone 50–200 mg** and a gluten-free diet.

Tropical sprue

This condition presents with diarrhoea and malnutrition due to malabsorption of two or more substances (particularly of fat and vitamin B_{12}). It occurs in residents in and visitors to affected tropical areas. There is partial villous atrophy of the mucosa throughout the small bowel. The cause is unknown. Most patients improve on leaving the sprue area and taking

folic acid 5 mg daily. **Tetracycline** 1 g daily for ~6 months is required by patients with more severe symptoms.

Bacterial overgrowth

Bacterial overgrowth of the small bowel occurs when there is intestinal stasis due to a structural or motility abnormality of the gut. Examples include jejunal diverticulosis, post-surgical intestinal blind loops, intestinal strictures or fistulae, and motility abnormalities such as autonomic neuropathy secondary to diabetes and radiation enteropathy. The diarrhoea is due to bacterial deconjugation and dehydroxylation of bile salts. Bacteria also metabolize B_{12}, which can cause a macrocytic anaemia.

Investigations

Investigation is with a **glucose-hydrogen breath test**, in which an orally ingested glucose load is given and expired hydrogen measured. Metabolism of the glucose in the small intestine by bacteria causes a characteristic early rise in breath hydrogen. A barium follow-through or small bowel MRI will exclude a structural abnormality of the small bowel.

Treatment

Underlying structural abnormalities should be corrected if possible. Rotating 2-week courses of antibiotics, usually **metronidazole** 400 mg 3 times daily, **co-amoxiclav** 250–500 mg 3 times daily and **ciprofloxacin** 500 mg twice daily, form the mainstay of treatment.

Bile salt malabsorption

Bile salts are synthesized from cholesterol and conjugated with glycine or taurine in the liver. They are excreted via the biliary tree into the duodenum, where they solubilize lipids in micelles, allowing fat absorption. They are reabsorbed in the distal small intestine and are later re-secreted by hepatocytes. Bile acid malabsorption usually occurs in patients who have undergone ileal resection but it is also occasionally encountered as a primary condition. Diarrhoea occurs, as the failure to reabsorb bile salts in the ileum leads to their accumulation in the colon, where they cause diarrhoea by reducing water and electrolyte absorption and increasing colonic motility.

Investigations

The SeHCAT test involves administering a fixed dose of radio-labelled ^{75}Se-homochoyl taurine, a bile acid analogue. A percentage retention at 7 days is calculated, with normal individuals retaining more than 15%.

Treatment

Treatment is with **colestyramine** 4–8 g daily in water, which forms an insoluble complex with bile acids. It should be taken 1 hour after or 4–6 hours before other drugs, as it can interfere with absorption. It is unpalatable and poorly tolerated, and causes constipation.

Massive intestinal resection (short-bowel syndrome)

This most often occurs following resection for Crohn's disease, mesenteric vessel occlusion, radiation enteritis or trauma. There are two common situations:

- Shortened small intestine ending at a terminal small bowel stoma. The major problem is sodium and fluid depletion, and the majority of patients with 100 cm or less of jejunum remaining will require parenteral supplements of fluid and electrolytes, often with nutrients. Sodium losses can be minimized by increasing salt intake, restricting clear fluids between meals and administering oral glucose–electrolyte mixture with a sodium concentration 90 mmol/L. Jejunal transit time can be increased and stomal effluent loss of fluids and electrolytes reduced by treatment with the somatostatin analogue **octreotide** 200 mcg SC 3 times daily, and to a much lesser extent with **loperamide**, **codeine phosphate** or **co-phenotrope**. There is no benefit to a low-fat diet, but fat assimilation can be increased on treatment with **colestyramine** and synthetic bile acids.

- **Shortened small intestine in continuity with colon.** Only a small proportion of these patients require parenteral supplementation of fluid, electrolytes and nutrients because of the absorptive capacity of the colon for fluid and electrolytes. Unabsorbed fat results in impairment of colonic fluid and electrolyte absorption, so patients should be on a low-fat diet. A **high carbohydrate intake** is advised, as unabsorbed carbohydrate is metabolized anaerobically to short-chain fatty acids (SCFAs), which are absorbed, stimulate fluid and electrolyte absorption in the colon and act as an energy source (1.6 kcal/g). Patients are often treated with **colestyramine** to reduce diarrhoea and colonic oxalate absorption.

INFLAMMATORY BOWEL DISEASE

Inflammatory bowel disease (IBD) comprises two major forms, Crohn's disease and ulcerative colitis. Both are idiopathic, lifelong, inflammatory diseases of the gastrointestinal tract. Microscopic ulcerative, microscopic lymphocytic and microscopic collagenous colitis also occur.

- **Crohn's disease** (CD) is characterized by chronic transmural granulomatous inflammation with a tendency to form strictures and fistulae. It can affect any part of the gastrointestinal tract, and often does so in discontinuity to form skip lesions. Most commonly it affects the terminal ileum and ascending colon (ileocolonic disease). CD is classified according to the site, extent and pattern of disease. These factors govern the clinical symptoms. Active CD characteristically produces the triad of abdominal pain, diarrhoea and weight loss, although the preponderance of each symptom (as well as malaise, fever and anorexia) will vary. Small bowel CD is often complicated by the development of luminal stenosis due to inflammatory or fibrotic strictures, leading to obstructive symptoms. Colonic CD is less often complicated by obstruction and tends to cause more severe diarrhoea. However, in contrast to ulcerative colitis, significant rectal bleeding is less common. Anal and perianal involvement is common.
- **Ulcerative colitis** (UC) is a more superficial inflammation than that of CD, and usually involves only the mucosa. It affects only the large bowel, although in rare cases there can be a 'backwash ileitis'. UC usually involves the rectum (proctitis) but extends proximally in continuity to a varying extent, often to affect the whole colon (total colitis). Bloody diarrhoea is the characteristic symptom of ulcerative colitis. During severe acute attacks systemic features such as anorexia, fever and malaise are also common. There is an increased incidence of cancer with pancolitis of over 10 years' duration.

Investigations

- **Blood tests.** Platelets, ESR and CRP are often raised in acute flares of CD but less so in UC. Low albumin levels occur with chronic active disease.
- **Colonoscopy.** This is useful both diagnostically and because it allows assessment of colitis and terminal ileal disease.
- **Imaging**
  - *Small bowel follow-through* is useful for diagnosing and assessing small bowel CD, particularly small bowel strictures.
  - *CT enterography* also detects pathology outside of the intestine.
  - *MR enterography* is being increasingly used, as it does not involve radiation. Pelvic MRI is used to assess perianal fistulae in CD.
  - *Capsule endoscopy* is a technique used to image the small bowel. It is useful in diagnosing small bowel CD when other tests have been negative, in assessing disease activity in known CD and in differentiating indeterminate colitis from CD.
  - *Labelled white cell scanning* involves radio-labelled white cells that are taken up preferentially by areas of inflammation. This technique is most useful in assessing the extent of disease involvement.
  - *Plain abdominal X-ray* is useful for assessing colonic dilatation in acute colitis and in excluding perforation.

Treatment

The aim of treatment is to induce and then maintain remission. It therefore depends on disease activity, with some treatment being used for acute flairs (corticosteroids), some for maintenance of remission (immunosuppressants) and some for both (5-aminosalicylates). All drug therapy has side-effects and patients should be warned of this and told to report any problems immediately to their doctor.

Drugs used in the treatment of IBD (Box 5.4)

Aminosalicylates

These comprise a range of different formulations, all of which deliver 5-aminosalicylate (mesalazine) in millimolar concentrations to the gut lumen. The site in the gastrointestinal tract at which the 5-ASA moiety is released determines the choice of agent.

- **Formulations**
  These drugs should be prescribed with their proprietary names stated as the different formulations are not interchangeable.
  - *Oral preparations.* These differ, depending on method of delivery.
    a) **Carrier molecules**: sulfasalazine is from the older generation of aminosalicylates. The 5-ASA moiety is linked to a sulfapyridine carrier molecule and is released after splitting by bacterial enzymes in the large intestine. **Olsalazine** (a dimer of 5-ASA) and **balsalazide** (a prodrug of 5-ASA) are without the sulfapyridine carrier molecule and therefore lack the sulphonamide side-effects. They are recommended for use in disease affecting the descending and sigmoid colon.
    b) **pH-dependent release mechanisms/resin-coated**: mesalazine. This type is recommended for use in colonic disease.
    c) **Time-controlled**: 5-ASA microspheres are recommended for use in ileocolonic disease.

Kumar & Clark's Medical Management and Therapeutics

> **Box 5.4** Options for medical treatment of Crohn's disease
>
> **Induction of remission**
> - Oral or IV glucocorticosteroids
> - Enteral nutrition
> - Oral glucocorticosteroids + azathioprine or 6-mercaptopurine (6MP)
> - Infliximab } being used as first-line agents in some centres
> - Adalimumab }
>
> **Maintenance of remission**
> - Aminosalicylates (colonic disease)
> - Azathioprine, 6MP, methotrexate, mycophenolate mofetil
> - Infliximab
> - Adalimumab
>
> **Second-line biological agents/cytokine modulators**
> - Certolizumab pegol
> - Natalizumab
>
> **Treatment of glucocorticosteroid/immunosuppressive therapy-resistant disease**
> - Methotrexate, mycophenolate mofetil
>
> **Perianal disease**
> - Ciprofloxacin and metronidazole

- *Topical preparations.* Mesalazine can be given as rectal suppositories to treat rectal disease (proctitis), and as liquid and foam enemas to treat sigmoidal and descending colonic disease (left-sided disease).
- Indications
  - *Maintaining remission.* There is little evidence to support 5-ASA use as maintenance therapy in **CD**, but as these compounds are generally well tolerated with few adverse effects they are often prescribed. Aminosalicylates are effective in maintaining remission in patients with **UC** and are first-line therapy. There are also weaker data to suggest that long-term 5-ASA use may reduce the long-term increased risk of colorectal cancer in UC. There are little comparative data between 5-ASA compounds and most generally seem to be equally effective. Choice depends on tolerability, cost and disease distribution. Once-daily dosing is now advocated with several compounds as maintenance treatment. Regular topical use may be required in left-sided disease or proctitis.
  - *Active disease.* There is little evidence to support the use of 5-ASA in acute **CD**. Mesalazine slow-release 4 g/day has been shown to be more effective than placebo in causing clinical improvement in patients with active Crohn's ileocolitis but clinical significance is debatable. Sulfasalazine may be useful in the treatment of mild colonic CD. There is good evidence to support the use of 5-ASA in active **UC**. Either starting with or increasing to high-dose mesalazine (> 3 g/day) induces remission in 50% of patients with mildly/moderately active UC. The addition of 5-ASA enemas to high-dose oral 5-ASA has been shown to increase remission rates further.

Suppositories 1 g once daily and enemas of mesalazine 1 g twice daily are useful in treating acute proctitis and left-sided disease.

- Adverse effects
  - *5-ASA* are generally well tolerated, with few adverse effects. Intolerance is 15%. Diarrhoea occurs in 3%, headache in 2%, nausea in 2% and rash in 1%. Renal impairment can rarely occur; blood disorders occur and patients should be advised to report unexplained bleeding, bruising or sore throat.
  - *Sulfasalazine* has more adverse effects than other 5-ASA due to the sulfapyridine carrier molecule. These occur in 10–45%. Minor effects include headache, nausea and diarrhoea. Hypersensitivity reactions are rare but other major effects include rash, fever, agranulocytosis, pancreatitis, alveolitis and toxic epidermal necrolysis. Reversible sperm count reduction can occur in males.

Corticosteroids

Corticosteroids are potent anti-inflammatory agents that reduce the production of inflammatory cytokines and promote apoptosis in various inflammatory cell types.

- Formulations
  - *Oral preparations.* **Prednisolone** is the most commonly used preparation. **Budesonide** is an oral steroid with a high first-pass metabolism. The low systemic availability leads to reduced systemic side-effects compared with oral prednisolone.
  - *IV preparations.* **Hydrocortisone** is the IV steroid formulation most commonly used in IBD (100 mg 4 times daily).
  - *Topical preparations.* **Prednisolone** is used as suppositories and liquid and foam enemas.
- Indications
  - *Maintaining remission.* There is no role for steroids in maintaining remission.
  - *Active disease.* Prednisolone 0.5–0.75mg/kg induces remission in approximately 60–80% patients with active **CD**. The starting dose is usually 40 mg orally once daily and it is then reduced by approximately 5 mg every 5–7 days. A more gradual dose reduction can be used for patients who have initially responded to prednisolone but have then relapsed on the lower doses. A starting dose of 60 mg is occasionally used for patients who have not responded to 40 mg, although the incidence of adverse events is significantly increased. Starting doses of < 15 mg are generally not effective. Budesonide is slightly less effective than prednisolone but is useful in moderately active terminal ileal/ascending colonic CD (3 mg 3 times daily) and, due to the lower frequency of long-term side-effects, longer courses can be given. IV steroids (hydrocortisone 100 mg 4 times daily) are used when the patient has either not responded to oral prednisolone or is so ill that hospital admission is required. Oral prednisolone induces remission in ~80% of patients with active **UC**. Dosing is similar to that used in Crohn's disease. Prednisolone can also be given topically in distal colitis and proctitis but is generally less effective than topical 5-ASA therapy. Sometimes topical 5-ASA and steroid therapy may be given in combination. As with CD, IV steroids are given to those who have not responded to oral steroids or who require hospital admission.

- Adverse effects (see Box 15.2, p. 585). Around 50% of patients report adverse effects with steroid use.
  - *Short term* — acne, moon face, oedema, sleep disturbance, agitation, increased appetite, weight gain and impaired glucose tolerance.
  - *Long-term* — associated with > 12-week use: osteoporosis and the rarer osteonecrosis of the femoral head, cataracts, myopathy and susceptibility to infection. DEXA scans for osteoporosis are performed every 2–5 years.
  - *Steroid withdrawal* — adrenal insufficiency (p. 582) if not withdrawn gradually, myalgia and malaise.

Thiopurines

Thiopurines are purine antimetabolites that inhibit ribonucleotide synthesis, leading to T-cell apoptosis.

- Formulations
  - *Azathioprine and 6-mercaptopurine.* Azathioprine is metabolized to mercaptopurine, which is in turn metabolized to 6-thioguanine, the principal active metabolite.
- Indications
  - *Maintaining remission.* Thiopurines have been shown to be effective in inducing and maintaining remission in **CD** and **UC**. Azathioprine is usually given at a dose of 2 mg/kg and mercaptopurine 1–1.5 mg/kg, although this will depend on blood monitoring (see below). In a Cochrane review the odds ratio for maintaining remission in CD was 2.2, with a number needed to treat of 7. Thiopurines are used as a steroid-sparing agent in steroid-dependent and steroid-resistant CD and UC. There is no absolute rule as to when they should be started but they are used in patients who have required two or more courses of steroids in 12 months or those who have relapsed within 6 weeks of a previous course. The duration of use is not clear-cut, but current guidelines suggest that thiopurines should be used for 3–4 years and then discontinuation should be discussed with the patient if there are no signs of active disease.
  - *Active disease.* Although thiopurines have been shown to be effective in active disease, the delay in onset of action (up to 3 months) limits their use as an immediate treatment.
- Adverse effects
  - *Minor:* **intolerance** — up to 20% of patients develop myalgia, headache, nausea or diarrhoea, usually within 2–3 weeks of starting thiopurines. This usually resolves without stopping the drug.
  - *Major:* profound **leucopenia** develops in 3% of patients. It can occur at any time during treatment, although it is commonest during the initiation phase. FBC monitoring is recommended, at least monthly for the first 2 months of treatment and 3–6-monthly thereafter. Leucopenia is commoner in individuals with deficiency of thiopurine methyltransferase (TPMT) activity, an enzyme involved in thiopurine metabolism. Many experts therefore advocate routine TPMT testing with 50% dose reduction in heterozygotes for TPMT activity and complete avoidance of use in homozygotes. **Hepatotoxicity** and **pancreatitis** occur in less than 5% of individuals. Liver biochemistry should be measured simultaneously with FBC.

Mycophenolate mofetil

This is an antiproliferative immunosuppressant agent and stops the proliferation of T- and B- lymphocytes. It is used in the same way as azathioprine.

Methotrexate

Methotrexate inhibits dihydrofolate reductase, an enzyme involved in purine synthesis and DNA/RNA synthesis.

- Indications
  - *Maintaining remission.* Methotrexate 10–20 mg orally **once weekly** has proven benefit as a **second-line steroid-sparing** agent in **CD** (40% of patients steroid-free at 3 months). There is less evidence for its use in **UC**.
  - *Active disease.* Slow onset of action (4–6 weeks) limits the use of methotrexate as a sole agent in the treatment of active **UC** or **CD**.
- Adverse effects
  - *Minor:* nausea, vomiting, malaise, fatigue and stomatitis. (The latter is reduced by co-prescription of folic acid 5 mg orally, given 24 hours after the methotrexate.
  - *Major:* **Hepatotoxicity (fibrosis/cirrhosis)** and leucopenia occur. Regular blood monitoring should be carried out weekly until the dose is stabilized, and then 3-monthly. **Pneumonitis** occurs rarely.

Ciclosporin

Ciclosporin, a calcineurin inhibitor, is a potent immunosuppressive agent preventing the clonal expansion of T-cell subsets.

- Indications
  - *Maintaining remission.* Oral ciclosporin is occasionally used as maintenance therapy in chronic active **UC**.
  - *Active disease.* **IV ciclosporin** 2 or 4 mg/kg/day is used as salvage therapy for patients with acute, severe **UC** whose only other therapeutic option is colectomy (p. 164). Initial response rates are ~60%, although the percentage of patients avoiding colectomy in the longer term is lower (30–40%).
- Adverse effects
  - *Minor:* occur in 30–50% and include tremor, paraesthesiae, malaise, headache and abnormal liver biochemistry.
  - *Major:* occur in 0–15% and can be life-threatening. These include neurotoxicity, renal impairment and infections. Risk of seizure is increased in patients with a low cholesterol (< 3.0 mmol) or low magnesium (< 0.5 mmol) and a reduced dose or oral preparation can be used in these circumstances. Mortality rates of 2% are reported. BP, FBC, renal function and ciclosporin concentration (trough 100–200 ng/mL) should be measured during therapy.

Biological agents/cytokine modulators

Infliximab is a chimeric (human/mouse) monoclonal antibody against tumour necrosis factor-alpha. It has potent anti-inflammatory actions and although the precise mechanism is unknown in IBD it is likely to involve apoptosis of T-cells. Adequate resuscitation facilities should be available.

- Indications
  - *Maintaining remission.* Regular 8-weekly maintenance infusions in both fistulizing and non-fistulizing **CD** are more effective then placebo in maintaining remission. Cost, however, may limit

Kumar & Clark's Medical Management and Therapeutics

availability of this strategy. Antibodies can develop to infliximab, limiting its efficacy, and are more common with sporadic use than with maintenance infusions. Maintenance infusions have been shown to be effective in maintaining remission in **UC** but are less commonly used than in CD.

- *Active disease.* Around 80% of patients with inflammatory **CD** refractory to 5-ASA, corticosteroids and/or immunomodulators respond to IV infusions of infliximab 5 mg/kg at 0, 2 and 6 weeks. Expert advice should be sought. Around 70% patients with refractory fistulizing CD respond to a course of 3 infusions at 0, 2 and 6 weeks (5 mg/kg).

    Between 50 and 70% of patients with chronic active refractory **UC** respond to infusions of 5 mg/kg at 0, 2 and 6 weeks, then 5 mg/kg every 8 weeks, although this is more controversial than in CD. Discontinue if there is no response after 1–2 doses. A single infusion of infliximab 5 mg/kg has also been shown to reduce colectomy rates in fulminant colitis compared to placebo and may be an alternative rescue therapy to ciclosporin.

- Adverse effects: **Infusion reactions** occur and respond to slowing infusion rate and treatment with antihistamines, paracetamol and corticosteroids. Patients should be monitored during infusions. Up to 60% of patients form antibodies against infliximab and this can shorten the duration of response and predispose to an infusion reaction. Risk from delayed hypersensitivity reactions increases if the drug-free interval is over 16 weeks. There is an increased incidence of **infection** and specifically disseminated TB. Active sepsis is therefore an absolute contraindication. All patients should be screened for TB, with history and CXR prior to treatment. Certain patients may require TB prophylaxis. **Development of anti-dsDNA antibodies and lupus-like syndrome** is a rare but recognized side-effect.

Adalimumab is a fully human IgG, anti-TNFα monoclonal antibody used for inducing and maintaining a clinical remission; it is given as for active CD as 160 mg at week zero and 80 mg at week 2, and 40 mg alternate weeks thereafter. Dose escalation to 40 mg weekly may be required in the longer term. Trials have shown similar efficiency to infliximab. Adalimumab is now being used as first-line biological therapy, as is infliximab.

Certolizumab pegol is a humanized anti-TNF Fab' monoclonal antibody fragment; it is attached to polyethylene glycol. It is used for inducing and maintaining a remission in moderate to severe active CD as a second-line biological agent.

Natalizumab, a humanized monoclonal IgG$_4$ antibody that binds to α_4 integrin, is effective in inducing and maintaining remissions and is used as a second-line agent.

Antibiotics

Antibiotics alter bacterial flora. Their beneficial action is consistent with the hypothesis that inflammation in IBD is driven by an inappropriate reaction to bacterial flora.

- Indications
  - *Active disease.* Both **metronidazole** 500 mg 3 times daily and **ciprofloxacin** 500 mg twice daily are established treatments for active perianal **CD**. They can be used in combination or in rotation for a relatively long course (4 weeks). Metronidazole has also been used to treat luminal CD, although it is now generally not recommended.

- **Adverse effects.** Peripheral sensory neuropathy can develop with long-term (> 4 weeks) use of metronidazole. Patients should avoid alcohol because of a disulfiram-like reaction causing facial flushing. For ciprofloxacin side-effects, see p. 83; for metronidazole, see p. 84.

Antidiarrhoeals

Antidiarrhoeals (p. 136) may be useful in certain patients but should not be used in patients with acute, severe disease.

Diet/lifestyle

- **Smoking.** All patients with CD should stop smoking.
- **Diet.** In general, patients with IBD should eat a normal diet and be encouraged to maintain a normal weight. Patients with small bowel strictures and symptoms of subacute obstruction should adhere to a low-residue diet.
- **Probiotics and pre-biotics.** Probiotics are live attenuated bacteria or bacterial products which, when ingested, modify the composition of the enteric flora. Pre-biotics are non-digestible food supplements that are fermented by host bacteria, stimulating their growth. Probiotics have been shown to be of benefit in pouchitis and may be useful in UC.
- **Haematinics.** Serum levels should be measured annually and replaced as necessary. Individuals with CD who have had a terminal ileal resection are at particular risk of B_{12} deficiency.
  - *Indications — active Crohn's disease.* Elemental diets (p. 126), when given as the sole nutritional source, achieve similar rates of remission to oral steroids. In paediatric patients they are particularly useful as an alternative to steroids, which cause growth retardation.
  - *Adverse effects.* Elemental diets are usually unpalatable and poorly tolerated.

Surgery

- Indications
  - *Maintaining remission.* Surgery is not performed for quiescent disease but may be of use in relieving stricturing disease. Colectomy is sometimes recommended in patients with UC and high-grade dysplasia.
  - *Active disease.* Surgery is generally only undertaken when other treatment options have failed, but nevertheless 80% of patients with CD will require an operation at some time during the course of their disease. The range of surgical options for CD is variable, reflecting the diverse nature of the disease. Local resection or stricturoplasty is performed for localized stricturing disease. Attempts are always made to preserve as much bowel as possible, as multiple operations may be required, which can culminate in intestinal failure (short bowel syndrome, p. 155) and a need for lifelong parenteral nutrition. Colectomy may be required for colonic disease but ileal recurrence is common. Abscess drainage and seton insertion are often required for perianal disease. Pan-proctocolectomy with ileo-anal pouch formation is the surgical procedure of choice for patients with UC that has proven refractory to medical therapy. This is usually performed as a two-stage operation, with initial removal of the colon with an ileostomy. The procedure is often performed semi-electively in individuals with chronic active disease but can be performed as an

emergency for patients with toxic megacolon who are at risk of per-foration. An ileo-anal pouch is then formed at further surgery some months later.

Pouchitis occurs in one-third of these patients with diarrhoea and bleeding. Treatment in severe cases is unsatisfactory but antibiotics for active disease (ciprofloxacin, metronidazole) and **probiotics** for maintenance of remission, e.g. lactobacilli, bifidobacteria, form the mainstay of treatment.

- **Adverse effects.** These are the same as for all abdominal surgery, although in addition patients with CD are at greater risk of forming post-operative fistulae.

Acute severe colitis

Acute severe colitis can occur in patients with UC and CD (but remember it can also occur with *C. difficile* infection). It presents with diarrhoea (> 6 stools/day), fever > 37.5° and tachycardia > 90 bpm. Investigations show an anaemia (< 10 g/dL), a high ESR and a low serum albumin (< 30 g/L). A plain abdominal x-ray can show a thin-walled dilated colon (> 5 cm, or 8 cm in caecum) that is gas-filled and contains mucosal islands (toxic megacolon) (Fig. 5.2). Daily X-rays are required, as perforation occurs, with a mortality of up to 25%.

Treatment

Treatment is urgent and should be supervised by an experienced physician and colo-rectal surgeon. Fluid and electrolyte imbalance should be cor-rected. IV hydrocortisone 100 mg 4 times daily is given. If there is no response in 48–72 hours and the CRP continues to be elevated > 45 mg/L, a second-line agent is commenced. **Ciclosporin** 2 mg/kg IV, accompanied by enteral nutrition for 5–7 days, can be used as a bridge to try to avoid surgery. Infliximab is used similarly (p. 161). The decision to proceed to surgery is often complex. In general, surgery is required if there is a toxic megacolon which does not respond rapidly to medical treatment, or if second-line treatment fails. If *C. difficile* infection is the cause of the severe colitis, do not treat with steroids and use vancomycin.

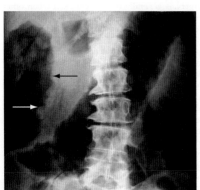

Fig. 5.2 Plain abdominal X-ray showing toxic dilatation. The arrows indicate mucosal islands.

Pregnancy and IBD

Women with inactive IBD have normal fertility. Active disease reduces fertility and increases the number of spontaneous abortions. Although the risk of exacerbations is not increased, if they do occur, they often occur in the first trimester and immediately post partum. Aminosalicylates, steroids and azathioprine are safe at the time of conception and pregnancy. Biological/cytokine modulators e.g. infliximab or adalimumab are thought to be safe in the first trimester. Methotrexate is completely contraindicated in pregnancy.

COLONIC AND ANAL DISORDERS

Acute colonic pseudo-obstruction

Acute colonic pseudo-obstruction (Ogilvie's syndrome) is a motility disorder characterized by massive colonic dilatation in the absence of an obstructing lesion. Around 90% of cases occur in association with other medical conditions such as sepsis or renal or respiratory failure, or after surgical procedures. Drugs, e.g. narcotic analgesics and tricyclic antidepressants, are often causative. The condition results in spontaneous perforation in 3–15% of cases, with an associated mortality of 40–50%.

Clinical features

Symptoms include abdominal distension, colicky pain, absolute constipation, and nausea and vomiting.

Investigations

- CT scan should always be used to exclude an **obstructing lesion**.
- A water-soluble contrast enema can both exclude obstruction and liquefy remaining stool.
- Colonoscopy can also be useful, both diagnostically and therapeutically (see below).

Management

- **Conservative therapy** resolves 75% of cases within 24–48 hours.
- **Nil by mouth** and a **naso-gastric tube** limit further gaseous distension and prevent vomiting, and **mobilization** measures include rolling the bed-bound patient regularly and encouraging the ambulatory patient to walk. **Electrolyte disturbances** (potassium, calcium, magnesium and phosphorus) should be corrected and **medications**, e.g. narcotics, antimuscarinics, sedatives or calcium channel blockers, should be stopped. **Total parenteral nutrition** is indicated in very protracted cases.
- **Neostigmine**, an inhibitor of cholinesterase given as an IV 2 mg bolus over 3–5 mins, leads to a resolution in 90% of cases. It can be repeated once if unsuccessful on the first occasion. Transient bradycardia can occur and patients should be monitored during drug administration.
- **Endoscopic colonic decompression** is indicated if the caecal diameter is > 9 cm or the patient has failed to respond to other therapies. It is technically difficult, with a perforation rate of 1–3%, but is initially successful in 70% of cases. Daily plain abdominal X-rays should be performed to detect recurrence.
- **Surgery** is indicated for those cases where there are signs of colonic perforation or when the patient has failed to respond to medical and endoscopic therapy and perforation is imminent (caecal diameter > 9 cm). Caecostomy is the procedure of choice.

Diverticular disease

Diverticula are pouches of mucosa that extrude through the colonic wall. They are almost ubiquitous in the Western world, possibly due to the low-fibre diet.

- **Diverticulosis** refers to the presence of diverticula and is asymptomatic.
- **Diverticulitis** refers to inflamed diverticula with associated intramural or extracolonic inflammation. It presents with left-sided abdominal pain and tenderness, as diverticula are commonest in the sigmoid colon in the developed world. A palpable tender mass may be present in the left iliac fossa. There may be altered bowel habit, and diverticulitis is usually associated with constipation. Patients may feel generally unwell and have a fever. Diverticula (particularly right-sided) are a cause of massive lower gastrointestinal bleeding (p. 152).

Investigations

- **Blood tests.** Diverticulitis is usually associated with a high white cell count and raised ESR and CRP.
- **CT scan.** This will show colonic wall thickening, diverticula and any pericolic collections and abscesses.
- **Colonoscopy.** Diverticula are usually diagnosed as a coincidental finding at colonoscopy. Colonoscopy is contraindicated if acute diverticulitis is suspected, due to the risk of perforation.

Treatment

Mild cases of diverticulitis can be managed with oral antibiotics (**cefalexin** 500 mg 3 times daily or **ciprofloxacin** 500 mg twice daily plus **metronidazole** 400 mg 3 times daily) and laxatives. Cases with systemic upset, fever and a raised white cell count should be admitted to hospital for **bowel rest** (patients are kept nil by mouth and hydrated with IV fluids — 0.9% saline with 20 mmol/L K$^+$) and **antibiotics** (**cefuroxime** 750 mg IV 3 times daily and **metronidazole** 500 mg IV twice daily). Once the acute attack has resolved, patients may be given laxatives (**ispaghula husk** 1 sachet twice daily) to avoid constipation and to reduce the likelihood of further attacks. Surgical intervention is only required for complications such as abscess or fistula formation, perforation and repeated attacks.

Ischaemic disease of the colon (ischaemic colitis)

Occlusion of the branches of the superior or inferior mesenteric arteries, often in the older age group, commonly presents with sudden abdominal pain and the passage of bright red blood from the rectum, with or without diarrhoea. The lesion usually affects the splenic flexure and settles with conservative management. A few patients need surgery.

Perianal disorders

Haemorrhoids

Haemorrhoids are engorged veins at the ano-rectal junction. They develop due to excessive straining at stool and can prolapse. Rectal bleeding is usually bright red and seen separate to the stool in the pan or on the toilet paper; pruritus ani and perianal pain occur. Proctoscopy shows haemorrhoids classically in the 3, 7 and 11 o'clock position. Haemorrhoids can thrombose and become acute, painful, tense, bluish lumps in the perianal area. Other more serious causes of rectal bleeding should be excluded with flexible sigmoidoscopy.

- Treatment
  - *Local anaesthetic creams* are often combined with **corticosteroids**. There are many different formulations available (e.g. **dibucaine** 0.5%, **hydrocortisone** 0.5%, **aluminium acetate** 3.5%, **hydrocortisone** 0.275% and **lidocaine** 5%).
  - *Stool softeners* are given to reduce straining at stool.
  - *Oral analgesics* may be required for thrombosed haemorrhoids (paracetamol 1 g 4 times daily).
  - *Injection* with phenol (5%) under direct vision acts as a local sclerosant; **band ligation** can also be performed.
  - *Haemorrhoidectomy* is reserved for cases where other measures have failed and symptoms are severe. Thrombosed haemorrhoids can be excised in severe cases.

Anal fissures

Anal fissures are acute tears in the skin lining the anal canal and are caused by the passage of hard stool. They usually heal in 2–3 weeks. They cause severe anal pain, particularly during defecation. On proctoscopy, fissures are usually seen as posterior elliptical tears. Local anaesthetic creams are available over the counter. **Glyceryl trinitrate** (0.4%) and **diltiazem** (2%) creams help to relax the sphincter spasm, facilitating healing. **Laxatives** in the form of stool softeners reduce symptoms.

Perirectal abscesses

These present as painful, indurated swellings in the perianal area. They can occur de novo or in association with inflammatory bowel disease. Examination under anaesthetic (EUA), MRI and endoanal US is used to outline the position and extent of the abscess. **Surgical drainage** is required for the majority, with **antibiotics** (**cefuroxime** 750 mg IV 3 times daily or oral **cefalexin** 500 mg 3 times daily and **metronidazole** 500 mg IV 3 times daily or 400 mg orally 3 times daily).

Perianal fistulae

These develop from perianal abscesses and present with chronic perianal discharge. Management of those associated with Crohn's disease is described on p. 162. MRI scan and EUA are usually required, followed by surgical treatment, with 90% being either laid open or excised.

FUNCTIONAL GASTROINTESTINAL DISORDERS

This term refers to a collection of overlapping disorders with symptoms attributable to the gastrointestinal tract but where no organic disease can be found. Investigations, if necessary, are performed to exclude relevant organic pathology, but many of the disorders can be diagnosed by the history alone. These disorders have been characterized by an international committee (Rome III 2006) into specific disorders but in clinical practice there is enormous overlap.

Functional oesophageal disorders (heartburn, chest pain of presumed oesophageal origin, dysphagia, globus)

Symptoms include heartburn (p. 139), chest pain and dysphagia. Dysphagia usually requires investigation with an endoscopy to exclude other oesophageal pathology. A barium swallow and **oesophageal manometry** help to exclude a motility disorder, e.g. achalasia. Globus describes an intermittent sensation of a lump in the throat.

Kumar & Clark's Medical Management and Therapeutics

Treatment

- PPI therapy (Table 5.1) may be beneficial in some patients, particularly those with heartburn (p. 59).
- Nitrates, e.g. **GTN spray**, and **calcium channel blockers**, e.g. **buccal nifedipine** 10 mg, occasionally help. A low-dose tricyclic antidepressant, e.g. **amitriptyline** 10 mg daily, has been shown to be effective in some patients, particularly those with associated depression. Antimuscarinic **side-effects** include constipation, dry mouth and urinary retention. Fatigue is also common and treatment should be taken at night.

Functional gastroduodenal disorders (dyspepsia, belching, nausea and vomiting, rumination syndrome in adults)

Dyspepsia is the second commonest functional disorder, causing upper abdominal discomfort, bloating, early satiety and nausea. Nausea is common in association with functional gastrointestinal disorders but vomiting is rare. Self-induced vomiting compatible with an eating disorder should be excluded. OGD is required in patients > 55 years of age with a short history or alarm features (p. 134). Nausea does not warrant investigation, particularly in the young and in patients with no alarm symptoms. Simple blood tests may help to reassure the patient.

Treatment

- Lifestyle changes may help, as many patients find their symptoms are exacerbated by certain foods and improve if these are avoided.
- Pharmacotherapy
  - *Antisecretory therapy*, e.g. PPIs, has been shown to have symptomatic benefit in some studies but is complicated by the high placebo response rates (20–60%).
  - H. pylori *eradication* is supported by some evidence to suggest that it provides symptomatic benefit, but the role of *H. pylori* testing and eradication in this condition remains controversial.
  - *Promotility agents* (**domperidone** 10 mg orally 3 times daily) may help with dysmotility-type symptoms.
  - *Antinausea drugs*, e.g. **hyoscine**, are sometimes helpful.
  - *Low-dose tricyclic antidepressants* − as above.

Functional bowel disorders (irritable bowel syndrome, bloating, constipation, diarrhoea)

Irritable bowel syndrome (IBS) is the commonest functional gastrointestinal disorder, with 1 in 5 people in developed countries reporting compatible symptoms. Many patients do not fulfil all the criteria but this should not prevent the diagnosis being made. The usual symptoms are lower abdominal pain relieved by defecation, increased frequency of defecation (> 3 per day) or constipation (< 3 per week), a variable stool consistency, and bloating and wind. These symptoms can be classified separately as constipation-predominant, diarrhoea-predominant or mixed IBS. In addition, non-intestinal symptoms are common, e.g. painful periods, dyspareunia, urinary frequency, back pain, fibromyalgia, fatigue and insomnia.

Treatment

- Reassurance and explanation of the symptoms are often all that is required.
- Pharmacotherapy is largely symptomatic and depends on the predominant symptom.

- *Antimuscarinics.* These are thought to relax intestinal smooth muscle and reduce pain but have little effect on stool frequency. The most commonly used preparation is **hyoscine butylbromide** 10 mg 3 times daily. **Dicycloverine hydrochloride** 10–20 mg 3 times daily is used less frequently due to its greater side-effect profile. Antimuscarinic **side-effects** include constipation, urinary urgency and retention, dry mouth, and rarely transient bradycardia and arrhythmias. These drugs are contraindicated in closed-angle glaucoma, paralytic ileus, myasthenia gravis and prostatic enlargement.
- *Antispasmodics.* Those used to treat IBS include **mebeverine** 135 mg 3 times daily and **peppermint oil** 1–2 capsules 3 times daily. **Side-effects:** allergy has been reported rarely.
- *Laxatives.* Constipation-predominant IBS may respond to simple laxatives, which are available both on prescription and over the counter (p. 137). Bulk-forming laxatives may exacerbate symptoms of bloating and in this situation osmotic laxatives may be more beneficial.
- *Antidiarrhoeal agents.* These may be effective in diarrhoea-predominant IBS (p. 136).
- *Tricyclic antidepressants.* Low-dose tricyclics, such as **amitriptyline**, have been shown to reduce symptoms in a number of randomized placebo-controlled trials. The mechanism of action is unknown but may involve a reduction in the sensitivity of enteral nerves. A meta-analysis indicated an odds ratio of 4 for benefit of these drugs compared to placebo. There is some evidence to suggest that they are more effective in diarrhoea-predominant IBS. Tricyclics are recommended for moderate to severe IBS with a predominant symptom of pain. They should be started at a dose of 25 mg. Doses < 30 mg seem most effective but the dose can be escalated to 100 mg if there is no response and providing they are tolerated. An attempt should be made to taper the dose after 12 months.
- *Selective serotonin reuptake inhibitors.* Good evidence to support their use is lacking. They should be reserved for when there is an active mood disorder or when tricyclics have failed. In constipation-predominant IBS, **paroxetine** 20 mg daily is helpful.
- *Non absorbable antibiotics.* **Rifaximin** has recently been shown to help IBS patients without constipation.
- *Other drugs.* 5HT4 agonists e.g. prucalopride improve colonic transit and can improve symptoms in constipation. Cisapride and tegaserod were withdrawn as they were not sufficiently GI selective in women and caused long QT syndromes. However the newer 5HT4 agonist, Prucalopride, is now licensed for the treatment of functional constipation and constipation predominant IBS. **Probiotics** (i.e. live or attenuated bacteria or bacterial products) and **pre-biotics** (i.e. non-digestible food substances that are fermented by host bacteria stimulating their growth) are also used. A trans-galacto-oligosaccharide pre-biotic has shown benefit in a small RCT. **FODMAPs** (**f**ermentable **o**ligosaccharides, **d**isaccharides, **m**onosaccharides **a**nd **p**olyols) are short-chain carbohydrates fermented in the colon, yielding large amounts of gas and causing bloating. Low-FODMAP diets have been helpful in some patients.
- **Dietary therapy.** Many patients find their symptoms are exacerbated by particular foods. The commonest identified are wheat-containing foods,

dairy products, alcohol and excess fibre. Patients are often able to identify and exclude particular food types independently or can be referred
to a dietitian for a more formalized exclusion diet.

● **Cognitive therapy.** Cognitive behavioural therapy (CBT), hypnotherapy
and relaxation therapy have all been reported as effective in small trials
of patients with IBS. Patients with anxiety and depression seem to
benefit more from these therapies.

PANCREATIC AND BILIARY TRACT DISEASE

Acute pancreatitis

In the developed world the majority of cases of acute pancreatitis are due
to gallstones or alcohol. Rarer causes include drugs (e.g. azathioprine,
corticosteroids), hyperlipidaemia and post-endoscopic retrograde cholangiopancreatography (ERCP) (5%). Severity ranges from mild self-limiting
episodes to severe disease with extensive pancreatic and peripancreatic
necrosis. Presentation is with upper abdominal pain, which is classically
epigastric and severe, and radiates to the back; it is often accompanied by
nausea and vomiting. Tachycardia, hypotension and oliguria are present
in severe cases.

Investigations

● **Serum amylase** is elevated if measured within 24 hours of the onset of
pain. A level three times the upper limit of normal is almost diagnostic.
Serum lipase is used in a similar way in some centres.
● **Ultrasound** is a useful test to detect gallstones.
● **Contrast-enhanced CT** allows assessment of the degree of necrosis and
detection of the complications of pancreatitis, such as collections and
pseudocyst development. It should be performed in all patients with
persistent organ failure or signs of sepsis 6–10 days after admission and
repeated as necessary to assess progress.

Assessment of severity

Multiple factors are used to develop scoring systems (Table 5.4). The
Ranson and Glasgow scoring systems have been developed to predict

Table 5.4 Factors during the first 48 hours that predict severe
pancreatitis*

Factor	Measurement
Age	>55 years
White cell count	>15 × 10⁹/L
Blood glucose	>10 mmol/L (>180 mg/dL)
Serum urea	>16 mmol/L (>45 mg/dL)
Serum albumin	<30 g/L
Serum calcium	<2 mmol/L (<8 mg/dL)
Serum LDH	>600 U/L
Serum aspartate transferase	>200 U/L
Pao₂	<8.0 kPa (60 mmHg)
CRP	>150 mg/L

*Three or more indicate a severe episode.

severe cases of pancreatitis with a sensitivity of 80%. The APACHE scoring system has also been used.

Treatment

The majority of cases are mild and can be treated symptomatically. Severe cases are best managed on an HDU and patients should be nil by mouth until free of pain. A naso-gastric tube may reduce vomiting and is used in patients with ileus. Avoid parenteral nutrition.

- **Fluid replacement.** Fluid losses can be large and so vigorous fluid replacement should be given with monitoring of urine output. CVP monitoring is also helpful. Measure electrolytes, calcium, urea and glucose daily. Hypocalcaemia and hyperglycaemia can occur but may not require correction.
- **Analgesia. Tramadol** 100 mg IV over 2–3 mins, repeated 6-hourly is the most commonly used analgesic. A patient-controlled analgesia (PCA) system can be used. **Morphine**-derived analgesics are usually avoided, as they can affect sphincter of Oddi function, but the evidence for this is weak.
- **Prophylactic antibiotics.** Although evidence to support their use is weak, prophylactic treatment is often given (**cefuroxime** 750 mg IV 3 times daily, **metronidazole** 500 mg IV 3 times daily).
- **Emergency ERCP.** Emergency ERCP with sphincterotomy and stone extraction is indicated for cases of **severe gallstone pancreatitis** and cholangitis, if performed within 72 hours of the onset of pain. This improves the outcome. After this time point the benefits are markedly reduced and the procedure should be reserved for cases that are not settling with conservative management. ERCP is of *no* value in cases of acute pancreatitis *not* associated with gallstones.

Complications

- **Necrotising pancreatitis.** This is defined as when > 50% of the pancreas is necrosed; it is associated with a poor prognosis. It is diagnosed by dynamic CT with IV contrast. Infection of the necrotic pancreas frequently leads to severe sepsis, which is poorly controlled with broad-spectrum antibiotics. Repeated CT scans are essential in the severe case. Surgical resection is often necessary for cases with extensive necrosis (30%) and evidence of infection on fine needle aspiration.
- **Pancreatic cysts.** Pancreatic fluid collections are common and the majority resolve spontaneously. A few form pseudocysts, which can cause persistent pain and be complicated by haemorrhage, infection and rupture. Asymptomatic small pseudocysts can be treated conservatively but larger cysts are usually drained endoscopically, radiologically or surgically.
- **Multi-organ failure.** Acute kidney injury (AKI) and pulmonary complications such as ARDS (p. 549) can develop.

Chronic pancreatitis

The vast majority of cases are due to alcohol abuse, although chronic pancreatitis also occurs in association with cystic fibrosis and rarely in an autosomal dominant inheritable form. Epigastric pain is the most common presentation and may radiate to the back. Steatorrhoea is due to failure of the exocrine function of the pancreas and diabetes is due to failure of the endocrine function of the pancreas.

Investigations

- Blood tests are unhelpful but a faecal elastase is decreased in the majority of symptomatic cases.
- Plain abdominal X-ray may show calcification.
- Contrast-enhanced CT shows calcification, atrophy and a dilated pancreatic duct, and is the best examination.
- Magnetic resonance cholangiopancreatography (MRCP) can detect subtle ductal abnormalities and has replaced ERCP as a diagnostic test.
- Endoscopic US may detect early disease. It is also used to assess complications, including pseudocysts.

Treatment

- Analgesia. Opiate analgesics (e.g. **tramadol** 50–100 mg 2–4 times daily) are usually required but may lead to dependence. If exocrine insufficiency is present, the addition of pancreatic supplements may improve pain. Alcohol abstinence is mandatory. Pain often improves with time but in severe cases coeliac plexus block or limited surgical resection may be required. ERCP with stenting can be used to treat pancreatic duct strictures or stones but with limited success.
- Enzyme replacement. Steatorrhoea due to exocrine insufficiency is initially treated with a low-fat diet (< 50 g/day). Pancreatic enzyme supplements should be taken with food and an H$_2$-receptor antagonist or PPI, which reduces gastric degradation, should be given 1 hour before. A starting dose should be given (**enteric coated Pancreatin** 1–2 capsules with meals) and increased until steatorrhoea is clinically improved. The most frequent **side-effects** are nausea and vomiting. Fat-soluble vitamin supplementation may also be required.
- Endocrine insufficiency. Diabetes occurs due to the destruction of islet cells and failure of insulin secretion. It is characteristically difficult to control due to coexistent failure of glucagon secretion. Treatment usually requires insulin therapy (p. 595).

Gallstones

Gallstones are common in the Western world, with a prevalence of 25–30% in the seventh decade. They are three times more common in women and prevalence increases with age. Around 80% are cholesterol stones and 20% pigment stones. The majority of gallstones are asymptomatic and are detected as a coincidental finding. About 20% of asymptomatic patients will develop complications over the next 10 years.

Acute cholecystitis

This is due to obstruction of gallbladder emptying caused by gallstones. This leads to an increase in biliary pressure, with ischaemia and inflammation of the gallbladder. Biliary pain is initially epigastric but becomes more localized to the right upper quadrant. There is often localized peritonism in the right upper quadrant and an associated fever.

Investigations

- Inflammatory markers. Acute cholecystitis is usually accompanied by a leucocytosis and a raised CRP.
- Liver biochemistry. This may be mildly deranged. More significant abnormalities suggest bile duct obstruction (see below).
- Ultrasound. US is very accurate and shows gallstones within the gallbladder and common bile duct. Thickening of the gallbladder wall and the presence of pericholecystic fluid suggest acute cholecystitis.

- Biliary scintigraphy. Biliary scintigraphy using technetium derivatives of iminodiacetate is an alternative imaging technique.

Management

The management of acute cholecystitis is with fluid replacement, analgesia, antibiotics and nil by mouth. Laparoscopic cholecystectomy should be performed within 5 days.

Long-term management of gallstone disease

- Laparoscopic cholecystectomy is the only treatment for symptomatic gallstones.
- Dissolution therapy or extracorporeal shock wave lithotripsy (ESWL) are no longer viable options.

Common bile duct stones and acute cholangitis

Biliary colic

This is due to temporary obstruction of the cystic or common bile duct by a gallstone migrating from the gall bladder. Biliary pain (the pain is usually not colicky) is in the epigastrium or right upper quadrant; it radiates to the right shoulder and lasts a few hours. The pain is constant and severe. Characteristically, it is often precipitated by a large meal with a high fat content and associated with nausea and vomiting.

Gallstones in the common bile duct most commonly present with biliary colic (see above). Complete occlusion of the common bile duct may occur, leading to jaundice of a variable degree. The presence of a fever in addition to biliary pain and jaundice indicates the presence of biliary sepsis (acute cholangitis).

Investigations

- Ultrasound rarely visualizes common bile duct stones, but is a sensitive technique for detecting dilatation of the biliary tree associated with obstruction and may also show stones in the gallbladder. Endoscopic US is particularly useful for small stones.
- CT is a sensitive technique for detecting biliary dilatation and allows exclusion of other causes of biliary obstruction, such as carcinoma of the pancreas.
- MRCP is a sensitive technique for visualizing common bile duct stones and assessing the biliary tree.

Management

Acute cholangitis can be treated with IV fluid replacement and broad-spectrum antibiotics (e.g. IV **cefotaxime** 2 g twice daily). However, mortality is high unless biliary decompression is achieved.

- ERCP. This is the initial therapy of choice for biliary decompression and duct clearance. Stones can be removed by balloon or basket and a temporary stent may be left in place to ensure biliary drainage.
- Percutaneous transhepatic cholangiography. If ERCP is unavailable or technically impossible, radiologically guided decompression of the biliary tree may be performed.

The **post-cholecystectomy syndrome** refers to right upper quadrant pain recurring some time after cholecystectomy. This is occasionally due to stones in the common bile duct and occasionally to sphincter of Oddi dyskinesia. Patients with a dilated common bile duct and abnormal liver biochemistry should have an endoscopic sphincterotomy performed. In many patients the pain is functional (p. 173).

Kumar & Clark's Medical Management and Therapeutics

Further reading

British Society of Gastroenterology: *Guidelines on the irritable bowel syndrome: mechanisms and practical management*, 2007.

BSG Endoscopy Committee: Non-variceal upper gastrointestinal haemorrhage: guidelines, *Gut* 51(Suppl IV):1–6, 2002.

European Crohn's and Colitis Organisation: *The second European evidence-based consensus on the diagnosis and management of Crohn's disease: current management*, 2010.

European Crohn's and Colitis Organisation: *Ulcerative colitis: current management*, 2008.

Itanauer SB, et al: Accent! Trial, *Lancet* 359:1541–1549, 2002.

National Institute for Health and Clinical Excellence: *Dyspepsia guideline*, 2004.

Rome III Gastroenterology 2006 *Supplement*.

Scottish Intercollegiate Guidelines Network (SIGN): *Management of acute upper and lower gastrointestinal bleeding*, 2008.

Whitcomb DC: Acute pancreatitis, *New Engl J Med* 354:2142–2150, 2006.

Further information

www.nice.org.uk

National Institute for Health and Clinical Excellence: Crohn's disease — infliximab and adalimumab

Liver disease 6

INVESTIGATIONS

Most of the tests designated as liver function tests (LFTs) are not direct measurements of 'liver function'. The only commonly used tests of synthetic function are the serum albumin and prothrombin time.

Routine serum liver biochemical tests

- Bilirubin is produced from the breakdown of red cells and a raised level indicates jaundice. In the serum, most of the total bilirubin is unconjugated. Gilbert's syndrome is the most common familial hyperbilirubinaemia, with isolated serum bilirubin levels of 17–102 μmol/L (1–6 mg/dL) (mostly unconjugated). **Unconjugated bilirubin** is also produced in haemolysis. It is not water-soluble so does not appear in the urine. Conjugated bilirubin is water-soluble and makes the urine dark.
- Serum enzymes
  - *Elevation of the serum aminotransferases* (aspartate aminotransferase (AST or SGOT) and alanine aminotransferase (ALT or SGPT)) occurs with hepatocellular damage from any cause. Mild elevations are a common finding at routine screening, often due to moderate alcohol consumption. ALT is more specific to the liver and only rises with liver damage, whereas AST is also elevated with muscle damage, e.g. myocardial infarction.
  - *Alkaline phosphatase* is present in the liver and many other tissues, e.g. bone, intestine and placenta. If there is an abnormality of the other liver enzymes, particularly the γ-GT, the alkaline phosphatase can be presumed to arise from the liver. The level is raised in cholestasis of any cause, whether intra- or extrahepatic, with infiltration of the liver, e.g. by metastases, and in cirrhosis, often without jaundice. Serum levels are higher than normal in children and adolescents (bone) and in pregnancy (placenta).
  - *γ-Glutamyl transpeptidase (γ-GT)* increases in the serum in parallel with the serum alkaline phosphatase in liver disease. γ-GT is an inducible enzyme and serum levels are elevated by alcohol and by drugs, e.g. phenytoin; when the liver tests are normal, this elevation does not indicate liver damage.

> ### Box 6.1 Abnormal liver biochemistry — how to proceed
>
> Always check the history and examine the patient for signs of liver disease.
>
> #### Mild–moderate rise in aminotransferases (ALT)
> - This occurs with liver cell damage
> - Measure:
>   - Hepatitis viral antibodies
>   - Serum ferritin for hereditary haemochromatosis
>   - Serum α_1-antitrypsin for deficiency
>   - Auto-antibodies for autoimmune hepatitis
>   - Serum caeruloplasmin in a young person for Wilson's disease
>
> #### ALT ↑ + raised MCV and high γ-GT
> - excess alcohol likely cause
>
> #### Raised serum alkaline phosphatase and γ-GT
> - This occurs with cholestasis
> - Measure:
>   - Mitochondrial antibodies for primary biliary cirrhosis
>   - US for infiltrative disease or biliary tract disease
>
> #### Raised bilirubin alone (without other abnormalities)
> - Probably Gilbert's disease (predominantly unconjugated bilirubin)
> - Exclude haemolysis
> - Measure:
>   - Reticulocyte count

- Markers of liver fibrosis
  - *Fibrotest/fibrosure tests* measure α_2-macroglobulin, α_2-haptoglobulin, γ-globin, apoprotein A_1, γ-GT and total bilirubin. These results are formulated to determine a **fibrosis index**. The index is sensitive and specific (> 90%) for the absence of fibrosis, and has 80% sensitivity and specificity for severe fibrosis.
- Liver function
  - *Serum albumin* falls in chronic liver disease and is a useful guide to prognosis. Because of its long half-life (20 days), the albumin level is often normal in acute liver disease.
  - *Prothrombin time (PT)* is a marker of synthetic function if vitamin K deficiency has been excluded by giving a 10 mg IV bolus of vitamin K and then rechecking the PT after 24 hours. The PT is used to predict outcome in fulminant hepatic failure. PT values vary in different laboratories and the International Normalized Ratio (INR), which is corrected by an international sensitivity ratio, is often used.

Box 6.1 shows an interpretation of abnormal liver biochemistry.

The role of imaging

- Ultrasound (US) examination is particularly useful in the jaundiced patient. Look for:
  - dilatation of the biliary tract — extrahepatic cholestasis
  - normal biliary tree — intrahepatic cholestasis.

US is useful for the detection of gallstones and for evaluation of hepatosplenomegaly and other abdominal masses. In focal liver disease, lesions > 1 cm can be detected and US is used to screen patients for hepatocellular carcinoma. Colour flow Doppler will show the direction of blood flow in the portal and hepatic veins. In **endoscopic ultrasound**, a small, high-frequency US probe mounted on the tip of the endoscope can accurately stage pancreatic tumours (particularly neuroendocrine) and also chronic pancreatitis.

- **Computed tomography (CT)** with IV contrast is useful for the evaluation of all liver diseases and can detect smaller lesions than US.
- **Magnetic resonance imaging (MRI)** avoids the use of irradiation and is very sensitive for the detection of liver masses. It cannot be used in patients with pacemakers, defibrillators and implanted metal objects.
- **Magnetic resonance cholangiopancreatography (MRCP)** allows non-invasive visualization of the bile and pancreatic ducts, thereby replacing diagnostic ERCP.
- **Endoscopic retrograde cholangiopancreatography (ERCP)** and **percutaneous transhepatic cholangiography (PTC)** are used to outline the biliary tree. ERCP also visualizes the pancreatic duct. Contrast is introduced into the lower bile duct through the ampulla of Vater using an endoscope (ERCP) or injected through the liver (PTC). Via **ERCP**, the biliary system can be drained by performing a sphincterotomy and inserting a stent. Stones can also be removed from the common bile duct at ERCP. Pancreatitis, with a raised serum amylase, can occur after ERCP (5%); bleeding is seldom serious. A broad-spectrum antibiotic, e.g. oral 500 mg ciprofloxacin ×2, should be given prophylactically to all patients with suspected biliary obstruction or a history of cholangitis. **PTC** is used when ERCP is not possible but sometimes the two techniques are combined, with PTC showing the biliary anatomy above the obstruction and ERCP showing the distal anatomy.
- **Scintiscanning** using an IV injection of ^{99m}-technetium colloid is less commonly used. In chronic liver disease most of the colloid is taken up by the spleen and bone marrow instead of the liver. Scintiscanning can also detect focal lesions. IV technetium-labelled iododiethyl IDA is excreted into the biliary system and can be used in the diagnosis of acute cholecystitis.
- **Elastography** measures hepatic stiffness (in κPa), which is a measure of liver fibrosis. It has a sensitivity and specificity of 80–90% compared with liver biopsy.

Liver pathology

- **Percutaneous liver biopsy** can be performed with or without US guidance for histological diagnosis. It is a safe procedure that can be carried out as a day case. Bleeding is the most common problem but is rarely serious. Biliary leaks occur rarely. **Contraindications** include ascites and extrahepatic cholestasis. If the PT is raised (by > 3 secs) or there is thrombocytopenia (< 80 × 10^9/L), a biopsy can be performed by the transjugular route, if this is really necessary.

JAUNDICE

Jaundice (Fig. 6.1) is due to intra- or extrahepatic cholestasis.

Kumar & Clark's Medical Management and Therapeutics

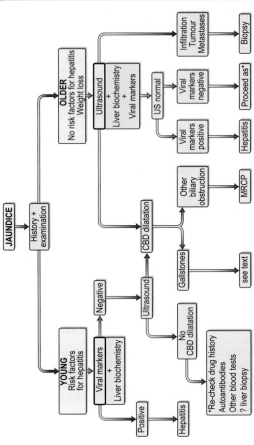

Fig. 6.1 Approach to the patient with jaundice.
CBD, common bile duct; MRCP, magnetic resonance cholangiopancreatography; US, ultrasound.

Approach to the patient

- **History** — risk factors for hepatitis, drugs (hepatotoxic), pain (biliary tract disease), weight loss (malignancy).
- **Examination** — signs of chronic liver disease (e.g. spider naevi, gynaecomastia, liver palms), hepatosplenomegaly, other abdominal masses.
- **Liver biochemistry** — raised bilirubin confirms jaundice. As a rough guide:
  - high transferases (> 300 U) — hepatitis picture
  - high ALP — cholestasis; if very high, more likely to be extrahepatic.
- **Viral hepatitis screen**
  - HAV IgM — diagnostic for acute HAV infection
  - Anti-HbcAg IgM — high titre — acute HBV infection.
- **Ultrasound** — not necessary if acute viral hepatitis.

VIRAL HEPATITIS

- Viral hepatitis (Table 6.1) is caused by hepatitis A virus (HAV), hepatitis B virus (HBV), hepatitis C virus (HCV), hepatitis D virus (HDV) and hepatitis E virus (HEV).
- In addition, 1–2% of viral hepatitis is due to non-A–E viruses, i.e. so far unidentified viruses, and occasionally is a feature of a recognized viral illness such as infectious mononucleosis (Epstein–Barr virus, EBV), cytomegalovirus (CMV), yellow fever or herpes simplex. Toxoplasmosis can also produce a similar picture to infectious mononucleosis.
- Hepatitis B, C and D may progress to chronic viral hepatitis, which implies the presence of persistent liver inflammation for at least 6 months.
- Co-infection of HBV and/or HCV with HIV is common — see p. 115.

Hepatitis A

This is the most common viral hepatitis worldwide, often occurring in epidemics, usually caused by the ingestion of contaminated food or water (e.g. shellfish). Overcrowding and poor sanitation facilitate spread (faeco-oral transmission), the virus being present in the faeces for up to 3 weeks from onset of the disease.

The main symptoms are general malaise and anorexia, followed by jaundice with raised serum transferases. It usually settles in 3–6 weeks. Less than 1% develop acute fulminant hepatitis.

An anti-HAV IgM in the serum confirms an acute infection; IgG antibody develops later and provides lifelong immunity.

Management

- **Supportive treatment.** If illness is not resolving, repeat bilirubin, AST, ALT, albumin and PT.
- **Vaccination.** Vaccination is recommended to all people travelling to endemic areas. Patients with chronic liver disease, people with haemophilia and workers in frequent contact with hepatitis cases should also be vaccinated. A formaldehyde-inactivated HAV vaccine is available and 0.5 mL is given into the upper arm, followed by a booster dose 6–12 months later. Immunity can then last for up to 10 years.
- **Hepatitis A immunoglobulin.** A single IM dose of immunoglobulin 0.02 mL/kg is given to anyone recently exposed to HAV who has not previously been vaccinated. If the patient has been vaccinated more

Kumar & Clark's Medical Management and Therapeutics

Table 6.1 Some features of hepatitis viruses

	A	B	D	C	E
Virus	RNA	DNA	RNA	RNA	RNA
Incubation	Short (2–3 weeks)	Long (1–5 months)	Long	Intermediate	Short
Spread					
Faecal/ oral	Yes	No	No	No	Yes
Blood/ IV drug use	Rare	Yes	Yes	Yes	No
Vertical	No	Yes	Rare	Occasional	No
Saliva	Yes	Yes	Yes	? No	?
Sexual	Rare	Yes	Yes (rare)	Uncommon	No
Age	Young	Any	Any	Any	Any
Carrier state	No	Yes	Yes	?	No
Chronic liver disease	No	Yes	Yes	Yes	No
Liver cancer	No	Yes	Rare	Yes	No
Mortality (acute)	<0.5%	<1%	–	<1%	1–2% (pregnant women 10–20%)

than once prior to exposure, no treatment is required. This dose gives protection for 3–4 months.

Hepatitis B

HBV is present worldwide, with an estimated 360 million carriers. The UK and the USA have a low carrier rate (0.5–2%), but this rises to 10–20% in parts of Africa, the Middle East and the Far East.

Vertical transmission from mother to child in utero, during parturition or soon after birth, is the usual means of transmission worldwide. This is related to the HBV replicative state of the mother (90% are HbeAg+, 30% HbeAg–ve) and is uncommon in Africa, where horizontal transmission (sibling to sibling) is common. HBV is not transmitted by breast feeding.

Horizontal transmission occurs particularly in children, through minor abrasions or close contact with other children, and HBV can survive on household articles, e.g. toys or toothbrushes, for prolonged periods so transmission may be possible.

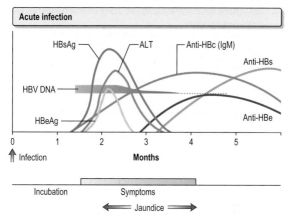

Fig. 6.2 Time course of the events and serological changes seen following infection with hepatitis B virus. ALT, alanine aminotransferase.

HBV spread also occurs by the IV route (e.g. by transfusion of infected blood or blood products, or by contaminated needles used by drug users, tattooists or acupuncturists) or by close personal contact, such as during sexual intercourse, particularly in men having sex with men (25% of cases in the USA). The virus can be found in semen and saliva.

Clinical features

● Acute. The symptoms are similar to those of hepatitis A and can vary from mild symptoms to a fulminant hepatic failure. Serum transferases are raised and jaundice occurs. Extrahepatic manifestations include cryoglobulinaemia, glomerulonephritis and polyarteritis nodosa.

● Chronic. Patients are usually asymptomatic for many years and may only be detected by abnormal liver biochemistry or later with symptoms of end-stage liver disease.

Viral markers

The **time course** of the events and serological changes seen following infection with HBV are as follows:

● Acute infection (Fig. 6.2)

  • *HBV DNA* appears in the serum following infection and decreases following recovery.

  • *Antigens:*

    – **HBsAg** appears in the blood from about 6 weeks to 3 months after an acute infection and then disappears.

    – **HBeAg** appears early and usually declines rapidly.

  • *Antibodies:*

    – **Anti-HBc** (HB core) is the first antibody to appear and high titres of IgM anti-HBc suggest an acute and continuing viral replication. It persists for many months. IgM anti-HBc may be the only serological indicator of recent HBV infection in a period when HBsAg has disappeared and anti-HBs is not detectable in the serum. IgG anti-HBc is seen in chronic stages, along with anti-HBs, and indicates past infection.

- **Anti-HBe** (i.e. seroconversion) appears after the anti-HBc and its appearance relates to a decreased infectivity and low DNA, i.e. a low risk. It is also seen in carriers with no HBV DNA in their serum.
- **Anti-HBs** appears late and indicates immunity. It is also found following immunization by HBV vaccines.

Treatment

HBV infection is mainly asymptomatic and the majority recover completely. Patients should have their HBV markers monitored. If HBcAg is persistent beyond 12 weeks, refer to experts, who may treat patients with nucleoside analogues. Around 1% of patients with acute hepatitis develop fulminant hepatitis (p. 187).

- Chronic hepatitis
  - *Inactive chronic HBV infection.* Approximately 1–10% of patients will not clear the virus following an acute HBV infection and develop an inactive chronic HBV infection. This occurs more in neonatal (90%) or childhood (20–50% below the age of 5 years) infection than when HBV is acquired in adult life (< 10%). There is a vast geographic variation in the incidence of inactive chronic hepatitis B. These patients have HBsAg in their serum and are HBeAg-negative, HBe antibody-positive with lower levels of HBV DNA in their serum. They have no evidence of active liver disease (normal or only slightly raised transferases) and are not highly infective. Most remain HBsAg-positive, but do not develop progressive liver disease. The spontaneous clearance rate of HBsAg is 1–2% per year.
  - *Active chronic HBV infection.* These patients have raised serum aminotransferases with evidence of HBV replication. This means that they have high levels of HBV DNA in their serum and are HBe antigen-positive (wild-type infection) or HBe antigen-negative (mutant strain). A liver biopsy shows chronic hepatitis. **Histologically**, there is a full spectrum of changes from near normal with only a few lymphocytes and interface hepatitis to a full-blown cirrhosis. HBsAg may be seen as a 'ground-glass' appearance in the cytoplasm on haematoxylin and eosin staining, and this can be confirmed on orcein staining or more specifically with immunohistochemical staining. HBcAg can also be demonstrated in hepatocytes by appropriate immunohistochemical staining.
  - *Chronic hepatitis — who to treat?*
    - Patients who are **positive for HBeAg**, HBsAg and HBV DNA (> 20 000 U/mL — for copies multiply by 5.6) with abnormal serum ALT (> 2 × normal) should be treated. Liver biopsy is not essential in this group.
    - Similar patients with HBV DNA levels > 20 000 U/L who have ALT values < 2 × normal should not be treated because the efficacy of therapy is low. A liver biopsy may help, as treatment is sometimes given if inflammation is marked.
    - Patients who are **negative for HBeAg** with an HBV DNA level of > 20 000 should also be treated. Those with DNA levels > 2000 should have a liver biopsy to help with the decision to treat or not.

The **aim of treatment** is the seroconversion of HbeAg (when present), i.e. the development of anti-HBe and the reduction of HBV DNA to undetectable levels by PCR. In addition, normalization of the serum ALT level and histological improvement in inflammation and fibrosis reflects a good response.

- Patients with **compensated cirrhosis** with HBV DNA > 2000 U/L should be treated and those with a DNA < 2000 should only be treated if the ALT is high.
- Patients with **decompensated cirrhosis** can also be treated but liver transplantation may be required.
- In patients in whom HBeAg disappears, remission is usually sustained. The patient remains a carrier with HBsAg present, although some will eventually become HBsAg-negative.

- *Hepatitis B mutants.* In hepatitis B associated with a mutant virus, HBeAg is not produced but the synthesis of HBcAg is unaffected. The presence of HBV DNA in the serum indicates viral replication. This must be measured, as e antigen cannot be used to indicate viral replication as the prevalence of mutant viruses increases. DNA polymerase mutants can also occur, particularly after lamivudine therapy.

Antiviral agents (Table 6.2)

- Pegylated α-2a interferon (180 mcg once a week SC) gives response rates of 25–65% (depending on genotype — A and B respond best) after 12 months of treatment. **Side-effects** of interferon treatment are many, occurring in up to 30% of patients, and the dose may have to be lowered; in 10% the treatment has to be discontinued.
- Nucleoside and nucleotide analogues
  - *Adefovir* 10 mg/day orally is also effective in HBeAg-positive and HBeAg-negative naive patients. Adefovir mutants are less frequent (20% at 4 years).
  - *Entecavir* 0–5 mg orally is more effective than lamivudine and reduces HBV DNA more quickly; there is much less viral resistance. Serum HBV DNA becomes negative in 67% (HBeAg-positive patients) and 90% (HBeAg-negative patients) by 48 weeks. It has been shown to reverse fibrosis in one study.
  - *Lamivudine* 100 mg/day given orally is well tolerated. It appears more effective than interferon, particularly in HBV DNA-positive individuals who have acquired the infection perinatally or in childhood. At 1 year, 50–70% of patients have normalization of their serum ALT and 30% have lost their HBe antigen with seroconversion in 15–20%. However, by 4 years, 80% develop viral resistance due to YMDD mutant (tyrosine (Y), methionine (M), aspartate (D)), which in itself causes hepatitis, but usually less severe than that due to the wild-type infection.
  - *Tenofovir* 300 mg per day orally is effective against lamivudine-resistant virus and, as monotherapy, has a similar potency to entecavir.
  - *Telbivudine* is a slightly more potent antiviral than lamivudine and adefovir. It has the same disadvantage as lamivudine in the production of mutants and is therefore not recommended.

Choice and duration of treatment

The duration of all treatment, and which combination of antivirals is optimal, are still being assessed. **In general**, current treatment for HbeAg-positive disease is with pegylated interferon or tenofovir or entecavir. Interferon should be given for 1 year. HBeAg-negative disease requires long-term (many years of) oral therapy. Older patients respond poorly to

Table 6.2 Drugs used and response rates after therapy in chronic hepatitis B

Drugs	Dose (oral unless stated)	Undetectable HBV DNA at 1 year of treatment (%)	Side-effects/Comment
Pegylated interferon (IFN) α-2a	180 mcg/week SC	25–63	Flu-like illness 6–8 hours after injection. Malaise, headache, myalgia. Depression, reversible hair loss. Bone marrow depression. Infection
Adefovir	10 mg daily	21–61	Negligible. Effective against lamivudine-produced mutants. Drug resistance (development of mutants) — 20% at 4 years
Entecavir	0–5 mg daily	67–90	Negligible. Most potent. Drug resistance very little. None at years 1–3; 1.2% at 5 years
Lamivudine	100 mg daily	40–72	Negligible. Well tolerated. More effective than IFN but drug resistance is a major problem — up to 80% at 4 years
Tenofovir	300 mg daily	76–93	Negligible. Most potent after entecavir
Telbivudine	600 mg daily	60–88	Well tolerated. High potency. High resistance and not now recommended. Monitor creatinine

(Adapted from Liaw YF, Chu CM 2009; Hoofnagle JH, et al 2007)

interferon and should be treated with nucleoside and nucleotide analogues.

Response rates

Factors predictive of a sustained response include a short duration of disease, high ALT levels, mild to moderate inflammation of the liver, low HBV DNA levels, absence of immunosuppression, female gender, delta virus-negative, adult acquirement and lastly the rapidity of response to oral therapy. Approximately 1% of patients will spontaneously clear the HbsAg annually. Between 5 and 10% of adults will develop chronic HBV, compared to 90% of children under the age of 5 years.

Active and passive vaccination for hepatitis B

Widespread vaccination in children is becoming more common. Vaccination is now recommended for all healthcare personnel, persons with multiple sex partners and those seeking treatment for STIs. People with haemophilia and patients with chronic kidney disease on dialysis units should also be vaccinated. A recombinant vaccine is safe and effective. Three injections of 1 mL are given at 0, 1 and 6 months into the deltoid muscle, giving good-term protection in over 90% of patients. A booster dose may be required 3–5 years later.

Combined prophylaxis, i.e. vaccination and immunoglobulin, should be given to all people with accidental needlestick injury if they have not been vaccinated, all newborn babies of HBsAg-positive mothers and regular HBV-negative sexual partners of HBsAg-positive patients. Adult dose is 500 U of specific hepatitis B immunoglobulin and the vaccines are given intramuscularly at different sites.

Hepatitis D

HDV is an incomplete RNA particle enclosed in a shell of HBsAg. It is unable to replicate on its own but is activated by the presence of HBV. Active HBV synthesis is reduced by HDV infection and patients are usually negative for HBeAg and HBV DNA.

Co-infection of HDV and HBV is clinically indistinguishable from an acute icteric HBV infection, but a biphasic rise of serum aminotransferases may be seen. Diagnosis is confirmed by finding serum IgM anti-D in the presence of IgM anti-HBc.

Superinfection results in an acute flare-up of previously quiescent chronic HBV infection. A rise in serum transferases occurs and the diagnosis is made by finding serum IgM anti-D in the serum.

Treatment
Peginterferon-alfa2a for 48 weeks produced a sustained clearance of HDV RNA in 25%.

Hepatitis C

HCV is transmitted by blood and blood products. Prevalence of infection is less than 0.02% in Northern Europe, 1–3% in Southern Europe and up to 6% in Africa. Incidence is high in IV drug users but sexual transmission is uncommon. Vertical transmission is rare. In 20% of cases, the exact mode of transmission is unknown.

Acute HCV infection is usually subclinical but a mild illness with jaundice may occur. HCV antibody is not detected for 6–8 weeks, although HCV RNA measured by PCR can be detected at 2 weeks.

Chronic hepatitis occurs in 80% of patients. It is often found in an asymptomatic individual who is discovered to have a mild rise in the serum transferase on routine screening. The diagnosis is confirmed by detecting antibody to HCV in the serum, and qualitative and quantitative PCR for HCV RNA would indicate the viral load. HCV genotype is useful to predict the success of treatment.

Treatment
- Acute. In cases due to needlestick injury, interferon is used to prevent chronic disease.
- Chronic. Treatment is appropriate for patients with chronic hepatitis on liver histology who have HCV RNA in their serum and who have raised serum aminotransferases for more than 6 months. Patients with persistently normal aminotransferases are also treated if they have abnormal

Kumar & Clark's Medical Management and Therapeutics

histology. The presence of cirrhosis is not a contraindication but therapeutic responses are less likely. The aim of treatment is to eliminate the HCV RNA from the serum in order to:

- stop the progression of active liver disease
- prevent the development of hepatocellular carcinoma.

Patients with decompensated cirrhosis should be evaluated for possible transplantation.

Trends are now going towards specifically targeted therapy (STAT). For example, patients with genotype 1 with a mutation in anti-viral IL-28B are targeted with **telaprevir** in addition to peg-INF and ribavirin.

Antiviral agents

Current treatment is combination therapy with **pegylated interferon**, which is interferon with a polyethyleneglycol tail (**α2a 180 mcg/week or α2b 1.5 mcg/kg/week**) and **ribavirin** (1000–1200 mg/day for genotype 1, 800 mg/day for genotype 2 or 3) in daily divided doses for 12 months for genotype 1, and 6 months for other genotypes. Efficacy is also determined by viral load, with HCV RNA ≥ 6 000 000 U/L less likely to respond. For the **side-effects** of interferon, see p. 184. Ribavirin is usually well tolerated but side-effects include a dose-related haemolysis, and pruritus and nasal congestion occur. Pregnancy should be avoided, as ribavirin is teratogenic. **Taribavirin** is a new alternative with less anaemia being reported.

Telaprevir is a specific inhibitor of the HCV protease. It is showing efficacy in clinical trials but a major adverse effect is rash.

Monitoring results

An **early virological response** is defined as becoming HCV RNA-negative or having at least a 2 log reduction in RNA following treatment in the first 12 weeks. This occurs in about 80% of patients tolerating full dosage. If this is not achieved, they are unlikely to respond and treatment should be stopped. If HCV RNA is undetectable at 4 weeks, treatment for patients with genotype 2 can be stopped at 12–16 weeks, and for genotype 1 (if HCV RNA < 600 000 U/mL at baseline) at 6 months.

A **sustained response** is clearance of HCV RNA at 6 months. It is a good surrogate marker for the resolution of the hepatitis. This is achieved in 40–50% of patients with genotype 1 and 80% in genotype 2 or 3. In sustained responders relapse is unlikely and histological progression is halted. For non-responders and relapsers, longer duration of therapy is being assessed.

Hepatitis E

HEV is enterally transmitted, usually by contaminated water, with 30% of dogs, pigs and rodents carrying the virus in many developing countries. Clinical features are similar to HAV hepatitis. There is no carrier state and it does not progress to chronic liver disease. An ELISA for IgG and IgM anti-HEV is available, although not always reliable. HEV RNA can be detected in the serum or stools by PCR. There is a high mortality, particularly in pregnant women (10–20%).

Prevention of hepatitis

Avoiding the risk factors is still necessary despite the availability of vaccination for HAV and HBV. Standard safety precautions in laboratories and hospitals must be enforced strictly. HAV and HEV infection in the community should be prevented by improving sanitation and overcrowding.

Fulminant hepatic failure (See Emergencies in medicine p. 708)

This is defined as severe hepatic failure in a patient with a previously normal liver in whom encephalopathy develops in under 2 weeks. It can occur from any cause of acute hepatitis, the commonest (worldwide) being viral hepatitis; paracetamol overdosage is commonly implicated in the UK.

Histologically there is multi-acinar necrosis involving a substantial part of the liver. The patient is encephalopathic and jaundiced; gastrointestinal haemorrhage, sepsis, hypoglycaemia and worsening of the encephalopathy occur. Patients require 10% glucose infusion, correction of any coagulopathy (with IV vitamin K, platelets, blood or fresh frozen plasma) and any electrolyte abnormality with potassium, calcium, phosphate and magnesium as appropriate. A proton pump inhibitor should be given intravenously to prevent stress ulcers. Prophylaxis against bacterial and fungal infections is not routine but given if there is advanced encephalopathy, refractory hypotension or the development of SIRS. Suspected infections should be treated with an appropriate antibiotic. Raised intracranial pressure requires 20% **mannitol** intravenously. Patients should be managed in a specialized unit (Box 6.2), as liver transplantation may be required. Prognostic variables are shown in Box 6.3.

> **Box 6.2** Transfer criteria to specialized units for patients with acute liver injury
>
> - INR > 3.0
> - Presence of hepatic encephalopathy
> - Hypotension after resuscitation with fluid
> - Metabolic acidosis
> - PT above normal (secs) > interval (hours) from overdose (paracetamol cases)

> **Box 6.3** Poor prognostic variables in fulminant hepatic failure indicating a need for liver transplantation
>
> **Non-paracetamol (3 of the following 5)**
> - Drug or non-A–E hepatitis
> - Age < 10 or > 40 years
> - Interval from onset of jaundice to encephalopathy > 7 days
> - Serum bilirubin > 300 µmol/L
> - PT > 50 secs (or > 100 secs in isolation)
>
> **Paracetamol**
> - Arterial pH < 7.3 (after resuscitation, 7.25 on N-acetylcysteine)
> Or
> - Serum creatinine > 300 µmol/L and
> - PT > 100 secs and
> - Grade III–IV encephalopathy

CIRRHOSIS AND ITS COMPLICATIONS

Cirrhosis results from the necrosis of liver cells followed by fibrosis and nodule formation. The liver architecture is diffusely abnormal and this interferes with liver blood flow and function. This derangement produces the clinical features of portal hypertension and impaired liver cell function. Serum albumin and PT are indicators of liver function, and the outlook is poor with a serum albumin level < 25 g/L. The PT is prolonged as the disease becomes more severe. Liver biochemistry is variable and not helpful in assessing function. Serum α-fetoprotein should be measured routinely every 6 months; a level > 400 ng/mL suggests hepatocellular carcinoma.

Prognosis

There are a number of prognostic classifications based on modifications of **Child's grading** (A, B and C). This is based on the presence of jaundice, ascites and encephalopathy, the level of serum albumin and the PT. Patients with good liver function (Child's grade A) do better than patients with poor liver function (Child's grade C: albumin < 30 g/L, bilirubin > 50 μmol/L and ascites).

The **M**odel of **E**nd-Stage **L**iver **D**isease (**MELD**) score is widely used as a predictor of mortality in transplant centres.

$$(3.8 \times LN \text{ bilirubin in mg/dL}) + (9.6 \times LN \text{ creatinine in mg/dL}) + (11.2 \times LN \text{ of INR}) + (6.4)$$

(LN = natural log)

To convert μmol/L to mg/dL: for bilirubin, divide by 17; for creatinine, divide by 88.4.

With a MELD score < 10, 1-year survival is 97%; with a score of 30–40, it is about 70%.

Complications

Variceal haemorrhage

Approximately 90% of patients with cirrhosis will develop gastro-oesophageal varices over 10 years and one-third of these patients will bleed from them. This is discussed in upper gastrointestinal haemorrhage, p. 149.

Ascites

Ascites is the presence of fluid within the peritoneal cavity and is a common complication of decompensated liver cirrhosis. Ascites occurs due to portal hypertension, low serum albumin and sodium retention.

- Diagnosis. Diagnostic aspiration should always be performed to exclude infection and to eliminate other causes of ascites.
- Management. The aim is both to reduce sodium intake and to increase renal excretion of sodium.
  - *Sodium and fluid restriction.* Dietary sodium restriction to 40 mmol (1 g in 24 hours) will still maintain an adequate protein and calorie intake with a palatable diet. Fluid restriction is not necessary unless the serum sodium is < 120 mmol/L.
  - *Diuretic therapy.* The aim should be to produce a net loss of fluid approaching 700 mL in 24 hours (0.7 kg of weight loss or 1.0 kg if peripheral oedema is present), and 60% of patients respond with this regimen. The aldosterone antagonist **spironolactone**, starting at 100 mg daily and increasing every 7 days to a maximum of 500 mg daily, is used. Chronic administration produces gynaecomastia.

Eplerone does not have this side-effect. **Amiloride** 5–15 mg daily is also used. A **loop diuretic**, such as furosemide 20–40 mg or bumetanide 1 mg daily, may be added if response is poor. These loop diuretics have several disadvantages, including hyponatraemia, hypokalaemia and volume depletion. Ascitic fluid is mobilized more slowly than interstitial fluid and diuretic dosage is lower in those without peripheral oedema.

- *Monitoring.* Check serum electrolytes and creatinine at the start and every other day of treatment; weigh patients and measure urinary output daily.
- *Electrolyte problems.* Diuretics should be temporarily discontinued if a rise in serum creatinine level occurs, representing over-diuresis and hypovolaemia. Hyponatraemia occurring during therapy almost always represents haemodilution secondary to failure to clear free water (usually a marker of reduced renal perfusion) and should be treated by stopping the diuretics if the sodium level falls below 120 mmol/L, as well as introducing water restriction. Diuretics should also be stopped if there is hyperkalaemia or the development of encephalopathy.
- *Paracentesis* is used to relieve symptomatic tense ascites and can also serve as a means of rapid therapy. Hypovolaemia can occur and IV albumin is infused (8 g per L of ascitic fluid removed).

Spontaneous bacterial peritonitis (SBP)

SBP is due to *Escherichia coli*, *Klebsiella* and enterococci. It should be suspected in any patient with ascites with evidence of clinical deterioration. Features such as pain and pyrexia are frequently absent.

- Diagnosis. Diagnostic aspiration shows a raised neutrophil count > 250 cells $\times$ 10^9/L in the ascitic fluid and is sufficient to start treatment immediately.
- Treatment. **Cefotaxime** IV 1 g twice daily, or **ceftazidime** IV 1 g 3 times daily, is used and modified on the basis of culture results. SBP has a mortality of 25% and recurs in 70% of patients. An oral quinolone, e.g. norfloxacin 400 g daily, prevents recurrence and prolongs survival. Patients are referred for possible liver transplantation.

Portosystemic encephalopathy (PSE)

PSE refers to a chronic neuropsychiatric syndrome secondary to chronic liver disease. PSE is seen in patients with cirrhosis, with portal hypertension that is due to spontaneous 'shunting', or in patients following a portosystemic shunt procedure, e.g. transjugular intrahepatic portosystemic shunting (TIPS). Encephalopathy is potentially reversible.

- Management consists of restriction of protein intake. Any precipitating cause, such as drugs, infection or electrolyte imbalance, is corrected. **Lactulose**, an osmotic purgative given 10–30 mL 3 times daily, and **rifaximin**, an unabsorbed antibiotic, are given to evacuate and sterilize the colon.

Hepatorenal syndrome

This occurs in a patient with advanced cirrhosis, jaundice and ascites. The urine output is low, with a low urinary sodium concentration due to a functional failure of the kidneys.

- It is precipitated by over-vigorous diuretic therapy, diarrhoea or paracentesis.
- Diuretic therapy should be stopped and hypovolaemia corrected. The prognosis is poor and liver transplantation is the best option.

Hepatocellular carcinoma

This is one of the ten most common cancers worldwide.

- It commonly follows HBV and HCV infection but can occur with other forms of cirrhosis, such as alcoholic cirrhosis and haemochromatosis.
- Patients present with weight loss, anorexia, fever and pain.

Diagnosis

- The tumour is either single or multiple, and can be detected by US and biopsy. Serum α-fetoprotein is raised.
- Screening for hepatocellular carcinoma should be carried out in patients with cirrhosis every 6 months with α-fetoprotein and US scan.

Treatment

Surgical resection is possible, with tumours < 7 cm having a 50% 5-year survival. Transarterial chemo-embolization is also used, with median survival > 2 years. **Sorafenib** has recently been shown to improve survival.

Liver transplantation

This is performed in patients with fulminant hepatic failure of any cause, the commonest being acute viral hepatitis and following paracetamol (aminophen) overdose. All patients with chronic liver disease and Child's grade C cirrhosis or MELD score > 15 should be assessed for transplantation.

- Transplantation in primary biliary cirrhosis is indicated when the serum bilirubin rises > 100 μmol/L.
- Patients with chronic hepatitis B with HBV DNA can be transplanted but recurrence of the hepatitis occurs despite the use of hepatitis B immunoglobulin and lamivudine.
- In chronic hepatitis C, the 5-year prognosis of the graft is good, although universal HCV reinfection occurs.
- Patients with alcoholic liver disease should have stopped drinking before being offered a transplant.

Prognosis

In low risk patients the 5 year survival is 70–80%.

CHRONIC LIVER DISORDERS

Autoimmune hepatitis

This disease is seen mainly in women in middle age presenting with fatigue and elevated levels of serum aminotransferases. The immunoglobulins are raised and antinuclear and anti-smooth muscle antibodies are present in the serum.

A younger group of women often present with an acute hepatitis and jaundice. The group may well have the clinical features of cirrhosis with hepatosplenomegaly, spider naevi and liver palms. They have similar biochemical features but anti-liver/kidney microsomal (anti-LKM1) antibodies are often present.

In both groups there may be features of other autoimmune diseases, such as pernicious anaemia, thyroiditis and Coombs-positive haemolytic anaemia.

- **Diagnosis** requires a liver biopsy, which shows variable interface hepatitis with plasma cell infiltration.
- **Treatment** is with **prednisolone** 30 mg daily for 2 weeks, reducing to a maintenance dose of 10–15 mg daily as the biochemical parameters improve. **Budesonide** is an alternative with less steroid side effects. **Azathioprine** 2 mg/kg is added as a steroid-sparing agent. This therapy induces remission in 80% of cases but relapses occur after stopping the therapy. Liver transplantation may be required.

Primary biliary cirrhosis (PBC)

This usually affects middle-aged women, with pruritus being the commonest symptom. There is progressive destruction of bile ducts with granuloma formation, eventually leading to fibrosis and cirrhosis.

- **Diagnosis.** Serum antimitochondrial antibodies are present in almost all cases. Of the mitochondrial proteins involved, the antigen M2 is specific to PBC. A high serum alkaline phosphatase is often the only abnormality in the liver biochemistry but the serum IgM may be very high with a raised serum cholesterol. US shows diffuse liver involvement with normal extrahepatic bile ducts.
- **Treatment:**
  - **Ursodeoxycholic acid** 10–15 mg/kg improves serum bilirubin and aminotransferase values, but it is not clear whether prognosis is altered.
  - **Vitamin supplementation** is required because of malabsorption of fat-soluble vitamins (A, D and K); when deficiency is detected, they should be given prophylactically in the jaundiced patient.
  - **Bisphosphonates** are required for osteoporosis. Hyperlipidaemia should be treated, usually with a statin.
  - **Colestyramine** 1 4 g sachet 3 times daily can be helpful for pruritus but this can be difficult to treat.
  - **Liver transplantation** is often necessary and should be performed when the bilirubin is 100 µmol/L.

Alcoholic liver disease

Ethanol is metabolized in the liver and 10–20% of people who drink heavily will develop serious liver damage.

Fatty change

The metabolism of alcohol invariably produces fat; this is minimal with small amounts of alcohol but with large amounts the hepatocytes become swollen with fat. Liver biochemistry shows mild abnormalities with elevation of the serum aminotransferases. The γ-GT is usually raised, and US or CT will demonstrate fatty infiltration. An elevated MCV indicates heavy drinking.

Alcoholic hepatitis

In addition to fatty change, there is an infiltration by polymorphonuclear leucocytes with hepatocyte necrosis. The clinical features vary from a few symptoms to an ill patient with jaundice and ascites. There is often a high fever and abdominal pain associated with the liver necrosis. In severe cases the mortality is at least 50%.

- Diagnosis. The serum bilirubin may be raised but there is always a rise in the serum transferases and serum alkaline phosphatase. The PT may be prolonged with a low serum albumin, indicating diminished liver function. A liver biopsy will confirm the diagnosis.
- Treatment. See below. This is often influenced by the **discriminant function (DF)**:

DF = [4.6 × PT above control in secs] + bilirubin (mg/dL)

Bilirubin μmol/L divided by 17 to convert to mg/dL.

A high DF of ≥ 32 suggests severe liver disease and the prognosis is poor.

Alcoholic cirrhosis

The symptoms are often related only to the complications. There is frequently hepatosplenomegaly with deranged liver biochemistry. **Diagnosis** is usually made with US or CT and is confirmed by biopsy if necessary.

Management and prognosis of alcoholic liver disease

All patients must stop drinking. A slow (over 30 mins) **IV** infusion of **thiamine 100 mg**, in a combined preparation with other vitamins, should be given to prevent Wernicke–Korsakoff encephalopathy. **Side-effects** include serious allergic reactions.

- Alcoholic hepatitis.
  - *Good nutrition is necessary* and this may need to be given via a fine-bore naso-gastric tube.
  - *Corticosteroids improve outcome* in severe cases (see above). The mortality is approximately 50% with a PT twice normal.
  - *Pentoxifyllene* 400 mg × 3 daily, an inhibitor of TNF synthesis, has been used with variable efficacy.
- Alcoholic cirrhosis. Management is that of the complications (p. 188). Abstinence from alcohol results in an improvement in prognosis with a 5-year survival of 90%, as opposed to 60% in those who continue drinking. Liver transplantation is being used more widely in those who have stopped drinking.

Non-alcoholic fatty liver disease (NAFLD)

This is the term used for patients who are found to have a fatty liver, either on US or on liver biopsy, and who do not drink alcohol to excess. It is often seen in the obese, patients with diabetes and those with raised serum lipids. If there is evidence of inflammation on the liver histology, as well as fatty change, the term **non-alcoholic steatohepatitis (NASH)** is used. The prognosis of a fatty liver on its own appears to be good but some patients with NASH and raised serum aminotransferases go on to develop chronic liver disease, with a few having cirrhosis and occasionally hepatocellular carcinoma.

Treatment

There is no specific effective therapy.
- Weight loss; strict control of diabetes and lipid levels.
- Thiazolidinediones, e.g. **pioglitazone**, these have shown improvement in fatty change and inflammation but benefits in the long term are unclear.
- Metformin has been used.

Hereditary haemochromatosis (HH)

HH is a common inherited disease characterized by excess iron deposition in various organs, leading to eventual fibrosis and functional organ failure.

Diabetes, arthritis, hypogonadism and cardiomyopathy are seen; the classic bronzed skin colour is rare. There is hepatomegaly with deranged liver biochemistry.

Diagnosis

- Serum iron is elevated (> 30 μmol/L), with a reduction in the total iron binding capacity (TIBC) and complete or almost complete transferrin saturation (> 60%).
- Serum ferritin is elevated (usually > 500 mcg/L or 240 nmol/L).
- Heterozygotes may have normal biochemical tests or only modest increases in serum iron or serum ferritin (usually > 400 mcg/L), with a transferrin saturation of > 50%. All patients and first degree relatives should be checked for a mutation in the *HFE* gene, which is strongly associated with HH.

Treatment

- Venesection prolongs life and may reverse tissue damage; the risk of hepatic malignancy still remains if cirrhosis is present and patients should be monitored with US and serum α-fetoprotein every 6 months. All patients should have excess iron removed as rapidly as possible, with venesection 500 mL (1 unit) performed twice weekly for up to 2 years, i.e. 160 U containing 250 mg of iron per U = 40 g of iron removed. During venesection, serum iron and ferritin and the mean corpuscular volume should be monitored. These fall only when available iron is depleted. Three or four venesections per year are required to prevent reaccumulation of iron, which is checked with a serum ferritin.
- Liver biopsy is useful to ensure removal of iron and to assess progress of hepatic disease.

Wilson's disease

This is a rare error of copper metabolism, which results in copper deposition in various organs, including the liver and the basal ganglion of the brain.

- Children usually present with hepatic problems, whereas young adults have neurological features such as tremor, dysarthria, involuntary movements and eventually dementia. A specific sign is the Kayser–Fleischer ring caused by copper deposition in Descemet's membrane in the cornea.
- The liver disease varies from an acute hepatitis, that can go on to fulminant hepatic failure, to chronic hepatitis or cirrhosis.

Treatment

- Lifetime treatment with **penicillamine 1–1.5 g daily** is effective in chelating copper but must be started early to prevent permanent damage.
- **Trientine 1.2–1.8 g/day** and **zinc acetate 150 mg/day** are used for maintenance therapy.
- Relatives should be screened for the *ATP7B* mutation.

α₁-Antitrypsin deficiency

This deficiency is sometimes associated with liver disease but more commonly causes pulmonary emphysema, particularly in smokers.

- The serum α₁-antitrypsin is low, and on electrophoresis most patients have the PiZZ phenotype. Liver biopsy shows the positive periodic acid–Schiff (PAS) globules in the liver, with fibrosis and cirrhosis.
- Liver transplantation is required for severe chronic liver disease.

Primary sclerosing cholangitis

This is a chronic disease due to fibrosing inflammation of intra- and extrahepatic bile ducts. Seventy per cent of patients have associated inflammatory bowel disease, usually ulcerative colitis. Primary sclerosing cholangitis is progressive and complicated by episodes of bacterial cholangitis and cholangiocarcinoma (20%).

- Diagnosis is supported by a raised alkaline phosphatase, a positive antineutrophil cytoplasmic antibodies (ANCA) and typical findings of strictures on ERCP or MRCP.
- Treatment. Episodes of cholangitis are treated with antibiotics. **Ursodeoxycholic acid** 250 mg 4 times daily has been used but liver transplantation is the only proven therapy.

Budd–Chiari syndrome

There is obstruction to the venous outflow of the liver due to occlusion of the hepatic vein. This occurs in hypercoagulability states and presents with abdominal pain, hepatomegaly and sometimes evidence of liver failure.

- Diagnosis. US (with Doppler), CT or MRI show the abnormalities in blood flow in hepatic vein.
- Treatment. Liver transplantation is the treatment of choice for chronic and fulminant cases.

Liver abscesses

Pyogenic abscess

These abscesses are uncommon but may be single or multiple. Aetiology is often unclear. The most common organism is *E. coli* but often the infection is mixed. Some patients are ill with fevers, rigors, anorexia, vomiting and abdominal pain, while others present only with malaise. US is the most useful initial investigation but a CT scan is diagnostic. Aspiration is usually attempted to obtain material for culture and broad-spectrum antibiotics such as IV **cefotaxime 1 g** every 12 hours are given and surgical drainage is not usually necessary.

Amoebic abscess

Entamoeba histolytica is carried from the bowel to the liver, producing inflammation and multiple microabscesses, which can develop into single or multiple large abscesses. An amoebic complement fixation test is always positive.

- Treatment
  - **Metronidazole** 800 mg 3 times daily for 10 days.
  - Aspiration is used in patients failing to respond, in multiple and large abscesses, and in those with abscesses in the left lobe of the liver.
  - **Diloxanide furoate** 500 mg 8-hourly for 10 days should be given subsequently to remove amoebae from the bowel.

DRUGS AND THE LIVER

- Many drugs are metabolized by liver enzymes and cause mild liver biochemical abnormalities.
- Some drugs can cause acute liver failure or chronic liver disease.
- Hepatotoxicity can be:
  - direct and dose-dependent; this is predictable, e.g. **paracetamol**
  - idiosyncratic and non-dose-dependent (Table 6.3): hypersensitivity; metabolic — due to altered drug clearance or increased hepatotoxic metabolics, e.g. **ketoconazole**.

Table 6.3 Liver damage produced by some drugs

Types of liver damage	Drugs
Zone 3 necrosis	*Amanita* mushrooms Carbon tetrachloride Cocaine Paracetamol Piroxicam Salicylates
Zone 1 necrosis	Ferrous sulphate
Microvesicular fat	Nucleoside reverse transcriptase inhibitors Sodium valproate Tetracyclines
Steatohepatitis	Amiodarone Nifedipine Synthetic oestrogens Tamoxifen
Fibrosis	Arsenic Maraviroc Methotrexate Other cytotoxic agents Retinoids Vitamin A
Vascular Sinusoidal dilatation	Anabolic steroids Oral contraceptives
Peliosis hepatis	Anabolic steroids, e.g. danazol Azathioprine Oral contraceptives
Veno-occlusive	Cytotoxics — cyclophosphamide Pyrrolizidine alkaloids (*Senecio* in bush tea)
Acute hepatitis	Atenolol Clonazepam Cytotoxic drugs Disulfiram Enalapril Isoniazid Ketoconazole Methyldopa Nevirapine Niacin Paracetamol (acetaminophen) overdose Paroxetine Pyrazinamide Rifampicin Ritonavir Statins Valproate Verapamil Volatile liquid anaesthetics, e.g. halothane

Table 6.3 Continued	
Types of liver damage	**Drugs**
Chronic hepatitis	Fenofibrate Infliximab (autoimmune) Isoniazid Methyldopa Nitrofurantoin

General hypersensitivity	Allopurinol
	Anticonvulsants, e.g.
	  Phenytoin
	Antithyroid, e.g.
	  Carbimazole
	  Propylthiouracil
	Diltiazem
	NSAIDs, e.g.
	  Diclofenac
	  Salicylates
	Penicillins, e.g.
	  Amoxicillin
	  Ampicillin
	  Co-amoxiclav
	  Flucloxacillin
	Quinine, e.g.
	  Quinidine
	Sulphonamides, e.g.
	  Co-trimoxazole
	  Fansidar
	  Sulfasalazine

Canalicular cholestasis	Azathioprine Chlorpromazine Ciclosporin Cimetidine/ranitidine Erythromycin Haloperidol Imipramine Nitrofurantoin Oral hypoglycaemics Sex hormones
Biliary sludge	Ceftriaxone
Sclerosing cholangitis	Hepatic arterial infusion of 5-fluorouracil
Hepatic tumours	Pills with high hormone content (adenomas)
Hepatocellular carcinoma	Danazol Oral contraceptives

The **'predictability' of drugs** to produce damage can be affected by metabolic events preceding their ingestion. For example, chronic alcohol users may become more susceptible to liver damage because of the enzyme-inducing effects of alcohol, or ill or starving patients may become susceptible because of the depletion of hepatic glutathione produced by starvation. Many other factors, such as environmental or genetic effects, may be involved in determining the 'susceptibility' of certain patients to certain drugs.

- The incidence is 14 per 100 000 population, with a 6% mortality.
- It is the most common cause of acute liver failure in the USA.
- Liver transplantation is used.

N.B. ⚠ *In any patient with liver dysfunction, ALWAYS ask about drugs taken (prescribed or unprescribed).*

Hepatic damage

The type of damage produced by various drugs is shown in Table 6.3. The diagnosis of these conditions is usually by exclusion of other causes.

- Most reactions occur within 3 months of starting the drug.
- Monitoring liver biochemistry in patients on long-term treatment, such as anti-TB therapy, is mandatory.
- If a drug is suspected of causing hepatic damage it should be **stopped immediately**.
- Liver biopsy is of limited help in confirming the diagnosis, but occasionally hepatic eosinophilia or granulomas may be seen.
- Diagnostic challenge with subtherapeutic doses of the drug is sometimes required after the liver biochemistry has returned to normal, to confirm the diagnosis.

Individual drugs

- Paracetamol. In high doses paracetamol produces liver cell necrosis. When ingested in small doses, most of it undergoes conjugation with glucuronide sulphate and the rest is metabolized by microsomal enzymes to produce toxic derivatives that are immediately detoxified by conjugation with glutathione. If larger doses are ingested, the former pathway becomes saturated and the toxic derivative is produced at a faster rate. Once the hepatic glutathione is depleted, large amounts of the toxic metabolite accumulate and bind irreversibly to liver cell membranes.
- Halothane and other volatile liquid anaesthetics. Halothane produces a hepatitis in patients having repeated exposures. The mechanism is thought to be a hypersensitivity reaction. An unexplained fever occurs ~10 days after the second or subsequent halothane anaesthetic and is followed by jaundice, typically with a hepatitic picture. Most patients recover spontaneously but there is a high mortality in severe cases. There are no chronic sequelae. Both **sevoflurane** and **isoflurane** also cause hepatotoxicity in those sensitized to halogenated anaesthetics but the risk is smaller than with halothane and remote with **desflurane**.
- Steroid compounds. Cholestasis is caused by natural and synthetic **oestrogens**, as well as **methyltestosterone**. These agents interfere with canalicular biliary flow by blocking the canalicular transporters (MRP2 and MDR3) and cause a pure cholestasis. Cholestasis is rare with the **contraceptive pill** because of the low dosage used. However, the contraceptive pill is associated with an increased incidence of gallstones, hepatic adenomas (rarely HCCs), the Budd–Chiari syndrome and peliosis hepatis. The latter condition, which also occurs with anabolic steroids, consists of dilatation of the hepatic sinusoids to form blood-filled lakes.

Kumar & Clark's Medical Management and Therapeutics

- **Phenothiazines.** Phenothiazines (e.g. **chlorpromazine**) can produce a cholestatic picture owing to a hypersensitivity reaction. This occurs in 1% of patients, usually within 4 weeks of starting the drug. Typically it is associated with a fever and eosinophilia. Recovery occurs on stopping the drug.

- **Anti-tuberculous chemotherapy. Isoniazid** produces elevated aminotransferases in 10–20% of patients. Hepatic necrosis with jaundice occurs in a smaller percentage. The hepatotoxicity of isoniazid is related to its metabolites and is dependent on acetylator status. **Rifampicin** produces a hepatitis, usually within 3 weeks of starting the drug, particularly in patients on high doses. **Pyrazinamide** produces abnormal liver biochemical tests and, rarely, liver cell necrosis.

- **Amiodarone.** This leads to a steatohepatitis histologically and liver failure if the drug is not stopped in time.

- **Sodium valproate.** This causes mitochondrial injury with microvesicular steatosis. IV carnitine should be used as an antidote.

Drug prescribing for patients with liver disease

The metabolism of drugs is impaired in severe liver disease (with jaundice and ascites), as the removal of many drugs depends on liver blood flow and the integrity of the hepatocyte. In general, therefore, the effect of drugs is prolonged by liver disease and also by cholestasis. This is further accentuated by portosystemic shunting, which diminishes the first-pass extraction of drugs. With hypoproteinaemia there is decreased protein binding of some drugs, and bilirubin competes with many drugs for the binding sites on serum albumin. In patients with portosystemic encephalopathy, care must be taken in prescribing drugs with a central depressant action.

Further reading

Czaja AJ, Manns MP: Advances in the diagnosis, pathogenesis, and management of autoimmune hepatitis, *Gastroenterology* 139:58–72, 2010.

Hoofnagle JH, Doo E, Liang TJ, et al: Management of hepatitis B: summary of a clinical research workshop, *Hepatology* 45:1056–1075, 2007.

Lange CM, Sarrazin C, Zeuzem S: Review article: specifically targeted antiviral therapy for hepatitis C, *Alimentary Pharmacology & Therapeutics* 32:14–28, 2010.

Liaw YF, Chu CM: Hepatitis B virus infection, *Lancet* 373:582–592, 2009.

Lucey MR, Mathurin P, Morgan TR: Alcoholic hepatitis: review, *N Engl J Med* 360:2758–2769, 2009.

Further information

http://www.gastrohep.com
Resource for gastroenterology, hepatology and endoscopy

http://www.aasld.org
Viral hepatitis (click on guidelines for management)

APPROACH TO THE PATIENT

Anaemia is present when the haemoglobin (Hb) level in the blood is < 11.5 g/dL in women and < 13.5 g/dL in men (reference ranges vary between laboratories). It is usually accompanied by a reduced red cell count (RCC) and packed cell volume (PCV). However, an increase in plasma volume (e.g. in massive splenomegaly) causes a low Hb level with a normal RCC.

Clinical features

- Symptoms are usually non-specific and vary with the speed of onset and severity of the anaemia. If the Hb falls slowly, symptoms are minimal, as there is time for haemodynamic compensation. Severe anaemia (e.g. < 8 g/dL) causes tiredness, light-headedness and dyspnoea; angina and intermittent claudication occur in those with atheromatous disease. If of sudden onset, anaemia with hypovolaemia causes syncope, tachycardia and visual impairment due to anoxia.
- Physical signs include pallor, tachycardia and a systolic flow murmur. Other signs are individual to the type of anaemia.

Investigations

- Blood count and blood film. The haemoglobin and **mean corpuscular volume** (MCV) help define the type of anaemia (Fig. 7.1). The **red blood cell distribution width** (RDW) is the ratio of the width of the red cell divided by the MCV, and is useful in the differential diagnosis of microcytosis but not macrocytosis. In a patient with microcytic anaemia, a raised RDW would favour iron deficiency and a normal RDW favours thalassaemia. The white blood cell count and platelet count can also be useful in the differential diagnosis. The **blood film** shows the red cell morphology (anisocytosis = variation in size; poikilocytosis = variation in shape). The **reticulocyte count** reflects marrow red cell activity; a high

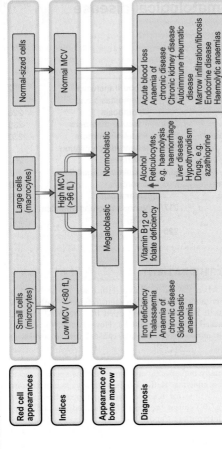

Fig. 7.1 Classification of anaemia. MCV, mean corpuscular volume.

Red cell appearances	Small cells (microcytes)	Large cells (macrocytes)		Normal-sized cells
Indices	Low MCV (<80 fL)	High MCV (>96 fL)		Normal MCV
Appearance of bone marrow		Megaloblastic	Normoblastic	
Diagnosis	Iron deficiency Thalassaemia Anaemia of chronic disease Sideroblastic anaemia	Vitamin B$_{12}$ or folate deficiency	Alcohol ↑ Reticulocytes, e.g. haemolysis haemorrhage Liver disease Hypothyroidism Drugs, e.g. azathioprine	Acute blood loss Anaemia of chronic disease Chronic kidney disease Autoimmune rheumatic disease Marrow infiltration/fibrosis Endocrine disease Haemolytic anaemias

count would be expected following haemorrhage or haemolysis and during the response to treatment with haematinics. A low reticulocyte count occurs with bone marrow failure and with deficiency of haematinics.

- **Additional tests.** Other tests may be necessary to confirm the diagnosis, e.g. ferritin, iron studies, serum B_{12}, red cell folate, Hb electrophoresis, glucose-6-phosphate dehydrogenase (G6PD) levels.
- **Bone marrow sampling.** This is not necessary for simple haematinic deficiencies, but can be useful for assessing iron stores and erythropoiesis. A bone marrow examination is indicated if bone marrow failure (e.g. myelodysplasia, aplastic anaemia, acute leukaemia) or infiltration is suspected from the blood count and blood film.

MICROCYTIC ANAEMIAS

Iron deficiency anaemia

In developed countries, menstrual blood loss or an increased iron requirement during pregnancy and lactation is a frequent cause in younger women. In males and post-menopausal females with no obvious sign of bleeding, occult blood loss from the gastrointestinal tract is the commonest cause. Malabsorption of iron can also occur, e.g. in coeliac disease, but dietary deficiency is relatively uncommon. However, in developing countries, inadequate diet associated with poverty, vegetarianism and parasitic infections are major factors. The most common cause worldwide is gastrointestinal blood loss from hookworm infection.

Investigations

- **Blood count.** The red cells are microcytic (MCV < 80 fL) and hypochromic (mean cell haemoglobin (MCH) < 27 pg).
- **Blood film.** There is poikilocytosis and anisocytosis (Fig. 7.2). Target cells are seen.

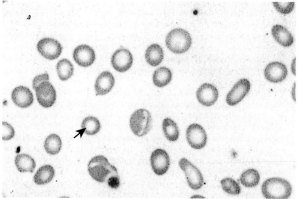

Fig. 7.2 Hypochromic microcytic cells (arrowed) on a blood film. Poikilocytosis (variation in shape) and anisocytosis (variation in size) are seen.

Kumar & Clark's Medical Management and Therapeutics

- Iron studies. A low **serum ferritin** (typical reference range in men 11.6–144 nmol/L (30–300 mcg/L) and women 5.8–96 nmol/L (15–200 mcg/L)) is diagnostic in uncomplicated iron deficiency, but because it is an acute-phase protein, a normal or even high serum ferritin does not exclude the diagnosis. **Serum iron** is usually low, and **total iron binding capacity** (TIBC) increased (these markers are less reliable indicators of iron stores). **Serum soluble transferrin receptors** are also increased.
- Bone marrow examination. This is not indicated unless other tests are unhelpful (e.g. normal/high ferritin in patients with inflammation) or coexisting causes of anaemia are suspected. Staining a bone marrow aspirate with Perls' reagent will demonstrate absence of iron stores.
- Other investigations. Investigations of the gastrointestinal tract (p. 153) for sources of bleeding or occult malignancy, or a gynaecological referral for menorrhagia may be appropriate, as directed by the history and examination.

Management

Identification and treatment of the underlying cause are essential. Oral iron is given to correct the anaemia and replenish stores.

- Oral iron. **Ferrous sulphate 200 mg** 3 times daily (180 mg ferrous iron in total) is best administered on an empty stomach before meals. An increase in Hb of 1 g/dL per week is usual and a rise in the reticulocyte count is seen in 7 days. Absorption is relatively inefficient, but improved by taking iron supplements with a source of ascorbic acid (e.g. fresh orange juice).
  - *Side-effects* are very common and include nausea, abdominal cramping, diarrhoea or constipation; therefore compliance can be a problem. Side-effects may be ameliorated by reducing the frequency or taking the iron with food.
  - **Ferrous gluconate** 300 mg twice daily can be prescribed as an alternative to ferrous sulphate, with fewer side-effects but a slower response (contains less elemental iron, 70 mg/day).
    Sustained-release or enteric-coated compounds are not recommended since they are expensive and poorly absorbed.
  - *Treatment* should be continued beyond correction of the Hb level, to ensure adequate replenishment of iron stores (typically 6 months). Common **causes of failure** to respond to oral iron include poor compliance, ongoing haemorrhage or incorrect diagnosis (e.g. thalassaemia trait).
- Parenteral iron. This should only be considered if oral therapy fails because of iron intolerance, in patients with severe malabsorption, or if rapid replenishment of iron stores is required, e.g. in pregnancy. Although replenishment of stores occurs more rapidly than with oral iron, the Hb level increases at the same rate. **Iron sucrose** (IV) and **iron dextran** (IV or IM) are the preparations available. The dose depends on iron deficit and body weight (consult product literature).
  - *Anaphylaxis.* **N.B.** Anaphylaxis (See Ch 20, p. 706) may occur with parenteral iron, so a small test dose should be given 1 hour before infusion. Facilities for cardiopulmonary resuscitation, including adrenaline (epinephrine), must be available.

The thalassaemias

This group of inherited anaemias is characterized by precipitation of excess globin chains in red cells (and their precursors) as a result of unbalanced α- or β-globin chain production (normally 1:1). This leads to ineffective erythropoiesis and haemolysis of mature red cells. The prevalence is high in parts of Africa, the Mediterranean, the Middle East, India and Asia.

α-Thalassaemia

α-Thalassaemia is caused by deletions or mutations in one or more of the four α-globin genes (two genes on each copy of chromosome 16), leading to an excess of β-globin chains. **Deletion of one gene** results in silent α-thalassaemia, which is of no clinical significance and the blood picture is usually normal. **Deletion of two genes** results in α-thalassaemia trait (microcytosis with or without mild anaemia but with normal serum iron and ferritin). Haemoglobin H (HbH) disease is caused by a **deletion of three α-globin genes**, and is characterized by a moderate haemolytic anaemia (Hb 7–10 g/dL) and splenomegaly. Regular transfusion is rarely required, but increased haemolysis may occur with oxidant drugs, as in G6PD deficiency (p. 216), and folic acid should be administered through-out pregnancy. If all **four α-globin genes are deleted** (Hb Barts), there is a complete absence of normal Hb production, which is incompatible with life outside the uterus (hydrops fetalis).

- Diagnosis is by α-globin gene analysis if required (e.g. pre-pregnancy genetic counselling), as Hb analysis by high-performance liquid chromatography (HPLC) or electrophoresis is normal.
- Genetic counselling of individuals with α-thalassaemia trait and HbH disease prior to pregnancy is mandatory.

β-Thalassaemia

β-Globin production is reduced (β⁺-thalassaemia) or absent (β⁰-thalassaemia) due to abnormalities in one or both β-globin genes, leading to precipitation of excess α-globin chains.

- *Thalassaemia minor (trait).* This is the asymptomatic heterozygous carrier state, associated with a mild hypochromic microcytic anaemia with a low MCV and MCH; it may be confused with iron deficiency but the RDW is normal. Iron stores are normal and iron should not be given.
- *Thalassaemia intermedia.* Thalassaemia intermedia is associated with moderate anaemia (Hb 7–10 g/dL) but patients are rarely transfusion-dependent. They may have splenomegaly, bone deformities and leg ulcers.
- *Thalassaemia major.* In thalassaemia major, both β-globin genes are severely dysfunctional, with extramedullary haematopoiesis leading to hepatosplenomegaly and bone expansion; the latter produces the classical thalassaemia facies. Disease presents in early infancy and results in severe transfusion-dependent anaemia.
- Investigations
  - *Blood count:* microcytic hypochromic anaemia. Iron studies normal. RDW normal.
  - *Hb electrophoresis or HPLC:* ↑ HbA₂ and/or ↑ HbF.
- Management of thalassaemia major
  - *Red cell transfusion* is required every 2–4 weeks in order to sup-press ineffective erythropoiesis and encourage normal growth and development throughout childhood. A 'trigger' Hb concentration of

Kumar & Clark's Medical Management and Therapeutics

around 9.5 g/dL is adequate, and lowers the rate of transfusional iron overload (transfusion haemosiderosis) associated with older 'hypertransfusion' regimens.

- *Iron chelation therapy* is essential in order to reduce damage to endocrine glands, liver, pancreas and myocardium caused by transfusion haemosiderosis.

  a) **Desferrioxamine** 20–50 mg/kg is administered by SC infusion over 8–12 hours on 3–7 nights per week, to chelate excess iron for excretion in the urine and faeces. Compliance is often a problem, especially in younger patients, so alternatively up to 2 g desferrioxamine can be administered intravenously alongside each unit of blood transfused (through a different IV line but using the same cannula). Local reactions occur and can be ameliorated by 2 mg of hydrocortisone added to the infusion bag. **Ascorbic acid 200 mg** daily increases the urinary excretion of iron in response to desferrioxamine, but should not be taken with food as it also increases iron absorption. **Complications** of long-term desferrioxamine therapy include cataracts, retinal damage, nerve deafness and infections, e.g. with *Yersinia enterocolitica*. The efficacy of iron chelation therapy should be periodically assessed by measurement of serum ferritin and hepatic iron stores. Visual acuity and hearing checks must be performed before long-term treatment and at 3-month intervals. Warn patients that desferrioxamine can turn their urine brown.

  b) **Deferasirox** (10–30 mg/kg daily) and **deferiprone** (25 mg/kg 3 times daily) are oral iron-chelating agents for use in patients with thalassaemia major who are unable to tolerate desferrioxamine. These oral agents are well tolerated, if taken dissolved in water or juice. They should be avoided in pregnancy; deferiprone is **contraindicated**, as it is teratogenic, and women of childbearing age should be advised to use appropriate contraception. There have also been reports of drug-induced neutropenia and hepatic damage with deferiprone, so it is not recommended as first-line therapy.

- *Long-term* **folic acid** *supplementation* is needed, as with all chronic haemolytic conditions (5 mg orally per day).

- *Splenectomy* is indicated in patients over the age of 6 years if transfusion requirements are increasing (there is an unacceptably high risk of sepsis associated with splenectomy in the under-6 age group). The spleen is the primary site of extravascular haemolysis. For postsplenectomy care, see Box 7.1.

- *Stem-cell transplantation (SCT)* is an option for young patients with an HLA-matched sibling donor, but the mortality increases significantly with age due to iron overload and hepatic dysfunction, and increasing alloimmunization by multiple transfusions (increasing the risk of graft rejection).

ANAEMIA OF CHRONIC DISEASE

A normochromic normocytic anaemia commonly occurs in association with chronic inflammatory and infective conditions (e.g. rheumatoid arthritis, malignancy, TB). The exact pathogenesis is complicated and contributing factors include a cytokine-mediated failure of iron utilization during erythropoiesis and high levels of hepcidin, which destroy

Vaccinate 2–3 weeks before elective splenectomy and record vaccination status clearly in patient case notes:
- 23-valent unconjugated pneumococcal polysaccharide vaccine repeated every 5 years
- Meningococcal group C conjugate vaccine
- Annual influenza vaccine
- *Haemophilus influenzae* type b (Hib) vaccine
- Long-term penicillin V 500 mg 12-hourly (or erythromycin)
- Meningococcal ACWY polysaccharide vaccine for travellers to Africa/Saudi Arabia, e.g. during Hajj and Umrah pilgrimages

ferroportin, limiting iron absorption in the intestinal cell. Red cell survival is decreased and there is an inappropriately low erythropoietin response for the level of anaemia. The MCV can be normal, or low in longstanding disease (resembling iron deficiency). The serum ferritin is usually normal or raised because of the inflammatory process. Iron is present in the bone marrow but not in developing erythroblasts.

Treatment
Address the underlying disorder, e.g. treat infection with antibiotics. **Red cell transfusions** may be necessary for symptomatic anaemia. Patients do not respond to oral iron, but coexisting iron deficiency should be identified and treated with parenteral iron (p. 202). **Recombinant erythropoietin therapy** at relatively high doses, e.g. 150–300 U/kg SC three times per week, is used, e.g. in rheumatoid arthritis, or intravenously in chronic kidney disease. **Pegylated (PEG) erythropoietin** is an alternative, administered once every 2 weeks.

Sideroblastic anaemias

The sideroblastic anaemias are uncommon disorders of iron metabolism characterized by refractory anaemia, with excess iron and ringed sideroblasts in the bone marrow.

Causes
Causes can be inherited or acquired. Acquired causes include drugs, such as anti-TB agents (isoniazid, pyrazinamide, cycloserine), chloramphenicol, D-penicillamine, progesterone; alcohol dependence; lead toxicity; myelodysplastic disorders; rheumatoid arthritis; and megaloblastic and haemolytic anaemias.

Treatment
Some inherited sideroblastic anaemias respond to oral **pyridoxine** 100–400 mg daily in divided doses. In acquired sideroblastic anaemia, treat the underlying cause if possible.

MACROCYTIC ANAEMIAS

Megaloblastic anaemia

Impaired DNA synthesis results in morphological abnormalities of blood cell precursors, characterized by delayed nuclear maturation

Kumar & Clark's Medical Management and Therapeutics

(nuclear-cytoplasmic asynchrony). All haematopoietic cell lines (and other rapidly dividing cells) are affected, and in severe cases there may be pancytopenia (i.e. anaemia, leucopenia and thrombocytopenia). Causes are predominantly those leading to B_{12} and folate deficiencies, although drugs (azathioprine, hydroxycarbamide, zidovudine), myelodysplasia and rare enzyme deficiencies affecting DNA synthesis (e.g. orotic aciduria) can also cause macrocytosis and anaemia.

- **Folic acid deficiency** develops over a few months, whereas B_{12} deficiency takes years to develop as B_{12} is stored in the liver. Folate deficiency is due to poor intake (elderly, excess alcohol use); increased utilization (pregnancy, haemolytic anaemia); malabsorption (e.g. coeliac disease); and drug therapy (anticonvulsants, trimethoprim, oral contraceptives, methotrexate, sulfasalazine, pyrimethamine), which can interfere with folate metabolism.
- **Vitamin B_{12} deficiency** can be caused by failure of intrinsic factor production in the stomach (pernicious anaemia, post-gastrectomy); malabsorption (pancreatic insufficiency, bacterial overgrowth); ileal lesions leading to B_{12} malabsorption (ileitis, e.g. inflammatory bowel disease); terminal ileal resection; and fish tapeworm (e.g. *Diphyllobothrium latum*). Vegans do not consume animal products and can become B_{12}-deficient, but will respond to oral B_{12} supplementation.

Clinical features

In **pernicious anaemia** the fall in Hb can be insidious and may not become symptomatic until the anaemia is severe. If the B_{12} is very low (e.g. < 60 ng/L (50 pmol/L)), neurological complications (e.g. symmetrical paraesthesiae in fingers and toes, early loss of vibration sense and proprioception) can occur. Very rarely, this is seen in the absence of significant anaemia.

If B_{12} deficiency is not corrected, subacute combined degeneration of the spinal cord can develop (combined spinal cord and peripheral nerve damage). Pernicious anaemia is frequently associated with other autoimmune diseases (e.g. hypothyroidism). Folate deficiency is not associated with neurological problems.

Investigations

- **Blood count.** This shows a macrocytic anaemia with anisocytosis, poikilocytosis and hypersegmented neutrophils (Fig. 7.3). Leucopenia and thrombocytopenia occur.
- **Serum B_{12} and red cell folate.** Samples must be taken before commencement of treatment. Red cell folate is a more accurate assessment of body stores than serum folate (which reflects recent intake).
- **Other investigations**
  - **Serum intrinsic factor auto-antibodies** are specific for pernicious anaemia but found in only 50% of cases. **Parietal cell antibodies** are less specific but are present in 90%. **Serum methylmalonic acid** (MMA) and **homocysteine** (HC) are raised in B_{12} deficiency. HC alone is raised in folate deficiency. **Bone marrow biopsy** is occasionally indicated to differentiate from myelodysplasia or malignancy, e.g. chronic myeloid leukaemia (CML).
  - Gastrointestinal investigations to exclude coeliac disease (p. 154), and imaging studies for inflammatory bowel disease (p. 157). Endoscopy

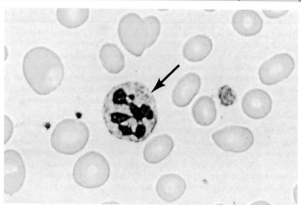

Fig. 7.3 Macrocytes and a hypersegmented neutrophil (arrowed) on a peripheral blood film.

is performed if there are gastric symptoms. The Schilling test to investigate B_{12} absorption is no longer routinely available.

Treatment

Transfusion should be avoided in chronic compensated anaemia (increased risk of congestive cardiac failure, especially in the elderly). Concurrent administration of vitamin B_{12} and folic acid may be necessary in severely ill patients while investigation results are awaited.

- Vitamin B_{12} deficiency. **IM hydroxocobalamin** 1 mg every 3–4 days is administered to a total dose of 5–6 mg. Thereafter, maintenance treatment with 1 mg IM every 3 months is usually necessary for life. A clinical improvement may be seen within 48 hours, and a peak reticulocytosis at 5–7 days. Hypokalaemia and iron deficiency can occur with the commencement of treatment and serum potassium should be checked. **Oral vitamin B_{12}** is absorbed by passive diffusion (1–2%) in the absence of intrinsic factor, so a 2 mg daily dose may be sufficient maintenance therapy for selected compliant patients.

- Folate deficiency. Oral **folic acid** 5 mg daily for at least 4 months is necessary to replenish stores in patients with folic acid deficiency. In pregnancy, all women are advised to take 400 mcg folic acid daily from at least 3 months prior to conception until the end of the first trimester, except where overt folic acid deficiency has been demonstrated (full-dose treatment required). **N.B.** Unless the serum B_{12} level is known to be normal, patients with megaloblastic anaemia should *never* receive folic acid replacement alone (risk of precipitating subacute combined degeneration of the spinal cord).

Other macrocytic anaemias

Macrocytosis in the peripheral blood with a normoblastic bone marrow is seen with alcohol excess, liver disease, hypothyroidism, reticulocytosis, some drugs (e.g. azathioprine) and aplastic anaemia.

— Kumar & Clark's Medical Management and Therapeutics

APLASTIC ANAEMIA

Aplastic anaemia is defined as pancytopenia with a virtual absence of reticulocytes and hypocellularity (aplasia) of the bone marrow. Causes of aplasia include drugs, e.g. chemotherapy (busulfan, doxorubicin), chloramphenicol, penicillamine, carbamazepine, phenytoin, chemicals (e.g. benzene), insecticides, ionizing radiation, viruses (e.g. hepatitis, EBV, HIV, erythrovirus B_{19} (previously parvovirus B_{19})), TB, paroxysmal nocturnal haemoglobinuria, myelodysplasia and primary bone marrow disease, e.g. leukaemia, myeloma, myelofibrosis.

Clinical and laboratory features

Symptoms of anaemia, bleeding and infection (especially of the mouth) occur. A bone marrow trephine biopsy is indicated to differentiate aplastic anaemia from other causes of pancytopenia and bone marrow failure, and characteristically shows hypocellularity with increased fat spaces. Further investigations should be directed at identifying secondary causes.

Treatment

For secondary aplastic anaemia, remove the cause if possible. Patients should be referred to a specialist centre as soon as possible for confirmation of the diagnosis and guidance on further management.

- Supportive care. This is the mainstay of therapy whilst awaiting bone marrow recovery (including stringent measures to prevent infection). Rapid treatment of infection with broad-spectrum parenteral **antibiotics** is essential, as for neutropenic patients (p. 261). **Red cell transfusion and platelets** should be kept to a minimum (p. 231, platelet transfusion thresholds) if SCT is being considered, as alloimmunization by donor blood products increases the risk of graft rejection.

- SCT. This is the treatment of choice for young patients with severe disease (characterized by the presence of two or more of the following: neutrophils $< 0.5 \times 10^9/L$, platelets $< 20 \times 10^9/L$, reticulocytes $< 40 \times 10^9/L$) and an HLA-identical sibling donor. For eligible patients (< 40 years of age), the search for a donor should begin as soon as the diagnosis has been made. Long-term survival and recovery of blood count to normal occurs in 75–90% of patients who have a sibling donor. Results with SCT from an unrelated donor are less favourable (5-year survival of 30%) due to a high incidence of graft versus host disease (GVHD), viral infection (e.g. cytomegalovirus reactivation) and graft rejection. Therefore, unrelated donor-SCT is often reserved for patients who do not respond to immunosuppressive therapy.

- Immunosuppressive therapy. A combination of **antithymocyte globulin (ATG)** and **ciclosporin** produces a response in 60–80% of patients, although there is a high relapse rate and risk of development of other clonal haematopoietic disorders. With treatment the 5-year survival is ~75%. **Rabbit ATG** (3.75 mg/kg/day for 5 days) is administered as an IV infusion into a central vein over 12–18 hours. **Horse ATG** was first-line therapy until recently but is no longer available. Profound immunosuppression and anaphylaxis can occur (a test dose is recommended before starting therapy). **Corticosteroids** have little activity in aplastic anaemia, but **prednisolone** is used to prevent serum sickness in patients receiving ATG (methylprednisolone 2 mg/kg/day given IV as a 30-min infusion before each ATG infusion, then oral prednisolone 1 mg/kg/day for 9 days from day 6 of therapy, tailed off over 5 days). Ciclosporin

5 mg/kg/day in a divided dose is commenced on the first day of ATG therapy (to maintain a trough blood level of 150–250 mcg/L for adults, 100–150 mcg/L for children). The dose of ciclosporin may need to be reduced if **itraconazole** is used for antifungal prophylaxis. Immunosuppressive therapy for aplastic anaemia should only be given under specialist supervision, and is contraindicated in the presence of active infection or uncontrolled bleeding.

- **Androgenic steroids. Oxymetholone** (1–5 mg/kg/day for 3–6 months) is sometimes effective in patients not responding to immunosuppression. Side-effects include hepatotoxicity and virilization.

Pure red cell aplasia is rare but can be due to persistent erythrovirus B_{19}. A thymoma is the underlying cause in about one-third of cases, and these patients may respond to thymectomy. An erythropoietin receptor agonist can correct the anaemia in those with anti-erythropoietin antibody.

MYELODYSPLASTIC SYNDROMES

The myelodysplastic syndromes (MDS) are a heterogeneous group of clonal haematopoietic stem-cell disorders, characterized by increased apoptosis of myeloid cell lines (red cells, granulocyte/monocytes and platelets), leading to ineffective haematopoiesis and peripheral cytopenias. They were reclassified by the WHO in 2008. Disease may be idiopathic, or secondary to previous chemoradiotherapy or exposure to environmental toxins. A small number of cases are associated with rare familial disorders, e.g. Fanconi's anaemia. Transformation to acute myeloblastic leukaemia (AML) occurs in one-third of patients.

Clinical features

The MDS most commonly affect the elderly (median age 69 years). Anaemia, bleeding and infection occur, depending on the degree and nature of the cytopenias.

Investigations

- Bone marrow histology is often hypercellular, despite cytopenias in the peripheral blood, but with gross morphological abnormalities. Ringed sideroblasts may be present (abnormal iron distribution in developing erythroblasts on Perls' stain). A high proportion of blast cells (> 5%) is associated with a poor prognosis. Bone marrow chromosomal analysis (cytogenetics) may show clonal abnormalities, which confirm the diagnosis and provide valuable prognostic information.
- Additional investigations (e.g. liver and renal biochemistry, CXR, ECG) are necessary to assess the level of co-morbidity before treatment decisions can be made, particularly in elderly patients.

Treatment

This is mainly supportive in patients with low-risk MDS (< 5% blasts in the bone marrow and ≤ one type of cytopenia) or in elderly patients with coexisting medical problems.

- Red-cell transfusions as required are used to treat **symptomatic anaemia**. Iron chelation with SC **desferrioxamine** or **oral therapy** (p. 204) should be considered once 25 U red cells (~5 g iron) have been transfused. Vitamin C 100–200 mg/day orally can be added after 1 month of therapy. **Neutropenic sepsis** requires urgent broad-spectrum IV antibiotics (p. 261). For **thrombocytopenia**, platelet transfusions are given to maintain a platelet count $> 10 \times 10^9/L$, or higher in patients with active bleeding.

- Erythropoietin (EPO) ± granulocyte-colony stimulating factor (G-CSF) may reduce or eliminate the need for red cell transfusion in some patients with MDS. Low-dose G-CSF may be appropriate in patients with severe chronic neutropenia, to maintain a neutrophil count of $> 1 \times 10^9/L$ (dose depends on product — refer to product literature).

- Immunosuppression with **antilymphocyte globulin (ALG)** as for aplastic anaemia can produce a sustained neutrophil and platelet response in hypoplastic MDS.

- 5-azacytidine 75 mg/m^2 SC for 7 days of a 28-day cycle, for 4–6 cycles, is an epigenetic therapy (hypomethylating agent) currently under scrutiny in clinical trials. Overall response rates of up to 47% have been seen in some subtypes of MDS, with a tendency towards increased overall survival.

- Lenalidomide (a thalidomide analogue) 10 mg daily for 21 days of a 28-day cycle is useful in the 5q- syndrome. **N.B.** Contraindicated in pregnancy; appropriate contraception *must* be advised. Neutropenia, thrombocytopenia and thromboembolism are all complications.

- Intensive chemotherapy regimes, as for AML (p. 284), are sometimes used for younger patients with high-risk MDS and good performance status. However, unless followed by an SCT procedure, there is little or no benefit in terms of overall survival for most patients.

- SCT offers the best chance of long-term remission in patients < 50 years with intermediate- or high-risk MDS, especially if an HLA-identical sibling donor is available. Matched unrelated donor SCT is associated with a high transplant-related mortality and is usually reserved for otherwise healthy intermediate-/high-risk patients under the age of 40, but the age limit is increasing with the introduction of reduced-intensity conditioning (RIC) protocols (p. 264).

HAEMOLYTIC ANAEMIAS

- Extravascular haemolysis occurs when red cells are phagocytosed and destroyed by macrophages in the reticuloendothelial system (mainly spleen and liver). A proportion of red cells are not completely destroyed and are released back into the circulation as spherocytes.

- Intravascular haemolysis occurs when red cells are lysed and release free Hb directly into the circulation. Most of the free Hb binds to plasma haptoglobins or is excreted in the urine, but some is deposited inside renal tubular cells as haemosiderin. This leads to raised levels of plasma haemoglobin, haemosiderinuria, very low or absent haptoglobulins and the formation of methaemalbumin (positive Schumm's test). Clinical features include fever and backache; renal failure can occur, depending on the aetiology.

Investigations

Investigation is to confirm that haemolysis is occurring and then to identify a mechanism, e.g. immune (indicated by a positive direct antiglobulin test (DAT)) vs. non-immune, intravascular vs. extravascular. A family history can be helpful.

Causes

Causes of haemolysis are shown in Figure 7.4.

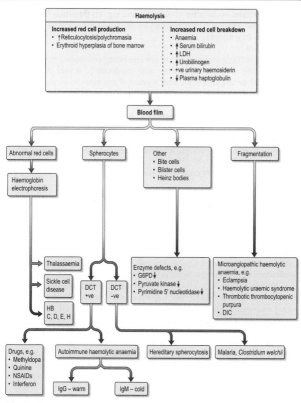

Fig. 7.4 Haemolysis. DCT, direct Coombs' test; DIC, disseminated intravascular coagulation; G6PD, glucose-6-phosphate dehydrogenase; LDH, lactate dehydrogenase.

Inherited haemolytic anaemias

Thalassaemias
See p. 203.

Hereditary spherocytosis
Hereditary spherocytosis (HS) is the commonest inherited cause of chronic haemolytic anaemia in Northern Europeans (1 in 5000 births). Inheritance is usually autosomal dominant but 25% of cases are due to spontaneous mutations. The red cells are poorly deformable due to abnormalities in the red cell cytoskeleton, so they become trapped in splenic sinusoids where they are destroyed. HS can present at any age (neonatal jaundice is common) and the clinical features are highly variable. Many patients are asymptomatic but features of chronic compensated haemolysis may be present, e.g. pigment gallstones, mild jaundice and splenomegaly. Aplastic

crises sometimes occur after viral infections, e.g. erythrovirus B_{19}. Investigations show anaemia and spherocytes on blood film, with evidence of haemolysis (see above).

● Treatment
  - *Splenectomy* removes the major site of red cell destruction and corrects the anaemia in patients with moderate to severe disease, but should be avoided until after 6 years of age because of the increased risk of overwhelming infection (Box 7.1, p. 205). Mildly affected patients may only require supportive treatment, but splenectomy is usually necessary in patients with hyperbilirubinaemia or symptomatic cholelithiasis.
  - **Oral folic acid** 5 mg daily is recommended for adults with moderate and severe HS to correct losses incurred by increased bone marrow turnover.
  - *Blood transfusion* may be necessary during aplastic crises.

Sickle syndromes

Sickle haemoglobin (HbS) is the result of a valine substitution for glutamic acid at position 6 in the β-globin chain, caused by a single-base mutation in the β-globin gene ($\alpha_2\beta_2^{6glu\rightarrow val}$). Two abnormal genes result in homozygous sickle cell anaemia (HbSS), and one abnormal gene results in the heterozygous carrier state, sickle cell trait (HbAS). Sickle cell disease is a collective term used to describe sickle cell anaemia and additional sickle syndromes caused by combined heterozygosity for HbS with other abnormal haemoglobins, e.g. HbC (HbSC disease), β-thalassaemia (HbS-β^0/ β^+-thalassaemia) or HbD (HbSD disease). At low oxygen tension, HbS forms an insoluble polymer, which irreversibly distorts red cells into the characteristic sickle shape. Sickle cells are poorly deformable and show abnormally increased adherence to vascular endothelium. Obstruction of small blood vessels leads to painful tissue infarction (sickle cell crisis). Most patients with sickle cell disease are of African descent, although the disease is also found in India, the Middle East and Southern Europe. The presence of HbS offers some protection against malaria; therefore the frequency of HbS carriers is high.

Sickle cell trait is usually asymptomatic, unless extreme circumstances lead to anoxia, such as travel in non-pressurized aircraft or problems with anaesthesia.

HbSC disease shares many clinical features with HbSS disease, but patients usually have higher baseline Hb, and there is an increased incidence of thromboembolic disease (especially during pregnancy) and retinopathy.

Sickle cell anaemia (HbSS)

Investigations

(See also demonstration of haemolysis, Fig. 7.4).

● Blood count and blood film (Fig. 7.5). Anaemia (Hb 6–8 g/dL) with normal MCV and MCH (unless coexisting thalassaemia), sickle cells, target cells and polychromasia (due to reticulocytosis). Adult patients will also have features of hyposplenism (basophilic stippling, Howell-Jolly bodies, Pappenheimer bodies).
● Sickle solubility test. Positive in the presence of HbS, but does not distinguish between sickle cell trait and sickle cell disease. Rapid screening solubility tests are available.

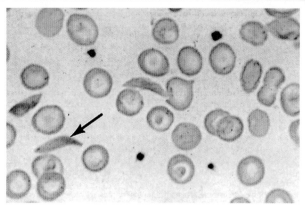

Fig. 7.5 Sickle cells (arrowed) and target cells.

- Hb electrophoresis. Required for confirmation of the diagnosis, and in homozygous sickle cell anaemia shows 80–95% HbS, with 2–20% fetal Hb (HbF). Normal Hb (HbA) is absent. Parents of an affected child will have features of sickle cell trait.

Clinical syndromes and management

- General management. Patients should be advised to seek urgent treatment for infections, and to minimize other factors that may precipitate a crisis where possible, such as dehydration, hypoxia and acidosis (e.g. from vigorous physical exercise) or exposure to cold temperatures. Multiple splenic infarctions over time result in autosplenectomy; therefore all patients should receive **appropriate antibiotic prophylaxis** and **vaccination** (Box 7.1, p. 205).

  - **Folic acid** *supplements* (5 mg daily) are recommended for all patients.
  - *Yearly ophthalmologic reviews* are necessary to detect and treat proliferative retinopathy.
  - *Psychological and social support* should involve a multidisciplinary team.
  - *Family counselling* should be offered as a basis for antenatal screening and diagnosis.
  - *Preventive therapy* includes **hydroxycarbamide (hydroxyurea)**, which reduces the frequency of painful crises and acute chest syndrome, and the need for **blood transfusions** (and iron chelation, p. 204) in adults with sickle cell disease. It increases the concentration of fetal Hb (HbF), which protects against sickling. The usual dose is 20–30 mg/kg/day orally. Long-term safety data suggest that there is a low incidence of secondary malignancy with prolonged use. Hydroxycarbamide is **contraindicated** during pregnancy and breast feeding, and should be avoided in both female *and* male patients who are trying to conceive. In an acute crisis, hydroxycarbamide must be stopped if platelets are $< 100 \times 10^9/\text{L}$, neutrophils $< 1 \times 10^9/\text{L}$ or reticulocytes $< 100 \times 10^9/\text{L}$.

Kumar & Clark's Medical Management and Therapeutics

- *SCT* is best reserved for children and adolescents younger than 16 years of age, who have severe complications (strokes, recurrent chest syndrome, or refractory pain) and an HLA-matched donor.

● **Anaemia.** Chronic haemolysis results in a steady state Hb of 6–8 g/dL, but symptoms of anaemia are mild because HbS releases oxygen to tissues more readily than normal Hb. Increased haemolysis can occur with certain drugs, acute infection and associated G6PD deficiency. Anaemia can also result from folate deficiency. A sudden drop in Hb is suggestive of aplastic or sequestration crisis (see below). Transfusion is not indicated for steady state anaemia, but if it is necessary a full antibody screen should be performed, and blood should be fully matched for Rh (C, D and E) and Kell antigens to reduce the risk of alloimmunization.

● **Vaso-occlusive crises.** Episodes of acute severe pain and fever due to bone marrow infarction and inflammation can present with variable frequency in patients with sickle cell disease. Dactylitis (painful swollen hands and feet) is common in young children, whereas severe pain in long bones, vertebrae, ribs and pelvis occurs in older children and adults.

- *Analgesia*
  - **Morphine** and **diamorphine** are the drugs of choice for severe pain (see Chapter 20).
  - **Antiemetics**, e.g. cyclizine 50 mg 3 times daily should always be given with these analgesics. **Inhaled nitrous oxide/oxygen** (50/50) is sometimes useful for initial pain control but should not be used for more than 60 mins at a time. Pethidine should not routinely be prescribed because the duration of the analgesic effect is much shorter than with morphine and there are concerns over safety (CNS and renal toxicity). With **opioid analgesia**, pain, respiratory rate and level of sedation should be monitored every 30 mins until the pain is controlled and every 2 hours thereafter. The dose should be reduced gradually (every 2–3 days) and replaced with oral analgesia as necessary. Regular **laxatives** should always be prescribed with opioids.
  - **Adjunctive oral analgesics, e.g. codeine, paracetamol or NSAIDs**, are effective and can be used alone for less severe pain, which is often managed in the community.
- *Supportive therapy.* This includes **IV fluids** and bed rest. If infection is suspected, empirical **antibiotic therapy** (e.g. a cephalosporin) should be started pending the results of blood, urine and sputum cultures. There is an increased risk of venous thromboembolic disease in patients with sickle cell disease, so prophylaxis with a low-molecular-weight heparin (LMWH, p. 243) should be given during an acute crisis. Blood transfusion is not indicated in uncomplicated crises.

● Acute chest syndrome (Box 7.2).
● This is a major cause of sudden death among patients with sickle cell disease. Chest pain, dyspnoea, fever, hypoxia and evidence of consolidation on physical and radiological examination are highly suggestive of chest crisis.
● It is a **medical emergency** requiring immediate admission to hospital and aggressive treatment.
● Precipitating causes include infection (e.g. *Streptococcus pneumoniae*, *Mycoplasma*, *Chlamydia*), pulmonary infarction and fat embolization from necrotic bone marrow.

Box 7.2 **Management of acute painful crisis in opioid-naïve adults with sickle cell disease.** Higher doses may be required for patients who have previously received opioids.

Morphine/Diamorphine:
- 0.1 mg/kg IV/SC every 20 minutes until pain controlled, then
- 0.05–0.1 mg/kg IV/SC (or oral morphine) every 2–4 hours
- Patient controlled analgesia (PCA) when pain controlled

Patient controlled analgesia (PCA) (example for adults >50 kg)

Diamorphine/Morphine:
- Continuous infusion: 0–10 mg/h
- PCA bolus dose: 2–10 mg
- Dose duration: 1 minute
- Lockout time: 20–30 minutes

Adjuvant oral analgesia:
- Paracetamol 1g 6 hourly
- +/− Ibuprofen* 400 mg 8 hourly
- or Diclofenac* 50 mg 8 hourly

Laxatives (all patients). For example:
- Lactulose 10 ml x 2 daily
- Senna 2–4 tablets daily
- Sodium docusate 100 mg x 2 daily
- Macrogol 1 sachet daily
- Lubiprostone

Other adjuvants:
Anti-pruritics:
- Hydroxyzine 25 mg x 2 daily as required

Antiemetics:
- Prochlorperazine 5–10 mg x 3 as required
- Cyclizine 50 mg x 3 as required

Anxiolytic:
- Haloperidol 1–3 mg oral/IM x 2 as required

*Caution advised with the use of NSAIDs in renal failure.
(Adapted from Rees DC et al. 2003.)

- *Management of acute chest crises*
- High-flow supplemental **oxygen**, **analgesia** and **antibiotics** — a broad-spectrum cephalosporin such as cefotaxime 1 g 12-hourly, and a macrolide such as **clarithromycin** 500 mg twice daily — should be commenced without delay.
- Continuous positive airway pressure (CPAP) ventilation may be beneficial, but transfer to ICU for ventilation should be arranged if the PO_2 on air cannot be maintained above 8 κP (approx < 60 mmHg) with $Fio_2 > 0.6$.
- **Exchange blood transfusion** (6 U out, 6 U in via IV line or using a cell separator where available) is essential if there is clinical deterioration despite CPAP or if the patient requires ventilation.

- **Sequestration crisis.** Vaso-occlusion and pooling of red cells within splenic sinusoids and liver can lead to sudden severe anaemia, hypovolaemia and death. It is commonest in children before autosplenectomy occurs, but may present in adults with composite heterozygous conditions (e.g. HbSC disease) where the spleen is still functional. **Emergency blood transfusion** and haemodynamic support are required, and **splenectomy** may be needed for recurrent episodes.

- **Aplastic crisis.** Viral infections (usually erythrovirus B$_{19}$) can trigger a sudden decrease in marrow production of blood cells. Bone marrow function usually recovers spontaneously within 1–2 weeks, but transfusional support is required in the interim.

- **Cerebral vascular event (stroke).** This is a relatively common occurrence in children under the age of 10 years and adults over 30. Yearly Doppler ultrasound is performed to look for significant arterial stenosis. Emergency exchange transfusion is indicated for acute stroke and the patient should be regularly transfused to maintain an HbS concentration of < 30% for at least 3 years; this reduces the incidence of recurrence. One-third of strokes are due to haemorrhage and this has a high mortality.

- **Priapism.** A persistent and painful penile erection due to vaso-occlusion occurs in over half of male patients at some time, and can lead to erectile dysfunction if left untreated for > 24 hours. Urgent referral to a urologist is necessary, and treatment options include exchange transfusion and surgical decompression.

- **Infections.** Hyposplenism and vaso-occlusion predispose patients to infection with organisms such as *Salmonella*, *Staphylococcus aureus* and *Strep. pneumoniae*. Osteomyelitis, pyelonephritis and pneumonia are common and should be treated with appropriate antibiotics.

- **Preparation for surgery.** Repeated transfusions over several weeks to reduce the proportion of circulating HbS to < 20% should prevent sickling for elective procedures. Exchange transfusion may be necessary before emergency surgery.

- **Pregnancy.** Painful episodes, infection and severe anaemia in the mother are more common, particularly in the third trimester, and are managed as for non-pregnant patients. Regular **transfusion** to reduce the proportion of circulating HbS to < 20% is occasionally necessary. Pre-eclampsia, spontaneous abortion and intrauterine growth retardation also occur more frequently in patients with sickle cell disease, but prophylactic transfusion does not improve fetal outcome.

Long-term problems

Repeated crises lead to **avascular osteonecrosis** (especially hip and shoulder joints — joint replacement often required), leg ulcers, pulmonary hypertension and chronic lung disease, cardiac and neurological problems, retinopathy, hepatic dysfunction, cholelithiasis, chronic tubulo-interstitial nephritis and delayed sexual maturation.

Glucose-6-phosphate dehydrogenase (G6PD) deficiency

G6PD deficiency is a common X-linked disorder prevalent in Africa, the Mediterranean, the Middle East and South-East Asia. G6PD-deficient red cells are more susceptible to oxidative damage and subsequent haemolysis in the spleen. Several different types exist, with varying degrees of enzyme deficiency and clinical severity.

Clinical and laboratory features

Rapid intravascular haemolysis with symptomatic anaemia, jaundice and haemoglobinuria occurs 1–3 days after ingestion of certain drugs (Box 7.3). Infection can also precipitate haemolysis but the anaemia is usually mild. Favism (severe haemolysis after ingestion of fava beans) occurs with the Mediterranean variant and can be rapidly fatal. Chronic non-spherocytic haemolytic anaemia (in the absence of a precipitating cause) and neonatal jaundice are also seen in some types of G6PD deficiency.

- The **blood count** and **blood film** are only abnormal during an acute episode, when 'bite' cells and Heinz bodies (on methyl violet staining) may be seen.
- Reticulocytosis and other features of haemolysis may be present (p. 210).
- Measurement of G6PD levels (during the steady state between attacks) and DNA analysis will confirm the diagnosis.

Treatment

Treatment includes withdrawal of precipitant drugs, treatment of infection and adequate hydration to maintain a good urine output. Blood transfusion may be required for severe haemolysis or symptomatic anaemia.

Pyruvate kinase (PK) deficiency

This is an autosomal recessive defect of red cell metabolism associated with chronic haemolytic anaemia and splenomegaly. The diagnosis can be confirmed by measurement of PK levels. **Treatment** is with blood transfusion as necessary (e.g. during infections and pregnancy) and folic acid supplementation. Splenectomy may be beneficial.

ACQUIRED HAEMOLYTIC ANAEMIAS

Autoimmune haemolytic anaemias

Autoimmune haemolytic anaemias (AIHA) can be caused by 'warm' or 'cold' autoantibodies, depending on the temperature (37°C or < 37°C) at which the antibody binds to red cells. In AIHA, opsonized red cells are phagocytosed by the reticuloendothelial system.

Warm AIHA

Warm AIHA most commonly occurs > 50 years of age and has a female preponderance, in common with other autoimmune conditions. It can be idiopathic or secondary to autoimmune rheumatological disorders (e.g. SLE); malignancy (lymphomas, carcinomas, chronic lymphocytic leukaemia, Hodgkin's lymphoma); or drugs (e.g. methyldopa). The clinical features are highly variable, ranging from acute severe anaemia with jaundice, to chronic compensated haemolysis. Splenomegaly is often present.

- Investigations show evidence of haemolytic anaemia (p. 210) with spherocytosis. The DAT, or Coomb's test, is positive for IgG (C3-positive or negative).
- Treatment is of the underlying cause. **Corticosteroids** (prednisolone 1 mg/kg/day) are effective in 80% of patients. **Splenectomy** and other **immunosuppressive drugs**, e.g. **azathioprine**, **cyclophosphamide** or **rituximab**, are used in those who fail to respond to steroids. **Folic acid** is also given.

Cold AIHA

Autoantibodies agglutinate red cells at temperatures < 32°C, causing cyanotic discoloration of the extremities in cold conditions. Complement

Box 7.3 Drugs causing haemolysis

In immune haemolytic anaemia

- Antihistamines
- Cephalosporins
- Chlorpromazine
- Dapsone
- Diclofenac
- Ibuprofen
- Interferon-α
- Isoniazid
- Levodopa
- Mefenamic acid
- Melphalan
- Methyldopa
- Penicillins
- Probenecid
- Procainamide
- Quinidine
- Quinine
- Ribavirin
- Rifampicin
- Sulphonamides
- Tetracycline
- Tolbutamide

In G6PD deficiency

Analgesics, e.g.
- Aspirin
- Phenacetin (withdrawn in the UK)

Antimalarials, e.g.
- Primaquine
- Pyrimethamine
- Quinine
- Chloroquine

Antibacterials, e.g.
- Most sulphonamides
- Nitrofurantoin
- Chloramphenicol
- Quinolones

Miscellaneous drugs, e.g.
- Vitamin K
- Probenecid
- Quinidine
- Dimercaprol
- Phenylhydrazine
- Dapsone
- Methylene blue

activation and intravascular haemolysis occur when coated red cells return to 37°C on re-circulation.

- Cold haemagglutinin disease (CHAD) is the most common syndrome, which can be acute and transient after infection (*Mycoplasma*, EBV) or chronic (idiopathic or secondary to a lymphoproliferative disorder). Red cell agglutination at room temperature may cause a spuriously low Hb and increased MCV if the FBC sample is not warmed prior to testing.
  - *Treatment* is of the underlying cause where possible. Exposure to cold should be avoided. The acute infection-related form is usually self-limiting, but if blood transfusion is necessary it should be administered via a blood warmer. **Corticosteroids** are usually ineffective. **Anti-CD20** monoclonal antibody **(rituximab)** or plasma exchange is occasionally useful.
- Paroxysmal cold haemoglobinuria is a rare but usually self-limiting cause of intravascular haemolysis, associated with common childhood infections, such as measles, mumps and chickenpox. The biphasic, cold-reacting IgG auto-antibodies are specific for P red cell antigens, and the diagnosis is confirmed by the Donath–Landsteiner test. Supportive **transfusions of warmed blood** may be necessary.

Drug-induced immune haemolytic anaemia

Interaction between certain drugs and the red cell membrane can sometimes stimulate antibody formation, which may lead to extravascular or intravascular haemolysis (Box 7.3). Treatment is by withdrawal of the responsible drug.

Alloimmune haemolytic anaemias

Haemolytic transfusion reactions are discussed on p. 226.

Non-immune haemolytic anaemia

Paroxysmal nocturnal haemoglobinuria (PNH)

This is a rare form of chronic haemolytic anaemia, characterized by episodic intravascular haemolysis and haemoglobinuria. It is due to mutations in the X-linked gene *PIG-A*, which result in defective binding of CD55 and CD59 proteins to the cell surface, and failure to inactivate complement. Venous thromboses in unusual sites (e.g. Budd–Chiari syndrome) are a common feature. Transformation to aplastic anaemia (p. 208) or AML (p. 284) occurs in a proportion of patients

- Diagnosis is by confirmation of intravascular haemolysis (p. 210), and flow cytometry to demonstrate the presence of a haematopoietic cell clone deficient in cell surface antigens CD55 and CD59.
- Supportive treatment with blood transfusion and thromboprophylaxis may be necessary. Long-term anticoagulation is required in patients with recurrent thrombosis.
- Eculizumab (monoclonal antibody; prevents cleavage of complement component C5) has been shown to reduce haemolysis and transfusion requirements in patients with PNH. Dose is IV infusion 600 mg once weekly for 4 weeks, then 900 mg on week 5. Maintenance 900 mg every 12–16 days. Vaccinate against *Neisseria meningitides* 2 weeks before treatment.
- SCT should be considered in young patients or if transformation occurs.

Kumar & Clark's Medical Management and Therapeutics

Mechanical haemolytic anaemia

Causes include artificial heart valves, march haemoglobinuria or long-distance running, and microangiopathic haemolytic anaemia. Treatment is directed at the underlying cause.

MYELOPROLIFERATIVE NEOPLASMS

Polycythaemia

Polycythaemia (or erythrocytosis) is defined as an increase in total red cell mass, as suggested by a raised haematocrit (HCT). The cause can be primary (polycythaemia vera, a myeloproliferative neoplasm), or secondary due to an **appropriate increase** in erythropoietin, e.g. high altitude, lung disease, right to left shunt. An **inappropriate increase** in erythropoietin occurs with renal, liver and endocrine (adrenal) tumours. A relative polycythaemia/erythrocytosis due to decreased plasma volume can be associated with dehydration, burns, smoking, alcohol, hypertension and obesity.

Polycythaemia vera (primary proliferative polycythaemia)

Primary polycythaemia vera (PV) is a clonal stem-cell disorder characterized by excessive proliferation of erythroid, myeloid and megakaryocytic progenitor cells. Most cases (> 90%) are due to a *JAK2 V617F* mutation (substitution of phenylalanine for valine in the Janus kinase (*JAK2*) gene, which stimulates erythropoiesis). A typical presentation is in patients over the age of 60 with non-specific symptoms (e.g. lethargy, headaches, dizziness). Pruritus after bathing and a burning sensation in the fingers and toes (erythromelalgia) are symptoms that are highly suggestive of PV. Physical signs include plethoric facies and hepatosplenomegaly. There may also be a history of gout as a result of increased cell turnover. The natural history of PV is progression to myelofibrosis (30% of patients at 20 years) and, less commonly, transformation to AML.

Diagnosis

This is based on the revised WHO criteria and requires either both major and one minor criteria, or the first major and two minor criteria.

- Major criteria
  - Hb > 18.5 g/dL in men, 16.5 g/dL in women or other evidence of increased red cell volume.
  - Presence of *JAK2 V617F* or other similar mutation.
- Minor criteria
  - Bone marrow biopsy showing hypercellularity for age with trilineage (erythroid, granulocytic and megakaryocytic) proliferation.
  - Serum erythropoietin level below reference range for normal.
  - Endogenous erythroid colony (EEC) formation in vitro.

Management

Treatment of PV minimizes the risk of complications, such as thrombosis, haemorrhage and hyperviscosity, but does not affect the rate of transformation into other myeloproliferative diseases or AML. Patients should also be advised to reduce other cardiovascular risk factors, such as smoking and obesity.

- Venesection. This is first-line treatment for most patients, with a target HCT < 0.45 (for males and females) to reduce the risk of complications. Rapid reduction of the HCT is desirable, e.g. 450 mL every 2–3 days in younger patients, smaller volumes or less frequently for older patients (isovolumetric replacement with 0.9% saline may be necessary). Maintenance venesection is then required with variable frequency, based on regular monitoring of the HCT. Once a patient with PV has become iron-deficient, it may be possible to reduce the frequency of venesection. Supplemental iron should not be given.

- **Cytoreductive therapy.** This is used when there is thrombocytosis or evidence of disease progression (e.g. increasing splenomegaly, weight loss, night sweats), or if the patient is unable to tolerate venesection.
  - *Hydroxycarbamide (hydroxyurea)* is administered continuously or intermittently, 10–30 mg/kg daily or 80 mg/kg every third day (see also p. 222); it is used as first-line cytoreductive therapy in patients > 40 years of age and second-line < 40 years of age.
  - *Anagrelide* is an inhibitor of megakaryocyte differentiation that can be used to control thrombocytosis in PV, but it has no effect on other cell lines or splenomegaly. The initial dose is 0.5 mg twice daily, increased at weekly intervals by 0.5 mg daily according to response. The maximum daily dose is 10 mg, divided into maximum single doses of 2.5 mg. **Side-effects** include headaches, dizziness, palpitations and fluid retention. Anagrelide is a positive inotrope and therefore contraindicated in uncontrolled congestive cardiac failure. Long-term use can accelerate myelofibrosis.
  - *Pegylated interferon α2b* 0.5 mcg/kg/week or **interferon-α** 3–5 MU 3 times per week by SC injection is suitable for patients refractory to other medications and those with intractable pruritus. Side-effects (Table 6.2 p. 184) are frequent and lead to poor compliance, but are less common with the pegylated formulation.
  - *Busulfan* 0.5–1 mg/kg orally can be administered as a single dose every 3–6 months to achieve adequate myelosuppression.
  - *Radioactive ^{32}P*
    - 2.3 mCi/m^2 as a single IV dose can control the disease for up to 18 months, but may be administered as often as every 3 months if necessary.
    - Busulfan and ^{32}P carry a significant risk of secondary acute leukaemia (5–10% at 10 years) and are used only in patients > 75 years of age.
  - *Specific JAK2 V617F inhibitors* are currently under investigation.
- **Low-dose aspirin.** 75 mg per day is recommended for all patients unless there is a contraindication. Higher doses are associated with an increased risk of haemorrhage.
- **Supportive treatment. Allopurinol** 300 mg nightly blocks uric acid production and prevents gout in patients with hyperuricaemia. **Antihistamines** or **H_2-receptor antagonists** (e.g. cimetidine) are occasionally effective for pruritus.
- **Surgery.** There is a high risk of severe haemorrhage in patients with uncontrolled PV; therefore treatment is recommended for at least 3 months before elective surgery. In emergencies, the HCT can be reduced by venesection with isovolumetric fluid replacement.

Essential thrombocythaemia (ET)

This disorder is closely related to PV, but is usually characterized by an isolated thrombocytosis (platelets > 600–1000 × 10^9/L) with a normal Hb and white cell count. It is diagnosed by exclusion of other causes of thrombocytosis, e.g. iron deficiency or infection. A mutation in the *JAK2 V617F* gene is present in only 50% of patients.

Treatment

Treatment is necessary for patients at high risk of thrombosis (i.e. with cardiovascular risk factors or age > 60) and is with **hydroxycarbamide (hydroxyurea)**, **anagrelide** or **busulfan** to control platelets to $< 400 \times 10^9/\text{L}$. All patients should receive low-dose aspirin (75 mg once daily), but caution is advised with platelet counts of > 1000 (increased bleeding risk as a result of reduced von Willebrand factor (VWF) activity).

Idiopathic myelofibrosis

Proliferation of a neoplastic stem-cell clone causes a fibrotic reaction in the bone marrow through cytokine release. Progressive bone marrow failure and extramedullary haematopoiesis in the liver and spleen are characteristic. Transformation from PV is seen in up to one-quarter of patients.

Clinical features

Symptoms include anaemia, weakness, weight loss, night sweats, bruising, bleeding and infections. Most patients will have symptomatic (often massive) splenomegaly and hepatomegaly. The blood count and film show features of a leucoerythroblastic anaemia and characteristic 'tear-drop' poikilocytes. A bone marrow trephine is often diagnostic, by showing patchy cellularity with increased reticulin fibrosis. Cytogenetic and molecular analyses are required to differentiate myelofibrosis from CML (p. 285).

Treatment

- Asymptomatic anaemia. This does not require treatment, but patients should be monitored for progression.
- Symptomatic anaemia:
  - *Red cell transfusions* are given, 2–3 U every 3–4 weeks. **Iron chelation** therapy after > 25 U have been transfused may be required (p. 209). Transfusion requirements may be decreased in some patients by oral **danazol** 200 mg 3 times a day, reduced gradually to the minimum effective dose, or **darbepoietin alfa (recombinant erythropoietin)** 150–300 mcg SC once a week.
  - *Corticosteroids*, e.g. prednisolone 30 mg per day, may ameliorate the marked decrease in red cell survival seen in some patients.
  - *Hydroxycarbamide or interferon-α therapy* (p. 221) can be used to treat painful splenomegaly.
  - *Allogeneic SCT* is the only potentially curative therapy, but SCT for myelofibrosis is associated with a particularly high incidence of transplant-related complications, which increases sharply with age, so the procedure is generally limited to younger patients with good performance status.

Prognosis

Without SCT, the median survival in patients with myelofibrosis is 5 years.

BLOOD TRANSFUSION

The transfusion of blood, blood components or blood products can reduce morbidity and mortality in a wide variety of clinical situations. However, there are significant risks associated with blood transfusion, and it is a limited and expensive resource.

Blood components

Blood components are prepared from single donations by simple separation methods. Component therapy (rather than use of whole blood) reduces the risks associated with transfusion of unnecessary blood constituents and makes the most economical use of each individual donation. Indications for blood components and suggested thresholds for platelet transfusion are listed in Box 7.4.

- **Red cells**, usually supplied as concentrates (plasma replaced by an additive solution), are stored at 4°C. There is no universal 'trigger' Hb level for red cell transfusion — the decision should be based on the indication and clinical state of the patient. Washed red cell concentrates are available for patients who have had severe recurrent urticarial or anaphylactic reactions.
  - 1 U (~330 mL) raises the Hb by ~1 g/dL in stable patients.
- **Platelet concentrates** are available as random-donor pools (separated and pooled from four blood donations) or from single donors (collected by apheresis). Single-donor units reduce the frequency of alloimmunization. Platelets can be stored for up to 5 days at 22°C with continuous gentle agitation to prevent aggregation.
  - A single donor unit or pooled donation can increase the platelet count by about $20–30 \times 10^9$/L in stable patients.
  - Platelets are more effective if they are compatible with the patient's ABO group.
  - Paracetamol and an antihistamine, e.g. chlorphenamine, are given if there have been previous transfusion reactions. Complications are similar to those of red cell transfusions.
- **Fresh frozen plasma (FFP)** is supplied in a pack that contains 180–400 mL and the usual dose is 10–15 mL/kg body weight, although higher doses may be required for severe bleeding. FFP should not be used for volume replacement.
- **Cryoprecipitate** contains factor VIII:C, VWF and fibrinogen, and is useful in disseminated intravascular coagulation (DIC) and other causes of hypo- or dysfibrinogenaemia. Two five-donor pools (equivalent to 10 single-donor units) is a typical adult dose, and contains 3–6 g fibrinogen in a volume of 200–500 mL. Treatment should be guided by the baseline fibrinogen, with the aim of maintaining a fibrinogen level of > 1 g/L. Cryoprecipitate is no longer recommended for haemophilia A and von Willebrand disease (VWD) because it is not virally inactivated.
- **Human albumin** is available as a 4.5% or 20% solution, and is indicated for the treatment of acute, severe hypoalbuminaemia and as a replacement fluid for plasma exchange. Albumin solutions should not be used as volume replacement. The 4.5% albumin solution contains 160 mmol/L of sodium and the 20% solution contains 130 mmol/L.

Procedure for red cell transfusion

- Pre-transfusion compatibility testing is performed on a blood sample taken from the patient after *careful* confirmation of the patient's identity.
  - The sample must be clearly labelled with sufficient details by the individual who performed the venepuncture.
  - Laboratory testing consists of blood grouping to determine the ABO and RhD groups of the patient, and screening of the patient's serum

Kumar & Clark's Medical Management and Therapeutics

Box 7.4 Situations in which blood component therapy can be used

Red cells

- Acute blood loss
- Bone marrow failure
- Inherited haemolytic anaemias
  - Thalassaemia major
  - Sickle cell disease
- Some acquired haemolytic anaemias
  - E.g. Haemolytic disease of the newborn
- Myelofibrosis
- Myelodysplasia

Fresh frozen plasma (FFP)

- Massive transfusion
- Disseminated intravascular coagulation (DIC)
- Thrombotic thrombocytopenic purpura (TTP)
- Reversal of warfarin therapy (only if severe bleeding)
- Liver disease/liver biopsy
- Factor V deficiency (no concentrate available)
- Sometimes justified in patients who are bleeding when no underlying cause can be determined

Platelet concentrates

- Bone marrow failure
  - Disease, e.g. leukaemia
  - Cytotoxic therapy
  - Irradiation
- Inherited or acquired platelet function disorders
- Massive transfusion
- DIC
- Cardiopulmonary bypass
- Immune thrombocytopenias
- Contraindicated in heparin-induced thrombocytopenia and TTP

Thresholds for platelet transfusion

10×10^9/L

- Prophylaxis in patients with bone marrow failure (higher threshold with concurrent sepsis, antibiotics or other haemostatic abnormalities)

50×10^9/L

- Most low-risk surgical procedures
- DIC
- Massive transfusion
- Bare minimum for lumbar puncture and epidural anaesthesia ($> 80 \times 10^9$/L preferred)

100×10^9/L

- High-risk surgery (e.g. neurosurgery or eyes)

or plasma for atypical antibodies to red cell antigens. If the antibody screen is positive, further testing is required to determine the blood group specificity of the antibody.

- **Selection of donor blood** is based initially on the ABO and RhD groups of the patient, but matching for additional blood group antigens is necessary for patients with clinically significant red cell antibodies, patients who require multiple transfusions (e.g. sickle cell anaemia) and women of childbearing age.
- **Crossmatching** involves testing the patient's serum or plasma against donor red cells using direct and indirect agglutination tests.
- **Maximum surgical blood ordering schedules (MSBOS)** are local guidelines produced by most hospitals to reduce unnecessary cross-matching in preparation for elective surgery. For many operations a '**group and save**' is sufficient and will avoid wastage due to the limited shelf life of blood. If the antibody screen is negative, blood can be made available quickly, if necessary, using saved serum or plasma. However, for patients with atypical antibodies, compatible blood should always be reserved in advance.
- **Emergency transfusion** may occasionally be needed. At least 45 mins will be required for full pre-transfusion testing by most laboratories. In extreme circumstances, O RhD negative blood or blood of the same ABO and RhD groups as the patient can be used until fully cross-matched blood becomes available.
- **Collection of blood from the blood bank refrigerator** is a common source of transfusion errors. Clear documentation confirming the patient's identity and location is required by the person responsible. One unit at a time should be collected from the blood bank to avoid potential wastage, unless rapid transfusion is required.
- **Prescription of blood** is the responsibility of a registered medical practitioner, and prescription sheets must be clearly labelled with full patient identification details. The prescription should include details of special requirements, (e.g. irradiated or cytomegalovirus-seronegative components). Transfusion details should also be clearly documented in the patient's case notes.
- **Administration** ⚠ involves a mandatory **meticulous final bedside check** before blood or blood component transfusion is administered.
  - The **patient's identification details** should be confirmed by direct questioning of the patient. These must be identical on the **patient's wristband**, the transfusion report form, the compatibility label on the blood pack, the prescription chart and the clinical record.
  - The **transfusion bag** itself should also be inspected for abnormalities (e.g. clots, turbidity) before transfusion.
  - Temperature, pulse and BP should be recorded before and every 15 mins during transfusion.
  - Transfusion should commence within 30 mins of collection from the blood bank and each unit should be infused over a maximum of 4 hours.

Complications and management of blood transfusion

Common complications

A temperature < 38°C and/or mild urticarial reactions are common. Providing the patient is stable, reduce the transfusion rate and give chlorphenamine 10 mg IV.

Kumar & Clark's Medical Management and Therapeutics

Immunological complications

- Immediate haemolytic transfusion reactions are the most serious complication of blood transfusion; they occur within minutes of commencing the infusion and are usually due to ABO incompatibility.
  - Complement activation as a result of the interaction between donor antigens and patient IgM antibodies leads to **massive intravascular haemolysis**.
  - *Management*
  - Stop the transfusion immediately and keep the line open with 0.9% saline after changing giving sets.
  - Start resuscitation. Check patient's identity against donor unit.
  - Maintain urine output above 1.5 mL/kg/hour, which will require infusion of 0.9% saline with additional furosemide. Monitor urine output with a catheter in severe cases.
  - Report reaction to transfusion laboratory immediately and send new blood sample from the patient. Check all documentation to identify source of error, including mislabelled samples or samples from the wrong patient, laboratory labelling, handling errors and collection/delivery errors. Return units to the laboratory.
- Delayed transfusion reactions occur in patients alloimmunized by previous transfusions or pregnancies (e.g. RhD).
  - The antibody level (IgG) is initially undetectable on pre-transfusion compatibility testing, but a secondary immune response occurs after transfusion.
  - The haemolysis is usually **extravascular**, and therefore haemoglobinuria and renal failure do not occur. Patients may be asymptomatic, or present with anaemia and jaundice 1–2 weeks after the transfusion.
  - The DAT is usually positive and compatibility tests should be repeated.
  - Transfuse fresh (crossmatched) blood if necessary.
- Non-haemolytic (febrile) transfusion reactions are less common since the introduction of universal leucodepletion of blood donations at source (to minimize the risk of variant Creutzfeldt–Jakob disease (vCJD) transmission).
  - They are usually caused by leucocyte antibodies in an alloimmunized recipient reacting with donor leucocytes.
  - **Fever** is less severe than for haemolytic reactions (< 40°C) but may be associated with chills and rigors.
  - *Management.* Reduce the infusion rate and administer antipyretics, e.g. paracetamol.
- Transfusion-related acute lung injury (TRALI). Antileucocyte antibodies, present in donor plasma (usually from multiparous women), can rarely cause a **severe pulmonary reaction** within 4 hours of a blood transfusion.
  - The clinical features are identical to ARDS (p. 549).
  - Management is similar to that of ARDS, except that diuretic therapy may actually be detrimental in patients with TRALI.
- Transfusion-associated graft vs. host disease (TaGVHD) is an almost invariably fatal but entirely preventable complication of blood transfusion.
  - Clinical features of rash, fever, diarrhoea, hepatic dysfunction and bone marrow failure typically appear 1–2 weeks after transfusion.

- It most commonly occurs in immunocompromised individuals (e.g. allogeneic SCT recipients) and is thought to be due to the presence of viable T-lymphocytes in the transfused blood component. It can also occur in immunocompetent individuals when there is a shared HLA haplotype with the donor (rare under normal circumstances, but frequent if the donor is a relative, e.g. mother to child).
- There is no effective treatment, other than supportive therapy (e.g. antibiotics, blood components). Prevention is by irradiation of all cellular blood products prior to administration, and patients at risk should carry an identification card.
- **Post-transfusion purpura** is a rare cause of severe thrombocytopenia and life-threatening haemorrhage that can occur 1–2 weeks after blood or platelet transfusion.
  - The recipient is usually human platelet antigen (HPA)-1a-negative, and develops allo-antibodies in response to transfusion from an HPA-1a-positive donor. Treatment is with high-dose IV immunoglobulin (IVIg) if there is bleeding. Plasma exchange (p. 233) is carried out if necessary. If platelet transfusion is required, there is no evidence to suggest that HPA-1a-negative platelets are superior to random donor platelets.
- **Anaphylactic reactions** occur in response to IgA in transfused blood components, when administered to an individual with IgA deficiency and anti-IgA antibodies.
  - Stop the transfusion immediately. Give **adrenaline (epinephrine) 0.5 mg IM** immediately (Fig. 20.3).
  - Future transfusions should be with blood components from IgA-deficient donors.

Non-immunological complications

- **Transfusion-transmitted infection (TTI)** is minimized in many countries by donor screening and by testing all donations for hepatitis B virus (HBV; risk still 1:900 000 units transfused), HCV (risk < 1:30 million Units), HIV (risk 1:8 million Units), human T-cell lymphotropic virus (HTLV)-1 and syphilis. Donor questionnaires should include recent travel to help exclude possible transmission risks.
  - Coagulation factor concentrates prepared from pooled plasma are now subjected to viral inactivation procedures such as solvent detergent treatments.
  - Bacterial TTI (e.g. *Yersinia enterocolitica*) is uncommon but nevertheless is a frequent cause of transfusion-associated death. The risk is increased with platelet concentrates, which are stored at 22°C. Inspect all platelet packs before administration for signs of turbidity.
  - vCJD transmission by red cell transfusion has been reported but the risk is diminished by universal leucocyte depletion of blood components.
  - Despite these stringent measures, it may never be possible to guarantee the absolute safety of donor blood.
- **Massive transfusion** is defined as complete replacement of the circulating blood volume within 24 hours.
  - Complications include thrombocytopenia and deficiency of coagulation factors, e.g. V and VIII.

- Clinical situations where massive transfusion is required (e.g. resuscitation after trauma) are also often associated with DIC, which causes further depletion of platelets, coagulation factors and fibrinogen (p. 239).
- Hypocalcaemia induced by the anticoagulant in stored blood, hyperkalaemia and hypothermia occur. Perform a platelet count, a coagulation screen (including a serum fibrinogen) and serum electrolytes at regular intervals.
- Transfuse platelet concentrates, FFP and cryoprecipitate as guided by frequent laboratory investigations (formula replacement is no longer recommended). Blood products should be administered via a blood warmer.

Alternatives to blood transfusion

- General measures. Stop drugs that inhibit haemostasis (e.g. aspirin, clopidogrel) and correct anaemia due to haematinic deficiencies prior to surgery. Antifibrinolytic drugs, e.g. tranexamic acid, may be used in major surgery.
- Autologous transfusion (use of the patient's own blood):
  - *Intra-operative and post-operative cell salvage.* Blood collected by approved methods during or after 'clean' surgical procedures may be retransfused. The operative site must be free of bacteria, bowel contents, fat, amniotic fluid and tumour cells.
  - *Autologous pre-deposit and pre-operative haemodilution.* These are no longer recommended by the UK National Blood Service (NBS).
- Artificial haemoglobin solutions and other blood substitutes are undergoing clinical trials but are not widely available.

HAEMOSTASIS AND THROMBOSIS

Normal haemostasis

Vascular injury leads to endothelial damage and exposure of collagen within the vessel wall.

- Primary haemostasis involves the immediate formation of a platelet plug, which is mediated by the binding of circulating VWF to exposed collagen. Activated platelets and damaged endothelium release mediators such as thromboxane-A2 and endothelin-1, which stimulate vasoconstriction and help to control bleeding by restricting local blood flow.
- Secondary haemostasis continues with the activation of factor VII (FVIIa) in plasma by tissue factor (TF) exposed as a consequence of vascular injury. The TF:FVIIa complex then activates a series of other coagulation factors in order to amplify local generation of thrombin, an enzyme that converts circulating fibrinogen to insoluble fibrin (Fig. 7.6). Fibrin strands cross-link with each other and retract around the platelet plug to strengthen and stabilize the developing clot.

Regulation of coagulation is mediated by naturally occurring anticoagulants such as antithrombin, protein C and its cofactor, protein S. These inhibitors target various proteins within the coagulation cascade, in order to control thrombin generation and to help localize the haemostatic response to the site of vascular injury. Activation of the fibrinolytic system in response to vascular injury provides an additional level of control. Circulating plasminogen is converted to plasmin, which breaks down

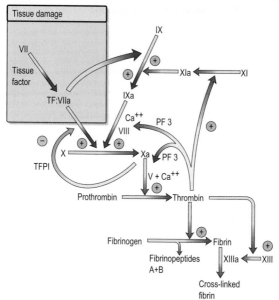

Fig. 7.6 The coagulation cascade. PF, platelet factor; TF, tissue factor; TFPI, tissue factor pathway inhibitor.

excess fibrin and fibrinogen into fibrin/fibrinogen degradation products (FDPs). One purpose of this mechanism is to recanalize blood vessels occluded by thrombus.

Approach to patients with bleeding disorders

Clinical features

Clinical features include spontaneous bruising, haemorrhage, and excessive bleeding after haemostatic challenges, e.g. tooth extraction, surgery, childbirth and minor trauma. A family history is essential.

- Platelet/VWF/vascular defects: bruising, and bleeding from mucous membranes.
- Coagulation factor deficiencies: joint bleeds, muscle haematomas and excessive bleeding after surgery or trauma.

Physical examination

Look at skin, mucous membranes and optic fundi for evidence of haemorrhage. Petechiae are pinpoint skin haemorrhages that do not blanch on pressure, whilst purpura (small) and ecchymoses (large) are areas of bruising.

Investigations

- FBC and blood film show the number and morphology of platelets, and the presence of blood disorders such as acute leukaemia. A spurious thrombocytopenia may be caused by platelet clumping due to EDTA anticoagulant — repeat the count with a fresh citrated sample. Reference range 150–400 × 10^9/L.

- Coagulation screen
  - *Prothrombin time (PT)* screens for defects in the coagulation pathway and is prolonged by warfarin therapy, vitamin K deficiency and liver disease. It is also prolonged by isolated abnormalities of coagulation factors VII, X, V, II or I, which are rare.
  - *Activated partial thromboplastin time (APTT)* (26–37 secs, depending on methodology) is prolonged by unfractionated heparin (UFH) and abnormalities of coagulation factors XII, XI, IX, VIII, X, V, II, I (Fig. 7.6).
  - *Thrombin time (TT)* is prolonged by quantitative/qualitative fibrinogen defects and inhibitors, e.g. heparin or fibrinogen degradation products.
  - *Correction tests* can be used to differentiate between various coagulation defects by the addition of normal plasma. The coagulation screen is repeated on a 50:50 mix of patient:normal plasma. Correction of prolonged PT, APTT and TT suggests coagulation factor deficiency. Partial or no correction suggests presence of an inhibitor, e.g. a lupus anticoagulant (p. 243).
  - *Bleeding time (BT)* is rarely performed as it involves a 1 mm deep, 1 cm long abrasion of the forearm with a sphygmomanometer cuff inflated to 40 mmHg. The lesion is blotted every 30 secs and bleeding should stop in less than 8 mins. The test can detect defects in platelet function (e.g. due to aspirin) and VWD. The laboratory-based **PFA-100** assay is now more commonly used to screen for these abnormalities.
- Further investigations include coagulation factor assays, VWF antigen and activity, fibrinogen, FDPs, platelet function and fibrinolysis assays.

VASCULAR DISORDERS

Diseases include **hereditary haemorrhagic telangiectasia (HHT)** with dilatation of the capillaries and small arterioles that produce characteristic small red spots in the skin and mucous membranes. Recurrent epistaxis and chronic gastrointestinal bleeding occur.

Easy bruising syndrome is a common benign disorder occurring in otherwise healthy people who present with bruises on the arms, legs and trunk on minor trauma.

Senile purpura and **purpura due to steroids** are both caused by atrophy of the vascular supporting tissue. **Henoch–Schönlein purpura** is described on p. 343. Episodes of inexplicable bleeding or bruising may represent abuse.

PLATELET DISORDERS

Thrombocytopenia

Increased bleeding does not usually occur at platelet counts above 50 × 10^9/L, unless there is a concurrent defect in platelet function (e.g. due to aspirin), and severe spontaneous bleeding is unusual with platelet counts above 20 × 10^9/L. Bone marrow examination can be helpful to distinguish between decreased platelet production and increased destruction.

- **Management.** Management of thrombocytopenia due to bone marrow failure (e.g. aplastic anaemia — p. 209), severe megaloblastic anaemia or infiltration (e.g. leukaemia, myelofibrosis, solid tumour infiltration and myeloma) is with platelet concentrates and treatment of the underlying cause.
- Asymptomatic patients with counts $> 20 \times 10^9/L$ do not usually require specific treatment.
- If the platelet count is very low ($< 10–20 \times 10^9/L$) or bleeding risk very high, then platelet concentrates (p. 223) should be transfused.
- If a patient requires urgent surgery, the count should be raised to $50 \times 10^9/L$, or to $100 \times 10^9/L$ for higher-risk surgery (e.g. neurosurgery, ophthalmic and some cardiac surgery).

Peripheral destruction of platelets

Immune thrombocytopenic purpura (ITP)

Platelets are opsonized by auto-antibodies binding to platelet surface antigens and are phagocytosed by reticuloendothelial cells.

- **Clinical features.** In children the presentation is often acute and spontaneous resolution usually occurs within 6–8 weeks. A precipitating cause, such as recent viral infection or immunization, can sometimes be identified. In adults the onset of ITP is more insidious, and is associated with other autoimmune diseases, malignancy (e.g. lymphoproliferative disorders) or viral infection. It is most common in women of childbearing age (female:male ratio 3:1). Spontaneous resolution in adults is rare.
- **Diagnosis.** Diagnosis is based on exclusion of other causes of thrombocytopenia.
- **Management.** Treatment is often unnecessary for children with ITP, but where indicated is similar to adult therapy. Adults with platelet counts of $> 30 \times 10^9/L$ do not usually require treatment unless they are bleeding or about to receive a haemostatic challenge (e.g. surgery, childbirth). Although the incidence of *Helicobacter pylori* (p. 144) is the same as in the general population, eradication therapy improves platelet counts, particularly in those patients with ITP of recent origin and those with less severe disease. Major haemorrhage (e.g. intracranial bleeding) is rare and associated with platelet counts of $< 10 \times 10^9/L$.
  - *First-line therapy*
    a) **Oral corticosteroids** are given, e.g. **prednisolone** 1 mg/kg daily for 2–4 weeks, tailing off very slowly. Relapse is common with dose reduction, and many patients require low-dose maintenance therapy to maintain an adequate platelet count. Long-term remission after completion of corticosteroid therapy is only seen in 10–20% of patients, and treatment should be rapidly tapered and stopped altogether in patients who fail to respond after 4 weeks.
    b) **IVIg** is used for a more rapid rise in the platelet count in patients with active haemorrhage and in preparation for invasive procedures (e.g. splenectomy) or childbirth. The response is usually only transient; therefore treatment should be repeated every 3–4 weeks. IVIg is usually administered over 2–5 days at 0.4 mg/kg/day; 1 g/kg as a single IV infusion on 2 days is equally effective, although **side-effects**, e.g. headaches and low-grade fever, are more common. The infusion should be commenced slowly at first and gradually increased, depending on tolerance, up to a

maximum infusion rate of 2 mg/kg/min. IVIg is contraindicated in patients at risk of renal dysfunction and in those with selective IgA deficiency.

- *Second-line therapy.* **Splenectomy** is used for patients not responding to or relapsing after medical therapy. An indium-labelled platelet scan can predict which are most likely to benefit. **IVIg** is administered 3–5 days prior to surgery, and pooled platelets should be available to control peri-operative bleeding complications if necessary. However, an immediate rebound thrombocytosis frequently occurs post-splenectomy (platelet count 600–1000 × 10^9/L), persisting for only 2–3 weeks in most patients but long-term in about 30%, so prophylaxis against thromboembolic complications should be given during this time (p. 243). A complete response to splenectomy occurs in about two-thirds of patients. Splenectomized patients are at risk of developing overwhelming infection by encapsulated organisms (particularly *Pneumococcus*), so appropriate vaccinations and antibiotic prophylaxis are required (Box 7.1, p. 205).

- *Chronic refractory ITP.* Treatment options include high-dose **corticosteroids** (e.g. methylprednisolone), high-dose **IVIgG**, or **immunosuppressive agents** such as azathioprine, ciclosporin, cyclophosphamide or vincristine. **Danazol** 400–800 mg daily for 1–3 months can be effective in ITP, but should not be used in young women. **Rituximab** (anti-CD20 monoclonal antibody) is also useful. **Eltrombopag**, a thrombopoietin receptor agonist, and **romiplostim**, a novel thrombopoiesis-stimulating protein, both significantly increase the platelet count in ITP and are very effective.

- *ITP in pregnancy.* **Oral corticosteroids** and **IVIg** should be administered if the platelet count is < 20 × 10^9/L; avoid immunosuppressant and cytotoxic drugs and splenectomy during pregnancy, as they are associated with a high rate of fetal loss. A platelet count of > 50 × 10^9/L is generally considered to be safe for vaginal delivery and caesarean section, but most anaesthetists would prefer a count of > 80 × 10^9/L before epidural anaesthesia is performed. **Fetal thrombocytopenia** can occur but the risk of intracranial haemorrhage during delivery is low. The neonate's platelet count should be monitored for several days post-delivery in case of delayed thrombocytopenia. **Gestational thrombocytopenia** is a common cause of mild thrombocytopenia in pregnancy, often presenting in the third trimester (platelet count typically 80–150 × 10^9/L). The fetus is unaffected, and the platelet count usually recovers spontaneously after delivery.

Other immune thrombocytopenias

Drug-induced thrombocytopenia

This is most commonly due to immune mechanisms (when drugs stimulate antibody production); it is often dose-dependent but may be idiosyncratic. Immune mechanisms include antibodies directly binding to platelet membrane proteins or hapten-dependent antibodies, which are antibodies against drugs covalently bound to platelet membrane glycoproteins. The mechanism is similar to that of drug-induced immune haemolytic anaemia (p. 219).

Drugs include methyldopa, quinidine, rifampicin, quinine, vancomycin, trimethoprim/sulfamethoxazole and heparin.

- Heparin-induced thrombocytopenia (HIT)/heparin-induced thrombocytopenia and thrombosis (HITT). This is an uncommon but serious complication of heparin therapy, which affects around 5% of patients receiving unfractionated heparin (UFH) for the first time, with a lower incidence seen after LMWH administration. It is due to the formation of immune complexes between IgG antibodies, heparin and platelet factor 4, leading to platelet activation and aggregation, and the formation of microthrombi. Venous and arterial thrombosis occurs in up to 15% of patients (HITT), which is associated with progressive gangrene, limb amputation and a high mortality. Minor decreases in the platelet count are common with heparin therapy, but a decrease of $\geq 50\%$ within 4–14 days after the first dose of heparin is suggestive of HIT.
  - All patients receiving heparin should have a baseline platelet count, with alternate-day platelet counts from days 4–14 in all patients receiving UFH and surgical patients receiving LMWH.
  - For patients exposed to heparin within the last 100 days, a repeat platelet count should be performed after 24 hours of therapy because the condition may develop earlier in patients with pre-existing antibodies.
  - Medical and obstetric patients receiving LMWH are considered low-risk and usually do not require routine platelet monitoring after the baseline count.
  - *Management.* Immediate cessation of all forms of heparin (including line flushes) and, if necessary, full-dose **anticoagulation** with an alternative agent should be commenced, e.g. **danaparoid sodium** or **lepirudin** (p. 245). Warfarin should not be commenced until the platelet count has recovered, and parenteral anticoagulation should be continued until a therapeutic INR has been achieved for > 48 hours. The diagnosis should be clearly recorded in the patient's **case notes** as a serious drug allergy.

Thrombotic thrombocytopenic purpura (TTP)

This is a rare but life-threatening condition characterized by profound thrombocytopenia, microangiopathic haemolytic anaemia (MAHA), fever, and neurological and renal impairment. There is a deficiency in the protease ADAMTS13 and ultra-large von Willebrand factor (UL-VWF) multimers are not broken down into smaller multimers in the circulation, which stimulate platelet aggregation and microvascular thrombus formation.

TTP can be idiopathic, congenital, or associated with pregnancy, oral contraceptives, SLE, infection (HIV and hepatitis) and some drugs (e.g. ticlopidine, clopidogrel, ciclosporin).

- Diagnosis. The blood count and blood film show typical features of MAHA (anaemia, thrombocytopenia, severe red cell fragmentation and spherocytosis). The coagulation screen is usually normal and the DAT is negative. LDH levels are markedly elevated (> 1000 U/L).
- Management:
  - *Daily single-volume plasma exchange.* This should be commenced within 24 hours, using **cryosupernatant** or **solvent-detergent treated plasma** if available (fewer high-molecular-weight VWF multimers), or **FFP**, both of which contain ADAMTS13. Daily exchanges should continue for ≥ 2 days following complete remission (i.e. normalization of platelet count and LDH levels). Electrolytes should be closely monitored throughout treatment.

- *Corticosteroids.* The British Committee for Standards in Haematology (BCSH) guidelines recommend **pulse methylprednisolone** 1 g IV for 3 days in order to achieve adequate immunosuppression with minimum long-term side-effects. Oral **prednisolone** 1–2 mg/kg daily is an alternative. **Low-dose aspirin** (75 mg daily) should be commenced as soon as platelets exceed $50 \times 10^9/L$.
- *Supportive treatment.* **Red cell concentrates** can be administered as necessary, but platelet transfusions are contraindicated in TTP unless there is life-threatening haemorrhage. **Folic acid** 5 mg orally daily and **hepatitis B vaccination** are recommended for all patients. Infections should be treated with **broad-spectrum antibiotics**, including cover for central venous access according to local policy.

Platelet function disorders

- Inherited causes are rare and include **Glanzmann's thrombasthenia**, **Bernard–Soulier syndrome** (failure of platelet aggregation/adhesion) and **storage pool disease** (poor platelet function due to failure of secretory activity).
- Acquired causes include myeloproliferative disorders, renal and liver disease, paraproteinaemias, and drugs such as aspirin or other antiplatelet agents. The diagnosis is suggested by increased mucocutaneous bleeding in patients with a normal or increased platelet count, but prolonged BT or PFA-100 closure time. Acquired causes often respond to treatment of the underlying cause (e.g. cessation of aspirin, dialysis for uraemia). For antiplatelet agents causing platelet dysfunction, see p. 239. **Desmopressin** (p. 235) and **red cell transfusion** or **erythropoietin** to increase the haematocrit to > 0.3 can decrease the BT in uraemic patients. Suspected inherited causes require further characterization with platelet aggregation studies and investigations to exclude VWD. **Platelet transfusion** is required for significant haemorrhage or if there is high risk of bleeding.

Thrombocytosis

- Reactive thrombocytosis is a common feature of the acute-phase reaction, e.g. malignancy, chronic infection, inflammatory disease or major surgery. Iron deficiency is also associated with an elevated platelet count. The platelet count in such conditions rarely exceeds $1000 \times 10^9/L$, and treatment of the underlying condition is usually all that is required. Low-dose aspirin (75 mg daily) can be prescribed for patients at risk of thrombosis. Thrombocytosis after splenectomy usually resolves spontaneously within 2–3 weeks.
- Essential thrombocythaemia (p. 221) and the other myeloproliferative disorders are discussed on p. 220.

INHERITED COAGULATION DISORDERS

Haemophilia A

Haemophilia A is an X-linked recessive disorder characterized by a low circulating FVIII:C level due to mutations in the factor VIII gene.

Clinical and laboratory features

Clinical features depend on the level of FVIII:C.

- Severe haemophilia A (FVIII level < 1 U/dL) usually presents in infancy or early childhood with frequent spontaneous haemorrhages, including haemarthroses and muscle haematomas. Inadequate treatment or repeated bleeding into a target joint may lead to arthropathy and long-term disability.

- Moderate haemophilia A (FVIII 1–5 U/dL) is associated with severe haemorrhage following injury but fewer spontaneous bleeds.
- Mild haemophilia A (FVIII > 5 U/dL) patients usually only bleed excessively after injury or surgery, which can delay the diagnosis until later in life.

Female carriers of haemophilia A are usually asymptomatic, with FVIII levels of around 50%, but levels can vary widely as a result of Lyonization (random inactivation of one X chromosome) in the fetus.

General management

- All patients should be registered at a comprehensive care centre for regular medical review and for social and psychological support.
- Blood group, liver biochemistry and baseline serology for HIV and hepatitis A, B and C should be determined at diagnosis, and hepatitis A and B vaccination administered to patients who are not immune.
- Antiplatelet drugs and IM injections should be avoided.
- Mild to moderate haemophilia A. Major bleeding episodes should be treated as for severe haemophilia A.
  - *Desmopressin* 0.3 mcg/kg SC or IV (in 50–100 mL 0.9% saline over 20–30 mins) may be sufficient for minor bleeding episodes, and can increase the baseline FVIII:C level by 2–5-fold. Alternatively, desmopressin can be administered intranasally (150 mcg in each nostril). Further doses can be administered every 12 hours but tachyphylaxis can occur, so the FVIII response should be monitored. A **slower IV infusion** over 60 mins will reduce side-effects, including vasodilatation, hypotension and facial flushing. Fluid overload and hyponatraemia may result from desmopressin therapy, so electrolytes should be monitored and adult patients should restrict fluid intake to 1.5 L/24 hours. Desmopressin should not be used in patients with heart failure.
  - *Oral tranexamic acid* 15–25 mg/kg 3 times daily is sometimes useful for minor cuts or dental extraction in patients with mild haemophilia A.
- Severe haemophilia A:
  - Bleeding episodes are managed with IV **FVIII concentrate**. Recombinant products are preferable but expensive; therefore some previously treated adult patients continue to receive plasma-derived FVIII.
  - Inpatient treatment can be guided by measurement of peak and trough FVIII:C levels, to ensure adequate haemostasis and avoid wastage. 1 U of **FVIII** per kg body weight typically raises the FVIII:C level by 2 U/dL. The half-life is 6–12 hours, so twice-daily treatment is required to maintain therapeutic levels. The FVIII:C level should be increased to 30–50 U/dL for minor spontaneous bleeds, and to > 50 U/dL for severe bleeding episodes.
  - Self-administration of FVIII concentrate at home enables many patients to begin treatment at the first signs of bleeding, which can reduce long-term joint damage and the need for hospital admission.
  - **Prophylaxis** from early childhood with 25–40 U/kg FVIII administered three times per week can prevent permanent joint damage and reduce the frequency of bleeding episodes.

- For **major surgery**, the goal should be to achieve a pre-operative FVIII:C level of 100 U/dL with maintenance above 50 U/dL until healing has occurred, often by continuous infusion.

Other treatments

- Inhibitors. Neutralizing allo-antibodies to FVIII:C develop in up to 30% of patients with severe haemophilia A, most commonly between the first 10–20 treatment exposures. They rarely occur in patients with mild or moderate haemophilia. The diagnosis should be suspected in patients who continue to bleed despite receiving standard doses of FVIII concentrate. The APTT is prolonged as expected, but fails to correct on mixing studies with normal plasma. Therapy is guided by monitoring inhibitory antibody titres. 'High responders' are so described because of a tendency to develop antibodies more rapidly with each repeat exposure to FVIII and are difficult to treat, whereas 'low responders' develop antibodies much more slowly.

  - *Conservative management* may be all that is required in low responders without bleeding symptoms, as the inhibitor titre may decrease over time.
  - *High-dose factor VIII* (50–200 U/kg every 8–12 hours) is often effective in low responders with minor bleeding. FVIII:C levels should be monitored immediately following administration and 3–6 hours after treatment.
  - *Bypassing agents*, such as recombinant factor VIIa (rFVIIa) or factor eight inhibitor bypassing agent (FEIBA), can achieve haemostasis in patients with inhibitors by direct activation of the final common pathway (Fig. 7.6) of the coagulation cascade without a requirement for FVIII. The usual dose of rFVIIa is 90 mcg/kg every 2–4 hours until bleeding has stopped; FEIBA is given in a dose of 50–100 U/kg every 6–12 hours (maximum daily dose 200 U/kg).
  - *Immune tolerance induction* by repeated FVIII injection over a period of months is used, particularly in younger patients. High responders may require high doses of factor concentrate for prolonged periods of time. **Immune suppression** with corticosteroids and cyclophosphamide may also be necessary.

- Carrier detection. A detailed family history, coagulation screen and factor assays should detect most carriers of haemophilia A. Confirmation by molecular genetic investigations is necessary. Antenatal diagnosis is possible by chorionic villus sampling at 11–12 weeks' gestation.

Prognosis

Viral infection with hepatitis B/C and HIV from pooled plasma products was common in people with haemophilia, but over the last 20 years the introduction of donor screening, viral testing and viral inactivation have dramatically improved the safety of plasma-derived concentrates. However, the theoretical possibility of new vCJD transmission by plasma-derived products still exists.

Haemophilia B (Christmas disease)

This is also an X-linked recessive condition but is caused by a deficiency of factor IX. The clinical features are identical to those of haemophilia A, but it is much rarer (1 in 30 000 males). The general management is similar to that for haemophilia A but desmopressin is not effective. Bleeding episodes should be treated with recombinant factor IX concentrates or pooled plasma products. 1 U of FIX per kg body weight raises the FIX level by 1 U/dL with a half-life of approximately 18 hours, so treatment and prophylactic doses are required less frequently than for haemophilia A. Inhibitor formation is rare, but where this does occur, bleeding episodes are managed with rVIIa as for haemophilia A.

Von Willebrand disease (VWD)

This is the most common inherited bleeding disorder worldwide (1–2% of the general population) and affects both sexes equally (autosomal inheritance). It is characterized by qualitative and quantitative deficiencies of von Willebrand factor (VWF), leading to defective platelet adhesion in primary haemostasis and FVIII:C deficiency on account of its secondary role as a carrier protein for FVIII:C in plasma. There are three main types of VWD; in general, types 1 and 2 are less severe than type 3. Bleeding from mucous membranes (e.g. epistaxis, menorrhagia) and easy bruising are common, and haemorrhages following minor trauma or surgery (e.g. dental extraction) can be life-threatening. VWF antigen (VWF:Ag) is commonly measured by ELISA, and VWF activity by the ability of patient plasma to agglutinate formalin-fixed platelets in response to the antibiotic ristocetin (ristocetin co-factor activity, RiCof).

- General management:
  - Aspirin and NSAIDs should be avoided. Oral **tranexamic acid** can be a valuable adjunctive therapy after procedures such as dental extraction (15–25 mg/kg 3 times daily or as a 5% mouthwash).
  - **Desmopressin** stimulates the release of VWF from intracellular storage sites, and may be sufficient therapy for bleeding episodes and minor surgery in patients with type 1 VWD (VWF molecule functionally normal but reduced in quantity). It is sometimes useful in type 2 VWD, but is contraindicated in type 2B (it increases platelet aggregation). Desmopressin is not effective in patients with type 3 VWD with complete absence of VWF. Individual patient responses to desmopressin can be assessed by measuring FVIII:C and VWF:RiCof before and 1 hour after a standard dose (p. 235).
- **Intermediate-purity FVIII concentrates.** These also contain VWF and are used to treat bleeding episodes or to cover surgery in patients with type 3 VWD. FVIII concentrate is also used if desmopressin is ineffective in patients with types 1 and 2 VWD, or to cover major surgery and severe bleeding episodes when desmopressin is insufficient. Different products vary in the amount of VWF they contain, so the product data sheet should always be consulted. As a general guide, 50 U (of VWF:RiCof activity) concentrate per kg body weight raises the patient VWF:RiCof activity to 100 U/dL. Treatment should be monitored by VWF:RiCof activity (or FVIII:C/VWF:Ag). For minor surgical procedures, levels of 50 U/dL for 1–3 days are usually adequate, but for major surgery the goal should be to obtain levels of 100% for 5 days and then maintain a level of > 50% until wound healing is complete (7–14 days post-operatively). Cryoprecipitate is no longer recommended as a source of VWF because it is not virally inactivated. Transfusion of platelet concentrates is sometimes useful in conjunction with VWF-containing concentrates for severe bleeding.
- **Menorrhagia.** The combined **oral contraceptive pill** or **tranexamic acid** (see above) taken prior to and during menstruation may reduce

Kumar & Clark's Medical Management and Therapeutics

excessive menstrual blood loss. **Oral norethisterone 5 mg** 3 times daily is sometimes useful for the acute management of menorrhagia. Insertion of a hormone-impregnated intra-uterine device (e.g. Mirena coil) can be a highly effective longer-term solution for some patients.

- **Pregnancy.** Levels of VWF and FVIII:C normally increase throughout pregnancy, and specific treatment during delivery may not be necessary if the VWF:Ag and VWF:Ac/RiCof is > 50 U/dL at 36 weeks. However, VWF levels fall rapidly after delivery and there is an increased risk of post-partum haemorrhage. Treatment is with **desmopressin or VWF-containing concentrates**, as above.

ACQUIRED COAGULATION DISORDERS

Vitamin K deficiency

Vitamin K is an essential cofactor for the γ-carboxylation of glutamic acid residues on coagulation factors II, VII, IX, X and anticoagulant proteins C and S. This post-translational modification step is necessary for the interaction of these factors with calcium and phospholipids during normal coagulation. Deficiency of vitamin K may be due to inadequate intake or stores (e.g. neonates, malnutrition), malabsorption states, sterilization of intestinal flora by antibiotics, or oral anticoagulant drugs (vitamin K antagonists). The PT and APTT are raised.

Treatment

- **Vitamin K. Phytomenadione** 10 mg can be administered orally, subcutaneously or by slow IV injection to correct deficiency in asymptomatic patients, and may be sufficient for minor bleeding episodes. There is a risk of anaphylaxis with IV administration. The PT should partially correct within 6–12 hours and fully after 48 hours. Patients with fat malabsorption (e.g. cholestasis) require an oral water-soluble preparation (10 mg daily as **menadiol sodium phosphate)** to prevent deficiency. The management of oral anticoagulant toxicity with vitamin K is discussed on p. 249.
- **Fresh frozen plasma.** FFP rapidly corrects the coagulation factor deficiencies in patients with active bleeding (p. 223). It does not correct the underlying abnormality, however, and so concurrent vitamin K therapy should also be administered. **Dried prothrombinase complex** concentrates (PCC), which contain only factors II, VII, IX and X, are also available.

Haemorrhagic disease of the newborn (HDN)

This is caused by vitamin K deficiency, because levels in the neonate are low, human breast milk is a very poor source, and there are few bacteria in the newborn gut to synthesize vitamin K. All neonates in the UK are offered a 1 mg IM injection immediately after delivery, which prevents HDN.

Liver disease

Liver disease leads to coagulopathy by a number of mechanisms, e.g. vitamin K deficiency secondary to malabsorption as a result of cholestasis, coagulation factor deficiency due to impaired synthesis, thrombocytopenia secondary to hypersplenism and portal hypertension, and functional abnormalities of platelets and fibrinogen. DIC (see below) may also occur in acute liver failure.

Management

Vitamin K should be given to all patients with liver disease because coagulation screening tests will not distinguish between vitamin K deficiency and intrinsic liver disease as the cause of the coagulopathy. FFP can be used to replace clotting factors in preparation for invasive procedures or to treat active bleeding in patients with prolonged coagulation times.

Disseminated intravascular coagulation (DIC)

DIC is a generalized intravascular activation of the coagulation cascade associated with a consumptive coagulopathy, widespread fibrin generation and deposition, platelet aggregation and activation of fibrinolysis. It is most often caused by release of tissue factor into the circulation after widespread endothelial damage, which occurs in many serious systemic conditions.

- The clinical picture is often masked by the underlying cause, but includes a mixture of generalized bleeding and bruising associated with end-organ dysfunction (e.g. renal impairment) from microvascular thromboses and ischaemia.
- Clotting times (PT, APTT and TT) are usually very prolonged and the fibrinogen level is markedly reduced.
- FDPs and D-dimers are raised due to increased fibrinolysis.
- Thrombocytopenia is often severe and there may be evidence of MAHA on the blood film.

Management

- The underlying condition should be treated.
- Supportive therapy should include maintenance of blood volume and tissue perfusion.
- In patients with haemorrhage, red cells, platelets, FFP and cryoprecipitate may be indicated, but replacement therapy should be guided by appropriate investigations. The aim should be to keep platelets $> 50 \times 10^9/L$, fibrinogen > 1 g/L, and PT/APTT < 1.5 times the upper limit of normal.
- Fibrinolysis inhibitors (e.g. tranexamic acid) are contraindicated.
- Antithrombin concentrates can be used in intractable shock or fulminant hepatic necrosis, and activated protein C concentrates in acquired purpura fulminans or severe neonatal DIC.

THROMBOSIS

Arterial thrombosis

This is usually associated with atheromatous plaque rupture and vessel occlusion, and is discussed further in the relevant sections (see coronary artery disease, p. 249; cerebral vascular disease, p. 628; and peripheral vascular disease). Drug therapy includes the use of antiplatelet drugs and thrombolytic therapy (Box 7.5). Anticoagulants are used occasionally.

Antiplatelet drugs

Platelet activation occurs at the site of vascular damage, leading to platelet aggregation and arterial thrombosis. The following drugs interfere with this process:

- Aspirin irreversibly inhibits the enzyme cyclo-oxygenase (COX), resulting in reduced platelet production of TXA_2 and inhibition of platelet aggregation. At the low doses (75–300 mg) of aspirin used in cardiovascular disease prevention and treatment, there is selective inhibition of

Kumar & Clark's Medical Management and Therapeutics

Box 7.5 Drugs used in the treatment of arterial thrombotic disorders

Antiplatelet
- Aspirin
- Dipyridamole
- Clopidogrel
- Prasugrel
- Ticagrelor
- Glycoprotein IIb/IIIa inhibitors, e.g. abciximab, eptifibatide, tirofiban
- Epoprostenol

Thrombolytic
- Streptokinase
- Alteplase (rt-PA)
- Reteplase
- Tenecteplase

the isoform COX-1 found within platelets. The inhibition is irreversible and is effective for the life of the circulating platelet (~1 week).

- Dipyridamole 100–200 mg 3 times daily inhibits platelet phosphodiesterase, causing an increase in cAMP with potentiation of the action of prostaglandin I_2 (a natural inhibitor of platelet aggregation). It has been used widely as an anti-thrombotic agent, but there is little evidence that it is effective. It is used with aspirin as secondary prevention following a TIA or ischaemic stroke.
- Clopidogrel 75 mg daily inhibits the adenosine diphosphate (ADP)-dependent activation of the glycoprotein IIb/IIIa complex on the platelet surface, leading to inhibition of platelet aggregation. It is metabolized by cytochrome p450 enzymes and is therefore slightly less effective in patients possessing the reduced function *CYP2C19* allele or in patients taking, for example, omeprazole (p. 134). It is similar to **ticlopidine** (no longer available in the UK) but has fewer side-effects. Trial evidence supports its use in acute coronary syndromes (p. 435).
- Prasugrel, a novel thienopyridine, is a pro-drug like clopidogrel. It is being trialled in acute coronary syndromes.
- Ticagrelor is similar but has a stronger, more rapid, antiplatelet effect.
- Glycoprotein IIb/IIIa receptor antagonists block a receptor on the platelet for fibrinogen and VWF. These drugs have been used as an adjunct in percutaneous coronary intervention therapies and as primary medical therapy in coronary heart disease. Excessive bleeding has been a problem. Three classes have been described:
  - a murine–human chimeric antibodies (e.g. **abciximab**, initial 250 mcg/kg IV injection over 1 min, then 125 ng/kg/min infusion)
  - synthetic peptides (e.g. **eptifibatide** IV injection 180 mcg/kg then by IV infusion 2 mcg/kg/min for 72 hours)
  - synthetic non-peptides (e.g. **tirofiban** IV infusion 400 ng/kg/min for 30 mins, then 100 ng/kg/min for 12–24 hours).
- Epoprostenol is a prostacyclin that is used to inhibit platelet aggregation during renal dialysis (with or without heparin) and is also used in primary pulmonary hypertension.

The indications for and results of antiplatelet therapy are discussed in the appropriate sections (pp. 435 and 632).

Thrombolytic therapy

- **Streptokinase.** This is a purified fraction of the filtrate obtained from cultures of haemolytic streptococci. It forms a complex with plasminogen, resulting in a conformational change that activates other plasminogen molecules to plasmin. Streptokinase is antigenic and the development of streptococcal antibodies precludes repeated use. Activation of plasminogen is indiscriminate, so that lysis of both free fibrinogen and fibrin within thrombus occurs, leading to hypofibrinogenaemia and an increased risk of haemorrhage.

- **Plasminogen activators (PA).** Tissue-type plasminogen activators (alteplase (t-PA), tenecteplase (TNK-PA) and reteplase (r-PA)) are produced by recombinant technology. They are not antigenic and do not induce allergic reactions. They are associated with a slightly higher risk of intracerebral haemorrhage.

- **Indications.** The use of thrombolytic therapy in coronary artery disease is discussed on p. 438. The extent of the benefit depends on how quickly treatment is given. They are also used in cerebral infarction (p. 629) and in massive pulmonary embolism. The main risk of thrombolytic therapy is bleeding.

- **Contraindications.** Treatment should not be given to patients who have had recent bleeding, uncontrolled hypertension or a haemorrhagic stroke, or who have undergone surgery or other invasive procedures within the previous 10 days.

VENOUS THROMBOEMBOLISM (VTE)

Venous thromboses usually occur in otherwise normal vessels (most commonly as a **deep venous thrombosis (DVT)** of the lower limb) in response to venous stasis and/or inherited or acquired hypercoagulable states ('thrombophilia'). The most serious risk from DVT is the potential for embolism, particularly to the pulmonary circulation (**pulmonary embolism (PE)**). Thromboembolic disease is a highly significant cause of adult mortality.

Common risk factors include surgery (particularly in the elderly), malignant disease, immobility, a previous history of thrombosis, obesity, oral contraceptive use, HRT and pregnancy. Venous thrombosis is also increased in some blood disorders, including polycythaemia, essential thrombocythaemia and inherited or acquired thrombophilia (p. 242).

Clinical features

The symptoms of a DVT in the lower leg are swelling, pain and discoloration of the calf or of the whole leg. A palpable venous cord may be felt, and the leg is swollen and warm with engorged superficial veins. Pitting ankle oedema may be present. The distal veins below the knee can be affected in isolation, but proximal extension of thrombosis to the ilio-femoral veins may be present or occur later in 20–30%, with signs remaining only in the calf area. In some patients presenting with PE, asymptomatic DVT is often detected later during the course of investigations.

The general risk factors for VTE are shown in Box 7.6.

> **Box 7.6** Risk factors for venous thromboembolism
>
> - Active cancer or cancer treatment
> - Age over 60 years
> - Critical care admission
> - Dehydration
> - Known thrombophilias
> - Obesity (BMI > 30 kg/m²)
> - One or more significant medical co-morbidities (e.g. heart disease; metabolic, endocrine or respiratory pathologies; acute infectious diseases; inflammatory conditions)
> - Personal history or first-degree relative with a history of VTE
> - Use of HRT
> - Use of oestrogen-containing contraceptive therapy
> - Varicose veins with phlebitis

Diagnosis

- **D-dimer.** A negative D-dimer (assuming the test has appropriate sensitivity) in conjunction with a low clinical probability score, has good negative predictive value (96% probability of no DVT). If the clinical probability is high, then the D-dimer should be repeated. An elevated D-dimer level alone is not specific for the diagnosis of a DVT, as it can be elevated in other conditions, e.g. infection.
- **B-mode venous compression ultrasonography.** This should be performed on all patients suspected of having a DVT. Ultrasonography has a sensitivity and specificity of 95% for an above-knee DVT. Below-knee thromboses are not detected reliably with this method but repeat testing improves the sensitivity. Venography is the best test for below-knee DVT.

Differential diagnosis of a swollen leg

DVTs are usually unilateral, unless they extend proximally up into the pelvic veins. The differential diagnoses include a calf haematoma, ruptured popliteal Baker's cyst, cellulitis, muscle injury or other causes of oedema, e.g. heart failure or lymphatic obstruction.

Investigation of inherited and acquired thrombophilia

Investigations should be performed when there is recurrent venous thrombosis, venous thrombosis in an unusual site (e.g. mesenteric or portal veins), a first venous thrombosis under the age of 40 years (no risk factor), a family history of thrombosis, a history of recurrent miscarriage (≥ 3), neonatal thrombosis, or unexplained arterial thrombosis under 50 years of age.

- General screening tests
  - A blood count and blood film are useful to exclude some acquired thrombophilic states, e.g. myeloproliferative neoplasms.
  - A coagulation screen should also be requested; a prolonged APTT that does not correct on mixing studies with normal plasma may indicate the presence of a lupus anticoagulant (see below).
  - Further screening investigations should be directed at identifying other possible causes of acquired thrombophilia, e.g. malignancy or PNH.

Investigation of inherited thrombophilia

Acute thromboses and anticoagulant therapy adversely affect some of the functional assays used for thrombophilia screening (e.g. protein C and S), and in any case the results almost never influence the initial management of a patient with VTE. Therefore, investigation before resolution of the thrombus and cessation of treatment is of little value, and a full investigation should only be undertaken at least 6 weeks after cessation of oral anticoagulant therapy. Tests include assays for protein C and S and for antithrombin deficiencies, and a coagulation-based assay for activated protein C resistance. If this is abnormal, genetic analysis for the factor V Leiden mutation is performed. The prothrombin gene mutation, *G20210A*, is a less common cause of activated protein C resistance.

Investigation of acquired thrombophilia

- Antiphospholipid antibody syndrome (APS) (p. 316) is diagnosed when arterial/venous thrombosis or recurrent miscarriages occurs in a patient with persistently positive tests for lupus anticoagulant.
- Lupus anticoagulant (LA) describes antiphospholipid autoantibodies that cause prolongation of phospholipid-dependent coagulation tests (such as the APTT), but which are associated with thrombosis and recurrent miscarriage rather than bleeding. The development of LA is a more frequent cause of thrombosis than heritable thrombophilic defects. The prevalence of LA in the general population is 1–2%. However, most individuals with LA will not experience an episode of thrombosis and it is often only a transient finding, e.g. after viral infection. In addition to a prolonged APTT that does not correct on mixing studies, the presence of LA must be confirmed with an alternative phospholipid-dependent coagulation test and correction procedure, and by demonstrating the presence of antiphospholipid antibodies (anti-β2-glycoprotein-I (β2-GP-I) and/or anticardiolipin (aCL)).
- Paroxysmal nocturnal haemoglobinuria – p. 219.
- Myeloproliferative neoplasms – p. 220. Molecular analysis for the *JAK2 V617F* and related mutations can be performed.

Prevention and treatment of VTE

Heparin

- Unfractionated heparin (UFH). This is a heterogeneous mixture of polysaccharide chains of varying length and molecular weight, derived from porcine mucosa. UFH has a rapid effect on coagulation by increasing the inhibitory activity of antithrombin, mainly against activated factor X (FXa) and thrombin (FIIa). Since the advent of low-molecular-weight heparins (LMWH), IV UFH has been used less frequently for the treatment of VTE because of its unpredictable bioavailability and the requirement for continuous monitoring by APTT. However, UFH is occasionally useful for the initial treatment of VTE where strict control of anticoagulation with the potential for rapid reversal is required (e.g. patients with recent VTE and a high bleeding risk), owing to the short half-life (45 mins to 2 hours; dose-dependent) and sensitivity to protamine sulphate. UFH can be administered intravenously or subcutaneously.
- Low-molecular-weight heparin (LMWH, e.g. **enoxaparin**, **dalteparin**). Controlled depolymerization of UFH fractionates polysaccharide chains into smaller pieces, generating LMWH. LMWH has greater inhibitory

Kumar & Clark's Medical Management and Therapeutics

Table 7.1 Low-molecular-weight heparins in DVT

Drug	Daily treatment	Prophylaxis	
		Moderate risk	**High risk, e.g. orthopaedic operation**
Bemiparin	115 U/kg SC	2500 U SC 2 hours pre- or 6 hours post-surgery; then 2500 U every 24 hours for 7–10 days	3500 U 2 hours pre- or 6 hours post-surgery; then 3500 U every 24 hours for 7–10 days
Dalteparin	200 U/kg SC	2500 U SC 1–2 hours pre-surgery, then 2500 U 24 hourly for 5–7 days Medical patients 5000 U SC every 24 hours	2500 U SC 1–2 hours pre-surgery, then 2500 U 8–12 hours post-surgery, then 5000 U 24-hourly for 5–7 days
Enoxaparin	1.5 mg/kg SC	20 mg (2000 U) 2 hours pre-surgery then 20 mg every 24 hours for 7–10 days Medical patients 40 mg (4000 U) every 24 hours for 6 days or until patient is ambulant	40 mg (4000 U) 12 hours pre-surgery, then 40 mg every 24 hours for 7–10 days
Tinzaparin	175 U/kg SC for at least 6 days	3500 U 2 hours pre-surgery, then daily for 7–10 days	50 U/kg 2 hours pre-surgery, then 50 U/kg every 24 hours for 7–10 days

N.B. Continue treatment until warfarin therapy is adequate — usually 5–9 days.

activity against FXa than against thrombin. It is administered subcutaneously and has a longer half-life than UFH (> 6 hours), so once-daily dosing is possible (Table 7.1). LMWH does not usually require monitoring because the bioavailability is more predictable than UFH, allowing the dose to be calculated according to body weight. However, weight-based dosing is unreliable in renal failure, pregnancy, gross obesity, neonates and infants, so LMWH therapy can be monitored by the anti-Xa activity assay in such patients. Heparin-induced thrombocytopenia (HIT) is less frequent with LMWH than UFH, but a baseline platelet count and coagulation screen should always be performed (p. 230).

- Relative contraindications to heparin therapy. These include bleeding disorders (e.g. haemophilia), thrombocytopenia (platelet count < 60 ×

10^9/L), peptic ulceration (unless cured by *H. pylori* eradication), recent cerebral haemorrhage, severe hypertension, severe liver disease, oesophageal varices, major trauma, and recent eye surgery or neurosurgery. Patients previously diagnosed with HIT/HITT should receive a suitable alternative to heparin (see below). In patients with hepatic and renal dysfunction, clearance of many parenteral anticoagulants is prolonged. There is a risk of osteoporosis with long-term heparin use.

Alternatives to heparin

- **Fondaparinux** is a synthetic pentasaccharide FXa inhibitor, used for prophylaxis of VTE in medical patients and in those undergoing major lower limb orthopaedic surgery, given subcutaneously 2.5 mg 6 hours after surgery and 2.5 mg daily thereafter. Fondaparinux can also be used for the treatment of DVT and PE (dosage by weight — see product literature).

- **Lepirudin** (recombinant hirudin) is an irreversible direct thrombin (FIIa) inhibitor, which is approved for use in patients with HIT. The therapeutic dose is 400 mcg/kg by slow IV injection, followed by continuous infusion of 150 mcg/kg/hour (to a maximum of 16.5 mg/hour). Lepirudin therapy is monitored with the APTT, 4 hours after the initial bolus (target APTT ratio 1.5–2.5 times control). Dose adjustment is necessary in patients with renal impairment. Caution should be exercised, as there is no effective antidote to lepirudin in patients who are bleeding. Lepirudin also prolongs the PT, so frequent PT monitoring is required when oral anticoagulant therapy, i.e. warfarin, is commenced.

- **Danaparoid** is a mixture of non-heparin glycosaminoglycans with a low cross-reactivity for heparin auto-antibodies, which can also be used in patients with HIT. Danaparoid is administered as an IV bolus followed by continuous infusion, dosed according to body weight (see product literature).

- **Bivalirudin**, a hirudin analogue, is a direct thrombin inhibitor and is used as an anticoagulant for patients undergoing percutaneous coronary intervention.

- **Two oral factor Xa inhibitors** have been recently licensed and approved by NICE for VTE prophylaxis following orthopaedic surgery. Caution is advised, as there is no effective antidote to either of these drugs in patients who are bleeding. However, they are oral, require no monitoring and in trials major bleeding has not been a problem.
  - *Dabigatran etexilate* 100 mg is given 1–4 hours after total hip or total knee replacement, then 220 mg daily. The dosage is halved for the elderly over 75 years. Continue for 9 days after total knee replacement, and 27–34 days following total hip replacement.
  - *Rivaroxaban* 10 mg daily after surgery and then continued 10 mg daily, for 3 weeks following total knee replacement and 5 weeks following total hip replacement.

These and other Xa inhibitors e.g. apixaban are being more widely used, e.g. in atrial fibrillation.

Vitamin K antagonists

Warfarin (a coumarin) is the treatment of choice for the secondary management of VTE in most patients, because it has few side-effects apart from bleeding. Vitamin K antagonists interfere with the synthesis of coagulation factors, II, VII, IX and X (and natural anticoagulants protein C and protein S). The anticoagulant activity is monitored using a PT-based assay. However, the reference range for the PT assay varies according to the method used, so in order to simplify the management of oral anticoagulation, calculation of the International Normalized Ratio (INR) allows comparison of PT results between laboratories.

- Warfarin can be commenced simultaneously with heparin.
- Heparin should be continued until a therapeutic INR has been achieved for ≥ 2 days (usually at least 4 days).
- Protein C levels initially fall on commencement of warfarin and can produce a temporary procoagulant state; thus in patients with protein C and S deficiency there is a theoretical risk of warfarin-induced skin necrosis.

An example nomogram for starting warfarin therapy is shown in Table 7.2.

- Anticoagulation for a period of 3 months (minimum 6 weeks for calf DVT) to a target INR of 2.5 (range 2–3) is recommended for patients

Table 7.2 Nomogram for starting warfarin (target INR 2.5)

Day	INR	Dose (mg)
1	< 1.4	10
2	< 1.8	10 (or 5*)
	> 1.8	Refer to haematology dept for advice
3	< 2	10
	2.0–2.3	5
	2.4–2.7	4
	2.8–3.1	3
	3.2–3.4	2
	3.5–4.0	1
	> 4.0	Refer to haematology dept for advice
4 onwards (maintenance)	1.6–1.7	7
	1.8	6 & 7 alternate days
	1.9	6
	2.0–2.1	5 & 7 alternate days
	2.2–2.3	5
	2.4–2.6	4 & 5 alternate days
	2.7–3.0	4
	3.1–3.5	3 & 4 alternate days
	3.6–4.0	3
	4.2–4.5	Miss 1 day, then 2 mg
	> 4.5	Refer to haematology dept for advice

*A lower starting dose may be required in patients with liver disease, excess alcohol users, body weight < 50 kg or congestive cardiac failure, and in the elderly.
(Adapted from Winter M, et al 2005.)

with temporary risk factors (e.g. recent surgery) and a low risk of recurrence. There is no evidence to suggest that patients with inherited or acquired thrombophilia should be anticoagulated to a higher target INR than patients without thrombophilia.

- A 6-month period of anticoagulation is recommended for *any* patient with either idiopathic VTE or permanent risk factors (e.g. thrombophilia).
- Longer-term anticoagulation in patients with thrombophilia depends on the individual case and should be based on clinical criteria such as family history (for inherited causes) or recurrent idiopathic events.
- For secondary thromboprophylaxis in patients with cancer and VTE, LMWH is superior to warfarin with lower recurrence rates and fewer bleeding complications.
- Target INR for most conditions is 2.5, 3.0 for an aortic mechanical prosthetic heart valve or prior to cardioversion, and 3.5 (range 3–4) for recurrence of VTE whilst on warfarin or some mitral mechanical prosthetic heart valves. Most patients with mechanical valves should receive long-term anticoagulation.

Initially, outpatient anticoagulation should be supervised in an anticoagulant clinic, but some patients may be suitable for self-management using near-patient testing devices. Standardized booklets are available nationally for recording INR results and anticoagulant doses, and should be issued to all patients. Once the recommended duration of therapy has been completed, warfarin can be stopped abruptly.

- **Contraindications to warfarin therapy.** These are generally the same as for heparin (see above), although oral anticoagulants can be used after initial therapy in patients with HIT/HITT. Oral anticoagulants are teratogenic and should be avoided in early pregnancy; specialist advice should be sought if anticoagulation in pregnancy is essential (p. 250). LMWH can be used as an alternative to warfarin where compliance is likely to be an issue (e.g. IV drug use).
- **Interactions with warfarin (Box 7.7).** Patients should be advised to notify the anticoagulation clinic whenever changes to regular medications are made, and will often require more frequent monitoring until the INR stabilizes again.
- **Management of over-anticoagulation due to warfarin.** This is summarized in Table 7.3.
- **Alternatives to warfarin.** Other coumarins (e.g. **acenocoumarol** and **phenindione**) generally have the same advantages and disadvantages as warfarin. However, they are occasionally useful in patients suffering an idiosyncratic adverse reaction to warfarin.

Prevention of VTE

- General measures. For all patients, early mobilization, elevation of the legs and compression stockings are used. Mechanical compression devices are used in many hospitals for pre- and post-surgical patients. Female patients with known inherited or acquired thrombophilia should be advised to use an alternative to the combined oral contraceptive and to avoid HRT. However, widespread thrombophilia screening in asymptomatic individuals before starting oral contraception or HRT is unnecessary.
  - *Low risk* (proximal vein thrombosis 0.4%; fatal PE < 0.2%) includes patients < 40 years undergoing major surgery (> 30 mins) with no

Box 7.7 Examples of warfarin interactions

Agents increasing the anticoagulant effect
- Alcohol
- Antibiotics
  - Macrolides, e.g. erythromycin, clarithromycin
  - Quinolones — some
- Anti-arrhythmics
  - Amiodarone
  - Quinidine
- Anabolic steroids, e.g. nandrolone
- Antifungal agents, e.g. miconazole, fluconazole
- Antidepressants, e.g. mirtazipine, tricyclics
- Disulfiram
- Hormone antagonists, e.g. tamoxifen, danazol
- NSAIDs, e.g. diclofenac
- Statins and fibrates, e.g. atorvastatin, gemfibrozil
- Proton pump inhibitors, e.g. omeprazole
- H_2-receptor antagonists, e.g. cimetidine
- Testosterone
- Thyroid hormones

Agents reducing the anticoagulant effect
- Antibiotics, e.g. rifampicin
- Antifungal, e.g. griseofulvin
- Anticonvulsants, e.g. phenytoin, carbamazepine, phenobarbital, primidone
- Antidepressants, e.g. tricyclics
- St John's wort

other risk factors, minor surgery (< 30 mins), trauma with no other risk factors but history of DVT or previous PE.
- *Medium risk* (proximal vein thrombosis 2–4%; fatal PE 0.2–0.5%) includes patients who have undergone major general, urological, gynaecological, cardiothoracic, vascular or neurological surgery and patients > 40 years or with one or more other risk factor(s), or patients with minor injury who have undergone plaster cast immobilization of the leg. Patients with a major acute medical illness requiring hospitalization are also included in this group. All medical patients are at increased risk if they have significantly reduced mobility for 3 days or more.
- *High risk* (proximal vein thrombosis 10–20%; fatal PE 1–5%) includes patients with a major fracture or who have had major orthopaedic surgery to pelvis, hip or leg, or major pelvic or abdominal surgery for cancer.
- Heparin prophylaxis for VTE. At times of increased risk, prophylaxis should be offered to *all* patients with a past history of VTE, and to the affected relatives of patients with heritable thrombophilia. If there is no previous or family history, then VTE prophylaxis should be offered to

Table 7.3 Management of bleeding and excessive oral anticoagulation

INR/severity of bleeding	Management
INR > 3.0 < 6.0 (target INR 2.5) INR > 4.0 < 6.0 (target INR 3.5)	1. Reduce warfarin dose or stop 2. Restart warfarin when INR < 5.0
INR > 6.0 < 8.0, no bleeding or minor bleeding	1. Stop warfarin 2. Restart warfarin when INR < 5.0
INR > 8.0, no bleeding or minor bleeding	1. Stop warfarin 2. Restart warfarin when INR < 5.0 3. If other risk factors for bleeding, give 0.5–2.5 mg vitamin K (phytomenadione) orally
Major bleeding	1. Stop warfarin 2. Give prothrombin complex concentrate (PCC) 50 U/kg, or fresh frozen plasma (FFP) 15 mL/kg 3. Give 5–10 mg vitamin K (oral or slow IV)

(Adapted from British Committee for Standards in Haematology 1998)

all medium- or high-risk medical and surgical patients. LMWH is the first choice for most patients, given subcutaneously once daily, e.g. enoxaparin 2–4000 U (20–40 mg) (Table 7.3). The recommended dose depends on the preparation used and level of risk, so the product literature must be consulted. Alternatively, UFH can be given, 5000 U SC every 8–12 hours (APTT monitoring is not required for UFH at prophylactic doses).

- Dabigatran and rivaroxaban. These drugs (p. 245) are now being used after lower limb joint replacement surgery, as they are as effective as LMWH and can be given orally for a longer period.

Treatment of established VTE

The aim of treatment is to prevent propagation and embolization of an existing venous thrombus until it resolves or organizes as a result of natural fibrinolytic activity. Initial therapy for the majority of patients is with LMWH, which has been shown to be at least as effective as UFH for the treatment of VTE, allows patients with DVT to be treated on an outpatient basis, and has a number of other advantages (p. 243). Differences in efficacy between LMWHs appear to be insignificant, so the choice of anticoagulant is usually guided by local policy. The recommended dose depends on the product used and patient weight, e.g. **enoxaparin** 1.5 mg/kg per day.

Where therapeutic anticoagulation with UFH is necessary, it is administered intravenously as a 75 U/kg bolus loading dose, followed by a continuous infusion of 18 U/kg/hour. The anticoagulant effect should be monitored by the APTT ratio 2–4 hours after the start of treatment or after a dose adjustment, and every 24 hours thereafter if no dose adjustment is required. The recommended APTT ratio is 1.5–2.5 times the control APTT (the sensitivity of reagents used between laboratories varies, so the APTT

Kumar & Clark's Medical Management and Therapeutics

needs to be locally calibrated against an anti-Xa assay to ensure accuracy and reproducibility of the results).

For continued management of the thrombotic episode until complete resolution of the thrombus, oral anticoagulant therapy, i.e. warfarin, can be commenced simultaneously with heparin (see below).

Insertion of an inferior vena cava (IVC) filter is sometimes useful where there is a contraindication to anticoagulant therapy, or in patients who develop PE despite adequate anticoagulation.

- Management of over-anticoagulation or haemorrhage. In patients receiving UFH, the infusion should be stopped, which may be sufficient because of the short half-life. If necessary, **protamine sulphate** can be administered, 1 mg IV for every 100 U heparin administered over the previous hour to a maximum dose of 40 mg. LMWH should be used with caution in patients with a high risk of bleeding complications, because of the long half-life and incomplete (~70%) neutralization by protamine sulphate. However, for life-threatening haemorrhage due to LMWH, there is limited evidence that recombinant FVIIa may be of benefit.

- Peri-operative management of anticoagulation
  - Minor procedures such as dental extraction can often be managed with 5% **tranexamic acid** mouthwash 4 times daily, without alteration of oral anticoagulant therapy.
  - Other minor surgical procedures may be performed at an INR close to 2.0, achieved by stopping or reducing the dose of oral anticoagulants and monitoring the INR pre-operatively.
  - Oral anticoagulants should be stopped at least 3 days prior to major surgery (the INR will fall to 1.5 after an average of 4 days), or alternatively a low dose of **vitamin K** can be given for more rapid reversal (e.g. 0.5–1.0 mg), although re-introduction of oral anticoagulants after surgery will take longer.
  - Further management depends on the level of thrombotic risk for the individual patient balanced against the risk of bleeding from the procedure. If necessary, anticoagulation can continue with LMWH until 24 hours before or UFH until 6 hours before surgery.
  - Very high-risk patients (e.g. recent thrombotic event) are managed peri-operatively with modified LMWH regimes in many hospitals, because there is far less experience with the safe and effective management of continuous UFH infusion amongst medical, nursing and laboratory staff since the introduction of LMWH. Where it is used, UFH is given by continuous infusion until 3 hours before surgery and restarted 12 hours after surgery with close monitoring of the APTT ratio. Warfarin can be re-introduced after 2–3 days, but UFH should be continued until the INR has been therapeutic for 48 hours.

- VTE in pregnancy. This is the commonest cause of maternal mortality in the UK, and the risk is greatest post-partum. Prophylaxis and treatment of VTE are usually with self-administered SC LMWH, but the bioavailability is less predictable in pregnancy and requires monitoring by anti-Xa activity. The dose and duration should be kept to a minimum where possible because of the risk of osteoporosis with long-term heparin use. Prophylaxis is usually offered to women with a past history of VTE or a family history of heritable thrombophilia, and should be continued until at least 6 weeks after delivery. LMWH at prophylactic doses can continue throughout labour and delivery, but therapeutic

LMWH should be reduced to a prophylactic dose as soon as labour commences. Epidural anaesthesia is contraindicated within 12 hours of a prophylactic dose of LMWH and within 24 hours of a therapeutic dose.

Further reading

Allford SL, Hunt BJ, et al: Guidelines on the diagnosis and management of the thrombotic microangiopathic haemolytic anaemias, *Br J Haematol* 120(4):556–573, 2003.

Baglin T, et al: Guidelines on the use and monitoring of heparin, *Br J Haematol* 133(1):19–34, 2006.

Blood Transfusion Task Force: Guidelines for the use of platelet transfusions, *Br J Haematol* Jul 122(1):10–23, 2003.

Bolton-Maggs PH, et al: Guidelines for the diagnosis and management of hereditary spherocytosis, *Br J Haematol* 126(4):455–474, 2004.

British Committee for Standards in Haematology (BCSH): *Guidelines on oral anticoagulation*, ed 3, *Br J Haematol* 101:374–387, 1998.

Campbell PJ, Green AL: Mechanisms of disease: the myeloproliferative disorders, *N Engl J Med* 355:2452, 2006.

Cazzola M, Malcovati L: Myelodysplastic syndromes — coping with ineffective hematopoiesis, *N Engl J Med* 352:536–538, 2005.

General Haematology Task Force: Guidelines for the investigation and management of idiopathic thrombocytopenic purpura in adults, children and in pregnancy, *Br J Haematol* 120(4):574–596, 2003.

George JW: *N Engl J Med* 354:1927–1935, 2006.

Hillmen P, et al: The complement inhibitor eculizumab in paroxysmal nocturnal hemoglobinuria, *N Engl J Med* 355:1233–1243, 2006.

Keel SB, Abkowitz JL: The microcytic red cell and the anaemia of inflammation, *N Engl J Med* 361:1904–1906, 2009.

O'Shaughnessy DF, et al: Guidelines for the use of fresh-frozen plasma, cryoprecipitate and cryosupernatant, *Br J Haematol* 126(1):11–28, 2004.

Rees DC, Olujohungbe AD, Parker NE, et al: Guidelines for the management of the acute painful crisis in sickle cell disease, *Br J Haematol* 120:744–752, 2003.

Rees DC, Williams TN, Gladwin MT: Sickle cell disease, *Lancet* 376:2018–2031, 2010.

Winter M, Keeling D, Sharpen F, et al: Haemostasis and Thrombosis Task Force of the British Committee for Standards in Haematology. Procedures for the outpatient management of patients with deep venous thrombosis, *Clin Lab Haematol* 27:61–66, 2005.

Malignant disease 8

CHAPTER CONTENTS

APPROACH TO THE PATIENT WITH CANCER

All efforts should be made to obtain a histological diagnosis of malignancy before anticancer treatment is commenced. A combination of clinical examination, imaging and biochemical tests is subsequently used to assess response to treatment.

Symptoms

Patients can present in a number of ways:

- Tumour site-specific symptoms, e.g. breast lump, hoarse voice of laryngeal carcinoma, post-menopausal bleeding typically seen with endometrial carcinoma, or progressive dysphagia of oesophageal carcinoma.
- Systemic symptoms
  - Weight loss, anorexia and fatigue.
  - Coagulopathy of malignancy. DVT and the associated complications may be due to pancreatic cancer or locally advanced pelvic malignancies.
  - Paraneoplastic syndromes (rare), e.g. hypertrophic pulmonary osteo-arthropathy of non-small cell lung cancer or ectopic endocrine syndromes, e.g. syndrome of inappropriate ADH secretion (SIADH) or ectopic ACTH secretion seen with small cell lung cancer.
- Complications of metastatic disease, e.g. back pain or spinal cord compression (common in lung or prostate cancer), hepatomegaly (often found with metastatic gastrointestinal cancer).

Risk factors

Smoking, obesity and alcohol are all risk factors for a variety of cancers. Some cancers also show a familial predisposition, e.g. familial adenomatosis or patients with *BRACA* mutations. The relatives of such patients should be referred to a geneticist.

Performance status

This is a measurement of a patient's overall functional status. It helps to predict how a treatment will be tolerated and also response to treatment.

Table 8.1 Eastern Cooperative Oncology Group (ECOG) performance status scale

Status	Description
0	Asymptomatic, fully active and able to carry out all pre-disease performance without restrictions
1	Symptomatic, fully ambulatory but restricted in physically strenuous activity, able to carry out performance of light or sedentary nature e.g. light housework, office work
2	Symptomatic, ambulatory and capable of all self-care but unable to carry out any work activities. Up and about > 50% of waking hours; in bed < 50% of day
3	Symptomatic, capable of only limited self-care, confined to bed or chair > 50% of waking hours, but not bedridden
4	Completely disabled, cannot carry out any self-care. Totally bedridden

Performance status is commonly measured using the Eastern Cooperative Oncology Group scale (Table 8.1) or the Karnofsky scale.

Investigations

These should be aimed at confirming the presence of malignancy and assessing the extent of spread (i.e. staging the tumour). Although tumours may have a characteristic radiological appearance, biopsy with histology should always be performed, as the prognosis and treatments of different cancers vary greatly. Different tumours are staged in different ways. The most commonly used staging system for solid tumours is the TNM (tumour, node, metastases) system, which is updated every few years (Box 8.6, p. 269).

The multi-disciplinary meeting

All cancer patients should be discussed with the appropriate multi-disciplinary team (MDT) — the cancer specialist, relevant physician and surgeon, radiologist, histopathologist, nurse specialists, palliative care team and psychologist. Further investigations for optimal treatment are coordinated. Information is then given to patients about their diagnosis, prognosis and treatment options. This enables the patient to make an informed decision about the proposed management.

Cancer treatment

Treatment may be in the form of surgery, systemic treatment (chemotherapy, hormonal treatment or targeted agents), radiotherapy or a combination of these. Surgery offers the best chance of cure in many cancers. However, this must be balanced against the potential loss of function and cosmesis.

● Aims of treatment. The patient and the other medical teams should be clear about the intention of treatment. This enables patients to be realistic and to have the opportunity to organize aspects of their life and obtain the appropriate support. Often, the intention of treatment may be palliative but the prognosis can vary from months to years dependent on tumour type.

> **Box 8.1** Definitions of response (RECIST)
>
> - Complete response — Complete disappearance of all detectable disease
> - Partial response — At least a 30% decrease in the sum of diameters of target lesions, taking as reference the baseline sum diameters
> - Stable disease — Neither sufficient shrinkage to qualify for PR nor sufficient increase to qualify for PD
> - Progressive disease — At least a 20% increase in the sum of diameters of target lesions, or the appearance of new lesions

- Types of treatment
  - *Adjuvant treatment.* Adjuvant treatment is given after complete surgical removal of a tumour. The risk of micrometastases is sufficiently high for therapy in the form of systemic treatment (chemotherapy, hormone therapy, targeted agents), radiotherapy or chemoradiation to be offered to reduce the risk of recurrent disease. These patients have no clinically detectable metastatic disease.
  - *Neoadjuvant treatment.* Chemotherapy and/or radiotherapy are given to downstage a tumour before surgery.
  - *Radical treatment.* Radical treatment in the form of chemotherapy and/or radiotherapy is given as primary treatment to a tumour. The intent of treatment is curative.
  - *Palliative treatment.* When cure is not possible, the aim of treatment is to improve quality of life. Improved survival may also be possible. Different tumours vary greatly in their prognosis.
- Measuring response to treatment (Box 8.1)
  - *Objective response to treatment.* This is measured radiologically using re-evaluation criteria in solid tumour (RECIST).
  - *Subjective response to treatment.* This is used mostly in palliative treatments to assess whether a patient perceives an improvement in symptoms. Measures of quality of life enable an assessment of the benefit of treatment compared to the side-effects.

PRINCIPLES OF RADIATION TREATMENT

Radiation is delivered to tissues by a variety of methods with the aim of causing cell death. The biological effect is achieved by X-rays causing direct or indirect damage to DNA.

The **unit of absorbed dose** is the Gray (Gy), which is equivalent to 1 joule absorbed per kilogram (1 J/kg) of absorbing tissue. Radiation dose is described by three factors: total dose in Gy, number of fractions, and duration of treatment (e.g. 50 Gy/25 Gy/5 weeks indicates that the total dose of 50 Gy is being given in 25 doses over 5 weeks) The effect of radiotherapy is also dependent on the volume irradiated and the radiosensitivity of the tumour and surrounding tissues.

Administration of radiotherapy

- External beam radiotherapy is the most commonly used form of radiotherapy. Treatment is with beams of ionizing radiation produced from a source external to the patient, most commonly a **linear accelerator**.

Kumar & Clark's Medical Management and Therapeutics

Box 8.2 Palliative benefits of radiotherapy

- Pain relief, e.g. bone metastases
- Reduction of symptoms associated with raised intracranial pressure from CNS metastases
- Relief from obstructive symptoms (oesophagus, bronchus)
- Improvement in symptoms of bleeding (bladder, cervix, endometrium)
- Reversal of neurological impairment from spinal cord compression or cranial nerve compression by metastases

Box 8.3 Potential side-effects of radiotherapy

Acute (during and up to 90 days)	
• Skin	Erythema, hair loss, dry desquamation, moist desquamation
• Gastrointestinal tract	Nausea, anorexia, mucositis, oesophagitis, diarrhoea, proctitis
• Genitourinary tract	Cystitis, urinary frequency, nocturia, urgency

Late (after 90 days)	
• Skin	Pigmentation, telangiectasia, atrophy
• Bone	Necrosis, sarcoma
• Mouth	Xerostomia, osteoradionecrosis
• Bowel	Diarrhoea, stenosis, fistula
• Bladder	Fibrosis, fistula
• Vagina	Stenosis
• Lung	Fibrosis
• Heart	Pericardial reactions, cardiomyopathy
• CNS	Myelopathy
• Reproductive	Infertility, premature menopause, impotence

Techniques are continually evolving to maximize dose to abnormal tissue while attempting to reduce dose to normal surrounding structures, e.g. conformal radiotherapy or intensity-modulated radiotherapy (IMRT). **Brachytherapy** is where the radiotherapy sources are placed within or close to the target volume, e.g. intracavitary (gynaecological, lung or oesophageal cancers), interstitial (tongue, floor of mouth, breast) or tumour surface (eye, skin).

- **Systemic radionuclides** are commonly used in oncology for diagnostic and therapeutic purposes. Therapeutic applications involve administering the radiopharmaceutical with the intent of selectively destroying diseased tissue, e.g. the radio-labelled tracer ^{131}iodine or ^{99}technetium is used in the treatment of benign thyroid disease and in follicular or papillary carcinoma of the thyroid after surgery.

Radiotherapy regimes

There are various radiotherapy regimes that can be used with curative or palliative intent, depending on the tumour and stage:

- **Radical radiotherapy** (e.g. skin, CNS, prostate, lymphoma).
- **Chemoradiation** (e.g. cervical cancer, anal cancer, oesophageal cancer and tumours of the head and neck).
- **Accelerated radiotherapy** (e.g. squamous cell tumours of head and neck, non-small cell lung cancers).
- **Adjuvant radiotherapy** (e.g. breast, endometrium).
- **Palliative radiotherapy.** For palliative treatments, a shorter course with a larger dose per fraction is used (Box 8.2).

Side-effects are shown in Box 8.3.

PRINCIPLES OF CHEMOTHERAPY

Chemotherapy drugs are preferentially toxic to rapidly dividing cells but have a less marked effect on non-proliferating cells. They target cancer cells at various stages of the cell cycle, e.g. 'phase-specific' (preference for a given phase) or 'cycle-specific' agents.

Chemotherapy drugs are commonly given in combination (Table 8.2); the rationale for this is two-fold. Firstly, if drugs with differing mechanisms of action are used, which act at differing stages of the cell cycle, this can maximize the number and types of cancer cells killed. In addition, some drug combinations may have synergistic effects. Secondly, the simultaneous use of multiple drugs reduces the risk of drug resistance developing and the survival chances of the tumour.

Table 8.2 Some common chemotherapy regimens

Malignancy	Regimen	Components
Hodgkin's lymphoma	ABVD	Doxorubicin, bleomycin, vinblastine, dacarbazine
	BEACOPP	Bleomycin, etoposide, doxorubicin, cyclophosphamide, vincristine, procarbazine, prednisolone
Non-Hodgkin's lymphoma	CHOP	Cyclophosphamide, hydroxy-doxorubicin, vincristine, prednisolone
Breast cancer	FEC	5-FU, epirubicin, cyclophosphamide
	FEC-T	5-FU, epirubicin, cyclophosphamide followed by docetaxel
	TAC	Docetaxel, doxorubicin and cyclophosphamide
Lung cancer	PE	Cisplatin, etoposide
	GC	Gemcitabine, carboplatin
Stomach cancer	ECF	Epirubicin, cisplatin, 5-FU
Colorectal cancer	FolFOx	Oxaliplatin, 5-FU, folinic acid
	OX	Oxaliplatin, capecitabine

Kumar & Clark's Medical Management and Therapeutics

Administration of chemotherapy drugs

- Chemotherapy drug doses are calculated on the basis of body surface area (BSA).
- Drug dosage may be modified during the course of treatment due to side-effects such as bone marrow suppression, stomatitis, renal insufficiency, hepatotoxicity and diarrhoea.
- Cytotoxic drugs are most commonly administered intravenously and should only be given by qualified personnel. **IV administration** may be via peripheral venous access or, in those who require repeated cycles of treatment, via indwelling venous catheter devices, such as Hickman, Groshong and peripherally inserted central catheter (PICC) lines. **N.B.** *Veins of the antecubital fossa and wrist should be avoided.*
- **Vesicant cytotoxic drugs** include **doxorubicin, epirubicin, vincristine, vinblastine, vinorelbine, mitoxantrone, paclitaxel** and **5-fluorouracil (5-FU).** Care is taken to prevent extravasation and phlebitis. Free flow of fluid to the vein and adequate flashback of blood in the cannula are mandatory before administration. **Dexrazoxane** 1 g/m^2 IV daily for 2 days can be used for anthracycline extravasation as soon as possible.
- Only trained personnel should administer **intrathecal chemotherapy**. It is used in meningeal carcinomatosis or as CNS prophylaxis, in certain patients with lymphoma, haematological malignancies and choriocarcinoma. Cytotoxic drugs that may be given intrathecally include **methotrexate, cytarabine** and **hydrocortisone. N.B. ⚠** *Never give vinca alkaloid drugs intrathecally.*

Available chemotherapeutic drugs

Cytotoxic drugs can be classified into the groups listed below according to their mechanism of action and chemistry.

- DNA-damaging agents
  - *Alkylating agents* (e.g. **chlorambucil, cyclophosphamide, ifosfamide** and **nitrosoureas**, e.g. **carmustine, lomustine, busulfan**). These contain an alkyl group and so act by forming covalent bonds with cellular DNA, RNA and protein molecules. Alkylation of DNA leads to cross-linking of DNA strands and deactivation of repair processes, which in turn causes single-strand breaks. These actions interfere with cellular synthesis of DNA and culminate in cell death. Cytotoxicity is cell cycle-non-specific.
  - *Non-classical alkylating agents.* **Platinum compounds** (e.g. cisplatin, carboplatin, oxaliplatin) cause inter-strand cross-links on the DNA helix and so block DNA replication. **Dacarbazine** (DTIC) is a purine analogue, which, following metabolism, acts in a similar manner to alkylating agents. **Temozolomide** is structurally related to **dacarbazine.**
- Antimetabolites. These compounds disrupt nucleic acid synthesis by falsely substituting for purines and pyrimidines, and may combine with vital enzymes required for cell division. Maximal cytotoxicity is seen in the S phase of cell cycle.
  - *Methotrexate* is a folic acid antagonist. It binds to the enzyme dihydrofolate reductase and so blocks the conversion of folic acid to folinic acid. This results in the inhibition of thymidine and purine synthesis and so arrests RNA and DNA synthesis. When high doses

of methotrexate are administered, folinic acid 'rescue' is given afterwards to protect normal tissues from prolonged exposure to methotrexate.

- *6-Mercaptopurine (6-MP)* is a purine antagonist.
- *Arabinosides* include **cytarabine (Ara-c)**, which acts by interfering with pyrimidine synthesis. A liposomal formulation of cytarabine is now available for intrathecal use in lymphomatous meningitis. **Gemcitabine** is another pyrimidine antimetabolite and **fludarabine** is an adenosine analogue.
- *5-Fluorouracil (5-FU)* blocks the enzyme thymidylate synthase, which is essential for pyrimidine synthesis and so inhibits DNA synthesis. **Folinic acid** is a cofactor necessary for thymidylate synthase and so is often given along with **5-FU** to potentiate its cytotoxic effects. **Tegafur** is a prodrug of **5-FU** and is used in combination with **uracil**.
- *Capecitabine* is an orally administered prodrug of **5-FU**, which is converted in tumours to **5-FU** through the intermediate doxifluridine. It has been shown to be of similar efficacy as the combination of **5-FU** and **folinic acid**.
- *Pemetrexed* inhibits folate-dependent enzymes, including thymidylate transferase.

- ● DNA repair inhibitors
  - *Cytotoxic antibiotics* bind to DNA by intercalating adjoining nucleotide pairs on the same DNA strand and inhibit DNA repair. They are cell cycle non-phase-specific. **Anthracycline antibiotics** (e.g. **doxorubicin**) have a cumulative toxicity to the myocardium, which can result in cardiomyopathy.
  - *Epipodophyllotoxins* (e.g. **topoisomerase I inhibitors**, e.g. **irinotecan**, **topotecan**; **topoisomerase II inhibitors**, e.g. **etoposide**, **teniposide**) act on the topoisomerase enzymes that regulate the 3-D structure of DNA by unwinding coiled double-stranded DNA. These drugs therefore indirectly cause the formation of single and double DNA strand breaks and have maximal effect late in S or G2 phases of the cell cycle.

- ● Anti-tubilin agents
  - *Vinca alkaloids* (e.g. vincristine, vinblastine) act by binding to tubulin and inhibiting microtubule formation, thereby preventing cell division. Due to their neurotoxicity they should never be given intrathecally.
  - *Taxanes* (e.g. paclitaxel, docetaxel) bind to tubulin dimers and prevent their assembly to microtubules.

Side-effects of treatment

- ● Nausea and vomiting are common side-effects of chemotherapy treatment, which can be prevented in up to 75% of patients with modern antiemetics. These symptoms may occur acutely (during the 24 hours following administration) or may be delayed (more than 24 hours after treatment and possibly lasting up to a week). The degree of emetogenicity is dependent on the drug and its dose (Box 8.4). Combination chemotherapy may also have greater emetogenicity than the sum of the single agents used alone. A stepped approach to antiemetic treatment depending on emetogenicity of the drug is used (Table 8.3). If the selected antiemetic regime is not sufficient, **lorazepam** 1–2 mg oral/sublingual

Box 8.4 Emetogenicity of common cytotoxic agents

Low (+); incidence <30%
- Bleomycin
- Fludarabine
- Vinca alkaloids
- Chlorambucil
- Docetaxel
- Etoposide
- Melphalan (oral)
- Methotrexate ≤ 500 mg/m^2
- Paclitaxel
- Mitoxantrone
- Topotecan
- Pemetrexed
- Mitomycin
- Gemcitabine
- Fluorouracil

Moderate (++); incidence 30–90%
- Cyclophosphamide < 1,500 mg/m
- Daunorubicin
- Doxorubicin
- Epirubicin
- Ifosfamide
- Cytarabine >1 g/m^2
- Methotrexate > 500 mg/m^2 to < 2 g/m^2
- Irinotecan
- Oxaliplatin
- Carboplatin

High (+++); incidence >90%
- Carmustine
- Cisplatin
- Cyclophosphamide $\geq 1,500$ mg/m^2
- Etoposide — high-dose
- Dacarbazine
- Dactinomycin
- Melphalan — high-dose
- Methotrexate ≥ 2 g/m^2

(particularly useful in anticipatory nausea and vomiting), oral **haloperidol** and **cyclizine** IV/SC/oral can be used.

- **Alopecia** (hair loss) is particularly troublesome with agents such as **cyclophosphamide**, **doxorubicin**, **etoposide**, **bleomycin** and **paclitaxel**. It usually begins 1–2 weeks following chemotherapy and becomes maximal 1–2 months later. Regrowth usually occurs shortly after treatment ends. Scalp cooling is sometimes used to reduce hair loss when the drug used has a short half-life, e.g. **doxorubicin**.

Table 8.3 Antiemetic recommendations

Emeto-genicity	On days of chemotherapy	Days after chemotherapy
Low	No antiemetic required routinely Metoclopramide 10 mg 3 times daily or domperidone 20 mg 3 times daily if the patient experiences nausea and vomiting	
Moderate	Metoclopramide 20 mg IV oral 3 times daily or domperidone 20 mg oral 3 times daily Dexamethasone 4–8 mg IV/oral daily	Metoclopramide or domperidone 20 mg 3 times daily for 3 days, then as required Dexamethasone 4 mg twice daily for 2 days
High	Granisetron 1 mg IV/ oral 1–2 times daily Dexamethasone 8–16 mg IV/oral daily (in 1 or 2 divided doses)	Metoclopramide or domperidone 20 mg 3 times daily for 3–5 days, then as required Dexamethasone 4 mg twice daily for 2–3 days Granisetron 1 mg twice daily for 2 days

- **Bone marrow suppression** is a common side-effect of many cytotoxic agents and is a dose-related phenomenon. It most commonly occurs 7–14 days following chemotherapy; however, some drugs can cause delayed myelosuppression (21–35 days after treatment), such as **chlorambucil**, **carboplatin**, **nitrosoureas** and **melphalan**.
    - *Anaemia* is managed with red cell transfusions or with **recombinant erythropoietin**. Patients are commonly transfused if they are symptomatic and if their haemoglobin is < 6–8 g/dL.
    - *Thrombocytopenia* ($< 10–20 \times 10^9$/L) is treated with platelet transfusions to prevent spontaneous haemorrhage from occurring.
    - *Neutropenic patients* are at high risk of fungal and bacterial infections, especially Gram-negative infections from enteric bowel flora. In addition, those patients with indwelling lines are at risk of infection with Gram-positive organisms. Neutropenic patients with a temperature > 38°C and $< 0.5 \times 10^9$ neutrophils should be treated immediately with **broad-spectrum antibiotics** until microbiological results are available, and should be closely monitored (Box 8.5). The use of **colony-stimulating haematopoietic growth factors**, such as granulocyte colony stimulating factor (GCSF) 5 mg/kg SC daily or pegfilgrastim 6 mg as a single dose 24 hours post-chemotherapy, can reduce the duration of neutropenia in patients on highly myelosuppressive chemotherapy regimes.

> **Box 8.5** Managing a febrile neutropenic patient
>
> - The patient should be reviewed promptly and treatment initiated without delay (see Fig. 20.6).
> - History and physical examination should be performed to help elucidate the source of infection, paying particular attention to indwelling lines.
> - Resuscitation should be carried out with IV fluids to restore circulatory function.
> - Cultures of blood (from indwelling lines and peripheral), urine, sputum, stool should be collected and a CXR performed.
> - Empirical IV antibiotic should be started, e.g.:
>   - Ceftazidime 2 g — followed by 1 g 3 times daily— *and* gentamicin 5 mg/kg IV daily (reduce dose in renal impairment).
>   - Piperacillin with Tazobactam 4.5 g x 3 daily + Gentamycin is an alternative
>   - If the patient clinically deteriorates and/or temperature is still elevated after 48 hours, the antibiotics should be changed according to culture results or changed to increase Gram-positive and negative cover, e.g. imipenem 500 mg 4 times daily and vancomycin 1 g twice daily IV
>   - If the patient fails to respond to second-line antibiotic treatment, fungal infection should be looked for with high-resolution CT scan of the chest. Antifungal agents, such as liposomal amphotericin, caspofungin or voriconazole, may be considered
> - Each time antibiotics are changed, blood and other cultures should be repeated and CXR performed.
> - Febrile neutropenic patients should be closely monitored and nursed in modified reverse isolation.
> - After 48 hours, if the patient has clinically improved, is afebrile and cultures are negative, antibiotics may be stopped and the patient observed closely.

- **Mucositis** is commonly seen with drugs such as methotrexate, 5-FU and high-dose melphalan, and reflects drug-induced mucosal sloughing. It can also be due to candidiasis secondary to the myelosuppressive effects of chemotherapy. If radiotherapy is administered simultaneously, mucositis can be more severe due to reduction in salivary secretions. Since the mouth is a potential portal for entry of enteric organisms, good oral hygiene is imperative in all cancer patients. Mucositis is best prevented using antiseptic mouthwashes such as **chlorhexidine gluconate** every 6 hours, along with prophylactic **nystatin** suspension or **amphotericin** lozenges. If mucositis is severe, IV fluid may be needed along with SC **diamorphine** for pain relief and **sucralfate** suspension orally. If there are any ulcers suggestive of herpes simplex virus infection, **aciclovir** should be prescribed. **Palifermin**, a human keratinocyte growth factor, is also helpful.
- **Cardiotoxicity** has been associated with anthracyclines such as doxorubicin and daunorubicin. It is dose-related, and can be avoided by

restricting the cumulative dose of **doxorubicin** to 450 mg/m^2. Unfortunately, once cardiomyopathy has developed, it is not reversible.

- Renal toxicity in the form of acute tubular necrosis can occur with agents such as cisplatin, methotrexate and ifosfamide. Renal function should be monitored during treatment and the patient should be adequately hydrated.

- Neurotoxicity occurs mainly with **vincristine**, **vinblastine**, **taxanes** and **cisplatin** (but less so with carboplatin). It is dose-related and cumulative. These drugs cause a peripheral sensory neuropathy and the dose should be reduced or the drug omitted before development of significant symptoms, as the neuropathy may potentially be permanent. Rarely, the plant alkaloids can lead to autonomic nerve dysfunction, which can in turn cause gastrointestinal aperistalsis. High doses of **cisplatin** can also cause ototoxicity, resulting in high-tone hearing loss and tinnitus. A dose-dependent encephalopathy can occur with **ifosfamide**; it can be reversed with 50 mg methylene blue in 2% solution by slow IV injection.

- Sterility in males and females can be caused by a number of drugs, such as **alkylating agents**, **vinblastine** and **procarbazine**. In males, storage of sperm should be offered in all patients treated with curative intent. In females, oocysts can be fertilized and cryopreserved.

- Secondary malignancies are one of the long-term complications of treatment since chemotherapeutic drugs have mutagenic potential. Acute leukaemia is the most common secondary malignancy and occurs 6–10 years after initial treatment. Solid tumours and lymphomas tend to occur more than 15 years after initial treatment and there is no time limit on the duration of risk. Drugs such as the epipodophyllotoxins and alkylating agents are particularly implicated in this complication.

- Tumour lysis syndrome can occur with chemosensitive tumours with rapid doubling times, as the result of a large cell kill following chemotherapy/steroid treatment. The sudden release of large amounts of intracellular contents into the bloodstream can lead to acute tubular necrosis. This is particularly associated with Burkitt's lymphoma, high-grade non-Hodgkin's lymphoma, lymphoblastic lymphoma and acute leukaemia. Patients are especially at risk if they have bulky disease, high uric acid levels and high levels of LDH prior to treatment. Tumour lysis syndrome comprises hyperkalaemia, hyperphosphataemia, hypocalcaemia and hyperuricaemia, and can lead to acute kidney injury, cardiac arrhythmias and tetany. At-risk patients should be treated prophylactically with **allopurinol 300–600 mg** orally or 200 mg IV, starting at least 24 hours prior to chemotherapy treatment and continued for the duration of chemotherapy treatment. Patients should be adequately hydrated, with IV fluids commenced prior to treatment and a fluid intake of at least 3 L daily maintained through chemotherapy treatment. **Rasburicase** 0.2 mg/kg/day for 5–7 days, starting on day 1 of chemotherapy treatment, is used if the patient is at very high risk or if significant tumour lysis develops despite prophylactic measures. U&E, urate, P_{O_4} and calcium must be monitored 6-hourly post chemotherapy and the renal dialysis used early if prophylactic measures prove unsuccessful.

Principles of high-dose therapy

In chemosensitive tumours, the administration of high doses of chemotherapy maximizes their cytotoxic effect, but their limiting effect is bone

Kumar & Clark's Medical Management and Therapeutics

marrow toxicity and susceptibility to infections. Haematopoietic stem cells are often infused into the patient to shorten the neutropenic period, which may last 2–3 weeks. The patient is reverse barrier-nursed in isolation, preferably in a negative air pressure-ventilated room.

The source of stem cells may be autologous (from the patient or an identical twin), allogeneic (from a non-identical donor) or umbilical cord blood.

Autologous stem cell transplantation/peripheral blood stem cell rescue (PBSCR)

This procedure involves the IV infusion of the patient's own stem cells as rescue from myelo-ablative therapy, resulting in minimal immunological disturbance and avoidance of a graft versus tumour effect. The peripheral blood stem cells are collected using leucopheresis following administration of growth factor GCSF. The cells are then re-infused intravenously following myelo-ablative treatment, some time having been allowed for the drugs to be cleared from the system. Autologous stem cell transplants are carried out in relapsed lymphoma, multiple myeloma, acute myeloid leukaemia, acute lymphocytic leukaemia and relapsed testicular tumours. The overall transplant-related mortality from autologous transplants is < 5%.

Allogeneic stem cell transplantation

In allogeneic transplantation a donor, ideally with fully matched major HLA antigens, e.g. siblings, acts as the stem cell source. Transplantation is highly toxic and the morbidity and mortality are related to the recipient's age and the donor's HLA compatibility. Transplant-related mortality for an HLA sibling-matched allograft is 15–30% but for volunteered unrelated donors can be as high as 45%. The first component of the transplant is myelo-ablative chemotherapy, often combined with total body irradiation (TBI). This has the dual effect of eradicating the malignancy and ablating the patient's immune system, allowing the graft to 'take'. A day following the conditioning treatment, the donor stem cells are then infused intravenously. It is thought that engraftment of the donor's immune system, along with anti-tumour activity (graft versus tumour), is responsible for the increased efficacy of this approach. In order to prevent graft rejection, **anti-T-cell antibodies** or a combination of immunosuppressants such as **ciclosporine**, **methotrexate** or **tacrolimus** may be given. Unlike with solid organ transplants, lifelong immunosuppressants are not required; they are usually continued for around 6 months. Allogeneic transplants have been used successfully in acute and chronic leukaemias, along with myeloma.

● **Non-myelo-ablative allogeneic stem cell transplantation/'reduced-intensity' transplantation.** In this form of transplantation the conditioning regime is not myelo-ablative but still has an immunomodulatory effect, produced by drugs such as **fludarabine**. The principle is that the anticancer effect of the allogeneic stem cells will still be present without the complications of a conventional transplant, particularly the severity of graft versus host disease (GVHD).

Transplant complications

Common side-effects associated with myelo-ablative conditioning regimens are nausea and vomiting, mucositis, oesophagitis, gastritis, abdominal pain, diarrhoea and reversible alopecia.

- **Infections.** The severe myelosuppression of the conditioning treatment renders the patient susceptible to a wide variety of potentially fatal infections with bacterial (Gram-negative and positive), viral (herpes simplex, herpes zoster, cytomegalovirus (CMV)), fungal (*Aspergillus*) and atypical organisms. Nearly all patients experience fever and require **broad-spectrum antibiotics** during this neutropenic period; GCSF is usually given, starting the day after transplant until neutrophil recovery. Despite recovery of their blood counts, patients who have undergone autologous transplantation do not recover full immune function for 3–6 months. Patients who have undergone allogeneic transplantation are affected, in addition to severe myelosuppression, by immune dysfunction that persists until their GVHD resolves. These patients are particularly susceptible to CMV disease secondary to reactivation. On testing positive for CMV, patients are treated with **ganciclovir** or **foscarnet**.

- **Graft versus host disease (GVHD).** This is secondary to the immune reaction of the donor cells against the normal host organs and affects 30–50% of allogeneic transplant recipients. GVHD is classified as being acute if it occurs in the first 100 days post transplant and chronic if it occurs after 100 days.
  - *Acute GVDH* is characterized by a rash, which may be either mild and maculo-papular, or severe, resulting in erythroderma and extensive desquamation. Other features include deranged liver biochemistry, fever, diarrhoea, failure of stem cell engraftment and viral reactivation, particularly by CMV.
  - *Chronic GVHD* can involve any organ system. Its clinical features include malabsorption with marked weight loss, hepatic dysfunction, sclerodermatous skin reaction due to excess collagen deposition, keratoconjunctivitis sicca, severe immunosuppression and features of autoimmune disease.

- **Veno-occlusive disease** usually presents in the first 2 weeks following allogeneic transplantation; it occurs in < 5% of patients. It is characterized by the triad of hepatomegaly, jaundice and ascites. Diagnosis is largely clinical but may be supported by hepatic Doppler US. Treatment is primarily supportive and thrombolysis is rarely used.

PRINCIPLES OF ENDOCRINE THERAPY

Breast cancer (p. 270)

- **Anti-oestrogens.** Oestrogen is the main hormone involved in the development of breast cancer and exerts its effects through the oestrogen receptor (ER), a ligand-activated nuclear transcription factor.
  - *Tamoxifen* acts as a competitive antagonist of the ER and so inhibits the growth of breast tumours. Its exact mechanism of action is complex, since it also has partial agonist effects, which are tissue-dependent. As a result, long-term administration is associated with an increased risk of uterine cancer and thromboembolism, but not with vaginal atrophy or osteoporosis. The usual dose is 20 mg daily.
  - *Fulvestrant* is a new type of anti-oestrogen with a different mechanism of action to tamoxifen; it acts as a pure ER antagonist and, as a result, reduces the risk of cross-resistance to treatment. In addition,

it down-regulates the cellular levels of ER, which results in a reduction in progesterone receptor (PgR) expression.

- Aromatase inhibitors. These include **anastrozole** 1 mg daily, **letrozole** 2.5 mg daily and **exemestane** 25 mg daily. In post-menopausal women residual oestrogen production is solely from non-glandular sources, in particular subcutaneous fat. Therefore, aromatase inhibitors should not be used in pre-menopausal women unless ovarian suppression has occurred. Aromatase inhibitors suppress oestrogen levels in these women by inhibiting or inactivating aromatase, the enzyme responsible for the synthesis of oestrogens from androgenic substrates; as a result the drugs have no partial agonist activity
- Gonadorelin analogues (gonadotrophin-releasing hormone (GnRH) agonists, e.g. **goserelin**). These exert their effect by binding to hypothalamic GnRH receptors in the pituitary, with the release of luteinizing hormone (LH) and follicle-stimulating hormone (FSH). These peptides are not released from their binding sites and receptor down-regulation occurs with suppression of LH release and FSH release and so oestrogen synthesis. The role of GnRH agonists in pre-menopausal women is controversial, with some trials demonstrating equivalence of GnRH administration when compared to older-style chemotherapy regimens. For pre-menopausal women with ER and/or PgR-positive metastatic or locally advanced breast cancer, ovarian ablation can be considered to facilitate the use of aromatase inhibitors. This may be in the form of oophorectomy, radiotherapy, or the use of GnRH agonists alone.

Prostate cancer (p. 276)

Hormonal treatment is commonly utilized in patients with prostatic metastatic disease, and also prior to and after radical radiotherapy for localized disease. Androgens are capable of stimulating the growth of prostate cancer cells and androgen removal can lead to apoptosis and tumour regression.

- GnRH agonists. The gonadorelin analogues, **leuprorelin acetate** and **goserelin acetate**, are administered SC as a monthly or 3-monthly depot preparation. As in breast cancer, these drugs exert their effects by suppression of LH and FSH release and also testicular androgen synthesis. Since these agents initially cause a transient rise in testosterone, their use should be covered with an anti-androgen. Anti-androgens are typically administered 2 weeks before and after the first GnRH agonist injection. **Side-effects** of GnRH agonists are similar to those of surgical castration and include loss of libido, impotence, hot flushes, gynaecomastia, mood disturbance, osteoporosis, metabolic syndrome and anaemia.
- Anti-androgens, such as **bicalutamide** and **flutamide**, work by competitively blocking the androgen receptor. In addition to their use in preventing tumour flare when initiating GnRH agonist therapy, they are also employed along with GnRH agonists in patients who develop disease progression despite medical castration. **Side-effects** are similar to those of GnRH agonists.

PRINCIPLES OF TARGETED TREATMENTS

The treatment of malignancy has been revolutionized by the advent of molecularly targeted treatments that inhibit the tyrosine kinase (TK) pathway. These treatments aim to exploit tumour-specific over-expression of epidermal growth factor receptors (EGFR), deranged and chaotic tumour vasculature and supporting extracellular matrix. Inhibition is achieved directly (using small molecules) or indirectly (using monoclonal antibodies). These treatments present an opportunity in the future to provide patient-specific treatment, reduce side-effect profiles and improve outcome.

Selective targets (Table 8.4)
Monoclonal antibodies

- *Trastuzumab* is a monoclonal antibody directed against Her2/Nu (human epidermal growth factor receptor 2), a member of the EGFR family. As well as modifying the immune response, it acts as an anti-growth factor and so increases the apoptotic response to cytotoxics.
- *Bevacizumab* is a monoclonal antibody that binds to vascular endothelial growth factor (VEGF), preventing activation of the VEGF

Table 8.4 Targeted therapies (cytokine modulation) used in cancer treatment

Drug	Target	Malignancy
Cetuximab	Anti-EGFR	Colorectal cancer Head and neck
Bevacizumab	Anti-VEGF	Colorectal cancer
Rituximab	Anti-CD20	Non-Hodgkin's lymphoma
Alemtuzamab	Anti-CD52	Chronic lymphocytic leukaemia
Trastuzumab	Anti-Her2	Breast cancer
Imatinib	Tyrosine kinase inhibitor	Chronic myeloid leukaemia Gastrointestinal stromal tumours
Gefitinib	Tyrosine kinase inhibitor EGFR	Non-small cell lung cancer
Erlotinib	Tyrosine kinase inhibitor	Non-small cell lung cancer Bronchoalveolar cancer
Dasatinib	Tyrosine kinase inhibitor	Chronic myeloid leukaemia
Sorafenib	Tyrosine kinase inhibitor	Renal cell cancer
Sunitinib	Tyrosine kinase inhibitor	Renal cell cancer
Nilotinib	Tyrosine kinase inhibitor	Chronic myeloid leukaemia
Bortezomib	Proteosome inhibitor	Myeloma
Panitumumab	EGFR	Metastatic colorectal cancer
Bexarotene	Retinoid X receptor agonist	Cutaneous T-cell lymphoma

EGFR, epidermal growth factor receptor; VEGF, vascular endothelial growth factor.

receptor TK and its downstream pathway. It has demonstrated significant activity in combination with chemotherapy in colorectal, lung and ovarian cancer.

- *Rituximab* is a humanized monoclonal antibody directed against the B-cell-specific antigen CD20. It is used in patients with low- and high-grade CD20-positive non-Hodgkin's lymphoma. It is given as an IV infusion and is usually administered weekly for 4 weeks. **Side-effects**: in patients with cardiovascular disease and those receiving cardiotoxic chemotherapy, exacerbation of arrhythmias and heart failure occur. Infusion-related side-effects are common and predominantly occur with the first dose. These include flu-like symptoms, nausea, flushing and, rarely, hypersensitivity reactions. Patients should therefore be given pre-medication with paracetamol and antihistamines; corticosteroids are also given.

Monoclonal antibodies may also be used as a carrier molecule to target toxins or radioisotopes to tumour cells.

- **Intracellular signal inhibitors.** Most of these TK inhibitors are small molecules and they compete with the ATP binding pocket of the catalytic domain of oncogenic TKs. They are administered orally and are often used in combination with chemotherapy drugs or radiotherapy. Patients can develop resistance to treatment and the agents are often only active in subgroups of patients. **Imatinib** is a TK inhibitor that specifically inhibits the fusion oncoprotein BCR-ABL. Further examples of TK inhibitors are listed in Table 8.4. Many other molecules with a role in inhibiting proteins involved in cancer cell signalling are under development. Examples include farnesyl transferase inhibitors, which inhibit ras proteins, drugs that target the proteosome, inhibitors of the platelet-derived growth factor receptor, and drugs that inhibit matrix metalloproteinase.

IMMUNOTHERAPEUTIC AGENTS

These agents exert their anti-tumour effects by modifying the host immune response. Interleukin and interferons were standard treatments in the management of renal cancer, but they are now used less commonly due to the advent of the TK inhibitors.

- **Interleukin(IL)-2 (aldesleukin)** is a cytokine used to activate T-cell responses, and the recombinant protein is often given in conjunction with interferon (IFN)-α, a B-cell activator. It is usually given by SC injection and is used in renal cell carcinoma and melanoma. High-dose IV IL-2 is now rarely used due to its acute toxicity, which may lead to the capillary leak syndrome with pulmonary oedema and hypotension.
- **Interferons** are naturally occurring cytokines that function by stimulating humoral and cell-mediated immune responses that can produce an anti-tumour effect. They also have antiproliferative activity in some tumours.
- **Tumour vaccines** may be used to activate the patient's immune system, using autologous and allogeneic tumour cells. A number of vaccine approaches have been investigated, including whole-tumour cell lysates, oncogenic peptides, genetically engineered antigen-presenting cells and solubilized cell surface antigens.

COMMON SOLID TUMOUR MANAGEMENT

Lung cancer

Lung cancer is the commonest cause of malignant death in men and women in the UK. Cigarette smoking is the main causative factor in up to 90% of cases; the disease is therefore preventable.

- Non-small cell carcinomas are staged according to the TNM system (Box 8.6) and have 5-year survival rates of < 6% overall.
- Small cell lung cancers are staged according to whether the disease is limited (tumour can be encompassed in a radical radiotherapy portal) or extensive (tumour is more extensive than limited-stage disease), and have a median survival of 12–24 months.

Treatment of non-small cell lung cancer

- Surgery in the form of lobectomy is curative in patients with operable non-small cell lung cancer. Any stage below and including IIIa is potentially operable, and should be discussed with a cardiothoracic surgeon at an MDT meeting. The patient needs to have sufficient pulmonary reserve and to be fit for surgery to be considered for this form of radical treatment.
- Radical radiotherapy is used for patients who are not suitable for surgery (usually due to co-morbidity) whose tumours can be encompassed in a radical radiotherapy field. Patients require an $FEV_1 > 1.5$ L and a transfer factor of > 50% to be considered for radical radiotherapy. Various methods have been used to improve the outcome. **Sequential chemotherapy** (platinum-based), followed by radiotherapy and concurrent chemoradiation, has demonstrated improvements over conventionally fractionated radiotherapy alone, although there is a preponderance of patients with locally advanced tumours in these trials.
- Chemotherapy with platinum-containing regimens can be given in patients being treated with radical intent. Neo-adjuvant chemotherapy

---

Box 8.6 TNM classification, as used for lung cancer

- Tx   Positive cytology only
- T1   ≤3 cm diameter
- T2   ≥3 cm/extends to hilar region/invades visceral pleura/ partial atelectasis
- T3   Involvement of chest wall, diaphragm, pericardium, mediastinum, pleura, total atelectasis
- T4   Involvement of heart, great vessels, trachea, oesophagus, malignant effusion
- N1   Peribronchial, ipsilateral hilar lymph node involvement
- N2   Ipsilateral mediastinal
- N3   Contralateral mediastinal, scalene or supraclavicular
- M0   No distant metastases
- M1   Metastases present

T, extent of primary tumour; N, extent of regional lymph node involvement; M, presence of distant metastases.

Kumar & Clark's Medical Management and Therapeutics

prior to surgery is currently being used in trials. Trials comparing surgery with surgery plus chemotherapy demonstrate a 13% reduction in risk of death and absolute benefit of 5% at 5 years. **Pemetrexed** is also used for maintenance therapy. **Erlotinib** (Table 8.4) is also used for locally advanced or metastatic disease after failure of chemotherapy.

● Palliative treatment
  ● *Chemotherapy* with platinum-containing regimens is used in patients with good performance status. Better response rates with increased 1-year survival and better palliation are seen when compared to best supportive care. Typical chemotherapy regimens include a **platinum agent** (**cisplatin** or **carboplatin**) with either **gemcitabine, vinorelbine** or **paclitaxel**. Second-line chemotherapeutic agents in use include **docetaxel** and **pemetrexed**.
  ● *Palliative radiotherapy* to the lung is used in any patient who is not suitable for radical radiotherapy. High-dose palliative regimens are used for patients who are fit but not suitable for radical radiotherapy, with variable results. Other fractionation regimens provide significant palliative benefit for patients with dyspnoea, haemoptysis or pain.
  ● *Targeted treatments* with **TK inhibitors**, such as **erlotinib** or **gefitinib**, are used (in patients with EGFR gene mutations) when chemotherapy regimens have been exhausted or a patient is not fit for them. A response rate of 19–33% was seen in a subgroup of patients who were female, were of Asian origin and have broncho-alveolar tumours. Gefitinib can also be used as initial treatment for pulmonary adenocarcinoma.

Treatment of small cell lung cancer

Chemotherapy with platinum (**carboplatin** or **cisplatin**) and **etoposide** forms the basis of treatment. Consolidation thoracic **radiotherapy** is given either concurrently or sequentially for limited-stage disease. If there has been a complete response at metastatic sites and at least a partial response in the thorax for extensive-stage disease, consolidation thoracic radiotherapy is also given. For limited-stage patients who achieve a complete response, prophylactic cranial irradiation is indicated; this has been shown to increase 3-year overall survival by 5.4% and reduce the incidence of brain metastases to 8% (from 22% in patients treated with chemotherapy alone).

Breast cancer

Presentation is usually with a painless lump that may be associated with skin changes and/or nipple symptoms. Many women who are referred for further investigation are asymptomatic but have had an abnormality identified on a screening mammogram.

Investigations

● Women should first be investigated by **triple assessment**. This comprises clinical examination, radiology (typically mammography and US but MRI if indicated) and fine needle aspiration cytology or core biopsy of the breast lump. The triple assessment is carried out in a dedicated one-stop clinic.
● Staging in early disease is surgical and is dependent on tumour size and the extent of loco-regional nodal involvement.

- Screening blood tests and CXR are routinely performed. Further investigations are performed to detect distant metastases depending on clinical suspicion; they include CT thorax and abdomen, breast MRI (lobular carcinoma), bone scan, liver US and PET CT.

Prognosis

Poor prognostic factors for breast cancer include positive lymph nodes, high tumour grade, young age, pre-menopausal status, hormone receptor-negative disease, Her2-positive disease and a large tumour.

In **early breast cancer** the prognosis can be predicted from the factors listed above, and the survival probability and benefit from adjuvant therapy by using the website www.adjuvantonline.com. The 10-year survival can vary from > 90% for small, low-grade, node-negative tumours to < 20% for large, high-grade tumours with more than three nodes involved, if no adjuvant treatment is given.

Local treatment

- Surgery. The type of surgery (wide local excision, mastectomy with or without reconstruction) is dictated by the tumour size and position, and patient preference. Surgical staging of the axilla is also performed by a sentinel lymph node sampling, in which a blue tracer, with or without a radiotracer, is injected around the tumour bed. The lymph node(s) (sentinel node) that picks up the dye or tracer is/are excised. If no lymph node metastases are identified in the histological sample, the patient can be spared the morbidity of a full axillary nodal dissection.
- Radiotherapy is indicated in all patients following breast-conserving surgery. It is also used following mastectomy in women who are at high risk of locally recurrent disease (large tumour, multifocal disease, skin involvement, more than four nodes involved). If an adequate surgical procedure to the axilla has been performed in women who are found to have positive lymph nodes, radiotherapy to the axilla can be avoided; otherwise the risk of lymphoedema significantly increases. In women who are node-positive (usually three or more nodes), radiotherapy to the supraclavicular fossa is offered in addition.
- Adjuvant systemic treatment
  - *Targeted treatments* This is indicated in women with hormone receptor-positive disease. Aromatase inhibitors are increasingly being used in post-menopausal women as first-line therapy in all but good-prognosis tumours. They can be used either alone for 5 years or sequentially with tamoxifen. Tamoxifen has a different side-effect profile to aromatase inhibitors. There is an increased risk of endometrial proliferation (and consequent malignancy), as well as thromboembolic problems with tamoxifen. The main **side-effects** of aromatase inhibitors are musculoskeletal, such as joint aches and reduction in bone density. Endocrine treatment should be given after completion of chemotherapy in a sequential manner.
  - *Chemotherapy.* The decision as to whether to offer adjuvant chemotherapy is based on an individual woman's risk of relapse. The consequent benefit of chemotherapy is therefore proportional to her risk of relapse. Optimal treatment regimes of combination chemotherapy include an anthracycline. A taxane is often added in node-positive women. The choice of combination offered depends on individual risk, co-morbidity and the toxicity profile of the combination. **Trastuzumab** is also given if a patient is confirmed as being Her2-positive.

Currently, standard practice is to give trastuzumab for 1 year in total but trials are ongoing to define the optimal duration. The main **side-effect** is reversible cardiotoxicity and trastuzumab is therefore not given concurrently with anthracyclines. During treatment, patients should undergo 3-monthly echos to monitor left ventricular function.

Treatment of metastatic breast cancer

The intention of treatment in this group of patients is palliation. Patients can have different patterns of metastatic disease, which have a significant impact on prognosis. Women with bone metastases alone have a much better prognosis than those with visceral (lung and liver) metastases. Combinations of **hormonal treatment**, **bisphosphonates**, **chemotherapy**, **radiotherapy** and **trastuzumab** are used judiciously, with the aim of maintaining a good quality of life for as long as possible.

- Endocrine treatment. Women who are oestrogen and progesterone receptor-positive are more likely to respond to endocrine manipulation. The choice of hormonal treatment is dependent on what was used in the adjuvant setting and the period since hormonal treatment was last used. Endocrine treatment is usually tried first in women who do not have immediately life-threatening disease. Remission of up to 2 years is seen and, on progression, alternate hormonal treatments can be used.
- Chemotherapy. This is used for patients with visceral metastases or rapidly progressive disease, or when all other treatment options are exhausted. Chemotherapy can provide good palliation and prolongation of survival. The choice of chemotherapy regimen is dependent on previously used regimes, Her2 status, fitness for treatment, and bone marrow and liver function.

  Commonly used regimens include: EC, AC (epirubicin or doxorubicin with cyclophosphamide), or FEC (5-FU, epirubicin and cyclophosphamide), docetaxel, docetaxel and capecitabine, vinorelbine, capecitabine, CMF (cyclophosphamide, methotrexate and 5-FU) and weekly paclitaxel.
- Targeted treatment. **Trastuzumab** is used in Her2-positive women, either concurrently or sequentially with chemotherapy; it is also used as monotherapy. It is given continuously, but may be stopped if there is significant cardiotoxicity or extensive progressive disease.

  Lapatinib is an oral TK inhibitor that inhibits both the EGFR and Her2 receptor. It can be given, together with capecitabine, to patients who have progressed on trastuzumab.

Gastrointestinal cancers

Colorectal carcinoma

Tumour stage at the time of diagnosis is the most significant prognostic factor. This is done histologically and is based on the penetration of the tumour through the bowel wall, along with the presence or absence of involved lymph nodes. Although the modified Dukes staging system is still used, the newer TNM system is becoming more widespread.

- Surgical resection. Surgery is the primary treatment modality for colonic cancer and removal of the primary tumour is possible in 90% of cases. The surgical procedure used is dependent on the tumour site and usually involves a right or left hemicolectomy or sigmoid colectomy. In patients with **metastatic disease**, palliative bowel surgery is recommended if there is evidence of bowel obstruction, significant luminal narrowing, and bleeding from the tumour. With rectal tumours, unlike in colon cancer, the ability to obtain wide resection margins may be limited by the bony pelvis and local recurrences are a greater problem (see below).

- Adjuvant treatment for colonic tumours: stage III disease. Despite adequate surgical resection, the 5-year survival in patients with stage III tumours is only 30–60%. Clinical failure is predominantly the result of clinical progression from previously undetected micrometastases. Studies have investigated the optimal treatment duration and established that 6–8 months of adjuvant treatment appears to be the most effective. Two treatment regimes are commonly used:
  - **Oxaliplatin** (FOLFOX4) with **5-FU** and **leucovorin** or **capecitabine** (CAPOX).
  - **Capecitabine**, an oral **fluoropyrimidine** as a single agent.
- Planned adjuvant treatment should commence within 6–8 weeks of primary resection. In patients with temporary stomas, stoma reversal can be performed prior to starting adjuvant treatment. Patients with low resections may find retaining the stoma helpful with regard to the control of chemotherapy-related diarrhoea. Chemotherapy may commence 2 weeks after an uncomplicated stoma reversal.
- Adjuvant treatment for colonic tumours: stage II disease. Chemotherapy is used e.g. in individuals with T4 tumours, poorly differentiated tumours, evidence of perforation, or lymphovascular or neural invasion, and those who may have been inadequately staged as a result of suboptimal lymph node examination (< 13 nodes in the surgical specimen). Other prognostic markers, such microsatellite instability and 18q loss of heterozygosity, may play a future role in patient selection.
- Rectal tumours
  - *Local trans-anal surgery.* This is used for early superficial rectal cancers.
  - *Total mesorectal excision (TME).* TME is used to remove the entire package of mesorectal tissue surrounding the cancer when a local trans-anal operation is inappropriate because of the extent of disease. A low rectal anastomosis is often possible; if not, abdomino-perineal excision can be performed but requires a permanent colostomy. TME combined with pre-operative radiotherapy reduces local recurrence rates in rectal cancer but has not been found to have a significant effect on survival. Post-operative 5-FU-based chemotherapy can be used in high-risk patients (lymph node-positive disease). If, on MRI, the circumferential margin appears involved or if the tumour is low within the rectum, long-course chemo-radiotherapy is given adjuvantly, followed by surgical resection 6 weeks later.
- Isolated colorectal metastates. Around 10–25% of patients present with metastatic disease isolated to the liver or develop liver disease as a recurrence after primary resection. Patients are eligible for hepatic resection if complete resection of the metastasis is possible

Kumar & Clark's Medical Management and Therapeutics

with tumour-free margins and if the functioning hepatic volume post resection is adequate. In a subgroup of patients in whom the predicted remaining functional hepatic volume is small, pre-operative selective embolization of the portal vein branches can be used, since it induces hypertrophy of the liver and so increases the functional hepatic volume. 'Down-staging' of liver metastases with neo-adjuvant chemotherapy is also used in those with potentially resectable lesions. Neo-adjuvant chemotherapy with **oxaliplatin** and **5-FU** is usually administered for 12–24 weeks dependent on response, and once surgery is deemed possible, it is scheduled for 3–4 weeks after chemotherapy is completed. The addition of **cetuximab** (for patients with wild-type *k-ras* gene) or **bevacizumab** (a humanized antibody against VEGF) to the chemotherapy regime may increase the number of patients suitable for resection and improve outcomes. Alternative options for isolated liver or lung metastases include local tumour ablation (such as radiofrequency ablation or regional hepatic intra-arterial chemotherapy or chemoembolization).

- Widespread metastatic colorectal tumours. Fluoropyrimidines (e.g. **5-FU**, **capecitabine**) as single agents, or more commonly in combination with either **irinotecan** or **oxaliplatin**, have become first-line therapy. When given to unselected patients in addition to combination chemotherapy, **panitumumab** (antibody specific to the EGFR and **cetuximab** (antibody against the EGFR) have been associated with worse toxicity and progression-free survival. However, they have been shown to be of benefit to those with the non-mutated (wild-type) *k-ras* gene.

Oesophageal cancer

The prognosis for oesophageal cancer is poor, with a 5-year survival rate of 7%. Thirty percent of patients have metastases at the time of diagnosis and adequate staging is essential.

- Patients with potentially resectable tumours should receive neo-adjuvant chemotherapy with **cisplatin** and **5-FU** for two cycles, prior to planned resection. This has been found to improve median survival by 3 months and 2-year survival by 11% (from 34 to 43%).
- The use of neo-adjuvant chemoradiation is controversial. Although a 25% complete pathological response rate can be seen, a survival advantage has not been consistently demonstrated.
- In patients with inoperable non-metastatic lesions, radical chemoradiation (with **cisplatin** and **5-FU**) should be used. The concurrent use of chemotherapy has been found to improve median survival by 5 months (from 9 to 14 months) and to be associated with a 5-year survival of 26%, versus 0% when compared to radiotherapy alone.
- Disease that is **not suitable for radical treatment** can be palliated in a number of ways. For dysphagia, placement of an oesophageal stent or palliative radiotherapy (or brachytherapy) can improve symptoms. Bleeding may be palliated by endoscopic laser treatment or radiotherapy. Palliative chemotherapy with epirubicin, cisplatin or oxaliplatin and 5-FU or capecitabine (ECF/EOX/ECX) can be used, and this provides a median 2-year survival of 14% and median survival of 9 months (as compared to 3–4 months with best supportive care).

Gastric cancer

- Surgery can be curative in the rare patient who presents with early-stage disease. However, fewer than 5% of patients present with such disease (T1N0 or T2N1). The type of surgery is dependent on the position of the tumour. The extent of lymphadenectomy varies.

- **Adjuvant chemoradiation** with **5-FU** and **folinic acid** has been shown to improve survival significantly. Median survival was 36 months for the adjuvant chemoradiation group, as compared to 27 months for the group undergoing surgery alone. This research has been criticized for a possible over-estimation of benefit due to inadequate surgical staging. Patients have to be extremely fit to receive this treatment, as it is associated with significant gastrointestinal morbidity.
- **Advanced disease** can be palliated in a similar manner to patients with oesophageal cancer (see above). In a subgroup of patients whose tumours over-express Her2, **trastuzumab** can be added.

Hepatocellular carcinoma

See p. 190.

Pancreatic cancer

The 5-year survival rate for carcinoma of the pancreas is 2–5%, with surgical resection offering the only chance of long-term survival.

Contrast-enhanced spiral CT is used to confirm the mass lesion, to exclude tumour invasion into vascular structures and lymph nodes, and to detect distant metastases.

Up to 20% of all cases have a localized tumour suitable for resection. Neo-adjuvant chemotherapy has shown no benefit.

Involvement of vessels, e.g. the superior mesenteric artery, and peripancreatic lymphatic involvement preclude surgery for these patients; treatment is controversial and there is little evidence of long-term survival. A combination of radiotherapy with **5-FU** or **gemcitabine** has shown short-term benefit. The role of adjuvant chemotherapy alone with 5-FU or gemcitabine is also under evaluation.

In the jaundiced patient stent insertion into the common bile duct relieves biliary obstruction and helps quality of life. For patients with metastatic disease, palliative chemotherapy with **gemcitabine**, either alone or in combination with **cisplatin**, can be used.

Gynecological malignancy

Epithelial ovarian cancer

Epithelial ovarian cancer is typically a disease of post-menopausal women. Most women present with disease that is locally advanced, as symptoms are non-specific (abdominal distension, discomfort, pain). The main prognostic factors are the stage at presentation and the amount of residual disease following surgery (quantified as no residual disease, less than 1 cm or more than 1 cm).

- **Surgery** has a major role in the treatment of ovarian cancer. It should involve a mid-line incision, total abdominal hysterectomy, bilateral salpingo-oophorectomy, lymph node sampling, omentectomy, peritoneal biopsies and washings, thorough inspection of the sub-diaphragmatic areas and removal of all the gross disease.
- **Platinum-based chemotherapy regimes** (with taxane for advanced disease) are given adjuvantly if the disease is early-stage but poorly differentiated, or if it is more advanced.
- **Treatment at relapse** depends on the time from end of completion of the last treatment. Patients may well be re-challenged with a platinum-based regimen, typically if relapse is after > 6 months. Other

chemotherapy agents used at relapse include paclitaxel, **oral etoposide**, **liposomal doxorubicin** or **topotecan**.

Endometrial cancer

This is usually considered a curable malignancy because the majority of patients present with stage I disease. However, endometrial cancer has a similar prognosis, stage for stage, as other gynecological malignancies.

- Hysterectomy and bilateral oophorectomy with peritoneal washings are the mainstay of treatment.
- Adjuvant radiotherapy (external beam and vault brachytherapy) is offered if the risk of nodal metastases is high, based on the pathology.
- Chemotherapy with **carboplatin** with or without **paclitaxel** are used adjuvantly in advanced-stage disease or on relapse.
- Progestogens are prescribed in metastatic disease, in women who are symptomatic and do not have a significant cardiac history.

Cervical cancer

- Wertheim's hysterectomy or chemoradiation is the ideal treatment. If there is lymph node disease, deep infiltration of the tumour or disease stage ≥ IB2, surgery should be avoided and the patient should be offered chemoradiation.
- External beam radiotherapy is given for at least $5\frac{1}{2}$ weeks, with intracavitary treatment given to boost the dose to the cervix.
- Cisplatin is also given concurrently, as this reduces mortality.

Genitourinary malignancies

Prostate cancer

Accurate histological tumour grading using the Gleason score, along with staging and prostate-specific antigen (PSA) level assessment can help determine prognosis and so aid in selecting the most appropriate treatment for the patient. The **Gleason grading** system is based on the degree of glandular differentiation. Since prostate tumours exhibit heterogeneity within tissue, two histological areas of the tumour are scored between 3 and 5. The overall scores are added, to give a score between 6 and 10.

- Treatment for localized disease

Watchful waiting with monitoring of PSA is used in patients with well-differentiated localized tumours, particularly if they are elderly, have an expected life expectancy of < 10 years or have significant co-morbidity. The **optimum management** for patients with localized tumours remains controversial. Treatment-related morbidity and quality of life issues are considerations and patient involvement in the decision-making process is essential. Prostatectomy patients are more likely to experience problems with urinary incontinence and erectile dysfunction than those undergoing radiotherapy, whereas radiotherapy patients are at increased risk of chronic bowel dysfunction.

- *Radical prostatectomy* involves the removal of the prostatic urethra and seminal vesicles, with lymph node dissection. Nerve-sparing procedures have reduced the incidence of erectile dysfunction.
- *Conformal external beam radiotherapy* has generally replaced conventional external beam irradiation, as the surrounding normal tissue receives less radiation. Intensity-modulated radiotherapy (IMRT) is increasingly used for prostate cancer, as this has the advantage of being able to shape the radiotherapy beam, enabling a higher

radiation dose to be given to the tumour but even lower doses to be received by surrounding tissue. **Brachytherapy** can involve the placement of either radioactive pellets into the prostate gland (for low-risk tumours) or temporary guidewire needles to facilitate high-dose rate treatment in locally advanced disease.

- *Hormonal therapy* may be given as a primary treatment in patients with localized disease, in whom surgery and radiotherapy are not appropriate. It is used with radiotherapy and also after radiotherapy in higher-risk patients.
- Treatment for metastatic disease
  - *Gonadorelin analogues or surgical castration.* Gonadorelin analogues (GnRH), e.g. **leuprorelin** or **goserelin**, which shut down the pituitary–gonadal axis, are given. Around 85% of patients are effectively palliated using hormonal therapy, with a median response of 18–24 months. Anti-androgens such as **flutamide** and **bicalutamide** act by competing with dihydroxytestosterone at the receptor level, and are always used when initiating GnRH therapy to prevent tumour flare.
- Second-line treatments. Despite continued androgen suppression most patients will develop progressive disease, with a median survival of 7–12 months.
  - *Maximal androgen blockade (MAB)* is achieved by the addition of an anti-androgen to GnRH treatment, and is used once there is evidence of progression on GnRH analogue alone.
  - *Hormone withdrawal* may be therapeutic in ~30% of patients who progress while receiving anti-androgen treatment, since anti-androgens may paradoxically stimulate the androgen receptor in these tumours.
  - *Other second-line hormonal therapies* may also be of palliative benefit such as low-dose **corticosteroids** and **diethylstilbestrol**.
  - *Radiotherapy* to bone metastases can provide excellent local pain relief in up to 75% of patients and in those with multiple painful bony sites; bone-seeking β-emitting isotopes may be useful. Studies have also demonstrated a reduced skeletal-related event rate using zoledronate, though currently it is not NICE-approved.
  - *Abiraterone* is a newer hormonal treatment that inhibits cytochrome p17. It has demonstrated encouraging results in clinical trials in patients with metastatic prostate cancer that had become castrate.
- Chemotherapy
  - *Docetaxel* in combination with prednisolone is now used as the first-line chemotherapy agent in hormone-refractory prostate cancer (HRPC). A 3-month overall survival benefit has been demonstrated as compared to mitoxantrone.
  - *Mitoxantrone* has been shown to palliate symptoms effectively and to delay time to disease progression when combined with prednisolone. However, no overall survival advantage has been demonstrated.

Bladder cancer

Urothelial cancers can arise at any site along the urothelial tract but are 50 times more common in the bladder than in the ureter or renal pelvis. Around 90% of these tumours are transitional cell carcinomas (TCC). Adenocarcinoma (5%) and squamous carcinomas (5%) also occur.

- **Superficial tumours.** Treatment is with cytoscopic resection and regular cytoscopic follow-up, since up to 70% of tumours recur. In patients with a high risk of recurrence, adjuvant intravesical chemotherapy utilizing **mitomycin-C** or **doxorubicin**, or intravesical immunotherapy utilizing **bacillus Calmette–Guérin (BCG)** is used.
- **Muscle-invasive disease.** Surgery in the form of a **radical cystectomy** with bilateral pelvic lymphadenectomy and/or **radical radiotherapy** is performed. The use of platinum-based neo-adjuvant chemotherapy has been shown to give a modest survival benefit. For high-risk patients with T3–T4 and/or N+ M0 disease, the 5-year survival after radical treatment is only 25–35%.
- **Metastatic disease.** MVAC (**mitomycin, vincristine, doxorubicin, cisplatin**) is associated with clinical responses in 50% of patients. The median survival with this combination is only 13 months, however, and is associated with moderate toxicity — particularly febrile neutropenia and mucositis. **Gemcitabine** and **cisplatin** (GC) are comparable to MVAC. In addition, GC has a more favourable side-effect profile and is easier to administer.

Testicular germ cell tumours

There are two main histological types of testicular germ cell tumour: seminoma and non-seminomatous germ cell tumours (NSGCT). Germ cell tumours may arise in extragonadal sites in the midline from the pituitary, mediastinum and retroperitoneum, but should be treated in a similar manner.

- **Inguinal orchidectomy.** This is performed prior to any further treatment, except in patients with life-threatening metastatic disease, who are treated with up-front chemotherapy.
- **Adjuvant treatments for stage I seminomas.** Seminomas are highly sensitive to chemotherapy and radiotherapy; as a result the cure rate in these patients is almost 100%. There are currently three treatment strategies for these patients:
  - *Adjuvant radiotherapy* is the most frequently used. There is a 15–20% risk of relapse after surgical treatment and adjuvant radiotherapy reduces this figure to 3–4%.
  - *Surveillance policy* with administration of chemotherapy or irradiation on relapse is also used. This involves regular follow-up and CT scanning to detect and treat early relapse. This approach takes into account the fact that 80% of patients do not need adjuvant radiation therapy, which is not without side-effects. Since relapses can occur up to 10 years after orchidectomy, follow-up is prolonged.
  - *Adjuvant carboplatin chemotherapy* with one cycle of **carboplatin (AUC-7)** has been shown to be as effective as radiotherapy. It carries the advantage of a shorter treatment time and has fewer secondary malignancies.
- **Adjuvant treatments for stage IIA/B seminomas.** Abdominal radiotherapy is the standard approach for these patients, with relapse-free survival at 6 years of 95% for stage IIA and 89% for stage IIB.
- **Adjuvant treatments for non-seminomas.** In **stage I** disease, vascular invasion of the primary tumour increases the rate of recurrence from 14–22% to 43%. Patients with vascular invasion are offered adjuvant chemotherapy with two cycles of BEP (**bleomycin, etoposide, cisplatin**). In patients with a low risk of relapse a surveillance policy is adopted.

- Treatment of patients with advanced disease
  - *BEP* is the gold standard chemotherapy treatment; 3–4 cycles are given, depending on prognostic stratification. Following chemotherapy treatment residual masses may remain despite normalization of tumour markers.
  - *In non-seminoma patients* residual masses > 1 cm should be resected, since they may contain residual active tumour or mature teratoma, the latter associated with a risk of late relapse secondary to malignant change over many years if not removed.
  - *In seminoma patients* residual masses should be closely followed with imaging and tumour markers.

Renal cell cancer (RCC)

- **Treatment of localized disease.** Laparoscopic radical nephroureterectomy is the primary treatment, unless bilateral tumours are present or the contralateral kidney functions poorly, in which case a partial nephrectomy may be considered. Most patients with localized disease treated surgically achieve complete disease control with local recurrence rates of less than 2–3%. At present, no adjuvant treatments are routinely used, even in high-risk patients.
- **Treatment of metastatic RCC.** In patients with isolated metastases suitable for curative resection, nephrectomy followed by metastectomy prolongs survival.
- **Systemic treatment of advanced disease.** Cytotoxic chemotherapy has virtually no activity in RCC.
  - *IFN-α* results in response rates of around 15% with a median survival benefit of 2 months, and is being superseded by new drugs (below), especially since increasing evidence shows that patients with intermediate and poor-prognosis disease derive no benefit from this form of treatment.
  - *Immunotherapy with high-dose IV IL-2* has overall survival rates similar to IFN-α treatment; however, in a small fraction of patients (7%) sustained remissions occur. The treatment is associated with considerable toxicity, secondary to a capillary leak syndrome, and studies have reported 4% of deaths to be treatment-related. Attempts are being made to identify which patients are most likely to derive benefit from this form of treatment.
  - *Sunitinib*, a TK inhibitor, has been shown to improve clinical outcomes in RCTs. It is now routinely used as a first-line agent.
  - *Sorafenib* targets the Raf/MEK/ERK pathway, which has been implicated in RCC. It acts by inhibiting Raf kinase and in addition has an anti-angiogenesis effect by targeting the receptor TKs, VEGF receptor 2 and platelet-derived growth factor receptor (PDGFR). Phase II and III studies of sorafenib in patients with advanced refractory RCC have demonstrated significantly prolonged progression-free survival. It is used in patients who have progressed following cytokine therapy.
  - *Bevacizumab*, a recombinant monoclonal antibody to VEGF, results in a prolonged time to progression of disease when used in combination with IFN-α but has not demonstrated any difference in survival.

There is evidence of non-cross-resistance between sorafenib and sunitinib, and of sunitinib after disease progression with bevacizumab. The second-line use of TK inhibitors should be considered.

Kumar & Clark's Medical Management and Therapeutics

- *Temsirolimus* is an inhibitor of the mammalian target of rapamycin (mTOR), which is downstream of the phosphoinositide 3-kinase and *Akt* pathways, and is regulated by the *PTEN* (phosphatase and tensin homologue) tumour suppressor gene. It therefore acts by inhibiting both angiogenesis and tumour cell proliferation. It has been shown to increase overall survival as a first-line agent in patients with poor-prognosis disease. **Everolimus**, an orally administered mTOR inhibitor, has been shown to increase progression-free survival in patients who have progressed after treatment with at least one anti-VEGF therapy.

Lymphoma

Lymphomas account for ~4% of all malignancies. They arise as a result of abnormal proliferation of the lymphoid system and so occur at any site where lymphoid tissue is found. Most patients present with lymphadenopathy, although primary extranodal presentations account for 20% of non-Hodgkin's lymphomas. They are currently divided into two major groups based on their histological appearance: Hodgkin's lymphoma and non-Hodgkin's lymphoma.

Hodgkin's lymphoma

Hodgkin's lymphoma describes a group of related disorders, which share some pathological and clinical features. It is an uncommon disorder and accounts for < 1% of all malignancies.

Classical Hodgkin's lymphoma (95% of cases) is classified into four histological subtypes based on morphological features. These correlate with prognosis:

- lymphocyte-predominant (LP)
- nodular sclerosing (NS)
- mixed cellularity (MC)
- lymphocyte-depleted (LD).

Treatment

The aim of treatment is to provide the best chance of a cure whilst minimizing acute and long-term treatment-related morbidity. Specific treatment is based on the anatomical distribution of disease (stage), its bulk and the presence or absence of 'B' symptoms.

The overall survival for patients with early-stage disease is > 85% and the 5-year survival for all patients with Hodgkin's disease is > 75%.

- Early-stage disease (I–IIA or B). The standard care for these patients is a combination of short-duration (2–4 cycles) chemotherapy, using ABVD (**doxorubicin, bleomycin, vinblastine, dacarbazine**), followed by involved field radiation (20–30 Gy). This regimen provides 10-year overall survival rates of about 95%, and reduces the risk of secondary malignancies and cardiotoxicity, when compared with alkylating agent-based regimes.
- Advanced-stage disease (III–IVA or B; I–IIB with bulky disease). The treatment of choice for these patients is combination chemotherapy with or without adjuvant radiotherapy.
  - *The 'gold standard' combination regimen* is ABVD given monthly for a total of 6–8 cycles, followed by involved field radiotherapy to all patients who presented initially with mediastinal bulk disease and to those with partial remission following chemotherapy. This approach is curative in ~50–60% of patients.

- *Long-term side-effects* associated with this regimen are lung and cardiac toxicity; secondary malignancy and infertility are less common than following regimes containing alkylating agents, which were the previous gold standard.
  - *Intensified chemotherapy regimens* such as escalated BEACOPP (**bleomycin, etoposide, doxorubicin, cyclophosphamide, vincristine, procarbazine, prednisolone**) are used in a small number of patients who do not respond to ABVD.
- Primary progressive and relapsed disease. Between 5 and 10% of patients with Hodgkin's lymphoma experience primary treatment failure and 30% of initial responders relapse. Treatment options for these patients depend on the initial treatment used and, in the case of patients with relapsed disease, on the length of remission following first-line treatment.
  - In patients who relapse after initial radiotherapy for early-stage disease, conventional chemotherapy is the treatment of choice.
  - In patients with primary refractory disease and in those who relapse < 12 months following initial treatment, second remissions are often achieved using non-cross-resistant chemotherapy regimes, the majority of which contain etoposide and an alkylating agent. It is conventional to consolidate remission in this group when possible with high-dose therapy (BEAM (**carmustine, etoposide, cytarabine, melphalan**) or CBV (**cyclophosphamide, carmustine, etoposide**)) and peripheral blood cell progenitor rescue (PBPCR). Registry data suggest that this may be curative in up to 50%, although follow-up does not extend beyond 15 years.
  - Patients who relapse after 12 months may be treated with radiation alone, if their disease is localized to a previously non-irradiated area and they are otherwise asymptomatic. Otherwise these patients may be treated with non-cross-resistant chemotherapy with or without radiation.

Late complications of treatment

- Patients cured of Hodgkin's lymphoma are at an increased risk of developing secondary tumours, particularly acute myeloblastic leukaemia.
- Patients who have received mantle radiotherapy are at increased risk of developing lung tumours, especially if they smoke, and breast cancer.
- Other long-term sequelae include a higher incidence of post-irradiation para-mediastinal fibrosis and coronary artery disease.
- Treatment-induced sterility is less marked with ABVD than with MOPP-containing regimes. Premature menopause is, however, more common in older females.

Non-Hodgkin's lymphoma (NHL)

These tumours collectively account for 4% of all malignancies and their incidence has increased over the last 20–30 years. The majority are of B-cell origin (70%), the rest being of mainly T-cell origin. The 2001 European-American Lymphoma WHO classification system categorizes these tumours in terms of their histological morphology, immunophenotype, and genetic and clinical features. The treatment used is very much dependent on the type of lymphoma.

Kumar & Clark's Medical Management and Therapeutics

Indolent B-cell non-Hodgkin's lymphoma

Follicular lymphoma is the most common and comprises 20% of all B-cell lymphomas. The other subtypes of indolent lymphoma are rare and include lymphoplasmacytic lymphoma, extranodal marginal zone B-cell lymphoma of MALT type, and nodal and splenic marginal zone B-cell lymphoma.

- **Follicular lymphoma (FL).** Although most patients present with minimal symptoms apart from lymphadenopathy, the disease is often disseminated and bone marrow involvement common. It is a remitting and recurring disease with a clinical course of a median of 10 years, during which there will be around three episodes of relapse. Chemotherapy has no major impact on survival and the disease outcome is independent of how early treatment is initiated. Death is secondary to either resistant disease or transformation to diffuse large B-cell lymphoma.
  - *Localized disease* (stage I and II) is seen in < 15%. Radiotherapy is the standard treatment and may result in long-term disease-free survival in a sizeable proportion of cases.
  - *Disseminated disease* with minimal symptoms follows a watch-and-wait period after diagnosis until the patient becomes symptomatic (B symptoms) or develops signs of advanced disease (organ impairment, i.e. bone marrow failure, bulky disease (lymph node mass > 10 cm), radiological progression documented on two scans 3 months apart). In this situation a repeat biopsy should be performed in case there has been histological transformation to large-B-cell lymphoma.
- **Treatment.** Chemoimmunotherapy with alkylating agents along with rituximab have become the standard treatment.

  The chemotherapy consists of an alkylating agent such as **chlorambucil** or an alkylating agent-containing combination such as **CVP** (**cyclophosphamide**, **vincristine**, **prednisolone**) or **CHOP** (**cyclophosphamide**, **doxorubicin**, **vincristine** and **prednisolone**). **Rituximab** is a monoclonal antibody directed against the B-cell-specific antigen CD20. It induces remission (partial) as a single agent in 30–70% of patients, with minimal toxicity. With chemotherapy there is an improved remission rate and freedom from progression, and one study has also reported a prolongation in survival.

Intermediate and high-grade lymphoma

Diffuse large B-cell lymphoma (DLBCL) is the **most common** lymphoma subtype and survival is limited in the absence of effective treatment, although over 50% of young patients are cured. Patients commonly present with rapidly progressive lymphadenopathy and progressive infiltration of many organs. The choice of treatment is dependent on stage and prognostic features, which are evaluated using the international prognostic index (IPI).

- The gold standard treatment is the cyclical R-CHOP regime (**rituximab**, **cyclophosphamide**, **daunorubicin**, **vincristine** and **prednisolone**). In patients with early-stage disease with good prognostic features, 60–70% are cured with either 6 cycles of treatment or 3 cycles followed by involved field radiotherapy. In patients with more extensive disease, 6–8 cycles are usually given and the cure fraction is around 45%.
- In poor-prognosis patients, CNS prophylaxis in the form of intrathecal chemotherapy may be given.

- First-line treatment failure has a very poor prognosis and despite second-line therapy < 10% of patients will achieve long-term disease-free survival.
- Patients who relapse after a prolonged disease-free interval are still curable, with prolonged survival in 25% of younger patients. Second-line agents include drugs such as **cisplatin**, **etoposide**, **gemcitabine**, **cytarabine** and **ifosfamide**.
- In suitable patients remission should be consolidated with high-dose therapy and PBSCR.

Burkitt's lymphoma

In the Western world Burkitt's lymphoma is rare, accounting for 2–3% of all non-Hodgkin's lymphomas. In patients with HIV, however, it accounts for 35–40% of lymphomas.

- **Treatment.** Typical chemotherapy regimens are CODOX-M/IVAC (**cytarabine** (intrathecal), **vincristine**, **doxorubicin**, **methotrexate** (IV-*high-dose* and intrathecal))/(**ifosfamide**, **etoposide**, **cytarabine**, **methotrexate** (intrathecal)). Up to 6 cycles of treatment are given at monthly intervals. The likelihood of tumour lysis syndrome correlates with tumour burden; as a result, adequate hydration and monitoring are essential. **Rasburicase** is a major advance (p. 263). The reported complete remission rate is high — 70–90%, depending on age, with very few recurrences after 1 year.

Primary extranodal lymphoma

- **Primary cerebral lymphoma** is an aggressive disease with a poor prognosis. Standard treatment is with radiotherapy and corticosteroids; despite this, median time to progression is less than a year. An alternative approach is high-dose methotrexate chemotherapy, with whole-brain radiotherapy reserved for disease recurrence.
- **Primary gastric MALT lymphoma (extranodal marginal zone B-cell)** is commonly associated with *Helicobacter pylori* infection. Generally these tumours are indolent; systemic spread and constitutional 'B' symptoms are uncommon. Treatment is with *H. pylori* eradication therapy (antibiotics and proton pump inhibitor), followed by endoscopic surveillance, and this results in complete tumour regression in 70–80% of patients. With disease progression, a further course of eradication therapy is recommended; other options include irradiation or alkylating agent therapy.
- **Primary cutaneous lymphoma** is usually of T-cell origin and includes the Sézary syndrome and mycosis fungoides. It is often multi-focal and other organs are usually involved late in the pathogenesis of the disease. Local treatment with topical steroids, topical nitrogen mustard and radiotherapy are used, along with immune-modulating photophoresis, PUVA photochemotherapy and oral retinoids.

MANAGEMENT OF LEUKAEMIA

Leukaemia is a rare disease with an incidence of around 10 per 100 000 per year. It may be subdivided into acute and chronic, myeloid and lymphoid types. The characteristic morphological appearance of leukaemic cells, along with the expression of cell surface antigens, cytochemistry and cytogenetic profile, allows the leukaemias to be subdivided into four main categories:

Kumar & Clark's Medical Management and Therapeutics

- acute myeloid leukaemia (AML)
- acute lymphoblastic leukaemia (ALL)
- chronic myeloid leukaemia (CML)
- chronic lymphocytic leukaemia (CLL).

Acute leukaemia

- Supportive treatment in the acute setting and during the course of the illness. If the patient is acutely unwell with signs of septic shock or is acutely haemorrhaging, cardiovascular and respiratory resuscitation should be implemented. Sepsis should be managed according to local neutropenic sepsis guidelines (Box 8.5). Leucopheresis may be required if the peripheral blast count is high or there are signs of leucostasis. Patients may require packed red cell transfusions, if anaemic, and platelet transfusions to prevent bleeding (platelet count $< 10 \times 10^9/L$ in the uninfected patient or $< 20 \times 10^9/L$ in the infected patient) or to control bleeding. In order to prevent infections, patients, relatives and staff should be educated about hand washing and isolation facilities. Selected antibiotics, antifungals and antiviral agents may be started prophylactically and good mouth care is obligatory.
- Specific treatment. Treatment depends on the leukaemic subtype, prognostic factors, and the patient's age and co-morbidity. Since potentially curative treatment for 'low-risk good-prognosis' leukaemia carries considerable morbidity and potential mortality and that for 'high-risk' leukaemia even more, it is essential that the 'risk–benefit' ratio be clearly addressed with patients. Curative therapy involves intensive chemotherapy treatment and admission to hospital for up to a month in the first instance, with subsequent shorter admissions over a period of up to 6 months. Palliative treatment includes palliative chemotherapy along with supportive measures as discussed above.

Acute myeloid leukaemia (AML)

AML is the most common acute leukaemia in adults (80%) and the incidence increases with age (median 60 yrs).

- Treatment
  - *Patients under the age of 60 years* are usually treated with **curative intent**; the approach used is based on the cytogenetic pattern, which determines a patient's 'risk'. The first stage is **induction chemotherapy**, which usually consists of 3 days of an **anthracycline** (e.g. **daunorubicin or idarubicin**) and 7 days of **cytarabine**, with treatment of CNS leukaemia using either intrathecal **cytarabine** or **methotrexate**. Remission rates of 70–80% are achieved. Once remission is achieved, **consolidative treatment** is required to reduce the undetectable burden of leukaemic cells, so that cure is possible. In young adults with favourable cytogenetics (e.g. t(8:21) or inv(16)), high-dose **cytarabine** is generally used. For **high-risk patients**, allogeneic stem cell transplantation provides the best chance of cure. For the remainder, treatment options include intensive chemotherapy, high-dose treatment with autologous stem cell rescue or sibling-matched allogeneic transplant. Using this approach, ~50% of those entering complete remission are cured (~30% overall).
  - *Patients over the age of 60 years* have a poor prognosis. They represent over half of patients and the choice of initial treatment is much more contentious. For the majority, treatment is **palliative**.

Options range from supportive care to low-dose chemotherapy (low-dose **cytarabine** or **hydroxyurea**), investigational agents as part of a clinical trial and high-dose chemotherapy (**anthracycline** or **mitox-antrone** and **cytarabine**).

- Acute promyelocytic leukaemia (APML). This AML subtype is uncommon and is typically associated with a coagulopathy, which is due to the release of thromboplastin by the promyelocytes. It is characterized by a translocation, t(15;17), which results in the production of a fusion protein, PML-RARα. These patients are treated with **all-trans retinoic acid** (ATRA) and an **anthracycline** in induction, with **ATRA/ anthracycline-based** post-remission therapy and a year of ATRA maintenance. Complete remissions and molecular remissions occur in at least 80% of younger patients. At least 60% of patients can expect to be cured.

Acute lymphoblastic leukaemia (ALL)

ALL is the commonest malignancy in childhood and the majority of cases occur between 2 and 10 years. It is uncommon in adulthood and prognosis is worse with advancing age.

- Treatment. Although specific treatment approaches differ according to subtype and risk, the overall strategy is based upon **remission induction therapy**, followed by **intensification (consolidation) therapy** and continuation treatment to eliminate residual leukaemia.
  - *Remission induction* commonly includes **dexamethasone, vincristine**, an anthracycline antibiotic (**doxorubicin**) and **asparaginase or cyclophosphamide** given in two phases. For patients with Philadelphia chromosome (ph)-positive ALL, imatinib is generally incorporated into their treatment.
  - *Choice of consolidation therapy*, once patients are in remission, is determined by the individual risk of recurrence. Allogeneic transplantation benefits certain very high-risk paediatric and adult patients, such as those with *BCR-ABL*-positive ALL (Philadelphia chromosome-positive) or those with a poor initial response to treatment.
  - *Maintenance treatment* is continued for 2 years and in most cases consists of **oral methotrexate** administered weekly and daily **mercaptopurine**. To prevent CNS recurrence, prophylactic intrathecal chemotherapy is given as soon as the blasts are cleared from the peripheral blood and, depending on risk, may be continued for 2 years. Intrathecal **methotrexate** or **cytarabine** and **hydrocortisone** are used. Cranial irradiation is reserved for patients at very high risk or who have known CNS involvement. An alternative is high-dose systemic **methotrexate** with intrathecal **methotrexate**.
- Prognosis for childhood ALL is now excellent, with 5-year survival rates of 70–83% and cure rates of ~80%. The experience with adult ALL has been much less satisfactory, with reported cure rates of < 40%, despite the use of allogeneic transplantation in high-risk patients. As with AML, recurrences occur within the first 3 years and the outcome is extremely poor.

Chronic leukaemia

Chronic myeloid leukaemia (CML)

CML is a clonal malignant myeloproliferative disorder, which originates from an early haematopoietic progenitor cell. The progeny of this stem cell proliferates over a period of months to years and when the leukaemia is diagnosed the peripheral blood white cell count is characteristically raised with granulocytes at all stages of development. CML accounts for 14% of all leukaemias and its peak incidence is at 40–60 years. It very rarely occurs in children. CML is characterized cytogenetically by a balanced transloca-tion between chromosomes 9 and 22, t(9;22)(q23;q11.2). The resultant chro-mosome is known as the Philadelphia chromosome (ph) and gives rise to a chimeric gene, *BCR-ABL*. This in turn translates into a fusion protein product with increased TK activity, which plays a pivotal role in the pathophysiology of CML.

The clinical course of CML is divided into a chronic phase, which lasts on average for 4–5 years, and an advanced stage, which is further subdi-vided into an accelerated phase and blast crisis. Without curative treat-ment, approximately one-third of patients with chronic-phase disease progress to an acute blast phase (blast crisis — 80% myeloid, 20% lym-phoid). The remaining two-thirds of patients transform gradually into an accelerated phase and subsequently progress to a blast crisis.

- Treatment
  - *Chronic phase.* **Imatinib** is an orally administered agent that specifi-cally inhibits the BCR-ABL tyrosine kinase, which is found in CML. It is first-line treatment for patients with chronic-phase disease, and has replaced IFN-α in this setting. Imatinib has been shown to induce haematological response rates of > 95%, and complete cytogenetic responses of around 80%. Imatinib treatment is generally well toler-ated. **Adverse effects** include oedema, rash, nausea, diarrhoea and muscle cramps. Patients receiving imatinib are monitored using a mixture of peripheral blood counts, cytogenetic analysis and real-time quantitative PCR (RQ-PCR) for *BCR-ABL* mRNA. Resistance to imatinib does occur and may develop through several mechanisms, the most common of which is reactivation of *BCR-ABL* kinase activity by either point mutation or gene amplification. In patients who have a suboptimal response to imatinib or who develop secondary resist-ance, second-generation tyrosine kinase inhibitors (TKIs), such as dasatinib or nilotinib, may be used. Imatinib dose escalation may be an alternative strategy for restoring responsiveness; however, its effect is unusually short-lived. **Allogeneic stem cell transplantation (SCT)** is commonly used in patients younger than 60 years of age who have incomplete cytogenetic responses to imatinib therapy and have suitable donors. In patients without suitable donors who are not suitable candidates for transplantation or are unable to take second-generations TKIs due to problems with QT prolongation, **IFN**, **cytarabine** plus **hydroxyurea** can be used. In patients who have had a good response to **imatinib** and have an HLA-matched donor, the decision is more difficult, since long-term survival data regarding imatinib treatment are not yet available. One option is to offer trans-plantation to patients at low risk of treatment-related death (young patients with sibling donors) and to reserve transplantation in higher-risk patients for when they show signs of disease progression. Since the graft versus leukaemia effect plays a role in SCT, reduced-intensity conditioning allogeneic transplantation may represent an improvement in the immunotherapeutic approach to CML. Initial reports have demonstrated high response rates with this approach but longer follow-up is needed.

- *Accelerated phase.* **Imatinib** treatment results in haematological responses in 82% of patients; cytogenetic responses, however, are only seen in 43%. Allogeneic transplantation in these patients has the potential for cure, though response rates are poor. Other options include autologous marrow transplantation to return the patient to a chronic phase, which in some cases is durable, **α-interferon**, high-dose **cytarabine** and **hydroxyurea**.

- *Blast phase.* **Imatinib** has demonstrated marked activity in patients with both myeloid and lymphoid blast crisis. Haematological responses of around 50% have been seen, with cytogenetic responses of 16%; however, 1-year survival with this approach is < 35%. Clinical trials are currently under way to evaluate the role of imatinib in combination with other drugs in this setting. Allogeneic SCT is successful in < 10% of patients, due to the high incidence of complications and risk of recurrence; nevertheless, in young patients with a suitable donor, it provides the only chance of a cure. Other treatment options include **vincristine** and **prednisolone** for patients with lymphoblastic transformation, or **cytarabine** and **daunorubicin** for patients with non-lymphoid blast crisis. Myeloid blast crisis is usually refractory to chemotherapy and these patients have a very poor prognosis.

Chronic lymphocytic leukaemia (CLL)

CLL is the type of leukaemia most frequently in the Western world and accounts for ~30% of all leukaemias. It most commonly affects elderly patients (median age 60 years), although 10–15% of cases occur in patients under the age of 50 years. CLL is invariably of B-lymphocyte origin (B-CLL) and is characterized by the clonal accumulation of malignant B-lymphocytes in the peripheral blood, with variable degrees of infiltration of the bone marrow, lymph nodes, spleen and liver. The survival of patients is highly variable; the median survival is 10 years, with some patients dying of other non-related causes and others dying soon after diagnosis.

- **Treatment** is dependent on stage and cytogenetic marker status. Early-stage, good-prognosis disease is typically managed expectantly, since there is no survival benefit for immediate versus delayed therapy in these patients. Treatment is instigated in these patients when they develop signs of disease progression, such as anaemia, recurrent infections, splenic discomfort or doubling of the lymphocyte count in < 6 months. Treatment is also recommended for those with advanced-stage disease and certain patients with intermediate-stage disease.

  - *Chlorambucil* with or without prednisolone achieves partial responses in 60–70% in previously untreated patients and successfully palliates the disease. Higher response rates have been seen with regimes combining anthracyclines and alkylating agents; however, these have considerably more toxicity and carry no survival advantage. Chlorambucil treatment is usually given for several months and then withheld until there is progression.

  - *Fludarabine* is a purine analogue, and alone or in combination with an anthracycline-containing regime has been found to result in higher remission rates and longer progression-free survival, than chlorambucil, but no survival benefit. It is, however, more toxic, with higher rates of infection (neutropenic sepsis, herpes simplex,

Pneumocystis), autoimmune haemolytic anaemia and persistent thrombocytopenia. The increased infection risk may persist for months to years after treatment with a purine analogue. Prophylaxis with **co-trimoxazole** for 6–12 months may therefore be given to prevent pneumocystic infection, and **aciclovir** prophylaxis to prevent herpes virus infection. According to NICE guidelines, fludarabine monotherapy should be offered as second-line treatment to patients who have failed first-line therapy with an alkylating agent.

- *Rituximab* added to chemotherapy combinations, such as **fludarabine** or **pentostatin** with **cyclophosphamide**, has recently been shown to result in significant improvements in response rates; long-term survival data are, however, awaited. **Alemtuzumab** (campath-1H), a monoclonal antibody directed at CD52, may be used as initial therapy in patients with a 17p deletion or as a second-line agent for those who have failed chlorambucil and fludarabine. Other treatments under evaluation include **myelo-ablative chemotherapy with autologous PBSCR and allogeneic stem cell transplantation** using myelo-ablative and non-myelo-ablative conditioning regimes.
- Treatment of disease complications
  - *Autoimmune haemolytic anaemia and/or thrombocytopenia* can occur in patients with any stage of CLL and initial therapy should be with corticosteroids. If haemolysis is refractory or recurrent, splenectomy is used.
  - *Infection* is common, especially in advanced disease, and includes organisms such as *Pneumocystis jiroveci* and *Candida albicans*. The early recognition of infections and institution of appropriate therapy are therefore critical in these patients. **IV immunoglobulin** can reduce the frequency of bacterial infections in patients with hypogammaglobulinaemia but is expensive and the long-term benefits are unproven.
  - *Patients with bulky disease* may benefit from radiotherapy, including irradiation to lymph nodes and spleen.
  - *Transformation to diffuse large B-cell lymphoma* can occur in advanced stages of the disease (< 3%) and is known as Richter's syndrome. It carries a poor prognosis, with a median survival of < 1 year.

Multiple myeloma

- This systemic malignancy peaks at 60–65 years of age and is characterized by the clonal proliferation and accumulation of malignant plasma cells in the bone marrow. These malignant plasma cells secrete paraprotein (M protein), mainly monoclonal intact IgG (55%), IgA (20%) and rarely IgD, and normal Ig production is impaired.
- Light chains (κ or λ) are excreted in the urine (Bence Jones proteinuria).
- About 20% of patients have no paraproteinaemia and only light chain secretion.
- **Plasmacytomas** (single lesions) may involve bone or soft tissue and about 25% of patients have a serum and/or urine M protein. They are treated with **radiotherapy** and should be closely followed up, as some will go on to develop classical myeloma.
- A minority of patients have a **monoclonal gammopathy of unknown significance (MGUS)**. This is characterized by the presence

of a monoclonal paraprotein of serum Ig in the absence of clinicopathological evidence of multiple myeloma. Around 25% of MGUS patients go on to develop myeloma over a 20–25-year period.

Diagnosis

Two out of three diagnostic features should be present:

- paraproteinaemia or Bence Jones protein in the urine
- radiological evidence of lytic bone lesions
- an increase in bone marrow plasma cells.

A low β_2 microglobulin and an albumin of about 35 g/L are of good prognostic value.

Treatment

Treatment selection depends on **patients' age**, their general health and the presence of complications of the disease. Treatment choice is generally dependent on whether the patient is eligible for a clinical trail or suitable for high-dose (HD) chemotherapy with PBSCR.

- Response to treatment. A complete remission is attained once there is an absence of monoclonal paraprotein in serum and urine using immunofixation for a minimum of 6 weeks; < 5% plasma cells in the bone marrow aspirate and trephine; no increase in number and size of lytic bone lesions; and/or disappearance of soft-tissue plasmacytoma.
- Patients eligible for HD chemotherapy and PBSCR
  - *Induction therapy* typically involves stem cell-sparing regimes such as **cyclophosphamide**, **thalidomide** and **dexamethasone** (CTD). Patients on thalidomide and dexamethasone are at increased risk of developing a DVT and antithromboembolic prophylaxis should be given. Around 50% of patients on thalidomide develop a sensory motor peripheral neuropathy. For those with primary refractory disease the combination of **bortezomib** (a proteasome inhibitor, which inhibits activation of NFκB and lowers IL-6 and VEGF levels), **doxorubicin** and **dexamethasone** (PAD) can be used. Following induction therapy peripheral blood stem cells are collected using either GCSF alone or with GCSF treatment during the recovery phase following high-dose **cyclophosphamide** treatment.
  - *Consolidation therapy* using high-dose **melphalan** and PBSCR is then undertaken. Another approach is the use of two sequential episodes of high-dose treatment and PBSCR, known as a tandem transplant. Early reports suggest that this approach has a better overall and event-free survival. Since a graft versus myeloma effect has been clearly demonstrated, non-myelo-ablative allogeneic stem cell transplant strategies are also under investigation.
- Patients ineligible for HD chemotherapy and PBSCR. Treatment regimes include attenuated **CTD** (CTDa), **melphalan, prednisolone** and **thalidomide** (MPT) or the combination of **cyclophosphamide** and **dexamethasone**. Chemotherapy is continued until there is a stable level of M protein in serum and urine and no evidence of progression.
- Relapsed disease. On first relapse the combination of **bortezomib** and **dexamethasone** can be used; with a subsequent relapse the combination of oral **lenalidomide** (a derivative of glutamic acid structurally similar to thalidomide but with less toxicity) along with **dexamethasone** may be used. If patients have not previously received thalidomide, a thalidomide-containing regime such as **CTD/CTDa** or **MPT** is used.

Kumar & Clark's Medical Management and Therapeutics

Treatment of complications

- Skeletal involvement may include bone pain, which may require analgesic treatment. **NSAIDs** are particularly effective but some patients may require local radiotherapy. **Bisphosphonates** (clodronate/zoledronic acid) are specific inhibitors of osteoclast activity and are used as an adjunct to chemotherapy, in patients with lytic lesions or osteopenia. Long-term administration has been shown to reduce the progression of bone disease.
- Spinal cord compression due to myeloma is treated with **dexamethasone followed by radiotherapy** or with surgical decompression.
- Vertebral body collapse and pathological fractures may require surgical treatment (kyphoplasty).
- Hypercalcaemia is corrected using **hydration** and **bisphosphonate** treatment. Factors responsible for renal impairment should be corrected, e.g. dehydration/hypercalcaemia. Patients with irreversible renal damage may require long-term peritoneal dialysis or haemodialysis.
- Symptomatic hyperviscosity may require plasma exchange.
- Infections should be promptly treated and patients should receive an annual influenza immunization.

ONCOLOGICAL EMERGENCIES

Neutropenic sepsis

See p. 261.

Spinal cord compression

This requires rapid diagnosis and treatment, with the aim of trying to salvage as much functional capacity as possible. Spinal cord compression is a medical emergency.

An urgent MRI of the whole spine is performed and high-dose **dexamethasone** 8 mg twice daily should be commenced with gastric protection (**omeprazole** 20 mg daily) once the diagnosis is suspected.

Neurosurgical opinion should be sought if the primary tumour is well controlled and metastatic disease is limited, if the compression is due to an unstable vertebral collapse or if a histological diagnosis is required to confirm malignancy. Radiotherapy is given following surgical decompression or within 24 hours of presentation, if used as the primary modality of treatment.

Superior vena cava obstruction

The superior vena cava (SVC) may be obstructed due to external compression or due to thrombus formation (which may be caused by compression or indwelling long lines). The commonest causes are lung cancer and mediastinal malignancies, such as lymphoma.

Patients who are very symptomatic should be referred for urgent SVC stenting (usually performed by the interventional radiologist or cardiologist). **Dexamethasone** 8 mg twice daily is prescribed, although there is little evidence of efficacy. As in spinal cord compression, starting corticosteroids may reduce peritumour oedema but in lymphoma they will have a direct anti-tumour effect. Definitive management is treatment of the underlying cause, e.g.:

- non-small cell lung cancer: radiotherapy (radical if tumour volume is small and localized)
- small cell lung cancer: chemotherapy
- lymphoma: chemotherapy.

Malignant hypercalcaemia

Malignant hypercalcaemia (see Box 15.3, p. 588) may complicate up to 10% of all cancers, especially breast, squamous cell carcinoma of lung and myeloma.

Patients present with a variety of symptoms, including gastrointestinal upset (nausea, vomiting, constipation), renal symptoms (polyuria, thirst) and neurological symptoms (lethargy, drowsiness, confusion, weakness). The mechanism of malignant hypercalcaemia is due to increased bone resorption (osteolysis) and/or humoral mechanisms (release of parathyroid hormone-related peptide).

Principles of **management** include rehydration with 3–4 L of IV 0.9% saline to establish a diuresis and bisphosphonates (e.g. **pamidronate 90 mg in 500 mL** of 0.9% saline over 90 mins) to inhibit osteoclastic bone resorption. **Zoledronic acid** 4 mg is an alternative.

Raised intracranial pressure

Around 50% of oncology patients with raised intracranial pressure have primary tumours (gliomas) and the remainder have secondary metastases. Patients with malignancy are also at risk of non-malignant causes of raised intracranial pressure (abscesses, haematoma) because of disruption of the blood–brain barrier.

High-dose corticosteroids (**dexamethasone** 8 mg twice daily) with gastric protection should be commenced when a patient presents with signs of raised intracranial pressure. Patients who are presenting without a past history of malignancy should be referred to the neurosurgeons for a biopsy, debulking or surgical removal. Those with solitary cerebral metastases and well-controlled extracranial malignant disease should also be referred for consideration of surgical removal usually followed by radiotherapy. In addition, patients with signs of hydrocephalus should be referred for consideration of a ventricular shunt. When the radiological diagnosis of cerebral metastases is clear, palliative radiotherapy is used. **Chemotherapy** is reserved for haematological malignancies.

Stridor

The term stridor refers to a high-pitched musical noise caused by turbulent flow through narrowed upper airways.

Patients should be resuscitated with oxygen, and high-dose corticosteroids (8 mg **dexamethasone**) should be commenced in an effort to reduce peritumoural oedema. Nebulized **adrenaline (epinephrine)** can also be given in severe cases; an emergency tracheostomy may be needed. Debulking of tumours obstructing the larynx can be carried out with laser surgery. For stridor secondary to mediastinal compression, the treatment is dependent on the underlying cause. For tumours such as small cell lung cancer, lymphomas and teratomas, chemotherapy should be started as soon as possible. Radiotherapy can be given in palliative cases and when the tumour is not very sensitive to chemotherapy.

Kumar & Clark's Medical Management and Therapeutics

Tumour lysis syndrome

See p. 263.

Hyperviscosity syndrome

This is defined as a very high white cell count ($> 100 \times 10^9/L$), platelet count ($> 1000 \times 10^9/L$) or very high haematocrit (> 50) seen in patients with untreated leukaemia or polycythaemia. Treatment is with leucopheresis or plasmapheresis.

PALLIATIVE CARE AND SYMPTOM CONTROL

The aim of palliation is to achieve the best possible quality of life for patients and their families by controlling physical symptoms, whilst recognizing psychological, social and spiritual needs. Palliative care is the active and total care of patients whose disease is not curable.

Palliative care teams have an essential role in the care of all cancer patients, not only terminally ill patients. They work together in an integrated manner with the MDTs, ideally being introduced to the patient early on in the course of the disease. Pathways used for the management of symptoms in terminal disease are also valuable in patients being treated adjuvantly or radically. These treatment courses are often extremely difficult, and careful attention to treatment-related symptoms is essential to minimize discomfort during treatment, lessen patient distress, reduce treatment breaks and maximize the chance of completing the proposed treatment schedule.

Pain

Around 70% of cancer patients experience moderate to severe pain during the course of their disease, but with conventional analgesia this can be well controlled in most. The principles of good pain management include careful assessment of the nature and cause of the pain, instigation of analgesics according to the WHO analgesic ladder and regular review of the effectiveness of the drugs prescribed (Fig. 8.1). WHO has developed a three-step analgesic ladder for cancer pain relief. If patients complain of pain, they should be started on medication as recommended on the first step of the ladder and then moved up to subsequent steps until their pain is under control.

● Step 1. Non-opioid drugs — such as paracetamol or aspirin and other NSAIDs, given regularly.
● Step 2. Weak opioid drugs — such as codeine, dextropropoxyphene, tramadol and combinations of codeine with paracetamol.
● Step 3. Strong opioid drugs — such as morphine, diamorphine, hydromorphone, oxycodone and transdermal fentanyl.

On whatever step of the ladder, the drug used should be administered regularly rather than on demand, and adjuvant co-analgesic drugs may be added at any step.

Strong opioid drugs

Morphine is the most commonly used strong opioid and is given by mouth. It is available as an oral solution or as an immediate-release tablet and is given regularly every 4 hours. When a patient commences morphine, a starting dose of 5–10 mg is commonly used; however, if it is replacing a stronger analgesic, a higher starting dose is necessary. If the

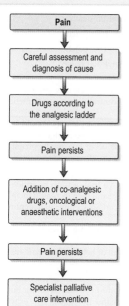

Fig. 8.1 Management of cancer pain.

patient's pain is relieved by morphine but the relief is not sustained until the next dose, the dose is increased by 50% until the pain is controlled. Once the patient's 24-hour morphine requirements have been established, this dose can be converted to a controlled-release preparation, which is then administered once or twice a day. For example:

20 mg morphine 4-hourly = 120 mg morphine over 24 hours

= 60 mg twice daily of a 12-hour preparation

or 120 mg daily of a 24-hour preparation

If patients suffer from pain in between their regular morphine doses, they should be prescribed with an additional dose of morphine as an oral solution or as standard formulation tablets; this is known as a 'breakthrough dose', which should be around one-sixth of the total daily dose of morphine. In situations where the patient is unable to take medication orally, e.g. if the patient has severe mucositis, is in bowel obstruction, has an altered level of consciousness or has uncontrolled nausea and vomiting, the opioid can be given subcutaneously. Diamorphine is the preferred drug and the dose used is around one-third of the oral morphine dose. It is available in the UK.

In some patients transdermal morphine preparations are used, most commonly in the form of fentanyl patches. Once a patient's 24-hour morphine requirement has been established, their prescription can be converted to fentanyl patches with oral morphine preparations for breakthrough pain. For example:

Morphine 24-hour total dose 90 mg = fentanyl '25' patch

Morphine 24-hour total dose 180 mg = fentanyl '50' patch

Morphine 24-hour total dose 270 mg = fentanyl '75' patch

Morphine 24-hour total dose 360 mg = fentanyl '100' patch

- Side-effects
  - *Nausea and vomiting* occur when morphine is initially prescribed but usually resolve after a few days. A centrally acting antiemetic may help relieve these symptoms.
  - *Constipation* is a common complaint and most patients should be commenced on laxatives at the same time as opioid analgesics.
  - *Confusion, nightmares and hallucinations* occur in a small percentage of patients; although distressing, they usually subside.

Co-analgesics

- Neuropathic pain: patients may benefit from a trial of tricyclic antidepressants such as **amitriptyline** 10 mg at night and then increased incrementally to 75–100 mg; other drugs such as carbamazepine, gabapentin and pregabalin are also used.
- Liver capsular pain: may be relieved by **prednisolone** 30 mg daily.
- Localized pain: nerve blocks are used.
- Transcutaneous electrical nerve stimulation: of help in some patients.

Gastrointestinal symptoms

- Anorexia and cachexia are common symptoms in advanced cancer but may also occur during adjuvant or radical treatment regimes. The exact mechanisms in advanced malignancy are poorly understood, although the production of endogenous cytokines (tumour necrosis factor and interleukins) plays a role in the aetiology. There is no specific treatment at present but general management requires addressing associated symptoms. Progestogens (**megestrol acetate**) and steroids (low-dose **dexamethasone**, e.g. 2 mg once to twice daily) can be used judiciously in the terminal phase of life. It is essential to enlist the help of a dietitian when anorexia can be predicted as a problem caused by treatment (e.g. radical chemoradiation of the head and neck when mucositis causes significant pain; radiotherapy to regions involving small bowel; highly emetogenic chemotherapy regimes) so that nutritional support can be used early.
- Nausea and vomiting are frequently encountered and can be treatment- or disease-related. Two-thirds of patients in the terminal phase of their disease will encounter nausea and vomiting. The treatment approach should be similar to that used for pain. A detailed history and examination will help to elucidate a cause for the nausea or vomiting. It may be necessary to administer the antiemetics parenterally until vomiting has stopped, to ensure adequate absorption. As with analgesics, antiemetics are most effective if prescribed regularly (Table 8.5).
- Constipation in cancer patients is due to many factors, such as medications (i.e. analgesia), anorexia and dehydration, immobility, hypercalcaemia, abdominal/pelvic malignancy or spinal cord compression. Patients should be encouraged to mobilize and advised to improve their diet and fluid intake. A stimulant laxative (**senna** 2 tablets at night) and stool softener (**sodium docusate** 200 mg twice daily) should be routinely prescribed with opiate analgesics. **Dantron** 5–10 mL at night,

Table 8.5 Management of nausea and vomiting

Cause	Antiemetic
Gastric stasis	Metoclopramide (10–20 mg 4 times daily)
Treatment-related (chemotherapy*, radiotherapy†)	Domperidone (20 mg 3 times daily), dexamethasone (4 mg twice daily), metoclopramide, ondansetron (8 mg twice daily), granisetron (1 mg twice daily), levomepromazine (3.175 mcg–25 mcg/24 hours)
Bowel obstruction	Cyclizine (50 mg 3 times daily), haloperidol (1.5 mg 1–2 times daily), levomepromazine (3.175 mcg–25 mcg/24 hours)

*Different chemotherapy regimes are classed as being of low, moderate and high emetogenicity. The type, combination and duration of antiemetic will be given prophylactically according to regime.
†If radiotherapy-induced nausea is due to small bowel being irradiated, a 5HT3 antagonist is usually necessary.

alone or with poloxamer, is used in terminally ill patients requiring both a stimulant laxative and a stool softener. **Methylnaltrexone** 0.15 mg/kg SC is used for opioid-induced constipation. For patients who are faecally impacted, an arachis oil enema should be used at night to lubricate and soften faeces, prior to administration of a phosphate enema in the morning. In patients who have chronic constipation usually with extensive constipation visible on a plain abdominal X-ray, macrogols (osmotic laxatives), in a maximum dose of 8 sachets/day for 3 days, are being used for severe cases.

● **Bowel obstruction** is a common complication of advanced abdominal/pelvic malignancy. Most patients will be managed medically, although some will be suitable for surgical intervention. Medical management of bowel obstruction is dependent on the symptoms.
  ● If nausea and vomiting occur, centrally acting antiemetics should be prescribed (**cyclizine** up to 50 mg 3 times daily or **haloperidol** 5–10 mg/day).
  ● Intractable vomiting due to high intestinal block may be relieved by naso-gastric tube. **Octreotide** is used to reduce intestinal secretions and vomiting at doses of 300–600 mcg/day, so reducing the volume of naso-gastric aspirate or vomit.
  ● For associated pain, an analgesic of adequate strength should be prescribed regularly (typically **diamorphine**).
  ● Intestinal colic may be relieved with **hyoscine butylbromide** SC infusion 20–60 mg every 24 hours.
  ● **Dexamethasone** is used in addition in an attempt to reduce the duration of the obstruction. For low obstructions, patients may be allowed to drink and eat a low-residue diet that is mostly absorbed in the proximal gastrointestinal tract.

Respiratory symptoms

Breathlessness can be a very distressing symptom in cancer patients and the underlying cause should be identified and treated if possible. Antibiotics may be used to treat respiratory infections, pleural and pericardial effusions may be drained and symptomatic anaemia transfused. Breathlessness at rest may be partly relieved by regular doses of oral morphine starting at 5 mg every 4 hours. If the breathlessness is associated with anxiety, diazepam 5–10 mg daily may also be of benefit. If there is significant bronchospasm or obstruction, corticosteroids are helpful. Excessive respiratory secretions occur frequently in the terminal stages of cancer and are sometimes referred to as the death rattle. For these patients SC infusion of **hyoscine hydrobromide** 0.6–2 mg/24 hours may be helpful.

Further reading

Benson JR, et al: Early breast cancer, *Lancet* 373:1463–1479, 2009.

Early Breast Cancer Trialists' Collaborative Group (EBCTCG): Effects of chemotherapy and hormonal therapy for early breast cancer on recurrence and 15-year survival: an overview of the randomised trials, *Lancet* 365(9472):1687–1717, 2005.

Elwood PC, et al: Aspirin, salicylates and cancer, *Lancet* 373:1301–1309, 2009.

Guppy AE, Nathan PD, Rustin GJ: Epithelial ovarian cancer: a review of current management, *Clin Oncol (R Coll Radiol)* 17(6):399–411, 2005.

Madoff RD: Rectal cancer: optimal treatments leads to optimal results, *Lancet* 373:811–820, 2009.

Sarssain C, et al: CNS complications of radiotherapy and chemotherapy-review, *Lancet* 374:1639–1651, 2009.

Rheumatological disease

APPROACH TO THE PATIENT

Bone, joint, muscle and soft-tissue structures all produce pain. This can be regional, when it is usually due to a local problem, or widespread, when it may be a manifestation of systemic disease. Clinical assessment is often all that is required for a diagnosis.

Clinical features in musculoskeletal assessment

- Articular disorders cause limitation of generalized movement (both active and passive) and joint line tenderness.
- Inflammatory articular disorders cause early morning joint stiffness (> 30 mins), warmth ± redness and boggy joint swelling. There may be a rapid response to anti-inflammatory drugs.
- Peri-articular (soft-tissue) disorders (e.g. tendon, ligament, bursa) cause limitation of active movement mainly in one direction. Resisted movement worsens pain.
- Non-inflammatory articular disorders produce pain that is worse with activity. There may be joint crepitus, firm joint swelling and joint locking.

Management

Management of all rheumatological conditions is multi-disciplinary and involves allied health professionals including physiotherapists, podiatrists, occupational therapists, as well as drug therapy and local injections.

DRUGS IN RHEUMATOLOGY

Simple and compound analgesic agents

Agents such as paracetamol (acetaminophen), aspirin (acetylsalicylic acid) or codeine compounds (or combination preparations), used when necessary or regularly, relieve pain and improve function. The side-effects are relatively infrequent, although drowsiness and constipation occur with codeine preparations and are worse in the elderly. Examples are **paracetamol** 500–1000 mg 6-hourly, **paracetamol with codeine** 1–2 tablets 6-hourly, and **paracetamol with dihydrocodeine** 1–2 tablets every 6–8 hours.

Table 9.1 Commonly used non-selective non-steroidal anti-inflammatory drugs (NSAIDs)

Agent	Typical dose	Anti-inflammatory effect	Side-effects
Propionic acids Ibuprofen	300–400 mg 3–4 times daily (max. dose 2.4 g)	+	+
Naproxen	500 mg twice daily (max. dose 1.25 g)	++	++
Acetic acids Diclofenac	75–150 mg daily in divided doses	++	++
Indometacin	50–200 mg daily in divided doses	+++	+++

Non-steroidal anti-inflammatory drugs (NSAIDs) (Table 9.1)

NSAIDs and paracetamol have comparable analgesic activities when given in single doses. However, with long-term use, NSAIDs also have an anti-inflammatory effect and therefore are more appropriate to use than either paracetamol or opioid analgesics in, for example, inflammatory arthritides such as rheumatoid arthritis. NSAIDs can also be used in osteoarthritis for soft-tissue problems or back pain. Paracetamol is preferred in the elderly for long-term usage.

The anti-inflammatory activity of individual NSAIDs is broadly similar but there is much variation in patient response and tolerance. Most (60%) will respond to a single NSAID, another can be tried if there is no response after 2 weeks. The analgesic effect will be achieved sooner than an anti-inflammatory effect, which may take up to 3 weeks.

NSAIDs are inhibitors of both cyclo-oxygenase 1 and 2 isoenzymes and thereby inhibit the prostaglandin pathway (Fig. 9.1). Typical agents used for rheumatological disorders are shown in Table 9.1, although there are many others.

- **Side-effects** (Box 9.1) are common, particularly in the elderly. Indigestion and gastric erosions occur and occasionally gastrointestinal haemorrhage. The risk increases from ibuprofen (low) to, for example, diclofenac, indometacin and piroxicam (intermediate/high). Piroxicam should therefore not be used as a first-line drug and the dose should not exceed 20 mg. Bronchospasm and urticaria occur due to type 1 hypersensitivity from release of leucotrienes. Fluid retention and an increase in blood pressure can occur. Although there is a reduction in renal blood flow, acute kidney injury is rare. **Avoid** in pregnancy and with breast feeding, even though the amounts in the milk are small.

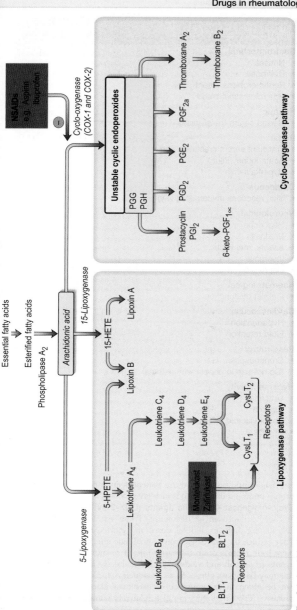

Fig. 9.1 Arachidonic acid metabolism and the effect of drugs. The sites of action of NSAIDs (e.g. aspirin, ibuprofen) are shown. The enzyme cyclo-oxygenase occurs in three isoforms: COX-1 (constitutive), COX-2 (inducible) and COX-3 (in brain). BLT, B leukotriene receptor; cysLT, cysteinyl leukotriene receptor; PG, prostaglandin.

> **Box 9.1** Side-effects of NSAIDs
>
> **Gastrointestinal**
> - Nausea
> - Diarrhoea
> - Peptic erosions/ulcers
> - Gastrointestinal bleed
>
> **Hepatic**
> - Raised serum transferases
>
> **Renal**
> - Transient serum creatinine rise
> - Acute kidney injury
> - Hyperkalaemia
>
> **Cutaneous**
> - Skin reactions (hypersensitivity)
>
> **Neurological**
> - Headache
> - Dizziness
> - Aseptic meningitis
> - Insomnia
> - Depression
>
> **Haematological**
> - Platelet dysfunction
>
> **Cardiovascular**
> - Hypertension
> - Fluid retention
>
> **Respiratory**
> - Bronchospasm
>   (Do not use in people with asthma)
>
> **Hypersensitivity**
> - Urticaria
> - Asthma
> - Anaphylactoid shock
> - Rhinitis

NSAIDs should not be used if a patient is on anticoagulants, unless a proton pump inhibitor (PPI) is also given.

- Cyclo-oxygenase-2 specific agents (COX-2 inhibitors) are equal in efficacy to naproxen or diclofenac. These agents include **celecoxib** 200–400 mg daily in divided doses and **etoricoxib** 30–120 mg daily. They reduce the risk of gastrointestinal side-effects by 50% but there have been reports of an increased rate of cardiovascular events; two agents (rofecoxib and valdecoxib) have already been withdrawn but this may be a class effect. As a consequence, COX-2 inhibitors should not be given in the presence of cardiovascular or cerebrovascular disease. COX-2 inhibitors are also relatively contraindicated in those with vascular risk factors (e.g. smoking, diabetes, hypertension, hypercholesterolaemia).

If the use of NSAIDs cannot be avoided in patients at high risk of gastrointestinal side-effects (those over 65 years of age, past history of peptic ulcer/bleed, concomitant steroid or warfarin use, or presence of serious comorbidity), use a non-selective NSAID combined with a PPI, e.g. **omeprazole** 20 mg daily. This is preferred to COX-2 inhibitors (see above). **Misoprostol** 200 mcg 2–3 times daily can also be used as a cytoprotective agent but causes diarrhoea.

NSAID should be used for the shortest possible time at the lowest effective dose.

Glucocorticoids

Systemic corticosteroids

These are potent anti-inflammatory agents.

- **Prednisolone** in doses up to 60 mg daily is used in many systemic rheumatic conditions, preferably taken in the morning after breakfast.
- **Methylprednisolone** 0.5–1 g IV for 3 days is used in severe organ-threatening disease in vasculitis, and 80–120 mg IM for acute flares of inflammatory arthritis, particularly rheumatoid.
- **Hydrocortisone** 50–250 mg IV is given short-term when oral prednisolone cannot be taken.
- **Side-effects** of steroids are many (Box 9.2) and include:
  - Insomnia, weight gain, thinning of the skin, bruising, hypertension, sodium retention, hyperglycaemia, cataracts and glaucoma.
  - Osteoporosis. This is a long-term problem, developing within 6 months on doses above 7.5 mg daily. It should be monitored with dual energy X-ray absorptiometry (DEXA scanning), which guides treatment with **calcium** 1–1.5 g/day and **vitamin D** 400 U daily, and a weekly **bisphosphonate** (p. 324). A proximal myopathy and avascular necrosis (often of the femoral head) can also occur.
- **Steroid reduction.** Patients who have taken low doses of prednisolone for less than 3 weeks may stop the drug immediately, as adrenal suppression will not have occurred in this time frame. Other patients, however, require a gradual reduction in the dosage, which can be fairly rapidly decreased to 20 mg and then more slowly down to 7.5 mg, equivalent to a physiological steroid dose.

Local corticosteroids

Steroids are often given intra-articularly in non-septic inflammatory monoarthritis and in osteoarthritis, particularly when associated with an effusion. Additionally, local soft-tissue injections are often indicated for patients with tenosynovitis, bursitis, enthesitis and carpal tunnel syndrome. In patients with an effusion, joint aspiration is required first.

Joint aspiration and injection for diagnosis and therapy (Box 9.3)

Aspiration

Aspiration should always be performed in patients with unexplained large joint effusions to obtain a diagnosis; for symptomatic relief in a patient

Box 9.2 Common steroid side-effects

General
- Anxiety
- Insomnia
- Weight gain
- Infection

Endocrine
- Hyperglycaemia
- Adrenal suppression
- Cushing's syndrome

Musculoskeletal
- Osteoporosis
- Myopathy
- Avascular necrosis

Gastrointestinal
- Peptic ulcer (little evidence)

Skin
- Bruising
- Thinning
- Acne

Ocular
- Cataract
- Glaucoma

Vascular
- Hypertension
- Sodium retention
- Hyperlipidaemia

Psychiatric
- Depression
- Psychosis

with known arthritis; and to monitor response to treatment in an infected joint.

- 'Normal' fluid is clear and non-inflammatory fluid is straw colour (high viscosity).
- Inflammatory and septic fluids are yellow and can be translucent or opaque. Opaque fluid suggests a high protein content and high white cell count, is of low viscosity and may clot.
- The fluid should be sent to the laboratory for a cell count, Gram strain and microscopic examination for crystals and culture.

N.B. Aspiration and injection of joints can be painful!

Joint injection

- Glucocorticoids. There are several preparations available; the dosages are variable and should be checked with the product literature. The

---

Box 9.3 Joint aspiration

This is a sterile procedure, which should be carried out in a clean environment.

Explain the procedure to the patient; obtain consent.

1. Decide on the site to insert the needle and mark it
2. Clean the skin and your hands scrupulously; remove rings and wristwatch. Put on gloves
3. Draw up local anaesthetic (and corticosteroid if it is being used) and then use a new needle
4. Warn the patient. Insert the needle, injecting local anaesthetic as it advances; if a joint effusion is suspected, attempt to aspirate as you advance the needle
5. If fluid is obtained, change syringes and aspirate fully
6. Examine the fluid in the syringe and decide whether or not to proceed with a corticosteroid injection (if fluid clear)
7. Cover the injection site and advise the patient to rest the affected area for a few days. Warn patients that the pain may increase initially but to report urgently if the pain persists beyond a few days, if the swelling worsens, or if they become febrile, since this might indicate an infected joint

---

'volume' injected varies with the size of the joint, e.g. small joints (hands and feet) 0.25–0.5 mL, larger joints (knees, shoulder) 1–2 mL. **Lidocaine** 1% solution can be mixed with the steroid in the syringe to make up to 1–10 mL depending on joint size.

- *Hydrocortisone acetate* (25 mg/mL) 0.5–1 mL, can be used for soft tissue injections and is the least likely to cause skin atrophy or depigmentation, as it is a short-acting preparation.
- *Methylprednisolone acetate* (40 mg/mL or 10 mg/mL) 0.5–2 mL, is often used for intra-articular injections.
- *Triamcinolone acetate* (40 mg/mL) 0.25–1 mL is an alternative to methylprednisolone acetate.

- Contraindications. These include infection over the site of needle insertion (absolute), and coagulopathy or bacteraemia (relative).
- Complications. Infection following procedure is rare but a serious complication (< 0.1%).

N.B. No more than three injections per joint should be performed in 1 year.

Disease-modifying anti-rheumatic drugs (DMARDs)

See p. 309 and Table 9.2.

Kumar & Clark's Medical Management and Therapeutics

Table 9.2 Disease-modifying anti-rheumatic drugs (DMARDs)

Drug	Usual dose	Side-effects	Miscellaneous
Sulfasalazine (SSZ)	500 mg–1.5 g twice daily (max. 3 g daily)	Gastrointestinal upset Cytopenias/hepatitis Rash, macrocytosis Reversible oligospermia	Use enteric-coated drug Monitor FBC/LFTs (monthly initially) Increase by 0.5 mg weekly to dose required
Methotrexate (MTX)	7.5–25 mg/week oral/SC/IM/IV for severe active disease	Well tolerated Gastrointestinal upset Cytopenias/hepatitis Alveolitis Nodules	Folic acid supplementation reduces side-effects Monitor FBC/LFTs Baseline CXR Avoid alcohol, trimethoprim Increase by 5 mg 6-weekly
Leflunomide	20 mg/day	Gastrointestinal upset Cytopenias/hepatitis Hypertension, hair loss, rash, headache	Monitor FBC/LFTs Monitor BP Long half-life
TNFα blockers			
Certolizumab	400 mg SC at 0, 2 and 4 weeks then 200 mg 2-weekly	As for etanercept	A fully humanised monoclonal TNF antibody given with MTX or as monotherapy
Etanercept	25 mg twice weekly or 50 mg weekly SC	Injection site reactions Other side-effects as for infliximab	A TNF-receptor protein given alone or with MTX
Adalimumab	40 mg alternate weeks SC	As for etanercept	A fully human monoclonal TNF antibody given with MTX (unless MTX is inappropriate)

Infliximab	3 mg/kg at 0, 2 and 6 wks, then 8-weekly IV	Infusion reactions Infections, including TB, cytopenias, auto-antibody formation, demyelination, lupus syndrome	A partly human monoclonal TNF antibody; co-administered with MTX to reduce production of neutralizing antibodies
Other biological agents			
Anakinra	100 mg/day SC	Injection site reactions Neutropenia Infections	An IL-1 receptor antagonist Monitor neutrophil count Usually used if anti-TNF therapy fails Used alone or with MTX
Rituximab	1 g IV on day 1 then day 15	Infusion reactions Infections	An anti-B cell antibody
Abatacept	IV 10 mg/kg on days 1, 15 and 30, then monthly	Nausea, vomiting, headaches	
Tocilizumab	IV 8 mg/kg infusion	Headaches, skin eruption, stomatitis, fever	A fully humanised monoclonal IL-6 receptor antibody
Other lesser-used therapies			
Azathioprine (AZA)	2.5 mg/kg/day	Gastrointestinal upset Cytopenias/hepatitis	Measure thiopurine methyltransferase (TPMT) first, initiate at 1 mg/kg after meal Monitor FBC/LFTs Decrease dose to 25% if on allopurinol

Table 9.2 *Continued*

Drug	Usual dose	Side-effects	Miscellaneous
Ciclosporin	2–3 mg/kg/day	Renal impairment Hypertension Hirsutism	A calcineurin inhibitor Monitor BP, renal function Specify brand because of differing bioavailability
Cyclophosphamide	0.5–1 g IV 2–4-weekly given in pulses or 1–2 mg/kg/day	Cytopenias Infertility Gastrointestinal upset Haemorrhagic cystitis Bladder cancer	Monitor FBC; maintain white cells > 3500/mm^3; monitor urine Consider *Pneumocystis* prophylaxis Give mesna with IV therapy — see text
Gammaglobulin	400 mg/kg/day IV for 5 days	Flushing, fever, myalgia, headache, dizziness, vomiting, anaphylaxis	Usually well tolerated Response short-lived (1–2 months)
Hydroxychloroquine (HCQ)	400 mg/day	Gastrointestinal upset Retinopathy rare	Take with food Monitor visual symptoms/acuity Well tolerated at < 6.5 mg/kg
Mycophenolate (MMF)	0.5–1 g twice daily	Gastrointestinal upset Cytopenias/hepatitis	Monitor FBC, LFTs

OSTEOARTHRITIS (OA)

Clinical features

This is a disorder of synovial joints characterized by degeneration of articular cartilage with reactive new bone formation at the articular margins. Clinical features are activity-related pain, stiffness, bony swelling, crepitus and deformity. Most patients are > 50 years of age. The most common joints involved are distal and proximal interphalangeal joints of the hands, cervical and lumbar spine, hips, knees and first metatarsophalangeal joint ('bunion'). In the knees there may be an effusion.

Investigations

- Blood tests are not usually helpful. Inflammatory markers, e.g. ESR, are normal but high-sensitivity CRP may be raised.
- X-rays show decreased joint space with subarticular sclerosis and marginal osteophyte formation. MRI shows early cartilage and subchondral bone change; IV gadolinium injection enhances inflamed tissue (Fig. 9.2).

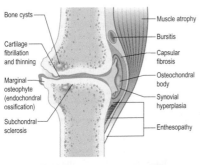

Bone cysts

Cartilage fibrillation and thinning

Marginal osteophyte (endochondral ossification)

Subchondral sclerosis

Muscle atrophy

Bursitis

Capsular fibrosis

Osteochondral body

Synovial hyperplasia

Enthesopathy

Fig. 9.2 X-ray of a knee showing early osteoarthritis. There is medial compartment narrowing owing to cartilage thinning, with subarticular sclerosis and marginal osteophyte formation (arrowed).

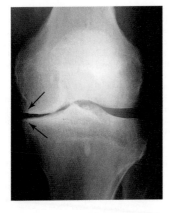

Management

- **General measures.** These are underused and include education and weight loss. Refer to physiotherapy for exercises (aerobic and muscle strengthening) and joint protection (e.g. lateral heel wedges for medial knee OA, patella taping, knee braces, shock-absorbing insoles and walking stick). Acupuncture is also used.
- **Drug therapy.** Drugs are overused.
  - *Paracetamol* up to 1 g 4 times daily should be trialled in all patients before trying alternative drugs.
  - *NSAIDs* are beneficial (topical or oral) for short-term pain relief.
  - *Capsaicin ointment* 0.025% topically has shown benefit for hand and knee OA but the full effect may take up to 4 weeks.
  - *Glucosamine sulphate* 1500 mg or chondroitin sulphate 800 mg daily have been used for hip and knee OA. Their value is unproven but some patients derive benefit.
  - *Intra-articular steroid injection* is often worthwhile in knee OA (particularly if there is an effusion) and in thumb-base OA.
  - *Hyaluronic acid* injections, provided as pre-filled syringes and given weekly for 3–5 weeks, are available for mild–moderate knee OA and can give a longer-lasting effect (up to 6 months) compared to steroid injections (up to 2 months).
  - *Total replacement arthroplasty* has transformed the management of severe OA. The safety of hip and knee replacement is now equal, with a rate of complications of about 1%; loosening and latent blood-borne infection are the most serious of these. Total hip or knee replacement reduces pain and stiffness, and greatly increases function.
  - *Arthroscopy and washouts* have no proven benefit.

INFLAMMATORY ARTHRITIS

Rheumatoid arthritis (RA)

Clinical features

RA is a chronic, systemic, inflammatory disorder of unknown aetiology. Any age can be affected but onset is generally between 30 and 60 years of age, with women affected three times more commonly than men.

- The characteristic feature is persistent (> 6 weeks) symmetrical polyarthritis affecting the hands (metacarpal phalangeal joints (MCPs), proximal interphalangeal joints (PIPs) and wrists) and feet (metatarsal phalangeal joint (MTPs)), although any synovial joint can be involved.
- Common extra-articular features include soft-tissue lesions, subcutaneous nodules, pleural effusions, carpal tunnel syndrome (CTS), systemic symptoms and Sjögren's syndrome.
- RA causes progressive damage, with > 90% having joint erosions within 3 years (Fig. 9.3). Early aggressive treatment is therefore warranted. Poor prognostic factors include extra-articular manifestations, poor scores on functional assessment, high inflammatory markers, a positive rheumatoid factor and early erosions on imaging.

Investigations

- Cyclic citrullinated peptide (CCP) antibodies have a high specificity for RA (90% with a sensitivity of 60%) and their presence indicates the development of more erosive disease compared to CCP-negative patients.

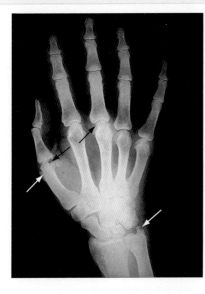

Fig. 9.3 X-ray of early rheumatoid arthritis. Typical erosions are seen at the thumb and middle MCP joints (arrowed) and at the ulnar styloid (white arrow on right).

- **Rheumatoid factor** is present in ~70% of cases.
- **ESR and CRP** are raised in proportion to the activity of the inflammatory process and are useful in monitoring treatment. X-rays in early disease only show soft-tissue swelling but MRI will show early erosions.

Management

This requires a multi-disciplinary approach based on early aggressive treatment with non-drug measures and drug therapy. The main aims are to reduce inflammation, maintain joint function, and prevent or slow the advancement of arthritis and deformity.

- **General measures.** Give education with reassurance; physiotherapy, i.e. exercises to maintain joint range and power; occupational therapy to help maintain normal function through the use of joint splints, gadgets and mobility aids; and podiatry for foot care.
- **Drug therapy.** In the first 6–12 weeks after disease onset, around 50% of patients will have negative auto-antibodies and normal X-rays. It may be difficult to differentiate RA from self-limiting post-viral arthritis during this time. One approach to treatment is to give an **IM injection of methylprednisolone** 120 mg (or 80 mg if < 60 kg), along with an NSAID, and review at week 12; a self-limiting polyarthropathy will have settled by this time. Persisting disease requires use of a DMARD (see below), the most common being **sulfasalazine** or **methotrexate**.
  - *Glucocorticoids* are potent anti-inflammatory drugs, which are used:
    a) to settle a disease flare; options are a short course of oral **prednisolone** < 20 mg daily, IM **methylprednisolone** 80–120 mg, intra-articular injections or IV methylprednisolone pulses of 500 mg

b) as an adjunct to DMARDs (see combination therapy below)

c) as the sole treatment when the risks of DMARD therapy outweigh potential benefit (e.g. in the very elderly) at a dose of prednisolone 5–10 mg daily. Doses > 7.5 mg may slow radiographic progression.

- *DMARDs (Table 9.2)* reduce inflammation (as reflected by a reduction of joint swelling and fall in plasma acute-phase reactants), slow the development of joint erosions and prevent irreversible damage. They act slowly and achieve disease remissions in up to 70% of patients. Combinations of 2–3 drugs may be necessary. These drugs are potentially dangerous in pregnancy and contraception should be used; manufacturer's advice should be followed.

- *Sulfasalazine (SSZ)* is a commonly prescribed agent. Radiological progression is reduced. Mild side-effects are common (30%), most occurring in the first 6 months. SSZ should not be used in glucose-6-phosphate dehydrogenase (G6PD) deficiency. There is a theoretical risk of neonatal haemolysis if it is used in pregnancy and folate supplements should be given.

- *Methotrexate (MTX)* is a folic acid antagonist. It is the most commonly prescribed initial DMARD. MTX can reduce radiological progression and clinical benefit is seen within 12 weeks. It is often preferred to SSZ due to a better benefit-to-toxicity ratio. It is given **once** weekly and this should be emphasized to all carers and the patient. Avoid in pregnancy and use contraceptives for at least 6 months after stopping treatment in men or women.

- *Leflunomide* is a pyrimidine inhibitor that is as effective as MTX and SSZ clinically and in inhibiting radiological progression. It is most commonly used if methotrexate is not tolerated or ineffective. *Do not use* in women or men planning pregnancy or in pregnancy. Use contraception for at least 2 years after stopping therapy in women and for 3 months in men, or alternatively washout with cholestyramine 8 g × 3 daily for 11 days before conception.

- *Anticytokine therapies* include the tumour necrosis factor (TNF) inhibitors (infliximab, etanercept, adalimumab and certolizumab) and other biological agents, including an interleukin-1 (IL-1) receptor antagonist (anakinra) and an anti-B-cell antibody, rituximab, which has been shown to be of significant benefit in MTX-resistant patients. These drugs should be avoided in pregnancy. Contraceptives should be used for 12 months after stopping therapy. These drugs all have a more rapid onset than MTX and are more effective at reducing the progression of radiological erosions. Although these drugs work well in early RA, they are costly and have a high complication rate, and hence are only used for active RA when two standard DMARDs (one of which is usually methotrexate) have failed. If one anticytokine fails, patients may respond to another. Reactivation of latent TB, often extrapulmonary, is a well-recognized complication of anti-TNF therapy, usually in the first 6 months. All patients must be screened for latent TB prior to treatment (p. 512). Cytokine inhibitors are contraindicated in pregnancy. However, if the potential benefit to the mother outweighs the risk of B-cell depletion in the fetus, it may be given. Contraception should be used during treatment and for 12 months after cessation of treatment in other circumstances.

- *Combination DMARD therapy* is used in patients who have had an incomplete response to monotherapy and also early in the disease in patients with poor prognostic factors. Early combination treatment should include methotraxate, short-term steroids and at least one other DMARD. Combination of methotrexate with anticytokine therapy in early RA leads to greater functional improvement and significantly less radiological damage compared to methotrexate monotherapy but because of cost it is not currently standard treatment.
- Drugs used less commonly
  - *Azathioprine (AZA)* antagonizes purine metabolism. It is not as effective as MTX or SSZ and thus not commonly used. A thiopurine methyl transferase estimation should be performed prior to starting the drug (p. 160). There is no evidence that AZA is teratogenic in pregnancy.
  - *Ciclosporin*, although clinically effective, is rarely used due to potential toxicity and unproven benefit radiologically. It is probably safe in pregnancy but needs careful monitoring.

Special situations

- Pregnancy. See Table 9.3.
- Surgery. Rheumatoid joint disease can be treated by surgical synovectomy to reduce the bulk of inflamed tissue and prevent damage. Excision arthroplasty of the ulnar styloid reduces pain and the risk of extensor tendon damage. Excision arthroplasties of the metatarsal heads reduce metatarsal pain and relieve pressure points. A major surgical

Table 9.3 Rheumatic drugs in pregnancy and breast feeding

Drug	Pregnancy	Breast feeding
Steroids	P	P
Hydroxychloroquine	P	A
Sulfalazine	P (stop in men 3 months before attempting conception due to oligospermia)	P
Methotrexate	A (stop 6 months prior to attempting conception)	A
Leflunomide*	A	A
Gold	A	A
Azathioprine	P	A
Ciclosporin	P	A
Anticytokine therapy	A (insufficient data)	A (insufficient data)
Cyclophosphamide	A	A
Mycophenolate	A (insufficient data)	A (insufficient data)
Rituximab	A	A

P, use permissible; A, avoid use. *Because of long half-life drug elimination, treat with colestyramine 8 g 3 times daily for 11 days prior to conception or starting another DMARD.

N.B. These drugs are all potentially dangerous. Follow manufacturer's advice.

— Kumar & Clark's Medical Management and Therapeutics

advance has been the development of total replacement arthroplasty of the hip, knee, finger joints, elbows and shoulders.

SERONEGATIVE SPONDYLOARTHROPATHIES

This group of conditions is characterized by:

- inflammation, mainly in spine and sacro-iliac joints
- an association with HLA-B27
- sero-negativity for rheumatoid factor
- asymmetrical large joint oligoarthritis (< 5) or monoarthritis
- enthesitis — inflammation at site of insertion of tendon or ligament into bone
- extra-articular features, e.g. uveitis, aortitis.

Ankylosing spondylitis (AS)

This condition tends to affect young adults, giving inflammatory low back pain associated with morning stiffness of > 1 hour, which improves with exercise. There can also be an asymmetrical lower limb arthritis and a uveitis. There is often a positive family history. Sacro-iliitis is demonstrable on X-ray or MRI and over 90% of Caucasians are HLA-B27-positive.

Psoriatic arthritis (PsA)

Between 5 and 8% of patients with psoriasis develop a type of arthritis: distal interphalangeal, arthritis mutilans (a destructive arthritis), symmetrical polyarthritis (resembling RA), asymmetric oligoarthritis (< 5 joints) of a spondyloarthropathy (similar to AS).

Reactive arthritis (REA)

An acute asymmetric lower limb arthritis occurs, usually in men, after a gastrointestinal or genitourinary infection. Enthesitis is common, causing plantar fasciitis or Achilles tendonitis. Other features include circinate balanitis, keratoderma blenorrhagica and conjunctivitis.

Enteropathic arthritis

Between 10 and 20% of patients with inflammatory bowel disease develop arthritis, which can be a spondylitis or sacro-iliitis similar to AS, or a large-joint (knee or ankle) arthritis.

Management

- **General measures.** All patients with spinal involvement should be referred to physiotherapy for instruction in a home exercise programme; this can decrease pain and improve function. Patients with AS should follow a regimen of exercise to slow progression. Smoking should be stopped, especially in AS, since respiratory problems are increased if obstructive lung disease compounds the restrictive lung disease that can occur in AS.
- Drug therapy
  - *NSAIDs* (Table 9.1) are often effective for the control of pain and stiffness. Commonly used agents are **indometacin** (25–50 mg 3 times daily or slow-release 75 mg twice daily) and **naproxen** (e.g. 500 mg twice daily).
  - *DMARDs* (Table 9.2). Patients who have peripheral arthritis are often treated with the same standard DMARDs used for RA if there is a failure to respond to NSAIDs or if there is radiological erosive disease. In AS, ReA and enteropathic arthritis, **SSZ** is often first-line, with **MTX** as an alternative therapy. In PsA **MTX** is first-line, as it is

also effective for skin disease; other options are **SSZ**, **leflunomide**, **ciclosporin** and **azathioprine**. However, unlike for RA, there are few well-controlled trials and the effect of these drugs on radiological progression in these disorders is unclear. The DMARDs listed above do not have an effect on spinal disease.

- *Anti-TNF therapy* has been shown to be effective for both peripheral and spinal disease in AS and PsA, and additionally can reduce radiological progression. Due to its cost and potential toxicity, use is currently restricted. AS patients who have active spinal disease despite sequential treatment with at least two NSAIDs are suitable for infliximab or etanercept; PsA patients with active peripheral disease, despite treatment with at least two standard DMARDs, are now given infliximab, etanercept or adalimumab.

CRYSTAL ARTHROPATHY

The three main types of crystal that can cause inflammatory disease are urate (gout), calcium pyrophosphate dihydrate (CPPD) (pseudogout) and hydroxyapatite. Joint aspiration allows identification of urate and CPPD crystals, but not hydroxyapatite, by polarized light microscopy.

Gout

Clinical features

- Acute gout is most common in middle-aged men and generally presents with an acute monoarthritis of the first MTP joint. Other frequently involved joints are foot, ankle, knee and wrist. There is extreme pain and erythema with acute synovitis. There may be an associated systemic upset. Precipitants include alcohol, dehydration, diuretics and intercurrent illness. The attack subsides within 1–2 weeks. Acute gout can also cause an acute bursitis (e.g. olecranon, pre-patellar). Most patients (90%) will have hyperuricaemia but not all individuals with a raised urate develop gout.
- Chronic gout can occasionally develop over time with polyarticular joint swelling (without erythema); hand involvement can mimic RA. There are often urate deposits (tophi) in or around joints, e.g. pinna of ears, olecranon and patellar bursa, and Achilles tendon. Patients may also develop a urate nephropathy.

Management

- General measures. These include weight loss, reducing alcohol (especially beer) and purine (red meat, shellfish) intake, and hypertension control, ideally avoiding diuretics. Ingestion of cherries and vitamin C can help reduce urate levels. Low-dose aspirin should be avoided. Asymptomatic hyperuricaemia does not require any treatment. Secondary causes of gout, e.g. myelo- and lympho-proliferative disorders, should be managed (p. 263).
- Drug therapy (Table 9.4). Acute gout can be treated in three ways:
  - *NSAIDs* in high dose (e.g. **indometacin** 50 mg 3 times daily, reducing to 25 mg 3 times daily after 4 days) are usually first-line and given for 7–10 days.
  - *Colchicine* 0.5 mg 4 times daily orally (higher doses often cause diarrhoea) is useful in patients with heart failure (no fluid retention, unlike with NSAIDs) and does not affect anticoagulation.

- *Steroids* (either intra-articular, oral (e.g. **prednisolone** 30–40 mg tapering over 10 days) or IM (e.g. **methylprednisolone** 80–120 mg) may be given.

Most patients will require long-term urate-lowering therapy as prophylaxis against further attacks, the goal being to reduce serum urate to normal.

- *Allopurinol*, a xanthine oxidase inhibitor and the most commonly used agent, is given at a dose of 300 mg daily, started 2–3 weeks after the acute attack has settled and gradually titrated up to a maximum of 900 mg to normalize uric acid levels. Hypersensitivity reactions, including a rash, can occur. Colchicine or an NSAID should be co-prescribed for 3 months to avoid an acute episode.
- *Febuxostat* 80 mg/day, a non-purine selective inhibitor of xanthine oxidase, is given where there is a contraindication or intolerance to allopurinol.
- *Sulfinpyrazone* (100–200 mg, increasing to 600 mg over 2–3 weeks and then reducing to a maintenance dose when uric acid level is normal), and probenecid (0.5–2 g daily) are both uricosuric drugs used in place of xanthine oxidase inhibitors if there is intolerance.

Calcium pyrophosphate (CPPD) disease

This causes an acute monoarthritis (pseudogout) in elderly patients, particularly in the knees and wrists. The precipitating factors are as for gout. X-rays may show chondrocalcinosis. Some patients, particularly those < 55 years of age or those with polyarticular involvement, may have an underlying metabolic disease (e.g. haemochromatosis, hyperparathyroidism or Wilson's disease). Crystal deposition can also cause chronic disease, most commonly mimicking symptoms or signs of OA but in unusual sites, e.g. MCP joints, shoulders, ankles and wrists.

Treatment

Management of pseudogout is as for acute gout. There is no prophylactic therapy for CPPD; chronic disease is managed as OA.

Hydroxyapatite deposition disease

Hydroxyapatite crystals can deposit in soft tissues and large joints. Patients may present with a calcific tendonitis or bursitis, most commonly around the shoulder. There is acute pain with peri-articular swelling, which gradually improves over 2–3 weeks. The typical patient is an elderly female. X-rays demonstrate soft-tissue calcification. Hydroxyapatite deposits in the shoulder joint can cause a destructive arthropathy (Milwaukee shoulder) associated with a bloody effusion, chronic joint pain and limitation, and rotator cuff tears.

Treatment

Treatment is as for acute gout.
- Additionally, needle aspiration of the calcific deposit may be helpful.
- Repeated joint aspiration is used.
- Supraclavicular nerve blocks and surgery may be needed.
- Intra-articular steroids are usually ineffective.

AUTOIMMUNE RHEUMATIC DISORDERS

These constitute a heterogeneous group of autoimmune disorders of unknown aetiology, but associated with antibodies to 'self' antigens.

Systemic lupus erythematosus (SLE)

This is a multi-system inflammatory disorder, most common in women of childbearing years. The disease is more common and has a worse prognosis in black and Asian people. The 10-year survival is 90%.

Clinical features

Symptoms include fever, fatigue, myalgia, mouth ulcers and Raynaud's phenomenon. Involvement of the skin includes a butterfly facial rash, a discoid rash being specific for SLE, and photosensitivity. An arthralgia is present in 90% of patients, with pulmonary involvement in 75%. Thrombocytopenia, haemolytic anaemia, pericarditis and coronary artery disease occur, as well as neuropsychiatric involvement giving headache, epilepsy, stroke, depression and psychosis. The course of the disease is variable and often episodic but with exacerbations and complete remissions that may last for long periods.

Diagnosis

- Autoantibodies to DNA and other nuclear antigens frequently occur.
- The presence of double-stranded DNA antibodies is specific for SLE.

Management

- General measures. Mild disease settles down with rest. Sunblock (at least factor 30) should be applied to reduce photosensitivity. Patients should be screened for cardiovascular risk factors (diabetes, hypertension, hypercholesterolaemia) and, if abnormal, managed appropriately. Patients should stop smoking. Influenza vaccination is given annually.
- Drug therapy (Table 9.4). Mild cases (i.e. those that are clinically stable **without major organ involvement**, e.g. fatigue, rash, arthralgia, serositis) can usually be managed with:
  - *NSAIDs.*
  - *Hydroxychloroquine* 200–400 mg/day. Patients should have pre-treatment visual acuity tested for each eye, followed by annual checks.
  - *Steroids*, topically for skin lesions, or low-dose oral prednisolone (< 10 mg daily). Patients **with major organ involvement** (e.g. glomerulonephritis, cerebral vasculitis, haemolytic anaemia, immune thrombocytopenia) require higher doses of oral prednisolone (1 mg/kg) or, if there is life-threatening involvement, IV methylprednisolone 0.5–1 g daily for 3 days followed by oral steroids. Oral steroids are tapered slowly according to response.
  - *Immunosuppressants*, such as **cyclophosphamide**, **azathioprine** or **mycophenolate mofetil**, will be required by patients with major organ involvement and those with mild involvement needing more than **prednisolone** 10 mg.
  - *IV cyclophosphamide*, given as boluses every 2–4 weeks, is generally used for severe disease, particularly diffuse proliferative glomerulonephritis and systemic vasculitis. **Mesna (mercapto-ethane sulphonic acid)** should be given (along with a high volume of fluids), as it reacts specifically with a metabolite of cyclophosphamide and ifosfamide, called acrolein, which is toxic to the urethra. It should be given concomitantly with IV therapy, or before if **cyclophosphamide** is given orally. Once disease remission is achieved, frequency of cyclophosphamide dosage is reduced (every 3 months) or patients are switched to less toxic therapies such as **mycophenolate mofetil**

Kumar & Clark's Medical Management and Therapeutics

Table 9.4 Urate-lowering drugs

Drug	Usual dose	Side-effects	Miscellaneous
Reduce uric acid production by xanthine oxidase inhibition			
Allopurinol	300 mg/day Start 100 mg Max. 900 mg/day	Hypersensitivity reactions, rash	Gradual dose increase lowers risk of acute attack; reduce in renal impairment
Febuxostat	80–120 mg daily	Abnormal liver biochemistry, rash	
Increase uric acid urinary excretion			
Probenecid (named patients only)	500 mg twice daily Start 500 mg/day Max. 3 g/day	Well tolerated	Avoid if renal disease or urate stones. Maintain good hydration (urine output > 1.5 L/day)
Sulfinpyrazone	100 mg 4 times daily Start 50 mg twice daily Max. 800 mg/day	Well tolerated	As for probenecid

(metabolized to mycophenolic acid) or azathioprine. In less severe disease, patients can be started on **azathioprine**, mycophenolate or, less commonly, **ciclosporin** instead of **cyclophosphamide**. Azathioprine is also commonly used as a steroid-sparing agent in patients who are steroid-dependent.

The anti-B-cell antibody, **rituximab**, has shown promise in early trials and has been used effectively in lupus nephritis unresponsive to standard agents.

Antiphospholipid syndrome (APS)

Clinical features

This syndrome causes arterial thromboses (most commonly strokes), venous thromboses (most commonly DVT of the legs ± pulmonary embolism), recurrent miscarriages and thrombocytopenia in the presence of antiphospholipid antibodies. Patients may have livedo reticularis. The syndrome can be primary or secondary, when the most common underlying disease is SLE.

Management

- **General measures.** Risk factors for hypercoagulopathy should be reduced, e.g. stopping the oral contraceptive pill and smoking. BP should be controlled and hypercholesterolaemia treated (p. 617).

- **Drug therapy.** Patients with thromboses generally require lifelong **anticoagulation** (p. 243). Those with an initial venous thrombosis can be warfarinized with an INR of 2.0–3.0; those who have recurrent venous thromboses or an arterial thrombosis should keep their INR between 3.0 and 4.0. Women who have had previous miscarriages but no thromboses should be started on **aspirin** 75 mg when they are planning pregnancy, and heparin (**low molecular weight heparin** (LMWH), e.g. **enoxaparin** 20–40 mg/day) should be added once pregnancy is confirmed. Those who are on warfarin due to thromboses before pregnancy should be switched to heparin (again LMWH) before week 6 of gestation, as warfarin is teratogenic. Heparin is withheld for the delivery and then continued to week 6 post-partum. Patients on heparin through pregnancy should have **calcium** and **vitamin D prophylaxis** to prevent osteoporosis. Therapy for patients with antiphospholipid antibodies but no thromboses or miscarriages is controversial, but a reasonable approach is aspirin 75 mg for those with lupus anticoagulant or moderate-/high-titre anticardiolipin antibodies.

Sjögren's syndrome

This is an autoimmune disorder that primarily causes lymphocytic inflammation in the exocrine glands, especially the salivary (dry mouth) and lacrimal glands (dry eyes). A third of patients have extraglandular manifestations, which include constitutional symptoms, arthralgia/arthritis, lymphadenopathy, Raynaud's phenomenon, vasculitis, peripheral neuropathy and occasionally pulmonary, gastrointestinal and renal disease. Lymphoma is a complication. Sjögren's syndrome can be primary (typically affecting middle-aged women) or secondary to RA or one of the other autoimmune rheumatic disorders.

Management

- Most patients will require only symptomatic treatment for dry eyes and dry mouth.
- Drugs with antimuscarinic properties, such as tricyclic antidepressants and neuroleptics, should be avoided.
- Dry and windy environments should be avoided and smoking stopped.
- Artificial tears can be prescribed, with liberal daytime use of low-viscosity drops such as **hypromellose 0.3%** and a higher viscosity agent such as **liquid paraffin** at night. In severe cases punctal occlusion can reduce tear drainage and a lateral tarsorrhaphy (suturing a portion of the eyelids together) can reduce the ocular surface area.
- Salivary flow can be promoted with sugar-free lozenges or chewing gum. Frequent sips of water and artificial saliva can give additional relief.
- Sugars, alcohol, caffeinated drinks and spicy foods should be avoided.
- **Pilocarpine**, a cholinergic agonist, 5 mg 4 times daily, can be helpful for both dry eyes and mouth but can cause flushing and sweating.

Management of associated features

Hydroxychloroquine 200–400 mg/day can improve arthralgia, myalgia and possibly fatigue. **NSAIDs** can help arthralgia. Severe manifestations, such as vasculitis, glomerulonephritis, neurological problems and interstitial lung disease, are treated in a similar way to SLE with major organ involvement (see above) using **steroids** (e.g. prednisolone 1 mg/kg) and immunosuppression with **azathioprine**, **cyclophosphamide** or **mycophenolate** (Table 9.2).

Systemic sclerosis (SS)

Clinical features

This is of unknown aetiology and is more common in women, with an onset usually between 30 and 40 years. There are two main subtypes: **limited and diffuse SS**. The latter is less common but is the more severe form, with more rapid onset and greater likelihood of internal organ involvement.

Management

There is no cure for SS and no drug has been proven to alter the natural course of disease. Therapy is symptomatic and directed towards the organ system involved. Regular exercises and skin lubricants may limit contractures.

- Skin-tightening. No treatment is of proven benefit but penicillamine is occasionally used and mycophenolate has shown promise in uncontrolled studies. Physiotherapy prevents joint contractures. Emollients can be helpful.
- Raynaud's phenomenon. Hand-warmers and peripheral vasodilators (most commonly nifedipine) are used.
- Pulmonary hypertension. Start warfarin, vasodilator therapy including calcium channel blockers (e.g. **nifedipine**), prostacyclin analogues (e.g. **iloprost** by inhalation 5 mcg 6–9 times daily), endothelin-receptor antagonist (**bosentan** 62.5–125 mg twice daily, **sitaxsentan** 100 mg daily) and oxygen; arrange a lung transplant if disease is severe.
- Pulmonary fibrosis. In the early stages, inflammatory alveolitis may respond to **steroids plus cyclophosphamide** or **mycophenolate**. Arrange a lung transplant if disease is severe.
- Dysphagia/reflux. Incline the bed, advise small meals, and give **PPIs**, give **metoclopramide** for dysmotility and bloating, and dilatation for strictures.
- Malabsorption. Antibiotics (e.g. **metronidazole**) may be useful for bacterial overgrowth.
- Malignant hypertension. Measures include bed rest, **ACE inhibitor**, **calcium antagonists**, **prostacyclin analogue** and dialysis. Use a prophylactic ACE inhibitor, e.g. ramipril, in all hypertensive patients. Avoid prednisolone (> 20 mg) as it may increase the risk of sclerodermal renal crisis.
- Arthralgia/myalgia. Arrange an exercise programme, and occasionally give NSAIDs; inflammatory myositis is treated as polymyositis (see below).

Raynaud's phenomenon/disease

Raynaud's phenomenon consists of spasm of the digital arteries, usually precipitated by cold and relieved by heat. If there is no underlying cause, it is known as Raynaud's disease. The vasoconstriction causes skin pallor, and cyanosis due to sluggish blood flow, followed by secondary hyperaemia, which is painful.

- Treatment. Avoid the cold, wear warm clothes and stop smoking. **Nifedipine** 5-mg × 3 daily reduces the frequency and severity of attacks. Vasodilators cause headaches.

Polymyositis/dermatomyositis

Clinical features

These disorders are characterized by an insidious onset of symmetrical proximal muscle weakness, often painless, with an increase in serum muscle enzymes, electromyographic changes and an abnormal muscle biopsy. Dermatomyositis is characterized by additional skin involvement (a red–purple rash, particularly over eyelids and knuckles). The disorders may be associated with other autoimmune rheumatic disorders (e.g. SLE, SS or Sjögren's syndrome) and with solid organ malignancies. Patients should be screened clinically for underlying malignancy, with more detailed investigations reserved for those at high risk (e.g. those with dermatomyositis, age > 45 years or vasculitis) and those not responding to treatment.

Management

- General measures. Rehabilitation should be started early, initially with passive exercises and stretching. Once inflammation is settling, active strengthening/stretching exercises are begun. Patients with dysphagia should be evaluated by a speech therapist. Sunblock is used for those with photosensitivity.
- Drug therapy. Most patients are started on **prednisolone** 1–2 mg/kg daily in divided doses (usually at least 60 mg/day). There is usually a clinical response and normalization of serum creatine kinase within 1–2 months. Prednisolone is then slowly tapered. During this period patients are monitored for disease flare-ups (recurrent weakness and rise in muscle enzymes) requiring intensification of treatment. All patients require osteoporosis prophylaxis. Immunosuppressants, typically methotrexate or azathioprine, are frequently necessary and are often added at onset as this reduces the time to steroid discontinuation. Patients presenting with severe manifestations, such as dysphagia and alveolitis, are initially treated with 3 days of **methylprednisolone** 0.5–1 g/daily and occasionally IV **gammaglobulin** (IV IgG) 400 mg/kg/daily for 5 days (Table 9.2).

VASCULITIS

The vasculitides are systemic disorders caused by vessel wall inflammation. Vasculitis should be considered in a systemically ill patient with unexplained involvement of two or more organ systems and in patients with unexplained ischaemia (e.g. claudication, myocardial infarction, stroke or cutaneous ischaemia). Vasculitis can be primary, or secondary to drugs (e.g. antibiotics), infections (e.g. hepatitis B or C, HIV, streptococci), connective tissue diseases (e.g. SLE, RA, Sjögren's syndrome) and malignancy (e.g. lymphoma, adenocarcinoma). Classification is based on vessel size involved.

Large-vessel vasculitis

Giant cell arteritis (GCA)

This usually affects Caucasians over the age of 50 years. Typical features include constitutional symptoms, temporal headache, jaw claudication and visual disturbance, including blindness. Temporal arteries may be thickened and pulseless. Polymyalgia rheumatica (discussed below) accompanies GCA in 40–50% of cases. The ESR is typically > 50 mm/hour; a temporal artery biopsy is usually diagnostic.

- Treatment
  - *Prednisolone* is started immediately at 40–60 mg daily. (Biopsy can be performed up to 7 days after steroids are started.) The higher dose is used if there is visual disturbance; if this is severe (particularly with unilateral visual loss), it can be preceded with 3 days of **IV methyl-prednisolone** (500 mg/day). Symptoms usually settle within 24–48 hours. Provided the disease remains in clinical remission and the ESR normalizes, steroids are slowly weaned over at least 2 years.
  - *Low dose aspirin* is recommended as there is evidence this may offer additional protection against ischaemic events.
  - *Calcium and vitamin D* supplements should be co-prescribed with steroids. Bisphosphonates should also be given.

Polymyalgia rheumatica (PMR)

PMR affects Caucasians over 50 years and is characterized by muscle pain around the neck, shoulder and pelvic girdle, accompanied by early morning stiffness lasting at least 30 mins. Patients may have constitutional symptoms and synovitis (e.g. shoulders, knees, wrists and hands). Approximately 10–20% have or can develop GCA, in which case management is as for GCA. The ESR is over 40 mm/hour in most patients. Temporal artery biopsies are positive in 10–30% and are useful in doubtful cases.

- Treatment. **Prednisolone** is started at 15 mg daily. There is usually a prompt response within a few days, which can be helpful diagnostically. This dose is maintained for 1 month and subsequently tapered slowly according to clinical response, initially by 2.5 mg weekly. **Calcium**, **vitamin D** and bisphosphonates are also co-prescribed for bone protection.

Takayasu's arteritis

This vasculitis, which affects the aorta and major vessels, is most common in Asian people and occurs mainly in women under 40 years of age. Clinical features include early systemic symptoms followed by vascular features (claudication, headaches, dizziness, syncope, hypertension), associated with asymmetrical pulses and high BP. Arterial imaging with CT, MRI, PET or angiography is diagnostic.

- Treatment. Treatment is with a **steroid**-reducing regimen, starting at 1–2 mg/kg (usually 60 mg/day) and weaning according to clinical response. **Methotrexate** weekly or **azathioprine** is used in refractory disease.

Medium-vessel vasculitis

Polyarteritis nodosa (PAN)

This rare disorder is most common in middle-aged men. Clinical features include systemic symptoms, myalgia, arthralgia/arthritis, skin lesions (livedo reticularis, ulcers, necrosis), peripheral neuropathy (particularly mononeuritis multiplex), abdominal pain, renal disease and hypertension. Up to one-third of patients have hepatitis B infection. Renal or mesenteric angiography may be diagnostic, avoiding the necessity for a tissue biopsy.

- Treatment. **Prednisolone** 1 mg/kg/day is first-line therapy, given as a gradually reducing regimen with the aim of withdrawal over 1 year. Some patients require long-term, low-dose prednisolone. Patients with major organ involvement (renal, neurological, gastrointestinal or cardiac) should additionally be given **cyclophosphamide** either orally

2 mg/kg/day or IV 2–4-weekly (Table 9.2). Once remission is achieved (usually 3–6 months), cyclophosphamide can be substituted with **methotrexate** or **azathioprine** for a total duration of treatment of 1–2 years. Relapses are rare. Concomitant modification of vascular risk factors is necessary (stop smoking; control BP, diabetes and hyperlipidaemia). Patients with hepatitis-associated PAN benefit from antiviral therapy. **Entecavir** plus **plasma exchange** is used with severe vasculitis over 2–3 months; if hepatitis is active, cyclophosphamide must not be used and prednisolone should be tapered quickly (2–3 weeks).

Small-vessel vasculitis

These disorders — Wegener's granulomatosis, Churg–Strauss syndrome and microscopic polyangiitis — are all associated with antineutrophilic cytoplasmic antibodies (ANCA) (90%, 60% and 80% respectively).

- **Wegener's granulomatosis (WG)** involves the upper respiratory tract, causing a bloody nasal discharge, oral ulcers and hoarseness. Lower respiratory tract symptoms also develop. A rapidly progressive glomerulonephritis and neurological involvement occur.
- **Churg–Strauss syndrome (CSS)** is asthma associated with an eosinophilia of > 10% of total white cells. Skin features (purpura), cardiovascular features (myocardial infarction), GI bleeding, polyneuropathy and strokes occur.
- **Microscopic polyangiitis (MPA)** is similar to Wegener's but without upper respiratory tract involvement.

Management

Management of these disorders is similar to that of PAN (see above). Most patients with WG or MPA will require **cyclophosphamide** in combination with **steroids** for induction of disease remission in view of renal involvement; in contrast, many (80%) with CSS can be managed only with steroids. For stable patients with WG or MPA without renal disease and mild involvement of other organs, **methotrexate** can be used with prednisolone from the initial stages. Although medication can often be discontinued within 2 years, relapses are common, particularly with WG, necessitating long-term follow-up and, if necessary, reintroduction of treatment. In WG, other measures include nasal saline irrigation and treatment of nasal superinfection (particularly *Staphylococcus aureus*) with antibiotics and sometimes with surgical drainage. Severe forms of CSS require **cyclophosphamide** followed by **azathioprine**.

SEPTIC ARTHRITIS

Non-gonococcal septic arthritis

Clinical features

This typically causes a monoarthritis of large joints, most commonly due to *Staph. aureus*, streptococcal species or, less commonly, Gram-negative organisms. The knee is the most common joint affected. Predisposing factors include immunosuppression and pre-existing structurally abnormal joints. Patients most often present with an acute monoarthritis, usually with erythema, marked limitation of movement and fever. Elderly patients may be apyrexial and have a normal white cell count. Blood cultures are positive in 50%. Joint fluid must be aspirated for Gram stain (60% positive) and culture (95% positive).

Table 9.5 Antibiotics used in septic arthritis and osteomyelitis

Organism	Antibiotic
Gram-positive organism (staphylococcus, streptococcus)	IV flucloxacillin 1–2 g 4 times daily and oral fusidic acid 500 mg 3 times daily If penicillin allergy — replace flucloxacillin by erythromycin 1 g IV 4 times daily or clindamycin 600 mg IV 3 times daily If MRSA suspected — use vancomycin to replace flucloxacillin
Gram-negative organism	Cefotaxime IV 1 g twice daily
No organism seen	IV flucloxacillin 1–2 g 4 times daily and oral fusidic acid 500 g 3 times daily, or cefotaxime IV 1 g twice daily in sexually active, ?gonococcus in immunosuppressed, elderly and IV drug users Penicillin allergy as above

MRSA, meticillin-resistant *Staphylococcus aureus*.

Management – See Chapter 20 (Emergencies in medicine p. 710)

- **Mobilization.** Initially the joint should be splinted for pain control but mobilization should begin within the first week with passive range-of-movement exercises, followed by strengthening exercises.
- **Drainage.** All septic joints should be drained, either by serial needle aspiration (may require daily aspiration) or surgically (e.g. arthroscopic).
- **NSAIDs.** These are given for pain control.
- **Empirical antibiotic treatment in septic arthritis.** IV antibiotics are started after joint aspiration and after the Gram stain result is known, but before culture results are obtained (Table 9.5). Discuss with a microbiologist.
- **Infected prostheses.** These should be removed.

Gonococcal septic arthritis

Neisseria gonorrhoeae typically causes a septic arthritis in young sexually active adults with normal joints. Presentation may be identical to that of non-gonococcal arthritis, but often there are associated migratory polyarthralgia, tenosynovitis and vesiculo-pustular lesions. Synovial fluid Gram stain is positive in only 25% and culture in 50%, but the organism may be isolated by culturing from other potential portals of entry, e.g. cervix, urethra or skin lesions. Nucleic acid amplification tests on urine are non-invasive and highly sensitive.

Management

Non-drug therapy is as for non-gonococcal septic arthritis but surgical drainage is rarely required.

- **Ceftriaxone IV 1 g/daily** for 24–48 hours is followed by oral **ciprofloxacin** 500 mg twice daily or, if the organism is penicillin-sensitive, **amoxicillin** 500 mg 4 times daily; in penicillin-allergic patients ciprofloxacin can be the initial IV agent. Treatment is for a total of 2 weeks.

- Patients should also be treated for silent *Chlamydia* (e.g. **doxycycline** 100 mg twice daily for 1 week). Sexual partners should be screened.

Other types of infective arthritis

Bacteria, viruses and fungi can cause arthritis.
- **Brucellosis (p. 38).** This usually causes a mono- or oligo-arthritis, which may be septic or reactive. Arthritis is more common in chronic infections.
- **Lyme disease (p. 40).** Around 25% develop an acute pauci-articular arthritis, which usually resolves. Another 20%, however, go on to develop a chronic arthritis. Treatment, which may take months, is with antibiotics and analgesics.
- **Viral infections.** A transient polyarthritis or arthralgia can occur before, during or after many viral illnesses. Treatment of the arthritis is symptomatic.

OSTEOMYELITIS

Clinical features

This is most common at the extremes of age and is usually due to staphylococcal infection; less common causes are Gram-negative rods, anaerobic organisms and TB. Patients generally have predisposing factors, such as open wounds, diabetes, IV drug use, immunosuppression or sickle cell disease. In adults the vertebral bodies are the most common site of infection. Patients usually have local bone pain/tenderness but fever is not invariable. Vertebral osteomyelitis can cause neurological signs.

Investigations
- ESR is generally raised but the white cell count may not be.
- X-ray changes of bone destruction and periosteal reaction take at least 2 weeks to develop but the bone scan, CT and MRI show early abnormalities.
- Microbiological diagnosis requires blood cultures (50% positive), wound cultures or bone biopsy (gold standard).

Management

In the acute stages the bone should be rested/immobilized. Many adults will require surgery to debride necrotic bone, to gain bone stability or to manage a discharging sinus or local abscess.
- **Drug therapy (Table 9.2).** Antibiotics are often given empirically to cover staphylococcal infection (e.g. **flucloxacillin** + **fusidic acid** or **vancomycin** if MRSA is suspected) until culture results are known. Gram-negative organisms should additionally be covered in the elderly. Subsequent antibiotic treatment should be guided by a microbiologist. Analgesia is required. For acute infection, antibiotics are given for 4–6 weeks with at least 2 weeks of IV therapy; for chronic osteomyelitis up to 6 months of antibiotics are required. TB requires anti-TB drugs for 12–18 months (p. 513).

OSTEOPOROSIS

This is a skeletal disease characterized by low bone mass and microarchitectural deterioration of bone tissue with consequent susceptibility to fractures. A variety of medical conditions and steroids can predispose to osteoporosis, but in most patients the main risk factors are post-menopause and age > 65 years. Patients are asymptomatic unless there is a fracture; the commonest sites are hip, thoracolumbar spine and wrist. Spinal fractures can be asymptomatic.

Management

- General measures
  - Stop smoking, avoid excessive alcohol consumption and take regular weight-bearing exercise (e.g. walking) — all can increase bone mass. Patients should maintain an adequate intake of **calcium** (1–1.5 g/day) and **vitamin D** (400–800 U) (e.g. dairy, fish, fortified cereals).
  - Falls risk should be minimized (e.g. corrective glasses, walking aids, avoidance of sedatives).
- Drug therapy. Drugs are used in the following situations:
  - a) osteoporosis confirmed on DEXA (i.e. T score < −2.5) unless < 65 years and no other risk factors when T-score should be < −3.0 for treatment
  - b) patients > 75 years with low-impact fracture (DEXA confirmation not essential)
  - c) current/anticipated steroid treatment > 3 months with either one additional risk factor or T score < −1.5.
    Table 9.6 shows the commonly used drugs and doses.
  - *Bisphosphonates* inhibit osteoclasts. **Alendronate** and **risedronate** are commonly prescribed first-line agents. The commonest

Table 9.6 Medications to reduce fracture risk: antifracture efficacy of interventions used in prevention of osteoporosis in post-menopausal women

Intervention	Vertebral fracture	Non-vertebral fracture	Hip fracture
Calcium and vitamin D 1.2 g + 800 U	ND	ND	+
Alendronate 70 mg weekly	+	+	+
Etidronate 400 mg daily for 14 days every 3 months	+	ND	ND
Ibandronate 150 mg monthly	+	+*	ND
Raloxifene 60 mg daily	+	ND	ND
Risedronate 35 mg weekly	+	+	+
Strontium ranelate 2 g daily	+	+	+*
Zoledronate — prescribe according to brand name	+	+	+
Teriparatide SC 20 mcg daily (max. 18 months)	+	+	ND
Parathyroid hormone (1–84) SC 100 mcg daily (max. 24 months)	+	ND	ND

*Demonstrated only in high-risk subgroup
ND, not demonstrated.

side-effects are gastrointestinal, the most serious being oesophageal rupture. Osteonecrosis of the jaw has been described with nitrogen-containing bisphosphonates but *not* in the low dosages used for osteoporosis. Contraindications are oesophageal disorders, pregnancy and a creatinine clearance < 35 mL/min. A low serum calcium should be corrected before use of bisphosphonate. The drugs are most effective taken upright $\frac{1}{2}$ hour before breakfast, as food decreases absorption. **Pamidronate** has an analgesic effect and is useful for acute fracture pain.

- *Strontium ranelate* 2 g daily (in water at bedtime, avoiding food for 2 hours before and 2 hours after) inhibits osteoclasts and stimulates osteoblasts. It is used when bisphosphonates are contraindicated or not tolerated. The commonest side-effects are gastrointestinal.
- *Denosumab* 30–60 mg SC 3–6-monthly is a potent suppressor of bone reabsorption. It is a monoclonal antibody to the receptor activator of NFκB ligand (RANKL). It can be used when there is a contraindication or intolerance to bisphosphonates.
- *Hormonal replacement therapy (HRT)* is rarely used due to limited fracture data from controlled trials and risks of long-term use. It is useful in women with early menopause and those with perimenopausal symptoms.
- *Raloxifine* is a selective oestrogen-receptor modulator, which does not have the cancer risk associated with HRT but does carry a small risk of thromboembolism.
- *Teriparatide*, a recombinant fragment of parathyroid hormone peptide 1–34 and recombinant parathyroid hormone 1–84 is currently limited to those over 65 years old who have failed on bisphosphonates and who have very low T-scores.
- *Calcitonin* can be given nasally or SC. It has an analgesic effect and is useful for acute fracture pain (e.g. 50–100 mg SC 3 times a week for 6 weeks).

OSTEOMALACIA

Clinical features

Osteomalacia (inadequate bone mineralization) is most commonly due to vitamin D deficiency as a result of inadequate sun exposure or dietary deficiency; some patients have malabsorption syndromes or chronic kidney disease. The commonest symptoms are diffuse aches and pains and occasionally proximal muscle weakness. Fractures can occur from secondary osteoporosis. Plasma calcium and phosphate can be normal or low; serum 25-hydroxy vitamin D_3 levels are low. Serum alkaline phosphatase is raised.

Management

- General measures. This involves dietary advice on vitamin D intake and increasing sun exposure.
- Drug therapy. Any underlying cause should be treated. Mild vitamin D deficiency can be treated with 800 U (20 mcg) **ergocalciferol** (vitamin D_2). This is usually given as a calcium/vitamin D combination tablet. Those with severe deficiency or intestinal disease require a higher initial dose, e.g. oral **cholecalciferol** (vitamin D_3) 50 000 U for 1–3 weeks or a single IM injection of **ergocalciferol** 300 000 U (7.5 mg), followed by replacement as above. Those with chronic kidney disease, who have a defect in 1-α hydroxylation of 25-hydroxy vitamin D_3, should be treated

with **1,25 dihydroxy cholecalciferol** (calcitriol) 0.5–2 mcg/day or α-calcitriol **1-α hydroxy cholecalciferol.** Therapy should aim to correct the level of 25-hydroxy vitamin D_3 to > 50 ng/mL.

PAGET'S DISEASE

Clinical features

This bone remodelling disorder is uncommon below the age of 40. Usually a number of bones are affected, most commonly pelvis, femur, spine, skull and tibia, but occasionally a single bone is involved. Most patients are asymptomatic and diagnosed incidentally on X-ray or found to have a raised serum alkaline phosphatase. Presentation can be with bone pain, adjacent joint pain due to secondary OA, or pathological fracture. There may be skeletal deformity and complications include cranial nerve compression and cardiac failure.

Management

- Drug therapy
  - Asymptomatic patients do not generally require treatment. Some asymptomatic individuals with active Paget's are treated prophylactically to prevent future complications, although there is no evidence base supporting this.
  - Clinical trials support the use of calcitonin or bisphosphonates for bone pain.
  - A single infusion of **zoledronate** 5 mg has a more rapid and sustained response compared to risedronate. **Risedronate** 30 mg daily for 2 months is commonly used.
  - Alternative bisphosphonates include **alendronate** 40 mg/day, **etidronate** 400 mg/day for 6 months or **pamidronate** infusions of 60–90 mg 3–12-monthly.
  - Subcutaneous **calcitonin** 50–100 U initially daily but later 2–3 times a week is reserved for patients who do not tolerate bisphosphonates.
  - Serum alkaline phosphatase levels are used to monitor treatment response.

Further reading

Little MA, Raza K, editors: Autoimmune rheumatic disorders, *Medicine* 38(2):67–124, 2010.

Mathews CJ, Weston VC, Jones A, et al: Bacterial septic arthritis in adults, *Lancet* 375:846–855, 2010.

Rosen CJ: Vitamin D insufficiency, *N Engl J Med* 364:248–254, 2011.

Scott DL, Wolfe F, Huizinga TWJ: Rheumatoid arthritis, *Lancet* 376:1094–1108, 2010.

Further information

http://www.rheumatology.org
American College of Rheumatology

http://www.rheumatology.org.uk/
British Society of Rheumatology

http://www.osteo.org/
US National Institute of Health's Bone Disease Resource Centre

CHAPTER CONTENTS

APPROACH TO THE PATIENT

The history should include a history of prior tests of renal function, previous urinary dipstick and BP recordings, and an obstetric (e.g. hypertension during pregnancy) and family history (e.g. inherited disorders).

Clinical presentations

Presentation with local symptoms

These include dysuria (infection, stones) and pain (loin pain, suprapubic pain, infection, stones, tumour, obstruction, sloughed papilla) from lower urinary tract symptoms including obstructive symptoms (poor stream, hesitancy, incomplete bladder emptying) and voiding symptoms (frequency, nocturia, urge incontinence).

Presentation with particular renal syndromes

Patients can present with the syndromes shown in Table 10.1.

Table 10.1 Presenting syndromes of renal disorders

Syndrome	Clinical findings
Asymptomatic proteinuria ± microscopic haematuria	Protein and/or blood on urine dipstick ± renal impairment
Nephrotic syndrome	Proteinuria +++ Hypoalbuminaemia Peripheral oedema
Nephritic syndrome	Microscopic haematuria and proteinuria Renal impairment Hypertension
Rapidly progressive glomerulonephritis	Rapidly worsening renal function with red cell casts in an active urinary sediment
Macroscopic haematuria	Visible bloody discoloration of the urine

Conditions that may be associated with renal disease

- **Hypertension** — may cause renal impairment and proteinuria, or be the consequence of renal disease.
- **Diabetes mellitus** — produces progressive proteinuria and renal impairment.
- Systemic lupus erythematosus (SLE) — lupus nephritis.
- Systemic vasculitis — rapidly progressive glomerulonephritis (RPGN).
- Hepatitis B or C — can cause glomerulonephritis.
- Drugs (NSAIDs, gold, penicillamine, antibiotics) — cause acute kidney injury, glomerulonephritis, tubulointerstitial nephritis.
- Ischaemic heart disease/peripheral vascular disease — ischaemic renal disease, renovascular disease.

Consequences of renal disease

- **Uraemic symptoms.** These do not develop until renal function is severely impaired (glomerular filtration rate (GFR) < 15 mL/min). Anorexia, nausea and vomiting, weight loss and loss of energy occur. Acidosis (with respiratory compensation) leads to shortness of breath. Confusion, fits and other neurological symptoms are signs of severe uraemia.
- Disturbance of salt and water homeostasis
  - *Salt and water overload* — hypertension, peripheral oedema, distended central veins. This may progress to overt pulmonary oedema, which commonly occurs as GFR falls.
  - *Hypovolaemia* — may be a cause of acute kidney injury in the context of acute illness. Polyuria is characteristic of tubulointerstitial diseases and may lead to hypovolaemia.

Examination of the urine

- **Specific gravity (SG).** SG is usually 1.003–1.035. As kidney disease progresses, the ability to concentrate the urine is lost. Urine may eventually have similar osmolality to plasma (which has SG = 1.010).
- **Proteinuria.** Normally the amount of protein in the urine should not exceed 150 mg/L, of which albumin should be < 20 mg/L. Significant proteinuria is a sign of glomerular disease, and usually consists predominantly of albumin (Bence Jones protein, as found in multiple myeloma, is an exception). 'Nephrotic range proteinuria' is a loose term, usually implying > 3 g/day of urine albumin loss and usually sufficient to cause hypoalbuminaemia. The urine dipstick is a sensitive marker of proteinuria. Quantification can be performed by measurement of:
  - *Microalbuminuria.* Normal individuals excrete < 20 μg of albumin per min (30 mg in 24 hours) but dipsticks only detect levels above 200 μg (300 mg in 24 hours). The level between these two is called microalbuminuria. This is an early indicator of glomerular disease and a useful prognostic marker for future cardiovascular disease. Kits are available for testing.
  - *Albumin/creatinine ratio (ACR)* can be tested on a random urine specimen. Because creatinine excretion is constant, correction by the creatinine concentration provides a correction for dilution. ACR may be useful in specific circumstances (e.g. early diabetic nephropathy). A ratio of 2.5–20 corresponds to albuminuria of 30–300 mg daily.

Protein/creatinine ratio (PCR) is commonly measured if the dipstick is positive for protein.

- *24-hour urine protein collection.* This is inconvenient for the patient, is expensive, and may be inaccurate due to incomplete urine collection.

- Haematuria. Red blood cells are not a normal finding in the urine. Between 5 and 10% of asymptomatic adults have microscopic haematuria. Causes include:
  - glomerular disease
  - infection
  - stone disease
  - renal or urological malignancies.

The urine dipstick is a sensitive detector of haem and if the dipstick is negative, blood is most unlikely to be present in the urine. If haematuria is found, then infection should be excluded (by sending a specimen of urine for culture) and the dipstick should then be repeated. **Urine microscopy** is useful to:

  - confirm the presence of red cells in the urine (not routinely necessary if the dipstick is positive) and to exclude myoglobinuria (absence of red cells with dipstick-positive haematuria)
  - diagnose red cell casts and dysmorphic red cells (normal morphology altered by passage through the renal tubules), pathognomonic of a glomerular cause of haematuria.

- Leucocyte esterase and nitrites. If white cells are present in the urine, then leucocyte esterase activity should be detectable. Nitrites are formed from nitrates by some bacteria. When both tests are positive, they are highly predictive of an acute urinary tract infection (UTI), with a sensitivity of 75% and specificity of 82%.

EVALUATION OF RENAL FUNCTION

Glomerular disease

Plasma is filtered by the glomerulus. Failing glomeruli filter progressively less of the plasma, leading to a fall in glomerular filtration rate (GFR). Filtered uraemic toxins accumulate and lead to the uraemic syndrome. Large molecules (such as proteins) and cells are not normally filtered, but may appear in the urine as proteinuria or haematuria if the glomerular filter is injured (as occurs in glomerulonephritis).

Measuring GFR

GFR is defined as the volume of plasma theoretically filtered in a unit of time (measured in mL/min). Normal GFR is 60–120 mL/min. Clinical estimation of GFR is by:

- *Serum creatinine concentration.* This provides a guide, but serum creatinine does not have a linear relationship with GFR. GFR will be as low as 50% of normal before the serum creatinine concentration rises above the upper limit of the 'normal' range.
- *Equations to estimate GFR.* Validated equations provide an estimated GFR (eGFR) and simplify the assessment of glomerular function. These are only appropriate for use in those with stable renal function (avoid in acute kidney injury). For the management of chronic kidney disease, eGFR is now the most useful measure of excretory renal function.

Kumar & Clark's Medical Management and Therapeutics

- Equations used to estimate GFR in clinical practice
  - *MDRD (Modification of Diet in Renal Disease) equation.* This calculates GFR from 4–6 variables (including age, sex, race, serum creatinine concentration ± urea, albumin). It is not valid for use in patients with malnutrition or following limb amputation. Interpret it with caution at extremes of body weight. The four-variable MDRD equation is the most widely used eGFR measurement in clinical practice.

$$\text{eGFR (mL/min per 1.73 m}^2) = 186 \times (\text{Creat}(\mu\text{mol/mL})/88.4)^{-1.154} \times (\text{Age})^{-0.203} \times (0.742 \text{ if female}) \times (1.210 \text{ if black})$$

  (MDRD calculator — see www.nephron.com). Creatinine in μmol/L to mg/dL, multiply by 0.0113.
  - *Cockcroft–Gault equation.* This is also well validated, but the formula requires an accurate weight.

$$\text{eGFR (mL/min per 1.73 m}^2) = \frac{1.23^* \times (140 - \text{age}) \times (\text{Wt in kg})}{\text{serum creatinine } (\mu\text{mol/L})}$$

  *For females, multiply by 1.04 rather than 1.23.
  - *Creatinine clearance by 24-hour urine collection*

$$\text{Creatinine clearance} = \frac{(\text{Urine volume} \times \text{Urine creatinine concentration})}{\text{Serum creatinine concentration}}$$

This equation corrects for normal creatinine turnover by the body and estimates GFR. It is inconvenient for the patient, requires a simultaneous blood sample and is often inaccurate due to incomplete urinary collection.

Tubular disease

In the tubules (proximal convoluted tubule, loop of Henle, distal tubule and collecting duct), solute reabsorption, maintenance of salt and water homeostasis, acid–base balance and excretion of some drugs occur. Tests of tubular function include:

- urine pH (renal tubular acidosis, p. 347)
- urine-concentrating defects (inappropriately dilute urine)
- glycosuria (despite normoglycaemia)
- phosphaturia, uricosuria and aminoaciduria (all markers of proximal tubular disease but rarely measured).

See p. 351 for the diagnosis and management of acute and chronic tubulointerstitial nephritis.

Imaging in renal disease

Many renal disorders are associated with normal imaging. The choice of imaging depends on the clinical presentation and on the information required.

- **Ultrasound (US)** is non-invasive and relatively simple to perform. It provides information about the renal size (normally 9–13 cm; small kidneys are a sign of chronic kidney disease) and the cortical thickness (thin cortices are a sign of chronic renal damage; irregular cortices may suggest that scarring has occurred). Obstruction is shown by a dilated ureter and renal pelvis, and a bladder US can assess for incomplete voiding. A US can pick up anatomical abnormalities, e.g. cysts (single or multiple, benign or malignant), polycystic kidney disease, congenital absence of a kidney and other congenital abnormalities.

- **Computed tomography of the kidneys, ureters and bladder (CT-KUB)** is sensitive in the detection of renal stone disease. It is used for the differentiation of benign and potentially malignant cysts or renal masses. In obstruction, it may show the level of obstruction and the cause (extrinsic compression, stone disease, sloughed papilla, ureteric, bladder or prostatic tumour). It is used to stage renal and bladder tumours.

- **Intravenous urography (IVU)** provides anatomical detail of the calyces, renal pelvis, ureters and bladder. After a single injection of IV contrast, serial X-rays are taken of the kidneys, ureters and bladder. IVU is used (with a control plain film) in the diagnosis of stone disease, to diagnose or rule out tumours in the kidney or ureter, and to rule out anatomical abnormalities in recurrent UTI. It requires contrast and is contraindicated in moderate–severe renal impairment. Multiple films involve high exposure to ionizing radiation. IVU is time-consuming and relatively expensive, and has now been largely superseded by CT, which provides similar or more information in less time.

- **Radio-isotope imaging** uses the radio-isotopes DMSA (di-mercapto-succinic-acid), DTPA (diethylene-triamine-pentaacetic-acid) and MAG-3 (mercapto-acetyl-triglycine) to obtain functional and anatomical information. It:
  - *Demonstrates scarring.* DMSA will fail to be taken up in scarred areas.
  - *Diagnoses obstruction.* DTPA or MAG-3 will be 'held up' on the obstructed side compared to the other side. This is useful if the US result is equivocal (a 'baggy' renal pelvis). Functional obstruction may be relieved after injection of diuretic, e.g. at the pelvi-ureteric junction.
  - *Compares split renal function.* This is necessary if nephrectomy is planned and asymmetrical renal function is suspected. It is also useful when assessing renovascular disease, in deciding whether intervention is justified.

    Renovascular disease may be suggested if uptake is slower in one kidney than the other. If repeated after administration of an **ACE inhibitor** ('captopril renography'), uptake may be reduced on the affected side.

- **Magnetic resonance imaging (MRI)** has a growing role in the assessment of renal tumours. It is useful in place of CT if contrast is contraindicated (renal impairment). MR angiography with gadolinium is a non-invasive, non-iodinated contrast used as an alternative to invasive angiography in the assessment of renovascular disease. Gadolinium should not be used in patients with renal insufficiency because of the risk of developing nephrogenic systemic fibrosis.

- **Renal angiography** is the gold standard investigation for renovascular disease. It can be combined with therapeutic angioplasty ± stent insertion. Complications include contrast-induced nephropathy (CO_2 angiography is an alternative, though images are not as clear) and cholesterol emboli, and may worsen renal function.

- **Plain KUB (kidneys, ureters, bladder) X-ray** centred on the umbilicus may be useful if stone disease is suspected (90% of renal stones are radio-opaque).

Uroradiology

- **Percutaneous nephrostomy** involves percutaneous placement under US guidance of a nephrostomy tube; it can relieve obstruction. It can be followed by a nephrostogram (injection of contrast down the nephrostomy tube, followed by X-ray) to diagnose the site of obstruction.
- **Urethroscopy, cystoscopy and ureteroscopy** will allow diagnosis and surveillance of bladder tumours and the placement of retrograde stents in obstruction.
- **Micturating cystourethrography** allows diagnosis of ureteric reflux in children.

Renal biopsy

Obtain written consent. Under US guidance and after infiltration of local anaesthetic, a spring-loaded biopsy needle is passed into the lower pole of one kidney via the loin. A sample of renal cortex is obtained for histological examination, immunofluorescence and electron microscopy (EM) examination for diagnosing kidney disease.

- **Complications** include bleeding (1% risk of requiring blood transfusion, 0.1% risk of death), clot colic with or without obstruction and pain (usually mild and transient).
- **Indications** include unexplained acute kidney injury, progressive chronic kidney disease where the cause is uncertain, nephrotic syndrome and nephritic syndrome.
- **Relative contraindications** include single (functioning) kidney, clotting or platelet abnormality (both should be checked pre-biopsy), small kidneys (likely to show end-stage glomerulosclerosis and tubulointerstitial fibrosis, and unlikely to result in any firm diagnosis or alter management) and uncontrolled hypertension, e.g. > 140/90 mmHg (increased risk of bleeding).

URINARY TRACT INFECTION (UTI)

Half of all women will have at least one UTI in their lifetime. Serious morbidity is unusual. Most patients have no anatomical abnormality of the renal tract and do not require further investigation, but patients with recurrent infections should be investigated. Renal stones, incomplete bladder emptying, duplex ureters, tumour or any other cause of disturbed urinary flow or stasis are predisposing factors, as are increasing age (loss of oestrogen in vaginal secretions) and recent or frequent intercourse. UTIs in men are unusual, and should always be investigated with imaging to look for abnormalities of urinary flow.

Lower urinary tract infection

Lower UTIs are diagnosed on history (dysuria, frequency, cloudy urine) combined with urine dipstick results showing positive nitrites and leucocyte esterase activity. Urine culture allows confirmation of the diagnosis, identification of the responsible organism and sensitivity to antibiotics, but uncomplicated patients can be treated without a urine culture. The most common organisms are *Escherichia coli* (70–90%), *Staphylococcus saprophyticus* (or *epidermidis*) (5–20%), *Klebsiella*, *Enterococcus faecalis* and *Proteus mirabilis*.

Upper urinary tract infection

Upper UTIs (acute pyelonephritis) present with systemic symptoms (fever, chills, nausea and vomiting) and loin pain. In the elderly the presentation may be non-specific with confusion.

Management

Uncomplicated lower UTIs should be treated with a short (3-day) course of antibiotic agents, e.g. **trimethoprim** 200 mg twice daily, **levofloxacin** 250 mg daily or a cephalosporin. The choice of antibiotic should be governed by local microbiological guidelines. Alternatively, a longer (7–10-day) course can be given. Complicated lower UTI (i.e. occurring in patients at risk of complications, e.g. immunosuppressed patients, renal transplant recipients, pregnancy or recurrent infection) and acute pyelonephritis should always be managed knowing sensitivity to antibiotics; a prolonged course may be required.

Recurrent urinary tract infection

Recurrent UTI is defined as more than four infections in a year. Imaging should be performed to exclude abnormalities of the renal tract. A high fluid intake should be maintained. Rotating prophylactic antibiotics are sometimes beneficial.

GLOMERULAR DISEASE

Nephritic syndrome

This can present insidiously or as rapidly progressive glomerulonephritis (RPGN), which is the most severe form of nephritic syndrome with rapidly progressing renal failure.

- **Presentation** is with haematuria (usually microscopic), proteinuria, red cell casts, renal impairment (often progressive), hypertension and fluid retention (puffy face), with or without oliguria. These findings indicate inflammation of, and damage to, glomeruli and this is usually immune-mediated. If this is not reversed, irreversible glomerular loss and chronic kidney disease occur. An urgent renal biopsy will demonstrate glomerular nephropathy (GN) and, if rapidly progressive, may contain crescents (macrophage invasion of Bowman's space, causing irreversible glomerular damage).
- **Causes** of the nephritic syndrome include vasculitis (e.g. ANCA-positive small-vessel vasculitis), SLE, antiglomerular basement membrane (GBM) disease (Goodpasture's syndrome), post-infectious (proliferative) glomerulonephritis, mesangiocapillary GN, IgA nephropathy and Henoch–Schönlein purpura.

Nephrotic syndrome

Nephrotic syndrome presents with:

- peripheral oedema
- proteinuria (> 3 g daily)
- hypoalbuminaemia
- hypercholesterolaemia (usually present)
- hypertension that accompanies the fluid overload
- microscopic haematuria (may or may not be present, depending on the cause).

Nephrotic syndrome is the result of damage to the glomerular filtration barrier. The barrier is made up of the endothelium, the GBM, and podocytes and their slit diaphragms. Both molecular size and charge affect the selectivity of the barrier, which is disrupted in the nephrotic syndrome.

- **Causes** of the nephrotic syndrome include minimal change disease, membranous GN, focal and segmental glomerulosclerosis, diabetic nephropathy, amyloidosis, light chain deposition disease, cryoglobulinaemia, HIV-associated nephropathy, mesangiocapillary GN and SLE.

Isolated microscopic haematuria

This is defined as non-visible blood in the urine, in the absence of proteinuria, renal impairment or hypertension. It is common (5–10% of the adult population).

- **Causes**
- Lower urinary tract causes, including stones and tumours, should be excluded.
- Once urological causes have been ruled out, then it can be assumed to be a benign glomerulopathy. Further investigation is not usually indicated; the prognosis is excellent without any treatment, though long-term follow-up is recommended.

Asymptomatic proteinuria

Presentation is incidental when urine is dipsticked as part of routine medical examination or in the context of another medical problem. Hypertension may be the cause or an associated cause. Poor BP control is likely to worsen the degree of proteinuria. By definition, the level of proteinuria is not sufficient to cause hypoalbuminaemia (< 3 g/day).

- **Causes** of asymptomatic proteinuria include IgA nephropathy, membranous GN, mesangiocapillary GN, hypertension, diabetic nephropathy and HIV-associated nephropathy.

Investigations of glomerular disease

- Urine dipstick: microscopy if haematuria demonstrated (?red cell casts). Quantify proteinuria (p. 328).
- Serum electrolytes, urea, creatinine (serial measurements — progressive disease requires urgent investigation), bone profile, liver biochemistry, protein electrophoretic strip, blood glucose and lipid profile. Urine for Bence Jones protein.
- Hb, white cell count, platelets.
- Markers of inflammation (ESR, CRP).
- Nephritic screen: ANA, dsDNA, C3, C4, ANCA, anti-GBM, hepatitis B and C serology, blood cultures if fever or suggestion of sepsis.

Other investigations to determine the cause of the glomerular disease

- Renal imaging.
- Renal biopsy is indicated (unless there is a compelling contraindication) to allow definitive management to be commenced.

Management of glomerular disease: general principles

- **Salt and water balance.** Accurate assessment of fluid balance is necessary (p. 368), as in severe nephrotic syndrome there may be intravascular depletion despite expansion of the extracellular compartment. **Hypovolaemia** should be corrected with oral or IV fluids. **Volume**

expansion should be managed with salt and water restriction, with or without diuretics. High doses of loop diuretics are often required to establish and maintain a diuresis, e.g. **furosemide** 40–250 mg twice daily.

- **BP.** Hypertension is usual in glomerular disease. Reducing BP leads to decreased intraglomerular pressure, and decreased levels of proteinuria, preservation of renal function and protection of other organs from hypertension-induced damage. ACE inhibitors and/or angiotensin receptor blockers (ARBs) have theoretical and evidence-based advantages over other agents, especially for those with significant proteinuria. **Target BP** should be 130/80 mmHg (120/75 mmHg if there is proteinuria).
- **Proteinuria.** ACE inhibitors or ARBs reduce intraglomerular pressure and proteinuria.
- **Lipids.** Statins are given to lower the serum cholesterol (< 4.5 mmol/L) (to convert mmol to mg/dL multiply by 38).
- **Dialysis.** This is required if renal impairment is severe. For indications for dialysis see p. 357. With definitive treatment and renal recovery, dialysis is discontinued after a period of time.
- **Diet.** A normal protein diet of 1.8 g/kg body weight is given.
- **Anticoagulants.** Risk of venous thromboembolism is high; give prophylactic anticoagulants (p. 247).
- Pneumococcal vaccination.

General principles for immunosuppressive treatment

- The decision to treat is based on balancing the potential benefits of the treatment with the potential risks. With potent immunosuppression, the side-effects may be life-threatening.
- A histological diagnosis is usually required before treatment.
- Many treatment regimes use the principle of induction (with a potent drug combination) to induce 'remission' and then maintenance therapy with less toxic treatment to prevent relapse.
- Monitoring must be appropriate and robust (e.g. weekly or fortnightly blood tests initially when on **cyclophosphamide** or **azathioprine**, checks of GFR and monitoring of serum levels when on **ciclosporin** or **tacrolimus**).
- Use adjunctive therapies to minimize the risk of side-effects whenever possible. These include:
  - Bone protection treatment for all on long-term steroids (yearly dual energy X-ray absorptiometry (DEXA) scans). Use a long-acting oral bisphosphonate (e.g. **alendronate** 5 mg daily) and/or calcium and vitamin D combinations (e.g. **calcium carbonate** 1.25 g and **cholecalciferol** 5 mcg).
  - **Co-trimoxazole** 480 mg twice daily as prophylaxis against *Pneumocystis jiroveci* infection for patients on cyclophosphamide.
  - **Isoniazid** 100 mg daily as anti-TB prophylaxis for at-risk patients (history of TB or TB exposure) on **cyclophosphamide**.
  - Statins (e.g. **atorvastatin** 20 mg daily) for steroid-exacerbated hyperlipidaemia.
- All immunosuppressive regimes have an associated risk of infections and, in the longer term, malignancy. Other common side-effects are shown in Table 10.2.

Kumar & Clark's Medical Management and Therapeutics

Table 10.2 Commonly used immunosuppressive drugs in glomerulonephritis

Drug	Dose regime	Mechanism of action	Indications for use	Common side-effects
Prednisolone	1 mg/kg per day (max. dose 60–80 mg), tapering to 5–7.5 mg daily by month 6	Modulates B- and T-cell action	Many glomerular diseases, either alone or in combination with other agents	Multiple, including osteoporosis, hypertension, diabetes, weight gain, poor wound healing, lipid abnormalities
Cyclophosphamide	Oral: 1.5–2 mg/day IV: 750 mg/m² monthly. Give mesna if dose > 2 g	Alkylating agent — inhibits DNA replication	Many GNs. Used to induce remission, with switch to less potent (and toxic) agents for maintenance treatment	Leucopenia Infertility (early menopause in females, azoospermia in males) Haemorrhagic cystitis and bladder cancer
Ciclosporin Tacrolimus	According to blood trough levels	Calcineurin inhibitors — affect interleukin (IL)-2-driven T-cell activation	Steroid-sparing agents used for many GNs. **N.B.** Tacrolimus has two different formulations	Renal impairment (monitor eGFR), hypertension, tremor, hirsutism, gum hypertrophy, impaired glucose tolerance
Mycophenolate mofetil	0.5–1 g × 2	Promotes T-cell-programmed cell death	As an alternative to cyclophosphamide or azathioprine in many GNs	Myelosuppression, diarrhoea
Azathioprine	1.5–2 mg/kg/day	Prodrug, converted to 6-mercaptopurine — inhibits DNA synthesis	Maintenance treatment for many GNs, acting as a steroid-sparing agent	Leucopenia, hepatitis
Rituximab	IV 500–1000 mg	Monoclonal anti-CD20 antibody — causes B-cell and antibody depletion	Promising results in lupus nephritis and some GNs. More evidence awaited	Infection including TB, septicaemia, hypersensitivity reactions, cytokine release syndrome

eGFR, estimated glomerular filtration rate; GN, glomerular nephropathy.

Specific glomerular diseases and their management

Minimal change disease

Minimal change disease presents as the nephrotic syndrome, often of sudden onset with no haematuria. It is most common in children (boys > girls) and accounts for > 95% of all cases of nephrotic syndrome in children, although it can occur at any age and accounts for up to 25% of all nephrotic syndrome in adults.

- Renal biopsy shows normal appearances on light microscopy with no immune complex deposition ('minimal change'). EM shows epithelial cell (podocyte) foot process fusion — a non-specific finding seen in any condition associated with the nephrotic syndrome.
- An immunological cause is suggested by the fact that the condition responds to immunosuppression. Production of a circulating factor (not yet identified) by T-cells or immature CD34-positive stem cells has been suggested.
- Renal function is usually normal, and does not normally deteriorate.
- Spontaneous remissions occur, so treatment should not be commenced unless hypoalbuminaemia and oedema are present.
- Management
  - *Start* with high-dose corticosteroids, i.e. **prednisolone** 1 mg/kg/day in adults or 60 mg/m^2 in children up to a maximum of 80 mg/day for 4–6 weeks, and then 40 mg/m^2 for 4–6 weeks. Remission may occur within days, but can take weeks.
  - *Once in remission*, **prednisolone** dose should be reduced slowly (cut dose by 30% after 4–6 weeks). Steroids should be tapered and the patient weaned off them over a total of 12 more weeks.
  - *Relapse* frequently occurs (but one-third of children will not relapse), especially if steroids are tapered too quickly, and this should be treated in the same way with prednisolone.
  - *Frequent relapsers* may be steroid-dependent (relapse when steroids are withdrawn) or steroid-resistant (fail to go into remission with steroids). **Cyclophosphamide** (1.5–2 mg/kg/day) for 8–12 weeks given with prednisolone 7.5–15 mg/day increases the likelihood of long-term remission. **Ciclosporin** (3–5 mg/kg/day aiming for trough blood level of 80–150 ng/mL) is an alternative but needs to be continued long-term to prevent relapse; it carries its own risks of nephrotoxicity so frequent monitoring of levels and kidney function is required. **Levamisole** 2.5 mg/kg (max. 150 mg) on alternate days has been found to be effective in maintaining remission in children.

Focal segmental glomerulosclerosis (FSGS)

FSGS usually presents with the nephrotic syndrome, often with microscopic haematuria. Hypertension and/or progressive renal impairment are often present.

- **Primary FSGS** is of unknown cause. A circulating permeability factor with serine protease activity has been implicated (the disease may recur after transplantation, often immediately). A renal biopsy is required to make the diagnosis, determine therapy and indicate prognosis. Segmental scleroses in affected glomeruli are seen, with other glomeruli looking normal on light microscopy. C3 and IgM may be present on immunofluorescence in affected segments. Mesangial hypercellularity may be present. Interstitial fibrosis and focal tubal atrophy are common. On

Kumar & Clark's Medical Management and Therapeutics

EM, affected glomeruli show capillary obliteration with hyaline deposits and lipids. Patchy foot process effacement is present, even on 'normal'-looking glomeruli. Five histological types are described by light microscopy:

- *Classic* — the glomerular changes may occur in any part of the glomerulus.
- *Tip lesion* — scleroses occur at the tubular pole of affected glomeruli, with foam cell-filled capillaries and adhesion of epithelial cells to the proximal portion of the tubule.
- *Collapsing FSGS* — with enlarged and vacuolated visceral cells, and collapsed capillary walls. This variant is often associated with HIV infection (especially in black people), when it is classified as HIV-associated nephropathy (HIVAN).
- *Perihilar variant* — with perihilar sclerosis and hyalinosis, frequently present in secondary FSGS (see below).
- *Cellular* — at least one glomerulus has segmental endocapillary hypercellularity, while other glomeruli may have changes similar to the classic form.

- **Secondary FSGS** occurs as a result of a loss of functioning nephrons of almost any cause, e.g. hypertension, obesity, previous nephrectomy or renal damage, with the remnant nephrons having to hyperfilter. This leads to hydraulic injury over time.
- **Management.** Mild to modest proteinuria should be managed with good BP control (**ACE inhibitors**), a **statin** and follow-up (Box 10.1). Overt nephrotic syndrome and/or progressive renal impairment (drop in eGFR of > 15% in 1 year or > 10% in 2 successive years) are risk factors for progression and indications for **immunosuppression**. **Prednisolone** 0.5–2 mg/kg/day should be continued for up to 6 months before steroid resistance is diagnosed. Commonly this is the case, and other disease-modifying drugs are required. **Ciclosporin** aiming for trough level 150–300 ng/mL may be effective, but relapse may occur when it is discontinued. **Cyclophosphamide** 1–1.5 mg/kg/day with high-dose prednisolone for 3–6 months, followed by maintenance treatment with prednisolone and azathioprine, may reduce proteinuria and slow progression, especially if there is mesangial hypercellularity and tip lesions. **Chlorambucil** has also been used with some success. Despite treatment, 50% progress to end-stage kidney disease within 10 years of diagnosis. HIVAN is managed with **anti-retroviral therapy**. Renal function may stabilize or improve.

Membranous glomerulonephritis

Membranous glomerulonephritis presents with nephrotic syndrome or asymptomatic proteinuria with or without renal impairment, microscopic haematuria and hypertension. It usually affects adults, mainly men. Spontaneous remission can occur. Specific treatment should be reserved for those with overt nephrotic syndrome and/or progressive renal impairment. Older age at presentation, male sex and heavy proteinuria are risk factors for progression.

- In 75% of cases no underlying cause is found. Causes include drugs (e.g. gold, penicillamine, NSAIDs), autoimmune disease (e.g. SLE, thyroiditis), infections (e.g. hepatitis B or C, schistosomiasis, *Plasmodium malariae*, leprosy) and neoplasia (e.g. solid organ tumours and lymphomas).

Kumar & Clark's Medical Management and Therapeutics

> **Box 10.1** Renoprotection in patients with CKD
>
> **Goals of treatment**
> - BP < 130/80 mmHg or < 120/75 mmHg if proteinuria and/or diabetes
> - Proteinuria < 1 g/24 hours or lower if possible
>
> **BP and proteinuria: treatment**
> - ACE inhibitor increasing to maximum dose
> - Add angiotensin receptor antagonist if proteinuria goals are not achieved (risk of hyperkalaemia — monitor serum potassium)*
> - Add diuretic to prevent hyperkalaemia and help to control BP
> - Add calcium channel blocker (e.g. **amlodipine** 5–10 mg daily) if goals not achieved
> - If another agent is needed, consider: β-blocker (e.g. **bisoprolol** 5–10 mg daily), α-blocker (e.g. **doxazosin** 4–16 mg daily), centrally acting agent (e.g. **moxonidine** 200–400 mg daily) or vascular smooth muscle relaxant (e.g. **minoxidil** 2.5–50 mg daily)
>
> **Additional measures**
> - Statins to lower cholesterol if high cardiovascular risk
> - Stop smoking (three-fold higher rate of deterioration in CKD)
> - Treat diabetes (HbA1c < 7%)
> - Attention to other cardiovascular risk factors (BMI, exercise, diet)
>
> *In type 2 diabetes start with angiotensin receptor antagonist.

- Pathology shows thickening of the capillary basement membrane on light microscopy and deposition of C3 and IgG on immunofluorescence. EM changes are detectable earlier in the course of the disease and mirror light microscopy changes, with electron-dense sub-epithelial capillary wall deposits. It is thought that immune complexes are formed in situ in the podocyte basement membrane and the target auto-antigen(s) in humans is the M-type phospholipase A_2 receptor (PLA$_2$R).
- Management (Box 10.1)
  - If an underlying condition is present, it should be treated. This may slow or halt the progression of disease.
  - In primary disease, spontaneous remission is common (up to 40%), so specific treatment should be withheld for up to 6 months unless there is progression. Even then, only those with severe proteinuria and/or progressive renal impairment should be treated with immunosuppression.
  - For such high-risk patients, steroids are ineffective if given alone. Combinations which have been used with some success include:
    a) **Prednisolone** 1 mg/kg/day on alternate days with cyclophosphamide 1.5–2.5 mg/kg/day for 6–12 months.
    b) **Chlorambucil** 0.2 mg/kg/day in months 2, 4 and 6 with prednisolone 0.4 mg/kg/day in months 1, 3 and 5.
    c) **Ciclosporin** 3.5 mg/kg/day for 12 months, with low-dose prednisolone.

Kumar & Clark's Medical Management and Therapeutics

d) **Rituximab**, an anti-CD25 antibody that ablates B lymphocytes; this has been shown to improve renal function and reduce proteinuria without significant side-effects in short-term studies. Long-term outcome is not yet known.

The effectiveness of the various drug regimens is unclear, and good controlled trials are lacking.

Amyloidosis

Amyloidosis is a systemic condition of abnormal protein folding, in which normally soluble proteins or fragments are deposited extracellularly. It may present with renal disease, usually nephrotic syndrome with or without renal impairment. Renal biopsy should be performed if renal involvement is suspected.

- There are two types:
  - *AA amyloid* is associated with chronic infections or inflammatory conditions (e.g. TB, bronchiectasis, IV drug use, rheumatoid arthritis, ankylosing spondylitis, familial Mediterranean fever, inflammatory bowel disease).
  - *AL amyloid* is associated with abnormal production of immunoglobulin light chains, and hence with haematological malignancies, especially myeloma.
- On renal biopsy, the mesangium is filled with abnormal eosinophilic deposits, which stain with the Congo red stain with apple green birefringence under polarized light. EM reveals the amyloid fibrils.
- The kidney is only one of the organs affected by amyloid. Serum amyloid protein (SAP) scanning can delineate the extent of involvement in other organs. Serial SAP scans are useful for documenting progression or regression.
- Management
  - Use renoprotective measures, as for all proteinuric renal disease (Box 10.1).
  - Remove/treat the underlying condition. The aim is to switch off production of the amyloid protein. In **AA amyloid**, infections or causes of chronic inflammation should be treated. **Eprodisate** is a drug that reduces deposition of the amyloid protein, and shows promise. In **familial Mediterranean fever**, **colchicine** 0.5–2 mg 3 times daily reduces the frequency of acute attacks and improves prognosis. In **AL amyloid**, treatments that reduce abnormal production of light chains can improve the renal prognosis and survival. Dexamethasone and melphalan are used. High-dose melphalan followed by autologous stem cell transplantation has also been used.
  - Despite this, specific treatment is often ineffective. Renal prognosis, once nephrotic-range proteinuria has developed, is poor. Survival depends mainly on the extent of involvement of other organs, especially the heart.

Diabetic nephropathy

This is the most common cause of chronic kidney disease in the developed world. Similar changes occur in both type 1 and type 2 diabetes. Thickening of the GBM and expansion of the mesangium are associated with glomerular hypertension and glomerular ischaemia, progressing to glomerulosclerosis with nodules (Kimmelstiel–Wilson lesions). Microalbuminuria progresses to overt albuminuria and then progressive renal impairment with or without nephrotic syndrome. **Renal biopsy** is usually not required unless there are grounds for doubt about the diagnosis (e.g. features suggestive of another cause of glomerulopathy).

- Management (Box 10.1)
  - *Tight glycaemic control* and lifestyle measures to reduce cardiovascular risk (stopping smoking, maintaining an ideal weight, healthy diet, regular exercise) and good BP control are the key to management in all patients with diabetes.
  - *Microalbuminuria and overt proteinuria* should be treated with an **ACE inhibitor** or **ARB**, irrespective of the BP. These drugs have been shown to slow the decline in renal function. **Combined ACE inhibitor and ARB** may reduce proteinuria further, usually under specialist supervision.
  - *BP targets* are more stringent if there is proteinuria, e.g. 120/75 mmHg.

Even with all of these measures, relentless progression is common.

Mesangiocapillary glomerulonephritis (MCGN)

MCGN may present with nephrotic syndrome, nephritic syndrome, or haematuria with hypertension. Progressive renal impairment may occur. Most cases progress to end-stage renal failure over several years. Histologically, all are associated with mesangial cell proliferation and basement membrane changes. Three sub-types are defined by appearances on EM:

- Type 1 — sub-endothelial immune deposits with 'splitting' of the GBM. Plasma C3 levels are reduced with normal C4, with activation of the classical pathway of the complement cascade. It is either idiopathic or associated with chronic infections, e.g. abscesses, infective carditis, or with cryoglobulinaemia and hepatitis C infection.
- Type 2 — electron-dense linear intramembranous deposits. C3 levels are also low, but with activation of the alternative pathway of the complement cascade. It may be idiopathic or associated with partial lipodystrophy.
- Type 3 — features of both type 1 and type 2, associated with activation with the final common pathway of the complement cascade.

Recurrence after transplantation is very common in type 2 (100%) and can occur in type 1 (25%), though rarely leads to graft loss.

- Management. Renoprotective measures (Box 10.1) are the key, especially BP control. Corticosteroids (prednisolone 40 mg/m^2 for 12 months) may be tried in children with progressive renal impairment but may not be effective. In adults, antiplatelet agents (aspirin 325 mg/day and dipyridamole 75 mg/day) may slow the rate of progression if there is renal impairment, and should be given for 6–12 months.

Cryoglobulinaemic renal disease

Cryoglobulins are immunoglobulins that precipitate with complement in the cold. Presentation is usually in fourth or fifth decade, and is more common in women than men. Renal glomerular changes resemble MCGN. Three types are described:

- Type I (10%): monoclonal immunoglobulin, associated with multiple myeloma and lymphoproliferative disorders
- Type II (50%): polyclonal IgG bound to a monoclonal IgA or IgM antiglobulin with rheumatoid factor properties
- Type III (40%): polyclonal IgG bound to a polyclonal IgA or IgM antiglobulin.

Recognized associations are as follows:

- viral infections: hepatitis B and C, HIV, cytomegalovirus (CMV), Epstein–Barr virus (EBV)
- fungal and spirochaete infections
- malaria
- infective endocarditis
- autoimmune rheumatic diseases: SLE, rheumatoid arthritis, Sjögren's syndrome.

- **Systemic features** include purpura, arthralgia, leg ulcers and Raynaud's phenomenon.
- **Specific treatment** for underlying diseases may halt renal decline. Renoprotective measures (Box 10.1) should be undertaken. For those with renal progression and or severe extra-renal disease, corticosteroids with intensive immunosuppression have been used. **Plasma exchange** (to remove circulating cryoglobulins) or **rituximab** may induce remission, but the evidence base is weak.

Lupus nephritis

SLE is an auto-antibody-mediated, T-cell-dependent and B-cell-mediated disease. Between 30 and 70% of patients with SLE develop renal involvement. Presentation is with proteinuria and/or haematuria and/or renal impairment. Early diagnosis and treatment improves prognosis, and hence all patients with lupus should receive regular checks of renal function, including urine dipstick and BP measurement.

- SLE is associated with characteristic serum immunological features. Auto-antibodies against cellular antigens include positive antinuclear antibodies, double-stranded DNA and anti-Ro, and serum complement components are reduced (C3, C4, C1q).
- Renal biopsy is *essential*, as it guides how aggressive treatment needs to be. Six histological types (International Society of Nephrology/Renal Pathological Society 2004) have been described:
  - Type 1 (normal glomeruli on light microscopy, mesangial immune deposits) just requires monitoring.
  - Type II (more deposits and mesangial hypercellularity and matrix expansion on light microscopy) does not usually progress.
  - Type III (focal proliferative, i.e. < 50% of glomeruli affected) and type IV (diffuse proliferative GN, i.e. > 50% glomeruli affected) have the worst prognosis and should always be treated with **immunosuppression**.
  - Type V (membranous changes) is treated if the nephrotic syndrome or type III or IV coexist.
  - Type VI shows advanced sclerosing lesions and progressive renal failure is invariably present.
- Immunofluorescence staining reveals positivity in the mesangium for C3, C4, C1q, IgM, IgG and IgA.
- Extraglomerular lesions may occur in SLE, including tubulointerstitial nephritis, and thrombotic lesions (renal vein or artery thrombosis, usually associated with antibodies against phospholipids, e.g. lupus anticoagulant or anticardiolipin).
- **Management.** Types I and II do not usually require immunosuppression. Types III and IV do. Most regimes include prednisolone and cyclophosphamide or mycophenolate for induction, with mycophenolate or azathioprine used for maintenance therapy. The use of mycophenolate for induction therapy is growing, though the evidence base for its use

in advanced renal disease is not (yet) convincing. For resistant disease, rituximab (anti-CD20 monoclonal antibody causing B-cell depletion) shows early promise, though long-term results are still awaited.

Post-infectious glomerulonephritis

This classically occurs in children 2–3 weeks after a Lancefield group A streptococcal throat infection and presents with acute nephritic syndrome. It is now rare in developed countries but can occur after infections, e.g. bacterial, malaria, schistosomiasis, viral infections and syphilis. Abscesses and deep-seated infections, including infectious endocarditis, may cause a similar clinical picture.

- Investigations may reveal renal impairment. There is a low C3 level with normal C4. Antistreptolysin O titres may be raised post streptococcal infection. Renal biopsy characteristically shows neutrophil infiltration in the glomerulus, with IgG and complement deposition (this is an immune complex disease). EM is consistent with this, with electron-dense deposits in the sub-epithelium of the capillary walls.
- Management
  - Active infection is treated aggressively.
  - The disease is usually self-limiting, so management is supportive with general measures including control of BP. A short course of steroids may be used if recovery is slow, provided the infection has been adequately treated.
  - Residual renal impairment and/or urinary abnormalities may occur, with increased risk of progression of chronic kidney disease in the future (though in children complete recovery is the rule).

IgA nephropathy

This is the most common GN, with a wide spectrum of presentation from asymptomatic, isolated microscopic haematuria with or without proteinuria to rapidly progressive renal failure and nephrotic syndrome. It may present with macroscopic haematuria (sometimes after an upper respiratory tract infection). It is commoner in children and young males. Hypertension is usual.

- Renal biopsy shows deposition of IgA in the mesangium, with or without mesangial cell proliferation. Crescent formation may occur.
- Management
  - **ACE inhibitors** and **ARBs** are used together if necessary, irrespective of BP, to reduce proteinuria to < 1 g/day and BP < 125/75 mmHg.
  - If there is modest proteinuria (< 1 g/day) with normal renal function, no specific measures improve outcome (which is likely to be good).
  - **Fish oil** 3 g 3 times daily may slow decline in renal function.
  - Steroids may be used if there is significant proteinuria 1–3 g daily, despite general measures and if renal function is preserved (**prednisolone 0.5 mg/kg** on alternate days).
  - Transformation to crescentic disease may occur, with rapidly declining renal function. Treat as for RPGN, with **prednisolone** and **cyclophosphamide** for 3 months followed by **prednisolone + azathioprine**, though the evidence base is not strong.

Henoch–Schönlein purpura

This vasculitis presents with a purpuric rash, usually in children. Renal pathology is identical to that of IgA nephropathy, as is management. The prognosis is good.

Rapidly progressive glomerulonephritis (RPGN)

Renal disease presents with acute nephritic syndrome and rapid deterioration of renal function (usually over several weeks). It may be limited to the kidney or there may be extra-renal disease. This includes a vasculitic rash or ulceration, arthralgia/arthritis, systemic symptoms (e.g. fatigue, anorexia, weight loss), gut or myocardial ischaemia, and pulmonary haemorrhage (may be life-threatening)

- Renal biopsy is essential to make the diagnosis and guide treatment. RPGN is characterized by inflammation and necrosis of the walls of small vessels, and by crescent formation (epithelial cells and macrophages that aggregate in Bowman's space). The pattern (or absence) of immune deposit deposition at biopsy is helpful in discriminating RPGN. Three staining patterns are seen:
  - linear immunofluorescence with IgG and C3, e.g. anti-GBM disease
  - granular immunofluorescence, e.g. idiopathic immune complex-mediated RPGN, associated with other primary GN, e.g. MCGN, IgA nephropathy, membranous GN, or associated with secondary GN, e.g. post-infectious GN, SLE, Henoch–Schönlein purpura, cryoglobulinaemia
  - negative immunofluorescence ('pauci-immune'), e.g. ANCA-positive vasculitis.

Anti-GBM disease

- (15–20% of all RPGN cases) is rare, usually presenting in men aged 20–30 or > 60 years (when male = female).
  - Antibodies against the α3 chain of type 4 collagen develop, which bind to the GBM with or without the alveolus (lung disease occurs only in cigarette smokers).
  - Lung haemorrhage occurs in ~66% of cases ('Goodpasture's syndrome').
  - Renal biopsy is mandatory, as is measurement of anti-GBM antibodies in the serum.
  - *Management*
  - *Plasma exchange* removes circulating pathogenic antibodies.
  - *Steroids* are used to suppress inflammation, e.g. **methylprednisolone** IV 500 mg daily for 3 days, followed by **prednisolone** 60–80 mg daily for up to 3 months, with gradual taper.
  - *Cyclophosphamide* is used to switch off antibody production.
  - *Ventilatory support and/or dialysis* may be required if pulmonary haemorrhage or severe renal failure are present.

The **renal prognosis** is poor if there is oliguria or the patient is dialysis-dependent. Recurrence does not occur, however, and immunosuppression can be tailed off and discontinued once anti-GBM titre is negative.

Antineutrophil cytoplasmic antibody (ANCA)-positive vasculitis

A group of small-vessel vasculitides are characterized by a positive ANCA titre. These include:

- Wegener's granulomatosis
- microscopic polyangiitis
- Churg–Strauss syndrome.

These diseases share a common pathology with focal necrotizing lesions that may be limited to the kidney or affect other organs, including the lungs (pulmonary haemorrhage), the dermis (vasculitic rash), and the nose and ear (vasculitic ulceration). Systemic symptoms may predominate (fever, weight loss, malaise) or be absent.

- **ANCA** are auto-antibodies directed against neutrophil antigens. They are sub-divided into two groups according to ELISA assays, binding either to proteinase 3 (PR3, or c-ANCA for cytoplasmic) or to myeloperoxidase (MPO, or p-ANCA for perinuclear). ANCA titres may be weakly positive in other autoimmune diseases or with some drugs.
- **PR3 ANCA** is associated with Wegener's granulomatosis and **MPO ANCA** with microscopic polyangiitis, but there is much overlap. It is more useful to group these disorders by clinical syndromes than ANCA (although ANCA may offer prognostic information regarding likelihood of relapse).
- Disease presents as RPGN with or without signs of small-vessel vasculitis affecting other organs (see above). Differential diagnosis includes anti-GBM disease and lupus, which should be excluded by measuring anti-GBM and anti-dsDNA titres. Drug-induced disease, e.g. propylthiouracil, hydralazine and penicillamine, is well described.
- The prognosis is very poor if disease is untreated, but better (80% 1-year patient survival) if treated aggressively and early, though dialysis dependence is common.
- Management
  - High-dose steroids are used (**IV methylprednisolone** 500 mg daily for 3 days for fulminant disease, and then **prednisolone** 60–80 mg/day reducing to 15 mg/day over 3 months).
  - Add **cyclophosphamide**. (Oral treatment appears to be associated with a lower rate of relapse, but IV treatment is better tolerated.)
  - Plasma exchange (3–4 L exchange daily for 14 days) is recommended if pulmonary haemorrhage or dialysis dependence is present at presentation, and may improve outcome in these circumstances.
  - Once remission is achieved, **azathioprine** should be substituted for **cyclophosphamide**. **Mycophenolate** or **methotrexate** is an alternative agent if azathioprine is not tolerated.
  - Treatment with **sulfamethoxazole/trimethoprim** reduces *Staphylococcus aureus* colonization of the upper respiratory tract and reduces the incidence of relapse.
  - Relapse is common (especially in Wegener's), and **low-dose immunosuppression** should be continued long-term.

Thrombotic microangiopathies (p. 231)

These are characterized by haemolysis, a low platelet count and tissue ischaemia secondary to thrombotic occlusion of small vessels. There are a number of causes, including:

- thrombotic thrombocytopenic purpura (p. 233)
- antiphospholipid syndrome
- haemolytic uraemic syndrome (HUS)
- malignant hypertension
- HELLP syndrome and pre-eclampsia
- SLE, rheumatoid disease, systemic sclerosis
- disseminated intravascular coagulation (DIC)
- metastatic malignancy.

The renal biopsy changes are similar, whatever the cause of the microangiopathy, with fibrin thrombi in glomerular capillaries and associated ischaemic changes.

Kumar & Clark's Medical Management and Therapeutics

- **Haemolytic uraemic syndrome** is characterized by intravascular haemolysis with red cell fragmentation, thrombocytopenia and acute kidney injury due to thromboses in small arteries and arterioles. Coagulation tests are normal, in contrast to DIC. HUS may follow a diarrhoeal infection (D+HUS) or occur spontaneously (D–HUS).
  - **D+HUS** usually follows gastroenteritis due to *E. coli* O157 (verocytotoxin). **Treatment** is mainly supportive, with fluid balance, antihypertensives and nutritional support; dialysis is often required. There is no evidence that plasma exchange has a role. There is a 5% mortality, and 30% go on to long-term renal damage.
  - **D–HUS** may be recurrent and may be related to abnormalities in the regulation of the complement cascade, e.g. factor H deficiency or membrane cofactor protein abnormalities. Plasma exchange or infusion is recommended.
- Other cases of HUS are related to drugs (mitomycin C, ciclosporin, cisplatin), infections (HIV, pneumococcus), malignancies, scleroderma and accelerated hypertension. Treatment is to address the underlying condition or remove the offending drug, and is otherwise supportive.
- **Malignant (accelerated) hypertension and systemic sclerosis** both cause similar renal histological changes with fibrin thrombi, fibrinoid necrosis and onion skin intimal thickening, and may precipitate acute kidney injury. Management consists of control of the BP. ACE inhibitors have a key role and should be used as first-line therapy; this has led to a significant improvement in renal outcome. Long-term follow-up is essential, as hypertension and chronic kidney disease often ensue. Prostacyclin infusion IV is sometimes used in severe systemic sclerosis, though its benefit for the kidneys is unproven.

Multiple myeloma

Acute or chronic kidney disease may occur, by one or more of the following mechanisms:

- cast nephropathy: deposition of light chains within the tubular lumen
- AL amyloidosis
- light chain deposition disease: Congo red-negative nodular glomerulosclerosis caused by deposits of (usually λ) light chains
- direct plasma cell infiltration
- hypercalcaemia
- hyperuricaemic nephropathy: may occur in the context of tumour lysis syndrome, with tubular deposition of urate crystals.

The management is to treat the underlying condition; renal management is supportive and dialysis may be required.

RENAL HYPERTENSION

Hypertension is both a cause and effect of renal disease, and a renal biopsy is often needed to ensure there is no other underlying condition. Many renal diseases are associated with hypertension. The mechanisms include activation of the renin–angiotensin system and salt and water retention. BP control is essential to prevent target organ damage and to improve renal prognosis. **ACE inhibitors** and/or **ARBs** have renoprotective effects over and above their effect on BP for many proteinuric renal diseases.

Renovascular disease

Renal artery stenosis leads to production of renin by the kidney and hypertension. Bilateral renovascular disease may cause renal impairment. Two groups of patients develop renovascular disease:

- **Atherosclerotic renovascular disease** occurs in older people, as with other diseases caused by atherosclerosis, and often alongside them. The stenosis tends to be at the ostium of the renal artery and may be bilateral. The diagnosis is suggested by the presence of vascular disease elsewhere, modest proteinuria, hypertension and asymmetrical kidneys on US. Confirmation of the diagnosis may be via MR angiography (if renal function is sufficiently preserved to allow the use of gadolinium) or CT angiography (though with the risk of contrast nephropathy). Arteriography is the gold standard investigation.
  - *Treatment* is aggressive management of risk factors for progression of atherosclerosis (BP, statins, aspirin, stopping smoking). **Angioplasty** ± stenting may be indicated if there is rapidly declining renal function, flash pulmonary oedema or resistant hypertension along with significant (> 75%) stenotic lesions. However, angiography may lead to cholesterol emboli and may worsen ischaemic renal disease. Further trials are needed to clarify which patients benefit most from this treatment.
- **Fibromuscular dysplasia** accounts for 30% of renovascular disease. It is not associated with atherosclerosis, occurring most commonly in young women. It presents with hypertension and usually with well-preserved renal function.
  - *Therapeutic angioplasty* may be curative and the prognosis is usually good.

RENAL STONE DISEASE

Stone disease affects 8–15% of the population. The male : female ratio is 2:1. Risk factors include living or working in a hot environment (and dehydration), hypercalcaemia, hypercalciuria, recurrent UTI, renal tubular acidosis, hyperoxaluria, hyperuricaemia, cystinosis and some drugs (loop diuretics, vitamins D and C, indinavir, sulfadiazine). Patients with polycystic kidney disease have an increased risk of stone formation. Many people have none of these and nevertheless develop stones ('idiopathic stone formation').

Over 90% of stones are calcium-based. Uric acid stones are radiolucent and occur in those with hyperuricaemia; uric acid is more likely to crystallize out in an acid urine.

Most stones are formed in the upper urinary tract but bladder stones may form when there is urinary stasis or abnormal flow (diverticula, surgical reconstruction, long-term catheterization).

Presentation is with loin pain (may radiate to perineum/testis), suprapubic pain, haematuria, dysuria and/or UTI. Signs may include loin or suprapubic tenderness and urinary dipstick abnormalities. Most stones are asymptomatic.

Investigations

These should include:

- **Imaging.** Carry out a plain X-ray (90% of stones are radio-opaque, urate stones are not). CT-KUB delineates anatomy and demonstrates opacifications in the renal tract. IVU is still widely used instead of CT.

- **Chemical analysis of stone.** Perform chemical analysis of the stone if one is passed. Also do U&E, Ca^{2+}, bicarbonate, urate and urine for culture.
- **24-hour urine analysis for Ca^{2+}, urate, citrate and oxalate.** This should be carried out in **recurrent stone-formers** (> 1 stone in 3 years). A spot urine should be sent for cystine.

Management of acute renal stone disease 75 mg by IV infusion

- Analgesia (NSAIDs, e.g. diclofenac, and/or opiate may be required).
- **Small** asymptomatic stones are managed conservatively.
- **Larger** stones (> 0.5 cm), especially if symptomatic, should be treated by:
  - *Extracorporeal shock wave lithotripsy (ESWL)*, which shatters the stone and allows the fragments to pass. A ureteric stent may be required to prevent fragments becoming lodged in the ureter.
  - *Retrograde removal* with ureteroscopy.
  - *Antegrade removal* via a nephrostomy tube for larger renal stones, e.g. stag-horn calculus.

Prophylaxis and prevention

- A daily urine output > 2 L/day should be maintained and any UTI treated aggressively.
- Hypercalciuric patients should eat a diet normal in calcium intake (30 mmol/day) and oxalate (oxalate absorption promotes calcium absorption). A thiazide diuretic can be added to reduce urine calcium excretion if necessary.
- Allopurinol and a high fluid intake may prevent formation of uric acid stones.
- Cystine stones are rare (1–2% of all stones), associated with cystinuria, and inherited in an autosomal recessive pattern. A urine output of > 5 L/day should be maintained. Penicillamine is effective in dissolving cystine stones.
- Hypocitraturia predisposes to calcium stone deposition (citrate has a calcium-chelating action). Potassium citrate is effective in increasing urinary citrate levels.

ACUTE KIDNEY INJURY

Acute kidney injury (AKI) is a deterioration in renal function over the course of days or weeks, which is usually (but not always) reversible. It occurs in 5–10% of all hospital admissions and up to 25% of all ICU admissions. AKI may not be easily distinguishable from chronic (or acute on chronic) kidney disease when the patient first presents.

The Acute Dialysis Quality Initiative group proposed the RIFLE (**r**isk, **i**njury, **f**ailure, **l**oss, **e**nd-stage kidney disease) criteria based on increases in serum creatinine or decreases in urine output (Table 10.3). They characterize three levels of renal dysfunction (R, I, F) and two outcome measures (L, E). These criteria indicate an increasing degree of renal damage and have a predictive value for mortality. The mortality of patients with AKI requiring dialysis is 50%.

The causes of AKI can be divided into pre-renal, renal and post-renal.

- **Pre-renal injury** results from impairment of renal blood flow leading to acute tubular necrosis (ATN). It accounts for > 80% of all AKI. This may be the result of hypovolaemia (e.g. haemorrhage, burns, diarrhoea),

Table 10.3 RIFLE classification of acute kidney injury

Grade	GFR criteria	UO criteria
Risk	SCr × 1.5	UO < 0.5 mL/kg/hour × 6 hours
Injury	SCr × 2	UO < 0.5 mL/kg/hour × 12 hours
Failure	SCr × 3 or SCr > 350 μmol/L with an acute rise > 40 μmol/L	UO < 0.3 mL/kg/hour × 24 hours
Loss	Persistent AKI > 4 weeks	
ESKD	Persistent renal failure > 3 months	

AKI, acute kidney injury; ESKD, end-stage kidney disease; GFR, glomerular filtration rate; SCr, serum creatinine; UO, urine output.

hypotension, changes in the effective circulating arterial volume (e.g. myocardial infarction, severe sepsis, congestive cardiac failure) or impairment of renal blood flow autoregulation by drugs (e.g. ACE inhibitors, NSAIDs).

- **Renal causes** include vascular lesions, e.g. large vessels (bilateral renal artery disease ± ACE inhibitor treatment, cholesterol emboli), small vessels and glomeruli (e.g. vasculitis, glomerulonephritis (p. 338, 341), accelerated hypertension), and tubulointerstitial disease (e.g. tubular interstitial nephritis, cast nephropathy (in multiple myeloma) and the tumour lysis syndrome).
- **Post-renal injury** is due to bilateral urinary tract obstruction, or obstruction of a single functioning kidney.

Clinical features

The history usually points clearly to the diagnosis. Diarrhoea, vomiting, nephrotoxic drug ingestion, symptoms of a multi-system disorder, inter-current illness or lower urinary tract symptoms may be present. Oliguria is not invariable. Polyuria occurs in other conditions, e.g. partial obstruction, tubulointerstitial disease. Clinical **examination** may reveal hypovol-aemia, signs of vasculitis (e.g. rash, fever) or a palpable bladder.

Investigations

- **Serum and urine samples** should be obtained for a full biochemical analysis of the blood and urine, including microscopy of the urine. If a **systemic disease** is suspected, the relevant test should be performed, e.g. dsDNA for SLE, hepatitis B and C serology. It can be difficult to differentiate between pre-renal and intrinsic causes of uraemia. A fluid challenge can be performed (see below). In pre-renal failure, there is a fractional excretion rate of sodium (FE_{Na}) of < 1%, as the kidney retains sodium, resulting in a low urine sodium concentration.

$$FE_{Na} = U_{Na}/P_{Na} \div U_{Cr}/P_{Cr} \times 100$$

- **Renal biopsy** is not required if the diagnosis is obvious. ATN can be presumed if there is a clear precipitating cause and no significant proteinuria.
- **Imaging** should include a US to exclude obstruction. AKI secondary to another cause is usually associated with normal-looking kidneys on US. Small kidneys (< 9 cm) imply chronic kidney disease. IV contrast should

---

> **Box 10.2** Indications for dialysis in acute kidney injury
>
> - Pulmonary oedema with oliguria unresponsive to diuretics
> - Hyperkalaemia (K^+ > 6 mmol/L if oliguria or if unresponsive to emergency measures)
> - Severe acidosis (but if hypovolaemic IV sodium bicarbonate can be given first)
> - Symptomatic uraemia (neurological symptoms, e.g. fits, twitching, confusion; pericarditis; vomiting)
> - Raised urea and creatinine — not an indication per se for dialysis, but if urea > 40 mmol/L for several days then symptoms are likely to develop.
> - Specific indications for removal of toxins, e.g. gentamicin, lithium, aspirin

---

be avoided, as the nephrotoxicity may exacerbate the ATN already present.

Management

- Managing fluid balance
  - Optimization of fluid balance is essential to allow renal recovery to occur and to maintain homeostasis for the rest of the body. If hypovolaemia is present, correct by giving IV 0.9% NaCl. A central line should be inserted. Give a fluid challenge of 200–300 mL and reassess clinical parameters if there is uncertainty about volume status (p. 368).
  - Pre-renal causes can coexist with established ATN, so beware persisting oliguria despite fluid replacement, leading to fluid overload.
  - Hypervolaemia should be managed with salt and water restriction (500 mL/day + losses). Diuretics do not improve outcome, but can sometimes simplify management by establishing some diuresis. High doses of loop diuretics are required (e.g. **furosemide** 80–250 mg/day).
  - Drugs that impair renal autoregulation (**ACE inhibitors**, **NSAIDs**) should be discontinued.
  - Hyperkalaemia requires urgent management (p. 376 and 711).
  - Dialysis may be required (Box 10.2).
- **Treatment of the underlying cause.** Any precipitating factor or cause should be removed. In addition, specific therapy should be given, e.g. immunosuppression for vasculitis (p. 321).

SOME RENAL CAUSES OF ACUTE KIDNEY INJURY

Acute tubular necrosis (ATN)

This is the most common cause of AKI, especially in hospital practice. Renal impairment secondary to pre-renal causes (p. 348) will progress to ATN if pre-renal factors are not corrected; patients may be oliguric or non-oliguric.

The cause is often multi-factorial, e.g. hypotension + sepsis + NSAIDs. Renal tubular cells are sensitive to hypoxia — hence necrosis occurs when the renal blood supply is impaired. ATN can also be the result of toxic damage, e.g.:

- myoglobin (rhabdomyolysis)
- haemoglobinuria (malaria, intravascular haemolysis)

- contrast media (see below)
- drugs (e.g. **gentamicin**, **amphotericin B** and **cisplatin**).
- **Management** is supportive until renal recovery occurs (usually within 6 weeks — prognostic renal biopsy is often performed at around this time if no recovery). Optimize fluid balance, avoid nephrotoxic agents, give dialysis if necessary (Box 10.2), and monitor urine output and serum biochemistry. Recovery is often accompanied by a brisk diuresis, which might even necessitate IV fluid replacement for a few days.

Acute tubulointerstitial nephritis (TIN)

TIN presents with AKI (caused by an intense inflammatory cell infiltrate into the renal interstitium), with modest or no proteinuria. There may be fever, arthralgia and a rash, reflecting the probable hypersensitivity reaction that is responsible for the renal damage.

- Causes include drugs (70%) and infections (15%), though no cause may be apparent. Non-infectious chronic inflammatory diseases may cause TIN, including SLE, sarcoidosis and Sjögren's syndrome (when renal tubular acidosis may also be present). They generally respond to management of the underlying condition.
- Drug-induced TIN is classically associated with an eosinophilia and eosinophils are seen in the infiltrate on renal biopsy. Common drugs include **penicillins**, **sulphonamides**, **NSAIDs**, **allopurinol**, **cephalosporins**, **rifampicin**, **diuretics**, **cimetidine** and **phenytoin**.
- Infectious causes include direct bacterial infection of the kidney with a neutrophil infiltrate. Systemic viral (HIV, measles, EBV) and bacterial (*Legionella*, *Leptospira*, *Mycoplasma*, *Brucella*, streptococcus) infections may cause an inflammatory infiltrate without evidence of direct bacterial invasion in the kidney. Treatment is to eradicate the causative organism.

Treatment

- Withdraw the offending drug(s) or treat the underlying infection/disease process. The prognosis is generally good, though residual renal impairment may result.
- Treat AKI as above.
- **Steroids,** e.g. **prednisolone** 30–60 mg daily, are often given for drug-induced TIN but there is no good evidence that steroids improve long-term outcome.

Contrast nephropathy

In patients with impaired renal function, e.g. from diabetes mellitus, heart failure or hypovolaemia, iodinated radiological contrast media may be nephrotoxic, possibly by causing renal vasoconstriction and producing a direct toxic effect on renal tubules. In many patients the effect is small but severe deterioration in renal function can occur in some. Pre-hydration with an infusion of 1 L of 0.9% **saline** during the 12-hour period before and also 12 hours after contrast exposure is helpful. Be careful not to overload susceptible patients when **furosemide** may be required. **N-acetylcysteine (NAC**; a potent antioxidant) given 48 hours prior to the radiological intervention may also prevent the worsening of the pre-existing renal disease.

N.B. Gadolinium used in contrast MRI causes nephrogenic fibrosing nephropathy (nephrogenic systemic fibrosis).

Kumar & Clark's Medical Management and Therapeutics

Post-renal AKI

Urinary tract obstruction

Complete obstruction occurs when there is no urine flow. **Partial** obstruction occurs when there is some urine flow, but increased pressure proximal to the obstruction. Both cause renal damage. Obstruction may be **bilateral** (as occurs in lower urinary tract obstruction) or **unilateral** (e.g. single ureter), when urine flow and serum creatinine are unaltered.

- Complete obstruction presents acutely with anuria. Depending on the cause and the level of obstruction there may be pain (full bladder, stones, associated infection). Examination can show a palpable bladder and/or loin tenderness/fullness. Serum biochemistry will show rising serum creatinine.
- Partial obstruction is often asymptomatic, or presents with similar signs and symptoms as complete obstruction. Tests of renal function may be normal. Symptoms of coexistent UTI may predominate.
- If the bladder is palpable, urethral catheterization should be attempted prior to imaging. Measurement of the residual urine volume makes the diagnosis.

Imaging

- US of the kidneys and bladder is quick, non-invasive and sensitive. It will show a dilated renal pelvis and collecting systems. The ureter is visualized and can show the level or cause of obstruction. Occasionally US is misleading, e.g. when ATN and oliguria are established and no dilatation is seen, in pregnancy and post renal transplant (in which cases the renal pelvis may be 'baggy' but not obstructed).
- Other imaging depends on the site and the cause of obstruction, e.g. CT for stone disease, CT-KUB for suspected PUJ or VUJ obstruction.

Management

- Relieving the obstruction
  - *Lower urinary tract obstruction* requires urethral catheterization. If a urethral stricture or prostatic obstruction is present, suprapubic catheterization is occasionally required.
  - *Upper tract obstruction* should be relieved from either above (with percutaneous nephrostomy) or below (with ureteric stenting).
  - *Complete obstruction* should always be treated without delay. Infection + obstruction is a medical emergency.
  - *A post-obstructive diuresis* often follows relief of bilateral obstruction. Measure urine output and replace fluid with IV 0.9% saline.
- Treating the underlying cause will relieve symptoms and preserve renal function. Bilateral ureteric stenting or long-term urethral catheterization is used if relief of obstruction is not possible.

Pelvi-ureteric junction (PUJ) or vesico-ureteric junction (VUJ) obstruction

This results from a functional disturbance of peristalsis at the PUJ in the absence of mechanical obstruction. Surgery (pyeloplasty) is indicated if loin pain is persistent or there is evidence of progressive kidney damage. VUJ obstruction also occurs in childhood but may only become evident in adult life. It is more common in males, presenting with a mega-ureter. Surgery (reimplantation of ureter) is indicated for children and adults with symptoms, recurrent UTI, stones or progressive kidney damage.

Retroperitoneal fibrosis (RPF) (peri-aortitis)

In this condition, the ureters become encased in fibrous tissue with result-ant obstruction. The cause is often unknown but drugs (**methysergide**, **ergot-derived dopamine agonists**, e.g. **cabergoline**) are causal; with an inflammatory aortic aneurysm, ceroid is thought to leak out from the atheromatous aorta and cause a fibrotic reaction. The male:female ratio is 3:1.

- **Investigations** show a raised ESR and a normochromic normocytic anaemia. CT scan makes the diagnosis, but biopsy is sometimes required to rule out lymphoma or other malignancy.
- **Management** is initially by ureteric stenting. Steroids (**prednisolone** 40–60 mg tapering over several weeks) may shrink the mass. Following this, options are surgical ureterolysis or permanent ureteric stenting. **Mycophenolate** and **tamoxifen** have also been used with some success. Monitor by ESR and CT scanning for recurrence.

Benign prostatic hypertrophy

Non-malignant enlargement of the prostate gland is a common cause of lower urinary tract symptoms with or without urinary obstruction in men. It is increasingly common in older age.

- **Management**
- Mild disease requires no specific treatment.
- Moderate disease can usually be managed medically with α-blockers (e.g. **tamsulosin**) with or without 5α-reductase inhibitors (e.g. **finasteride**), which block conversion of testosterone to dihydrotestosterone (the androgen primarily responsible for prostate growth).
- Acute urinary retention should be managed with a bladder catheter. With the above drugs a successful trial without the catheter may be possible.
- Transurethral resection of the prostate is reserved for those in whom medical therapy fails or is inadequate.

CHRONIC KIDNEY DISEASE

Chronic kidney disease (CKD) is a longstanding condition with (usually) a progressive impairment of renal function; it is common, up to 5% of the adult population having CKD.

The loss of glomeruli is associated with hyperfiltration in the remaining glomeruli. Local activation of angiotensin II and cytokine release cause mesangial cell activation and progressive fibrosis and sclerosis. Protein in the proximal convoluted tubule also stimulates cytokine activation and inflammation, eventually causing peritubular fibrosis. Hypertension worsens hyperfiltration injury and proteinuria. CKD is usually (but not invariably) associated with hypertension. Once established, whatever the cause, CKD tends to progress.

CKD can occur from any kidney disease, either congenital or acquired, or from post-renal causes. Acute on chronic deterioration in renal function sometimes occurs due to:

- decreased renal perfusion
- drugs
- urinary tract obstruction or infection
- renal vein thrombosis.

Table 10.4 Classification of chronic kidney disease

	GFR (mL/min)	Description
1*	> 90	Normal kidney function
2*	60–90	Mild reduction of kidney function, with other evidence of kidney damage
3	30–60	Moderately reduced kidney function
4	15–30	Severely reduced kidney function
5	< 15	End-stage or approaching end-stage kidney disease

*eGFR of > 60 is normal, unless there is other evidence of kidney disease, e.g. proteinuria, haematuria.

Classification
The US National Kidney Federation Dialysis Outcomes Quality Initiative classification of CKD has been universally adopted (Table 10.4).

Clinical features
- **History.** The history often elicits the cause; previous tests of renal function, BP and urinalysis help document the decline in renal function. Previous surgery, drug treatment or medical history may point to the diagnosis. CKD is often asymptomatic, especially in the early stages, with symptoms and signs of advanced CKD occurring in stage 4 of disease.
- **Assessment of renal function.** Serial measurement of eGFR is practical and useful. If a sudden or non-linear decline in renal function is detected, a cause for that decline should be sought. As a guide, eGFR decline should be < 5 mL/min/year in a CKD patient with well-controlled BP.
  - *Urinalysis.* Significant proteinuria and/or haematuria suggest a glomerular cause. UTI may cause a more modest proteinuria. Haematuria may reflect bleeding from a renal tract tumour and should be investigated unless another cause is known. Red cell casts on urine microscopy indicate a glomerulonephritis.
  - *Urine culture.* This will exclude infection. Sterile pyuria suggests TB; send early morning urine samples for TB culture.
  - *Haematology.* Anaemia is a feature of more advanced CKD (see below). Raised ESR may suggest multiple myeloma or vasculitis.
  - *Immunology.* Antibody screening for autoimmune conditions and viral infections is performed.
- **Imaging.** Renal US provides details of renal size and anatomy, and usually excludes obstruction. Small kidneys with thin cortices imply that the process is chronic (months or years). CT (e.g. for diagnosis of retroperitoneal fibrosis) or MRI (for assessment of renovascular disease) is sometimes indicated.
- **Renal biopsy.** This should be performed for all unexplained progressive renal failure with normal-sized kidneys, unless there is a contraindication.

Complications of CKD

- Anaemia
  - The causes are multifactorial but the major cause is decreased production of erythropoetin as renal function declines. Iron deficiency and blood loss also contribute.
  - If the GFR is < 45 mL/min and Hb < 10 g/dL, then a therapeutic trial of **erythropoetin** should be commenced (IV or SC 50 U/kg epoetin alfa or beta) over 1–5 mins 3 times weekly. Check iron indices, B_{12} and folate first and correct if abnormal. **Darbepoetin alfa** is given weekly and **pegzerepoetin alfa** is given monthly.
  - Most patients on erythropoetin require supplementary iron treatment with a ferritin > 100 mg/L and transferrin saturation > 20% to optimize response to EPO, e.g. **ferrous sulphate** 200 mg 3 times daily. Those who do not respond to or do not tolerate oral iron should receive IV iron replacement, e.g. **iron sucrose** 200 mg IV weekly for 3 weeks.
  - BP, Hb and reticulocyte count should be measured every 2 weeks and the dose adjusted to maintain target Hb of 11–12 g/dL. An increase in stroke on treatment has been reported and therapy continues to be evaluated.
- Renal bone disease
  - The kidney is the site of 1α-hydroxylation of 25-hydroxy vitamin D. Renal failure leads to loss of this function, in turn leading to secondary hyperparathyroidism.
  - Decreased renal excretion of phosphate in renal failure leads to hyperphosphataemia.
  - Secondary hyperparathyroidism leads to increased and uncontrolled bone turnover and eventually cyst formation and bone marrow fibrosis.
  - Derangement of calcium and phosphate metabolism and secondary hyperparathyroidism have non-skeletal effects as well, including increased arterial calcification, left ventricular hypertrophy and cardiac fibrosis, with increased risk of cardiovascular morbidity and mortality.
  - *Management of renal bone disease*
    - *Hyperphosphataemia* should be treated by dietary restriction of phosphate with or without the use of phosphate binders (Table 10.5). Phosphate binders bind phosphate in the stomach, preventing gastrointestinal absorption.
    - *Hyperparathyroidism* (parathyroid hormone (PTH) level 3 times normal) should be treated with activated vitamin D, e.g. **calcitriol**, **alfacalcidol** 0.25–1 mcg daily orally. Hypercalcaemia may result and may limit treatment — aim to keep serum calcium in the lower half of the normal range. Vitamin D may worsen hyperphosphataemia, so serum phosphate should be controlled first. The calcium-phosphate product correlates with the risk of ectopic calcification and hypercalcaemia should be avoided. Concern over high calcium loads (with use of calcium-containing phosphate binders) exists; alternative binders are often used first-line for this reason.
    - *Calcimimetics* (e.g. **cinacalcet**, a calcium-sensing receptor agonist 30–180 mg daily orally) mimic the effect of calcium on the parathyroids, thus driving down PTH production without causing

Table 10.5 Phosphate binders used in chronic kidney disease

Preparation	Limitations	Side-effects
Calcium salts, e.g. **calcium acetate** 500 mg 3 times daily	Calcium load may worsen or precipitate arterial calcification	Hypercalcaemia
Sevelamer 2.4–12 g in divided doses chewed with meals 3 times daily	Only used in dialysis patients	GI disturbances
Lanthanum 1.5–3 g in divided doses chewed with meals 3 times daily	Only used in dialysis patients	GI disturbances
Aluminium hydroxide 475 mg tabs, 1–3 times daily with meals	Aluminium toxicity: avoid except for short-term use	

hypercalcaemia. Cinacalcet has a role in patients on dialysis with secondary hyperparathyroidism, when hypercalcaemia prevents further increase in activated vitamin D doses.

- *Surgical parathyroidectomy* may be necessary when optimal medical therapy fails to suppress PTH. Low PTH levels are associated with adynamic bone disease, decreased bone turnover and increased ectopic calcification. This may occur after parathyroidectomy or with over-treatment with vitamin D.

- Cardiovascular disease
  - This is the biggest killer of patients with chronic kidney disease. Cardiovascular disease is 16 times as prevalent as in the normal population.
  - The reasons include increased arterial stiffness and calcification, left ventricular hypertrophy, hypertension, calcium and phosphate abnormalities and high levels of oxidative stress.

Management of patients with CKD (Box 10.1)

- Underlying cause. Treat the underlying cause of CKD if possible.
- BP control. Poor control of BP accelerates progression and also imposes adverse cardiovascular risk.
  - Target BP should be 130/80 mmHg, or 120/75 mmHg if significant proteinuria and/or diabetes is present.
  - If proteinuria is present, ACE inhibitors are the first-line treatment, as they reduce proteinuria over and above their antihypertensive effects in both diabetic and non-diabetic renal disease. Proteinuria is an independent marker for progression and must be treated.
  - ARBs are an alternative, with similar effects on proteinuria and prevention of progression.
  - Combined ACE inhibitors and ARBs have a synergistic effect on proteinuria. Use both if necessary to reduce proteinuria to < 1 g/24 hours.
  - Patients with CKD often need three or more agents to achieve BP control, and should be warned of this (Box 10.1).

- In stages 4 and 5 CKD, salt and water retention may be significant factors in hypertension. Manage with loop diuretics, e.g. furosemide 40–250 mg per day in divided doses.
- **Diet.** Dietary protein restriction may slow progression, but malnutrition is a significant risk and a normal protein diet (0.8–1 g/kg/day) is recommended. Dietary education is necessary as renal failure progresses and includes the following:
  - An adequate energy intake (carbohydrates and lipids) is essential.
  - Restriction of sodium to < 5–6 g/day helps to control fluid overload, hypertension and thirst.
  - Potassium restriction is almost always necessary as CKD becomes advanced, especially if taking ACE inhibitors and/or ARBs. Avoid potassium-sparing diuretics in these circumstances.

Preparation for renal replacement therapy

- Less than 5% of all patients with stage 3 CKD reach end-stage renal disease (most patients die with their CKD rather than from it).
- Once the eGFR is < 30 mL/min, dialysis should be discussed with the patient. Timely preparation for dialysis improves outcome. The patient needs to understand and be prepared for:
  - what dialysis involves for the patient
  - which modality of dialysis is most suitable for the individual
  - insertion of a peritoneal dialysis catheter or creation of an arteriovenous fistula
  - whether kidney transplantation is feasible; if so, whether there is a suitable living donor (consider pre-emptive transplant).
- Specialized clinics for pre-dialysis preparation and conservative management facilitate management and are recommended. Dialysis should be commenced before uraemic symptoms supervene.

Non-dialysis management of end-stage renal failure

Some patients may make an informed decision not to commence dialysis, as survival on dialysis in patients with high co-morbidity is often measured in months rather than years. Dialysis can be arduous, especially if the patient is frail with co-morbidity at the outset. Non-dialysis management may keep such patients at home and with a better quality of life, with little or no reduction in the length of life.

The decision not to dialyse should always be made by the medical team and patient (with carers if appropriate) together. No patient should have dialysis withheld against his/her wish or knowledge.

RENAL REPLACEMENT THERAPY

Approximately 100 white individuals per million population in the UK commence renal replacement therapy (RRT) each year (the figure for blacks and Asians is 3–4 times higher, mainly because of the higher incidence of hypertensive and diabetic nephropathy in these groups).

RRT is delivered either by dialysis (haemodialysis or peritoneal dialysis) or by renal transplantation. The aim of dialysis is to mimic the functions of the normal kidney, including fluid and electrolyte balance and excretion of nitrogenous wastes. Erythropoietin production and hydroxylation of vitamin D are not affected by dialysis and require additional treatment.

Table 10.6 Composition of dialysate (mmol/L)

	Haemodialysis	Peritoneal dialysis
Sodium	130–145	130–134
Potassium	0.0–4.0	0.0
Calcium	1.0–1.6	1.0–1.75
Magnesium	0.25–0.85	0.25–0.75
Chloride	99–108	95–104
Lactate	35–40 (or acetate 35–40)	35–40
Glucose	0–10	77–236
Total osmolality		356–511 mOsm/kg

Haemodialysis

Blood is removed from the circulation and passed across a semi-permeable membrane. On the other side of that membrane flows dialysate in a counter-current fashion. Dialysate (Table 10.6) consists of ions at physiological concentrations, allowing homeostasis to be maintained/restored by dialysis treatment by diffusion and equilibration across the membrane. Water (and salt) removal can be controlled by controlling the trans-membrane pressure.

Blood flow required is typically 200–350 mL/min. The most reliable method of achieving such flow is by creation of an arterio-venous fistula (surgical anastomosis of an artery to a vein, usually the cephalic vein to the radial or brachial artery). The high flows and pressures thus created in the vein allow needles to be inserted and removed at the beginning and end of each treatment. If no suitable vein exists, a polytetra-flouroetheylene (PTFE) graft can be inserted between artery and vein. For emergency dialysis, a dual lumen catheter inserted into the jugular vein allows satisfactory blood flows. Tunnelled catheters may be used in place of an arterio-venous fistula in patients unsuitable for fistula creation, but are associated with a high incidence of sepsis and may cause venous stenosis. Anticoagulation (usually with heparin) is required to prevent the blood clotting.

Haemofiltration

Haemofiltration involves removal of plasma water and electrolytes by convective flow across a high-flux semi-permeable membrane, with replacement by a solution of physiological biochemical composition. Haemofiltration is rarely used as treatment for chronic kidney disease, but is useful in acute kidney injury in critically ill patients. Continuous low-volume haemofiltration (e.g. 1 L/hour) is a gentler treatment than intermittent dialysis and confers greater cardiovascular stability.

Haemodiafiltration

Haemodiafiltration combines the principles of dialysis and filtration. Long-term outcome trials are awaited, but clearance of 'middle' molecules appears to be improved, with a reduction of β_2-microglobulin deposition, leading to reduced dialysis amyloid-associated carpal tunnel syndrome and possibly other more significant benefits.

Prescription and adequacy of haemodialysis

- **Dry weight.** Each patient should have an ideal dry weight established, i.e. that weight at which salt and water balance is optimal. The dry weight should be attained during the dialysis session by removal of salt and water.
- **Dialysate composition.** A high dialysate sodium concentration may stimulate thirst and hypertension. High calcium in the dialysate may lead to hypercalcaemia. Low calcium may worsen secondary hyperparathyroidism. The buffer used is usually bicarbonate (or acetate).
- **Frequency.** Unless there is significant renal function, most patients need to dialyse at least 3 times per week for 4–5 hours per session to allow adequate clearance of small molecules and control of fluid status. More frequent dialysis leads to better control of BP, serum phosphate and other biochemical parameters.
- **Membranes.** Biocompatible membranes are superseding cellulose-based membranes, as they cause less activation of inflammatory cascades.
- **Adequacy.** Insufficient dialysis is associated with increased morbidity and mortality. Measures of dialysis adequacy (measuring the amount of urea removed per session) should occur regularly for all patients on chronic dialysis treatment.

Complications of haemodialysis

These include hypotension, which can be avoided by careful management of fluid balance, infection of indwelling lines (treat with IV antibiotics) and thrombosis of vascular access. Long-term complications include an increase in cardiovascular disease, bone disease and dialysis amyloid.

Peritoneal dialysis

The **peritoneum** is a semi–permeable membrane. If dialysis fluid is infused into the peritoneal cavity, equilibration occurs between the **dialysate** and the extracellular fluid of small molecules, ions and water.

A peritoneal dialysis catheter is inserted into the peritoneal cavity. This single-lumen tube is usually inserted through the midline and tunnelled subcutaneously to exit on the anterior abdominal wall. **Dialysate** (Table 10.6) can be infused into the peritoneal cavity using gravity, and after a period of time drained out (again using gravity). Typically the peritoneal cavity can accommodate 1.5–2.5 L of dialysate at any time. Attention to sterile technique is essential.

- Chronic ambulatory peritoneal dialysis (CAPD) involves regular exchanges of dialysate through the day (typically 6 hour dwells, with 4 exchanges per day). Automated peritoneal dialysis (APD) is the process in which a machine automatically drains fluid in and out; it is usually performed at night, with multiple exchanges overnight (e.g. 2-hour dwells).
- Variation of the amount of glucose in the dialysate allows the osmolar 'pull' of the dialysate to be varied, and hence the amount of water removed with each dwell (Table 10.6).

Adequacy of peritoneal dialysis

- Urea clearance can be measured. In addition, the 'transporter' status of the peritoneum can be assessed. 'High transporters' have rapid equilibration of ions and small molecules across the membrane. Fluid removal is less efficient as the osmolar gap is less pronounced. 'Low transporters' clear small ions and molecules less efficiently, but fluid removal is easier.

- For patients with little residual renal function, peritoneal dialysis alone frequently provides inadequate dialysis. Loss of membrane function (see below) with loss of residual function necessitates a transfer to haemodialysis.

Complications of peritoneal dialysis

- **Peritonitis.** This is the most common serious complication of peritoneal dialysis. It presents with abdominal pain, fever and cloudy dialysate (microscopy shows white blood cells). Organisms are usually staphylococci (*epidermidis* or *aureus*) or Gram-negative bowel organisms. Diagnosis is by culture of peritoneal fluid with or without blood. **Intraperitoneal or IV antibiotics** (p. 64) are usually effective. Failure to resolve after 48 hours usually requires removal of the peritoneal dialysis catheter. Reinsertion may be possible after a few weeks.
- **Drainage problems.** Constipation, catheter malposition or fibrin clots may all contribute. Plain abdominal X-ray may facilitate management. Occasionally surgical repositioning is required.
- **Membrane failure.** Eventually the peritoneal membrane becomes thickened and less efficient. Factors contributing to this are sepsis and high glucose concentrations. Falling dialysis adequacy and less effective fluid removal require more intensive dialysis and may eventually necessitate transfer to haemodialysis. Sclerosing peritonitis is caused by sepsis and/or prolonged exposure of the peritoneal membrane to high glucose concentrations. Thickening of the peritoneal membrane leads to recurrent small bowel obstruction, pain and malnutrition. Peritoneal dialysis should be abandoned in this situation.

RENAL TRANSPLANTATION

Renal transplantation is the most effective form of renal replacement therapy. It replaces all the functions of the kidney, and is associated with longer and better quality of life compared to dialysis.

- **Cadaveric transplantation** involves the removal of the kidney from a brain-dead donor (either heart-beating if brain death is diagnosed on a ventilator, or non-heart-beating if criteria for brain death diagnosis are not met). The organ is immediately cooled with ice and cold perfusate. After cross-matching with the recipient is completed, the organ is implanted into the recipient. Transplant outcome is best if 'cold ischaemic time' (the time from removal to implantation) is minimized, and should certainly be kept below 24 hours.
- **Living donor transplantation** involves the removal of a kidney from a healthy living donor, usually but not always a family member. Donors require assessment to ensure that they are fit and both kidneys are functioning normally. In the UK, donation can only be on altruistic grounds and no material or financial gain to the donor should be involved.

Graft survival is now typically 80% 5–10-year survival. Around 50% of grafts can be expected to last 10–30 years. Graft outcome is better after living donor transplantation, mainly because the cold ischaemic time is shorter.

Immunosuppression in renal transplantation

The most commonly used drugs are shown in Table 10.7. Immunosuppression is tailored to the individual, balancing the risks of rejection with those of over-immunosuppression and other side-effects. There are many different combinations of drugs used, varying by patient and by transplant unit, and with trial data continually leading to modifications and refinements in regimes. Monotherapy is unusual — most patients are on 2–3 different immunosuppressive drugs, e.g. **ciclosporin** (or **tacrolimus**) + **mycophenolate MMF** (or **azathioprine**) + **prednisolone**. Steroid-free regimes (or early withdrawal of steroids) and calcineurin-free regimes exist and may be suitable for those at highest risk of side-effects from these drugs. In addition, induction agents (e.g. **daclizumab, basiliximab, anti-thymocyte globulin**) are often given to those at higher risk of rejection at the time of transplantation.

Early complications of transplantation

Surgical complications

- **Renal vein thrombosis.** This presents in the first few days after surgery with pain, shock and a tender graft. Urgent nephrectomy is required.
- **Urine leak.** This is usually from the vesico-ureteric anastomosis. A ureteric stent is often placed at the time of surgery to allow healing of the anastomosis (removed after a few weeks).
- **Lymphocoele.** Asymptomatic fluid collections around the graft are common. Drainage is required if persistent infection or mechanical compression affects renal function or urine flow.
- **Ureteric stenosis.** Ureteric stenosis at the site of the anastomosis often requires reimplantation of the ureter.
- **Wound infection.** This usually responds to antibiotics.

Medical complications

- **Delayed graft function.** The transplant may produce urine and clear waste products immediately, or ATN may take days or weeks to resolve. A biopsy every few days may be required to ensure that rejection is not occurring as well. Delayed graft function is associated with prolonged cold ischaemic time and with less good outcome.
- **Acute rejection.** This presents with a rise in creatinine from baseline and is diagnosed by transplant biopsy. Treatment is usually with steroids (e.g. **methylprednisolone** 500 mg IV daily for 3 days) with or without intensification of the ongoing immunosuppression regime. Severe rejection may require treatment with anti-thymocyte globulin.
- **Infections.** Infections are common and can be life-threatening:
  - *Bacterial infections,* e.g. UTIs, chest infections. Immunosuppression increases the risk and steroids may mask the presentation. A low index of suspicion is required.
  - *Viral infections.* CMV infection is common and tends to occur 1–6 months after transplantation (though can occur at any time). Prophylaxis with **valganciclovir** (dose depends on level of renal function) for the first 3–6 months after transplantation is common in high-risk patients (those receiving grafts from CMV-positive donors). Diagnosis is by recognition of the clinical presentation (fever, neutropenia, graft dysfunction, liver dysfunction), coupled with PCR of blood to demonstrate viraemia. Treatment is with **IV ganciclovir** or **oral**

Table 10.7 Immunosuppressive drugs used in renal transplantation

Class	Mechanism of action	Examples	Clinical role	Side-effects
Calcineurin inhibitors	Disrupt T-cell signalling	Ciclosporin Tacrolimus	Mainstay of most regimes	Nephrotoxicity (monitor levels), hypertension, diabetes, hirsutism, virilization
Inhibitors of purine synthesis	Inhibit purine synthesis and hence active proliferation of cells (especially lymphocytes)	Azathioprine Mycophenolate mofetil (MMF)	Used in most regimes	Neutropenia, pancytopenia, deranged LFTs (azathioprine), diarrhoea (MMF) Interaction with allopurinol (azathioprine)
Steroids	Inhibition of cytokine-regulated T-cell signalling	Prednisolone (oral) Methylprednisolone (IV)	Used in most regimes. Dose tapers over first few weeks IV methylprednisolone used on induction and to treat acute rejection	Multiple, including osteoporosis, hypertension, diabetes, weight gain, poor wound healing, lipid abnormalities
Rapamycin (Sirolimus)	Inhibits cytokine-dependent cell proliferation	Alternative to calcineurin inhibitors	Role still being explored	Delayed graft function, myelosuppression, impaired wound healing, thrombocytopenia Levels should be monitored
Anti-CD25 antibodies	Monoclonal antibody, blocking the IL-2 receptor	Daclizumab Basiliximab	Given on induction. Usually used in patients with medium-high risk of rejection	Well tolerated
Antibodies causing T-cell depletion	Targets and destroys T-cells	Anti-thymocyte globulin (ATG) = polyclonal. OKT3 = monoclonal anti-CD3 antibody	For steroid-resistant rejection (7–10-day course). May be used as induction agent for patients at high risk of rejection	Severe T-cell depletion (risk of sepsis) Late development of malignancy, esp lymphoma
Anti-CD52 antibody	Depletes both T- and B-cells	Alemtuzumab	Used as induction agent	Over-immunosuppression, risk of sepsis and malignancy in longer term Long-term outcome data awaited

valganciclovir. BK virus has been recently recognized as a significant cause of graft loss. Treatment is reduction of immunosuppression.

Late complications of transplantation

- Chronic allograft nephropathy. There is progressive renal dysfunction. This may be multi-factorial, and graft biopsy should be performed to guide management. Calcineurin toxicity may contribute, and these drugs may be withdrawn in favour of other agents. ACE inhibitors may improve outcome if proteinuria and/or hypertension are present.
- Malignancy. Skin malignancies are common (sun protection advice is vital) and should be screened for regularly. Post-transplant lymphoproliferative disease (PTLD) is a B-cell lymphoma, usually associated with EBV infection. Treatment is by reduction of immunosuppression with or without chemotherapy; the response depends on sub-type. Other solid organ tumours may occur, more frequently than in the general population.
- Cardiovascular disease. There is an increased risk of cardiovascular disease, especially if there has been a significant period of time on dialysis pre-transplant. Risk is exacerbated by steroid therapy, hypertension (common post-transplant) and hyperlipidaemia, which must be treated aggressively.

POLYCYSTIC KIDNEY DISEASE

This inherited condition affects 1 : 800 live births in an autosomal dominant inheritance pattern (a more severe and rarer juvenile form is autosomal recessive). It is characterized by the development of renal cysts, which increase in size and number over time. The abnormal mutation is in the genes *PKD-1* (chromosome 16) or *PKD-2* (chromosome 4). Both genes alter the structure of polycystin, a membrane protein affecting the proliferation of collecting duct epithelial cells. The end result is the development of innumerable renal cysts. Gradually progressive chronic kidney disease and hypertension are usual. Management is supportive, with tight control of the BP, thus minimizing the rate of progression. Experimental therapies aimed at preventing cyst formation are in the pipeline.

TUMOURS OF THE RENAL TRACT

Renal cell carcinoma

Adenocarcinoma accounts for 80% of all renal tumours. The male : female ratio is 4 : 1, the average age of presentation is 55, and smoking is a significant risk factor. The classic triad of presenting features is loin pain, haematuria (macro- or microscopic) and a palpable mass, though patients may present with symptoms related to metastatic disease.

- Diagnosis is usually made by US and then CT scan (a solid renal mass is a tumour until proven otherwise, and percutaneous biopsy is usually avoided as there is a risk of seeding along the biopsy track). Radiological staging is by CT (local spread, lung or liver involvement) and bone scan, with or without MRI (invasion of renal vein). Prognosis is closely related to stage; most local tumours can be cured with surgery, while advanced tumours have a 5-year survival of < 10%.
- Treatment is by nephrectomy where possible. Partial nephrectomy (nephron-sparing surgery) may be appropriate if the other kidney is

functioning poorly, if there are bilateral tumours, or if there is a genetic predisposition, making further tumours in the future likely (as occurs in von Hippel–Lindau syndrome). Even if metastases are present, removal of the primary tumour is recommended, as regression of metastases has been reported. Patients unfit for surgery may receive radiofrequency ablation.

- **Metastatic disease** can be treated with interleukin 2; a minority of patients gain significant benefit. Interferon has been used, but this has been supplanted by newer therapies, including **temsirolimus** or **everolimus**, specific inhibitors of rapomycin kinase; **bevacizumab**, an antibody to vascular endothelial growth factor; and **sunitinib** or **sorafenib**, tyrosine kinase inhibitors.

Urothelial tumours

Over 90% of bladder tumours are transitional cell carcinomas, the male : female ratio being 3 : 1 and peak prevalence at over 60 years of age. Presentation is with lower urinary tract symptoms with or without haematuria, or with symptoms of metastatic disease.

- **Diagnosis** is made by imaging, and then cystoscopy and biopsy.
- **Treatment** is by local transurethral excision for superficial tumours. Locally advanced tumours require more invasive surgery with radical cystectomy, or radiotherapy if surgery is not appropriate.
- **Local recurrence** is common and can be reduced by intravesical treatment with BCG, mitomycin or doxorubicin. Long-term follow-up and surveillance are essential, as prognosis depends heavily on stage of disease.

Prostatic carcinoma

This accounts for 7% of all male cancers, incidence increasing with age. Many are undiagnosed and incidental diagnosis in elderly men at postmortem is common, showing that many men die with this disease rather than from it.

- **Diagnosis** is made by transrectal US-guided biopsy. The presentation may be with lower urinary tract symptoms or with symptoms of metastatic disease. Measurement of serum prostate-specific antigen (PSA) may help, with significantly elevated levels being diagnostic. PSA testing does not (yet) fulfil the criteria for a national screening programme, as there is insufficient clarity as to what its benefit would be.
- **Optimal management** of this condition remains unclear. For disease confined to the gland itself, surgery with radical prostatectomy is often curative, as is radical radiotherapy. The prognosis depends on the stage and grade (measured by the Gleason score); those with a low grade may benefit most from a watchful waiting policy, especially if they are elderly or have co-morbidity. At present the optimal approach for the individual patient is not always clear.
- **Advanced and metastatic disease** is treated with hormonal therapy (anti-androgens or oestrogens) or bilateral orchidectomy.

DRUGS AND THE KIDNEY

Many drugs are predominantly or completely excreted by the kidneys. In practice, for many drugs the therapeutic range and the toxic ranges are so widely spaced that dose reduction is not necessary, even in severe renal failure.

- Drugs that require dose reduction include those with a narrow therapeutic index, in which the risk of toxicity is significant at levels comparable to therapeutic levels.
- A fall in GFR may precipitate toxicity, e.g. **digoxin**, **lithium**, **aciclovir**.
- If renal toxicity is a side-effect of the drug, a vicious circle of worsening renal function and rising drug levels may ensue e.g. **aminoglycoside toxicity**, **ciclosporin/tacrolimus**.

In practice:

- When prescribing drugs to patients with renal impairment, always consider whether it is necessary to adjust the dose according to the eGFR.
- Drugs known to be nephrotoxic should be avoided if possible.
- The amount of sodium or potassium a drug contains may be relevant when the GFR is reduced (risk of precipitating salt and water overload).
- Monitoring for drug toxicity is by measurement of clinical effects, e.g. hypotension and/or measurement of drug levels in the blood. Drug level monitoring is not useful if the metabolites rather than the drug itself are responsible for toxicity, e.g. **opioids**.

Further reading

Scrier RW: *Renal and Electrolyte Disorders,* ed 7, Philadelphia, 2010, Lippincott Williams & Wilkins.

Worcester EM, Cole FL: Calcium kidney stones, *New Engl J Med* 363:954–963, 2010.

Water, electrolyte and acid-base balance

11

CHAPTER CONTENTS

INTRODUCTION

The human body is mainly water. Total body water in litres is calculated as $0.6 \times$ weight (kg) in men, and $0.5 \times$ weight (kg) in women. Water is compartmentalized in the body, two-thirds within the intracellular space and one-third as extracellular fluid (ECF) (of which one-third is plasma and two-thirds are in the interstitial space).

Osmotic pressure maintains the tonicity of any compartment:

- Within cells, K^+ determines osmotic pressure confined by the hydrophobic cell membrane.
- Within the extracellular space, Na^+ acts as the principle osmotic determinant. Intravascular protein, as well as Na^+, allows plasma (separated by relatively permeable capillary walls) to maintain an osmotic gradient against tissue.

SALT AND VOLUME DISTRIBUTION

Na^+ retention and excretion control extracellular volume (water will passively follow salt). Systemic baro-receptors (carotid sinus, aortic arch) 'sense' changes in arterial tone (a function of cardiac output and systemic vascular resistance). A **fall** in effective arterial blood volume (EABV) activates the sympathetic nervous system, leading to Na^+ retention by the kidney. With an **expanded** EABV, increased renal Na^+ loss occurs.

Oedema

Oedema is a clinically noticeable increase in the interstitial component of the ECF (apparent after > 2 L fluid gain, obvious in dependent areas such as the ankles). For this to occur, salt and water must be retained and capillary permeability permits fluid shifts into the interstitium, e.g. in acute kidney injury.

Any cause of a fall in EABV leads to salt and water retention through the activation of the renin–angiotensin–aldosterone system and this releases antidiuretic hormone (ADH, vasopressin). If prolonged, over time this net gain in sodium and water presents as oedema, e.g. in heart failure and hepatic cirrhosis. This mechanism plays a bigger role than a fall in intravascular oncotic pressure (if plasma proteins such as albumin are reduced, e.g. in the nephrotic syndrome), leading to water loss into the interstitium. Endothelial dysfunction, or 'leaky capillaries', is often present in addition to falling arterial tone.

Water and volume

- Hypothalamic osmoreceptors, which sense osmolality rather than volume, increase thirst, and pituitary ADH release in response to falling total body water (TBW). ADH regulates free water absorption in the renal collecting ducts to reverse this.
- With **water overload** (and a falling osmolality), thirst and ADH release are suppressed, with dilute urine being passed.
- For **normal water** homeostasis, the body requires a normal hypothalamus, access to water, a functioning pituitary (ADH release) and responsive collecting ducts.

Assessing volume status

Thirst is a symptom of dehydration; oedema indicates increased volume.

- Examine pulse rate and BP, both lying and standing; a postural drop in BP is a good indicator of hypovolaemia.
- The JVP is helpful; it is high in increased circulating volume and low in decreased volume.
- A fluid challenge done accurately by yourself gives accurate information with a central vein catheter in place (Fig. 11.1).
- Daily weights and assessment of peripheral perfusion are also helpful in assessing volume status.
- Re-assess frequently and get a CXR for further evidence of fluid overload. Treatment of oedema is discussed under renal disease (p. 334), hepatic cirrhosis (p. 188) and heart failure (p. 426).

Fluid therapy in hospital

Two common circumstances necessitate fluids as therapy (Table 11.1) in hospital:

- Patients who cannot drink for any reason require maintenance fluids. This may be given by intravenous infusion (IVI) for short periods, but

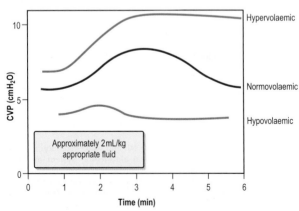

Fig. 11.1 The effects of rapid administration of a 'fluid challenge' to patients with a central venous pressure (CVP) within the normal range (Based upon Sykes MK 1963).

Table 11.1 IV fluids in general use for fluid and electrolyte disturbances

	Na⁺ (mmol/L)	K⁺ (mmol/L)	HCO₃⁻/ lactate (mmol/L)	Cl⁻ (mmol/L)	Indication (see footnote)
Normal plasma values	142	4.5	26	103	
Sodium chloride 0.9%	150	–	–	150	1
Sodium chloride 0.18% + glucose 4%	30	–	–	30	2
Glucose 5% + potassium chloride 0.3%	–	40	–	40	3
Sodium bicarbonate 1.26%	150	–	150	–	4
Compound sodium lactate (Hartmann's)	131	5	29	11	5

1. Volume expansion in hypovolaemic patients. Rarely to maintain fluid balance when there are large losses of sodium. The sodium (150 mmol/L) is greater than plasma and hypernatraemia can result. It is often necessary to add KCl 20–40 mmol/L.
2. Maintenance of fluid balance in normovolaemic, normonatraemic patients.
3. To replace *water*. Can be given with or without potassium chloride. May be alternated with 0.9% saline as an alternative to (2).
4. For volume expansion in hypovolaemic, acidotic patients alternating with (1). Occasionally for maintenance of fluid balance combined with (2) in salt-wasting, acidotic patients.
5. Also has 2 mmol/L Ca⁺. Used post-operatively and when hypokalaemia is likely to occur.

use the enteral route if possible. If fluids are required for > 5 days, a naso-gastric tube with water and/or enteral nutrition provides more physiological replacement than IV fluids.

- Patients who are dehydrated or hypovolaemic require replacement or resuscitation fluid, usually intravenously. *Always check* patients' renal and cardiac function before prescribing a fluid regimen.

The volume administered varies according to the state of hydration; in otherwise well 'nil by mouth' patients with no losses, aim for 2 L/24 hours of saline (0.18%) and glucose (4%), usually with added potassium

20 mmol/L. Post-surgical fluid therapy should reflect the nature of the surgery (and the likely ongoing losses).

SODIUM

Disorders of sodium are more accurately disorders of water than of sodium, as disturbances of sodium concentration are mainly caused by a disturbance of water balance. The danger posed by a low or high serum Na^+ comes from both the electrolyte abnormality *and* its correction; the skull does not allow the brain to change in volume, so movement of water into the CNS risks increased intracranial pressure (and eventually tentorial herniation). Equally, movement of water out of the brain can lead to sudden and irreversible osmotic injury (central pontine myelinolysis (CPM)).

Hyponatraemia

Hyponatraemia (plasma $Na^+ < 135$ mmol/L) is common in hospitalized patients, but symptomatic hyponatraemia is very much less common — and more dangerous.

Clinical features
Clinical features of hyponatraemia are due to cerebral swelling, and include headaches, apathy, and confusion progressing to coma and seizures (encephalopathy). These tend to occur with a serum sodium of:
- <125 mmol/L if **acute** (< 48 hours, usually post-operative) *or*
- <110 mmol/L if **chronic**

Certain patients are more at risk for the neurological complications of hyponatraemia: the elderly, malnourished or alcoholic patients, premenopausal women (oestrogen may enhance the body's response to ADH) and those whose hyponatraemia is caused by thiazide diuretic use.

Always exclude pseudohyponatraemia. Around 93% of plasma is water; conditions that increase the 7% of plasma made up of protein and lipids (e.g. hyperlipidaemia, hyperglycaemia, myeloma proteins) artefactually reduce the water phase in which Na^+ is assayed, falsely reducing the measured sodium.

Investigations
- Repeat serum Na^+, K^+, HCO_3^- and glucose.
- Measure/calculate blood and urine osmolality.
- Perform renal, adrenal and thyroid function tests.
- Assess volume status (p. 368). Hyponatraemia with a normal, decreased or increased extracellular volume has different causes and different therapy (Fig. 11.2).

Hyponatraemia with a normal extracellular volume
Excess body water results from an abnormally high intake.
- **Excessive use of 5% glucose IV infusions** without sodium is the commonest situation in hospital.
- **Absorption of sodium-free bladder irrigation fluid** after prostatectomy is another possible cause.
- **Psychogenic polydipsia** occurs usually in psychiatric patients who drink > 12 L a day (above the renal excretion capacity).
- **The syndrome of inappropriate antidiuretic hormone secretion (SIADH)** Where hypotonic fluid administration has been excluded, the syndrome of inappropriate anti-diuretic hormone secretion (SIADH) is

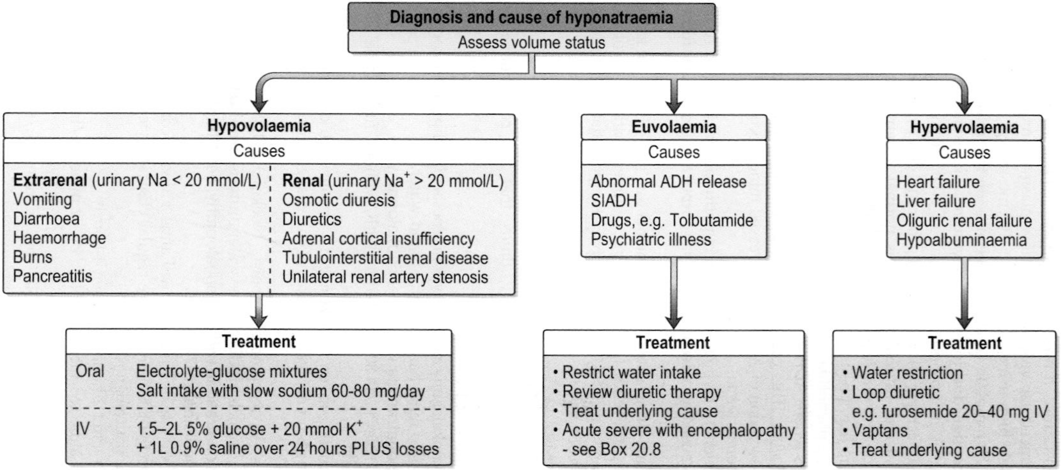

Fig. 11.2 Diagnosis and causes of hyponatraemia.

Diagnosis and cause of hyponatraemia
Assess volume status

Hypovolaemia

Causes

Extrarenal (urinary Na < 20 mmol/L)	**Renal** (urinary Na⁺ > 20 mmol/L)
Vomiting	Osmotic diuresis
Diarrhoea	Diuretics
Haemorrhage	Adrenal cortical insufficiency
Burns	Tubulointerstitial renal disease
Pancreatitis	Unilateral renal artery stenosis

Treatment

Oral	Electrolyte-glucose mixtures
	Salt intake with slow sodium 60–80 mg/day
IV	1.5–2L 5% glucose + 20 mmol K⁺
	+ 1L 0.9% saline over 24 hours PLUS losses

Euvolaemia

Causes

Abnormal ADH release
SIADH
Drugs, e.g. Tolbutamide
Psychiatric illness

Treatment

• Restrict water intake
• Review diuretic therapy
• Treat underlying cause
• Acute severe with encephalopathy
  – see Box 20.8

Hypervolaemia

Causes

Heart failure
Liver failure
Oliguric renal failure
Hypoalbuminaemia

Treatment

• Water restriction
• Loop diuretic
  e.g. furosemide 20–40 mg IV
• Vaptans
• Treat underlying cause

the commonest cause. It produces a hyponatraemia, normal or slightly increased extracellular volume, and a low plasma osmolality with an inappropriately high urine osmolality (> 100 mosm/kg). Urine sodium excretion > 30 mmol/L continues because of the release of atrionatriuretic peptide due to increased volume. This syndrome occurs because there is inappropriate secretion of ADH from the posterior pituitary or an ectopic source, resulting in renal free water excretion. Renal, adrenal and thyroid function is normal. **Common causes** of SIADH include tumours (e.g. small cell carcinoma of the lung), pulmonary disorders (e.g. pneumonia), neurological causes (e.g. meningitis) and drugs (e.g. phenothiazine).

- Other causes where ADH secretion occurs inappropriately include:
  - *Adrenal failure.* This causes cortisol deficiency, which leads to an increased secretion of ADH and decreased mineralocorticoids which cause hyponatraemia.
  - *Hypothyroidism.* Hyponatraemia in hypothyroidism is due to ADH secretion caused by a decreased cardiac output and glomerular filtration rate.
  - *Drugs.* Many drugs cause hyponatraemia due to ADH release (antipsychotics, tricyclics, carbamazepine, antineoplastics, narcotics). Some drugs, e.g. NSAIDs, chlorpropamide, potentiate the antidiuretic action of vasopressin. Stress, e.g. post-surgical, also causes vasopressin release.
- General principles of management
  - Stop drugs and hypotonic IV fluids that are contributing to hyponatraemia.
  - Restrict fluid to < 1 L/day.
  - Correct hypokalaemia and/or hypomagnesaemia (if present); correction improves renal handling of salt and water.
- Treating hyponatraemia *without* encephalopathy
  - Give oral NaCl 40–80 mmol/day with/without furosemide 20–40 mg/daily.
  - Asymptomatic proven SIADH may be treated with demeclocycline 150–300 mg 6-hourly (causes nephrogenic diabetes insipidus and free water loss).
  - Aquaretics (V_2 receptor antagonists blocking ADH's action), e.g. conivaptan, which produce a free water diuresis, are also being used.
- Treating hyponatraemia *with* encephalopathy, see Chapter 20, Emergencies in medicine, p. 711
  - A serum Na^+ rise of 5 mmol/L will almost always control seizures.
  - Transfer to the HDU and ensure regular clinical review.
  - Document neurology regularly.
  - Repeat Na^+ after 2 hours and then 4-hourly.
  - If *acute*: aim to increase Na^+ by 2 mmol/L/hour or until asymptomatic.
  - If *chronic*: aim to increase Na^+ by 0.5 mmol/L/hour or until asymptomatic.
  - *Never* correct by > 10 mmol/L/24 hours. CPM often takes a few days to develop; it causes a spastic para-/quadriparesis and mental disturbances, and can lead to death. MRI is useful in diagnosis.
  - *Calculation:*

    Na^+ deficit = total body water $\times$ [desired Na^+ – actual Na^+]

- For practical purposes total body water can be calculated as 50% of weight in kg.
- 3% NaCl (hypertonic saline) contains 1 mmol NaCl per 2 mL (513 mmol in 1 L). Acute and chronic hyponatraemia require different hourly correction rates (see above)

For example, a 50 kg woman has a serum sodium of 115 mmol/L. She requires 10 mmol to correct to 125 mmol/L. Thus, $10 \times$ half of the body (i.e. 25) = 250. Thus, she requires 250 mmol of 3% NaCl, which is 500 mL. This should be given slowly over 4–6 hours via a central vein.

Hyponatraemia with a decreased extracellular volume

A decreased volume stimulates thirst and vasopressin release, which in turn inhibits water excretion. Losses from the kidney occur in tubulointerstitial disease, the recovery phase of acute tubular necrosis, unilateral renal artery stenosis, excessive use of diuretics, adrenocortical insufficiency and osmotic diuresis (e.g. hyperglycaemia, severe uraemia). Losses from the gastrointestinal tract are due to vomiting, diarrhoea, naso-gastric suction and haemorrhage (Table 11.2). Losses can also occur from the skin (burns), pericarditis and peritonitis.

- **Management.** The underlying diagnosis is usually apparent. Urinary Na^+ will be very low (< 10 mmol/L) unless the sodium loss is renal in origin. Replace salt and water with oral rehydration fluid (p. 59) or IV 0.9% NaCl. If the patient is encephalopathic (depressed level of consciousness, fitting), hypertonic 3% sodium chloride is given slowly as above.

Hyponatraemia with an increased extracellular volume

In this situation there is evidence of volume overload with a decreased circulatory volume, e.g. oedema. This leads to a reduced glomerular filtration rate with avid reabsorption of sodium from the proximal tubule. This in turn leads to a reduced delivery of chloride to the diluting ascending loop of Henle. There is thus an inability to excrete dilute urine.

- **Causes** include heart failure, liver cirrhosis and the nephrotic syndrome, in which there is evidence of fluid overload that exceeds the increase in sodium so that a dilutional hyponatraemia occurs.

Table 11.2 Average concentrations and potential daily losses of water and electrolytes from the gut

	Na^+ mmol/L	K^+ mmol/L	Cl^- mmol/L	Volume (mL in 24 h)
Stomach	50	10	110	2500
Small intestine				
Recent ileostomy	120	5	110	1500
Adapted ileostomy	50	4	25	500
Bile	140	5	105	500
Pancreatic juice	140	5	60	2000
Diarrhoea	130	10–30	95	1000–2000+

- Management
  - *Fluid* is restricted to < 1 L intake per day.
  - *A loop diuretic* such as furosemide 20–40 mg IV 8-hourly leads to a diuresis of water in excess of salt.
  - *In encephalopathy* (depressed level of consciousness, fitting), hypertonic 3% sodium chloride is given slowly as above.
  - V_2 *antagonists*, e.g. tolvaptan, are now being used.

Hypernatraemia

Defined as a serum Na^+ > 145 mmol/L, hypernatraemia is almost always due to a water deficit. As osmolality increases, water leaves cells, including the cells in the brain. The brain compensates over time by retaining organic solutes, increasing cellular tonicity and so reducing water loss into the hyperosmolar ECF. Sudden correction may lead to a rapid gain of water with intracranial expansion of the brain and tentorial herniation. Symptoms and signs include thirst, weakness and confusion progressing to coma and fits.

Causes
Water deficit is due to the following:
- Renal water loss as seen in diabetes insipidus (DI), either pituitary (failure of ADH secretion) or nephrogenic (failure of response to ADH), or due to an osmotic diuresis.
  - *Pituitary DI* occurs from pituitary tumours, infections, infiltration, post-surgical, post-radiotherapy, trauma or vascular causes.
  - *Nephrogenic DI* is due to renal tubular acidosis, hypokalaemia, hypercalciuria, drugs — lithium or glibenclamide (glyburide) — or sickle cell disease. Osmotic diuresis is seen with a diabetic hyperosmolar state.
- Non-renal water loss as seen in diarrhoea and also with increased insensible losses through the skin or lungs.
- Excessive administration of sodium when hypertonic sodium solutions are used (e.g. 8.4% sodium bicarbonate after cardiac arrest), excess of 0.9% saline, particularly if accompanied by renal loss (diabetic ketoacidosis) or ingestion of drugs with high sodium content, e.g. piperacillin.

Hypernatraemia is accompanied by increased plasma osmolality, which is a potent stimulus to thirst, and hypernatraemia does not occur unless thirst is impaired or water unavailable.

Investigations
- Simultaneous urine and plasma osmolality and sodium measurement is carried out.
- A water deprivation test is used in DI; the administration of desmopressin will correct pituitary DI but not nephrogenic DI.

Management
Always treat underlying cause.
- **Acute hypernatraemia** (< **24 hours' duration**, usually due to hypertonic IV solutions) is safe to correct quickly. Aim to lower the Na^+ by 1 mmol/L/hour, checking Na^+ after 2 hours then 4-hourly, and *re-assess your patient regularly*.
- **Chronic hypernatraemia** (> **24 hours**) should be corrected *slowly* to avoid cerebral oedema.

- Fully assess and document neurological status.
- Aim to lower Na^+ by not more than 1 mmol/L every 2 hours, or < 10 mmol/L/day; correct 50% of the water deficit in the first 12–24 hours and the remaining water deficit over next 24–48 hours.
- Check serum Na^+ after 2 hours then 4-hourly.
- Calculate water deficit (include ongoing losses!).
- Calculate TBW (p. 368):

$$\text{Water defect (L)} = \frac{\text{plasma } [Na^+] - 140}{140 \times \text{TBW}}$$

So, in a 50 kg female with a serum Na^+ of 155 mmol/L:

$$\text{Water deficit (L)} = \frac{155 - 140}{140 \times 25} = 2.5 \text{ L}$$

Include ongoing losses in the deficit (allow 1 L insensible losses/day).

- The fall in N^+ per litre of correction fluid = ([Na^+] in fluid − plasma [Na^+])/TBW + 1. Administer an appropriate volume of replacement fluid for the desired drop in [Na^+] per hour/day. Replacement fluid is either 0.18% saline with 4% glucose or 5% glucose alone. K^+ must be added as required.

POTASSIUM

Most of the total body K^+ (about 3500 mmol) is intracellular, with only 2% (or 70 mmol) in the extracellular space. Total body K^+ is kept in strict balance; dietary intake amounts to about 100 mmol/day, with 90 mmol/day lost in the urine (and the rest in stool). This gives a normal range for serum K^+ of **3.5–5.5 mmol/L**; this is, however, a poor indicator of total body potassium.

Abrupt changes in K^+ can be life-threatening, so a number of **compensatory mechanisms** exist to maintain serum K^+ within the normal range.

- Extracellular K^+ can be 'shifted' rapidly into or out of cells. Transmembrane Na^+/K^+-ATPases pump K^+ into cells (and Na^+ out) under the influence of insulin or β_2 receptor stimulation by catecholamines. By moving K^+ into cells, transient hyperkalaemia can be accommodated, even though total body K^+ is unchanged.
- Total body K^+ is controlled by modifying urinary losses (which can vary from < 10 mmol/day to > 200 mmol/day).
- Fine control of urinary K^+ secretion is regulated mainly by aldosterone (but also by high tubular sodium delivery and pH). Aldosterone acts in the distal nephron to promote Na^+ retention and K^+ losses (hyperkalaemia stimulates aldosterone release). With a well-maintained urine output, renal K^+ losses can be profound, correcting a raised total body K^+ within days. The kidney is less efficient in response to hypokalaemia; although aldosterone secretion is suppressed, hypovolaemia will override this mechanism (to conserve Na^+).

History and examination

These may suggest an underlying cause. *Always* take a full drug history and review the drug chart.

Investigations

Repeat any abnormal serum K^+. Check Na^+, renal function, bicarbonate, glucose, serum Mg^{2+}, urinary K^+ and thyroid function if hypokalaemic. Do an ECG to exclude cardiac toxicity. Monitor urine output and re-measure serum K^+ repeatedly to assess response to therapy.

Hyperkalaemia

Always exclude spurious hyperkalaemia — usually due to haemolysis after phlebotomy, particularly with abnormal cells. Hyperkalaemia is a relative state; patients with longstanding renal impairment can tolerate K^+ of up to 7 mmol/L, while those accustomed to low–normal K^+ may develop dangerous arrhythmias if K^+ is about 6.0. It is *never* safe to ignore a $K^+ > 6.5$ mmol/L.

Causes

Causes of hyperkalaemia are **decreased excretion** due to renal failure and drugs, e.g. amiloride, triamterene, spironolactone, NSAIDs, ACE inhibitors and ciclosporin, **increased release of K^+ from cells**, diabetic ketoacidosis, rhabdomyolysis, digoxin poisoning, tumour lysis and **increased extraneous load** of oral potassium chloride, salt substitutes or transfusion of stored blood.

Clinical features

Cardiotoxicity is the most serious effect and an ECG is performed. Muscle weakness occurs due to partial depolarization of the cell membrane impairing membrane excitability. This produces weakness and a flaccid paralysis. Respiratory muscle involvement can cause hypoventilation and metabolic acidosis occurs due to impaired acid excretion, as hyperkalaemia inhibits both the synthesis of ammonia in the proximal convoluted tubule and reabsorption in the loop of Henle.

Management (See Emergencies in medicine p. 711)

- Re-check K^+ and stop all K^+-sparing drugs.
- Check the ECG for electrical signs of hyperkalaemia; tall, tented T waves progress to P wave loss and a prolonged PR interval, then widening of the QRS complex to ventricular fibrillation (Fig. 11.3).
- **Protect the heart:** calcium (10 mL 10% calcium gluconate or 5 mL 10% calcium chloride) given as a slow IV bolus over 5 minutes usually normalizes cardiac membrane excitability, preventing or reversing arrhythmias. Its effect only lasts 15 minutes but the dose can be repeated.
- **Shift K^+ into cells:** 10 U short-acting insulin in 50 mL of 50% glucose will activate trans-membrane Na^+/K^+-ATPase, lowering serum K^+ by 1 mmol/L about 4 hours. This can be repeated, if need be. Monitor capillary blood glucose.
- **Encourage a good urine output** if possible (often not if underlying kidney disease): keep well hydrated with 0.9% saline, and give furosemide 20–40 mg oral/IV as a potassium-wasting diuretic. Aim for urine output > 2 L/day.
- Other agents
  - *β_2 agonists* such as salbutamol will also pump K^+ into cells (by activating trans-membrane Na^+/K^+-ATPase), but are *not* additive to insulin and glucose; they may provoke cardiac instability and arrhythmias.
  - *Sodium bicarbonate* corrects acidosis, with the net effect of driving K^+ into cells. This may help in severe acidosis (pH < 7.2), but causes hypocalcaemia (in turn arrhythmogenic) and gives a large salt load.

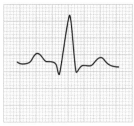

(a) Normal

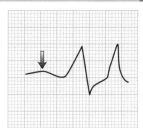

(c) Reduced P wave (arrow) with widened QRS complex

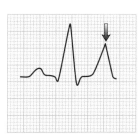

(b) Tented T wave (arrow)

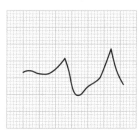

(d) 'Sine wave' pattern (pre-cardiac arrest)

Fig. 11.3 Progressive ECG changes with increasing hyperkalaemia.

- *K^+-binding resins* exchange luminal K^+ for resin-bound calcium in the gut. They are slow to have an action (24 hours) and cause constipation (limiting a route of K^+ excretion).
- *Haemodialysis* will rapidly control resistant hyperkalaemia within 20–30 minutes.

Hypokalaemia

Causes

- **Increased renal excretion** is the commonest cause of hypokalaemia, usually due to the use of diuretics, both thiazides and loop diuretics. Increased aldosterone secretion, either primary (Conn's syndrome) or secondary to ECF depletion, cardiac failure, hepatic cirrhosis or the nephrotic syndrome, causes increased sodium reabsorption in the collecting ducts and K^+ loss. Type 1 distal renal tubular acidosis and, in the diuretic phase following renal damage or obstruction, hypokalaemia occur.
- **Reduced intake,** particularly if associated with vomiting or severe diarrhoea, with loss of potassium via the gastrointestinal tract, causes hypokalaemia.
- **Redistribution into cells** decreases serum K^+ without affecting total body K^+. This occurs with insulin therapy for ketoacidosis or following β-adrenergic stimulus.

Kumar & Clark's Medical Management and Therapeutics

Clinical features

Hypokalaemia of > 3 mmol/L is usually well tolerated. Symptoms, predominantly apathy, myalgia and weakness, are all due to a neuromuscular disturbance. It can progress to life-threatening cardiac arrhythmias if $K^+ < 2.5$ mmol/L. Eventually an areflexic paralysis may also occur. A spot urinary K^+ will rapidly differentiate renal losses from extra-renal losses (when urinary $K^+ < 20$ mmol/L). Patients prescribed digoxin or other anti-arrhythmics are at particular risk of arrhythmias from hypokalaemia.

Diagnosis

The causes of hypokalaemia can usually be found in the history but urine K^+ is helpful, as well as an assessment of acid–base balance.

Management of asymptomatic or mild hypokalaemia (K > 2.5 mmol/L)

- Stop diuretics if prescribed, or change to a potassium-sparing diuretic.
- Start oral potassium chloride (KCl) supplements as 1–3 g 3 times daily (limited by gastrointestinal tolerability). It is always safer to give orally than intravenously, which is only used in severe hypokalaemia.
- Re-check K^+ within 1 week, and more frequently if renal impairment is present.

Management of symptomatic or life-threatening hypokalaemia (K < 2.5 mmol/L)

- Check the ECG for electrical signs of hypokalaemia (Fig. 11.3): small T waves, the presence of a U wave (after the T wave) and an increasing PR interval (poor correlation with serum K^+ levels).
- Check magnesium, and if low, correct (p. 379).
- Add 20–40 mmol KCl to 1 L 0.9% saline and infuse at 20 mmol KCl/hour.

MAGNESIUM

Magnesium contributes to all energy (ATP)-requiring reactions, as well as cell membrane function, nerve conduction and muscle contraction. Plasma Mg^{2+} is tightly controlled by the kidney (modifying urinary losses) within a normal range of 0.75–1.1 mmol/L (1.5–2.2 mEq/L).

History and examination

These may suggest an underlying cause. *Always* take a full drug history and review the drug chart. Check K^+, Ca^{2+}, Na^+ and renal function. Obtain an ECG to exclude cardiac toxicity.

Hypomagnesaemia

This is common in undernourished hospitalized patients. Hypomagnesaemia presents with the symptoms of hypokalaemia and hypocalcaemia, both of which occur as a result of a low plasma Mg^{2+}.

Clinical features

Irritability, tremor, ataxia, hyper-reflexia, confusion and fits may be present.

Causes

Causes are decreased absorption; increased renal excretion, e.g. drugs (diuretics); and gut losses, e.g. excessive purgation, diarrhoea, prolonged naso-gastric suction or acute pancreatitis.

Management

Withdraw any causal agents. ECG evidence of hypomagnesaemia includes prolonged PR interval, broad flattened T waves and a widening QRS complex leading to fatal ventricular arrhythmias. Oral magnesium is poorly absorbed and tolerated. Even mild hypomagnesaemia (> 0.4 mmol/L) should be treated with IV magnesium sulphate (20–60 mmol/day in 0.9% saline). Acute or severe hypomagnesaemia is associated with torsades de pointes (p. 409). Give 2–4 mL 50% magnesium sulphate as a bolus.

Hypermagnesaemia

Hypermagnesaemia only usually occurs in patients with impaired renal function (unable to excrete Mg^{2+}) given magnesium (usually as an enema). It presents as neuromuscular depression (depressed reflexes, respiratory weakness and bradyarrhythmias).

Management

Discontinuing Mg^{2+} (if urine output is well maintained) will usually safely lower levels. Giving 10 mL 10% calcium gluconate antagonizes magnesium's cardiotoxic effect. Haemodialysis rapidly corrects severe hypermagnesaemic toxicity.

PHOSPHATE

Phosphate is essential to almost all biochemical systems, and its control is closely linked to that of calcium. Active vitamin D_3 increases dietary phosphorus absorption, with most (80%) total body phosphate (the inorganic fraction of phosphorus) found in the skeleton. Sodium–phosphate co-transporters in the kidney retain phosphate (depending on oral phosphorus intake) for a normal plasma range of 0.8–1.4 mmol/L (3.0–4.5 mg/dL) (higher in children). Parathyroid hormone and phosphatonins inhibit renal reabsorption to encourage phosphate wasting in response to a rising plasma phosphate.

Check Ca^{2+}, Na^+, K^+, renal function and bicarbonate, glucose and parathormone levels.

Hypophosphataemia

Phosphate depletion is common in the critically ill, often presenting with symptoms as limited reserves are redistributed to provide energy or synthesize protein in response to treatment. Acutely, symptoms include respiratory and proximal muscle weakness, ileus and cardiac depression. Spontaneous muscle breakdown and acute confusion may follow. Prolonged hypophosphataemia leads to osteomalacia.

Causes

Causes include decreased intake and intestinal absorption, e.g. dietary factors, vomiting, malabsorption and alcohol withdrawal. Renal losses occur with renal tubular defects and with diarrhoea. Redistribution into cells (similar to K^+) is probably the major cause in hospital and is seen in the treatment of diabetic ketoacidosis, in refeeding after malnutrition and in respiratory alkalosis. It is also seen after parathyroidectomy.

Management

- Mild hypophosphataemia (> 0.5 mmol/L) rarely needs treating. Generally, increase dietary phosphorus (or phosphate in total parenteral nutrition (TPN)). Oral phosphate supplements are poorly tolerated (diarrhoea) but may be useful in chronic depletion.

- Symptomatic hypophosphataemia should be treated with IV phosphate at no more than 9 mmol/12 hours in TPN or 5% glucose.
- Phosphate infusion may precipitate hypocalcaemia – check Ca^{2+} repeatedly.

Hyperphosphataemia

Chronic hyperphosphataemia leads to vascular and soft tissue calcification, as the [calcium × phosphate] product exceeds the limit of solubility.

Causes

The cause is usually renal failure but hyperphosphataemia is also seen in hypoparathyroidism, tumour lysis syndrome and rhabdomyolysis, or after excess phosphate administration.

Management

- Acute hyperphosphataemia rarely needs treating (rhabdomyolysis, tumour lysis).
- Chronic hyperphosphataemia is almost always associated with renal impairment. Limit the dietary phosphorus intake, and use oral phosphate binders (e.g. calcium carbonate 0.5–1 g 3 times daily) with meals to limit phosphorus absorption.

ACID–BASE DISORDERS

The concentration of hydrogen ions $[H^+]$ is tightly regulated in all body compartments. In extracellular fluid (including blood), the normal range is 7.38–7.42 (pH = negative log of $[H^+]$). To maintain pH within this narrow range, buffering systems work in concert with the lungs and kidneys to minimize sudden changes in $[H^+]$.

Physiological buffers

- **Bicarbonate** (HCO_3^-) $H^+ + HCO_3 \leftrightarrow H_2CO_3 \xleftrightarrow{\text{Carbonic anhydrase}} CO_2 + H_2O$
- **Bone salts** (calcium carbonate and calcium phosphate)
- **Blood proteins** (haemoglobin).

Normal dietary acid intake is about 70 mmol/day. Any acid load is rapidly buffered by bicarbonate (normal serum range 22–26 mmol/L). As the bicarbonate buffering system does not reduce the *total* acid load, the kidney excretes H^+ to maintain homeostasis. To achieve this, bicarbonate must be and is efficiently reabsorbed in the proximal tubule, with acid excretion occurring in the collecting duct. Under the influence of aldosterone, Na^+ is reabsorbed, leaving the tubular lumen increasingly electronegative. To maintain electrical neutrality, H^+ (and K^+) is secreted into the lumen. H^+ is rapidly buffered in the urinary space by titratable acids (H^+ incorporated to form phosphoric or sulphuric acid) or ammonia (to form NH_4^+), and passed out as acidified urine (pH < 5 in the face of acidosis).

Diagnostic tests

- **Arterial blood gases.** Acid–base disorders are grouped as metabolic, respiratory or mixed in nature, depending on the principal contributor to the derangement (Fig. 11.4 and Table 11.3).
  - *Metabolic acidosis* is due to either bicarbonate loss or the accumulation of acid. Hyperventilation leads to a primary decrease in plasma bicarbonate and a compensatory fall in P_{CO_2}.

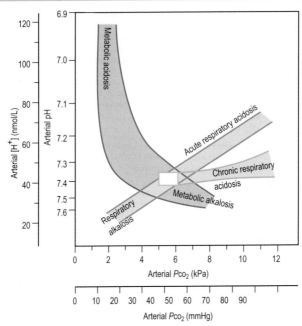

Fig. 11.4 The Flenley acid–base nomogram.

Table 11.3 Changes in arterial blood gases, pH and bicarbonate

	pH	$P_a co_2$	HCO_3-
Respiratory acidosis	N or ↓	↑↑	↑ (compensated)
Respiratory alkalosis	N or ↑	↓↓	↓ (slight)
Metabolic acidosis	N or ↓	↓	↓↓
Metabolic alkalosis	N or ↑	↑ (slight)	↑↑

- *Metabolic alkalosis* is due to hydrogen iron loss or bicarbonate gain, leading to an increase in plasma bicarbonate. There is a compensatory rise in Pco_2.
- *Respiratory acidosis* is caused by retention of CO_2 with a rise in Pco_2 and [H^+], partly compensated by a rise in bicarbonate.
- *Respiratory alkalosis* is caused by hyperventilation, with a fall in Pco_2 or metabolic acidosis.
- **Plasma anion gap (AG).** Measurement is helpful in the diagnosis of metabolic acidosis. It is calculated by subtracting measured cations from anions:

$$AG = [Na^+ + K^+] - [Cl^- + HCO_3^-] = 8 - 16 \text{ mmol/L in health.}$$

Kumar & Clark's Medical Management and Therapeutics

This should be corrected for hypoalbuminaemia by adding $0.25 \times (44 - \text{serum albumin})$. In AG each 1 g/L of albumin has a negative charge of $0.2 - 0.28$ mmol/L. A high AG is seen in renal failure (increase of sulphate and phosphate) or an accumulation of organic acids, e.g. lactate, ketones. A low AG occurs, e.g. in hypoalbuminaemia and hyperlipidaemia.

- **Urinary anion gap (UAG).** Measurement is useful in distinguishing a renal tubular acidosis from an extra-renal bicarbonate loss such as in diarrhoea. Again, it is the difference between the major measured anions and cations:

$$\text{UAG} = [Na^+]_u + [K^+]_u - [Cl^-]_u$$

In diarrhoea, urinary ammonium chloride (NH_4Cl) is high, giving a negative UAG. A positive (or zero) UAG is seen in renal disease and distal renal tubular acidosis (low urinary NH_4 production).

Metabolic acidosis

Metabolic acidosis (Fig. 11.4) is defined as a fall in systemic pH to < 7.35 with a primary decrease in plasma bicarbonate. It may be caused by excess generation or retention of acid, or by increased bicarbonate losses.

Metabolic acidosis is often associated with serious underlying disease, and history and examination should be directed toward a global patient assessment, with particular attention to haemodynamic stability and excluding sepsis.

If the systemic pH falls < 7.2, acidaemia leads to impaired cardiac contractility, vasodilatation, resistance to catecholamines and ineffective oxygen delivery. This reflects the severity of the associated insult.

- Check Na^+, K^+, Ca^{2+}, glucose and renal function. Obtain a venous or arterial blood gas.
- Measure the AG.
- If normal AG: *urinary* pH, ketones and electrolytes are helpful.
- If high AG: blood lactate, toxicology screen, urine for oxalate crystals (found with ethylene glycol poisoning) are measured.

Metabolic acidosis with normal AG

- **Causes.** Metabolic acidosis with a normal AG is caused by increased gastrointestinal bicarbonate losses, e.g. diarrhoea, ileostomy, and increased renal bicarbonate loss. This occurs in proximal (**type II**) renal tubular acidosis, hypoparathyroidism, tubular damage due to drugs and with **acetazolamide**. Increased renal hydrogen ion secretion occurs in **type I** and **type IV** renal tubular acidosis. Increased hydrochloride production occurs rarely with ammonium chloride ingestion and increased catabolism of lysine and arginine. In all these conditions plasma bicarbonate decreases. It is replaced by chloride to maintain electroneutrality. These conditions are sometimes referred to collectively as 'hyperchloraemic acidosis'.
- **Management**
  - If possible, correct the underlying cause.
  - Chronic mild acidosis should be treated with bicarbonate replacement therapy to prevent long-term osteomalacia, muscle wasting and anorexia. Use oral $NaHCO_3$ as 1.5–4.5 g in 3 divided doses.
  - Severe acidosis (pH < 7.2) in an unwell patient may require IV $NaHCO_3$ if there is real concern that acidaemia may be affecting cardiac performance; 200–500 mL 1.26% should be given over 1–4

hours. Always be aware of the Na^+ load. Ventilation needs to be increased to remove the CO_2 generated.

Metabolic acidosis with high AG

● Causes

- *Chronic kidney disease* is a frequent cause of chronic acidosis, caused by failure to excrete the fixed acid load of sulphate, phosphate and organic ions. Acidosis also occurs when functioning nephrons decrease, so there is an inability to excrete ammonia and hydrogen ions in the urine. Tubular disease may cause bicarbonate wasting.

- *Diabetic ketoacidosis* causes a high anion gap acidosis with the accumulation of organic acids, aceto-acetic acid and hydroxybutyric acid, owing to their increased production and decreased peripheral utilization (p. 608).

- *Lactic acidosis* occurs when there is increased production because of abnormal cellular respiration, either due to lack of oxygen in the tissues (**type A**) or a metabolic abnormality such as may be induced by a drug (**type B**). The most common cause in clinical practice is **type A** lactic acidosis, occurring in septic or cardiogenic shock.

Metabolic acidosis commonly occurs, e.g. in cholera, when there is an expected normal AG acidosis owing to massive gastrointestinal losses of bicarbonate but the AG is often increased owing to renal failure and lactic acidosis as a result of hypovolaemia.

● **Clinical features.** There is stimulation of respiration, leading to air hunger or Kussmaul respiration. Acidosis increases delivery of oxygen to the tissues by shifting the oxyhaemoglobin dissociation curve to the right but it also leads to inhibition of 2,3DPG production, which returns the curve towards normal. Cardiovascular dysfunction is common, as acidosis is negatively ionotropic. Severe acidosis is often associated with confusion and fits.

● Management

- *Always* treat the underlying cause, rather than the acidosis.

- The use of $NaHCO_3$ is highly controversial; theoretically, rapidly raising the pH may worsen the accompanying intracellular acidosis, decrease plasma ionized calcium (which itself impairs cardiac contractility) and abolish protective conditioning that acidosis may confer against hypoxia.

- Correction is only rarely required (if systemic pH < 6.9 in patients with poor cardiac performance); use 1.26% or 1.4% $NaHCO_3$. Aim for a pH > 7.1 or a plasma bicarbonate > 10 mmol/L, then review.

- The occasional use of 8.4% $NaHCO_3$ should be reserved for the management of patients in cardiac arrest.

Metabolic alkalosis

The retention of bicarbonate or loss of H^+ leads to a metabolic alkalosis (Fig. 11.4), usually due to primary chloride or potassium depletion. Any significant loss of Cl^- (vomiting, diuretics) will lead to HCO_3^- retention to maintain electrical neutrality. Any cause of secondary hyperaldosteronism (e.g. hypovolaemia) will lead to Na^+ retention, and potassium and H^+ depletion. Hypoventilation may buffer an evolving alkalosis to a degree, and modest elevations of P_{CO_2} are usual.

Kumar & Clark's Medical Management and Therapeutics

Clinical features

Exclude diuretic use and gastric losses (naso-gastric drainage; vomiting, which may be surreptitious). Symptoms are usually associated with other electrolyte abnormalities or the underlying disease.

Check Na^+, K^+, Cl^-, bicarbonate, Ca^{2+}, renal function and blood gas estimation. Also do a spot urine K^+ and Cl^-, with a urinary diuretic/laxative screen, renin and aldosterone if indicated.

- Interpreting urinary electrolytes (in mmol/L)
  - Urinary Cl^- < 10 with gastric losses (including surreptitious vomiting) but > 30 with diuretic therapy (abuse).
  - Urinary K^+ > 30 with diuretics and hyperaldosteronism, but < 20 with extra-renal K^+ losses.

Causes

- Chloride depletion from gastric acid losses with vomiting is the most common cause.
- The administration of diuretics, both thiazide and loop diuretics, may be responsible.
- Diarrhoea may be the cause, particularly with villous adenoma, which depletes both potassium and chloride.
- Although the sodium and potassium loss in the gastric juice is variable, obligate urinary loss of these cations is intensified by the bicarbonaturia that occurs.

Management

- Treat the underlying cause; stop diuretics (or convert to a potassium-sparing agent such as spironolactone); give an antiemetic and a proton pump inhibitor if naso-gastric ongoing drainage is indicated.
- If the patient is volume-deplete (as is often the case), replace with 0.9% NaCl. If volume-overloaded, treat with potassium as below.
- If the patient is hypokalaemic, give KCl as described on p. 378, and continue until alkalosis (rather than potassium) normalizes.
- In critically unwell patients (hepatic encephalopathy, arrhythmias, seizures) with pH > 7.6, consider IV HCl as acid replacement.

Further reading

Schrier RW: *Renal and electrolyte disorders*, ed 7, Philadelphia, 2010, Lippincott Williams and Wilkins.

Sykes MK: Venous pressure as a clinical indication of adequacy of transfusion, *Ann R Coll Surg Engl* 33:185–197, 1963.

Cardiovascular disease 12

CARDIAC ARRHYTHMIAS

APPROACH TO THE PATIENT

History

Arrhythmias can cause palpitations, shortness of breath, chest pain, dizziness and syncope. They are a cause of sudden death.

- **Palpitations.** Ask if these are regular (sinus tachycardia) or irregular (ventricular ectopics, atrial fibrillation (AF)). Ask the patient to tap the rhythm out on the table. Ask how rapid (rapid irregular beats suggest paroxysmal AF). Ask if the palpitations are terminated by breath-holding or the Valsalva manœuvre (supraventricular tachyarrhythmia is more likely).
- **Chest pain.** Chest pain sometimes occurs with palpitations or can be ischaemic in origin.
- **Syncope. Stokes–Adams attacks** are a sudden loss of consciousness unrelated to posture due to intermittent high-grade atrio-ventricular

(AV) block, profound bradycardia or ventricular standstill. The patient falls to the ground without warning, and is pale and deeply unconscious. The pulse is usually very slow or absent. After a few seconds the patient flushes brightly and recovers consciousness as the pulse quickens. Ask about history of previous heart problems (e.g. ischaemic heart disease (IHD), cardiomyopathy), familial congenital problems (e.g. congenital long QT syndrome, cardiomyopathy) and general medical conditions (e.g. thyrotoxicosis).

Examination

- What is the heart rate? Is it normal, slow (i.e. bradycardia) or fast (i.e. tachycardia)?
- Has the patient collapsed? Is the patient compromised by the abnormal heart rate?
- Is the pulse regular or irregular?
- Are canon 'a' waves present on the jugular venous pulsation? These occur when atrial contraction occurs against a closed tricuspid valve. This indicates AV dissociation and is seen in complete heart block and in ventricular tachycardia.
- Are there signs of underlying cardiac disease? For example:
  - heart failure, tachycardia, raised venous pressure, third heart sounds, basal crackles or peripheral oedema
  - cardiomyopathy — a young person with:
    a) double apical pulsation (forceful atrial contraction producing a fourth heart sound)
    b) jerky carotid pulse because of rapid ejection and sudden obstruction to left ventricular (LV) outflow during systole
    c) ejection systolic murmur due to LV outflow obstruction late in systole; it can be increased by manœuvres that decrease afterload, e.g. standing or Valsalva, and decreased by manœuvres that increase after-load and venous return, i.e. squatting
    d) pan-systolic murmur due to mitral regurgitation
    e) fourth heart sound (if not in AF).

Investigations

Twelve-lead electrocardiogram (ECG)

This test provides a three-dimensional snapshot of the electrical activity of the heart and is a useful screening tool. The sum of the depolarization (activation) and repolarization (recovery) potentials of the atrial and ventricular myocardium gives rise to the ECG waveform (Fig. 12.1).

Potentials are recorded in the frontal or coronal plane by the six limb leads and in the transverse plane by the six chest leads. Deflections on the ECG are positive if the depolarization wavefront spreads towards the positive pole of a lead. The converse is true if the wavefront spreads towards the negative pole. If the wavefront is orthogonal to the lead's axis, the deflection will be equally positive and negative, i.e. biphasic.

Atrial depolarization spreads from the sinus node inferiorly and to the left, producing a P wave that is usually positive in lead II and negative in aVR. Ventricular activation begins with depolarization of the interventricular septum from left to right, producing a small, positive R wave in lead V1 and a small, negative Q wave in lead V6. Depolarization of the remaining ventricular mass is usually dominated by the more massive left ventricle and therefore directed to the left and posteriorly. This results in

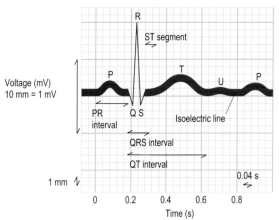

Fig. 12.1 The waves and elaboration of the **normal ECG**.

Box 12.1 Normal ECG intervals	
P wave duration	120 ms or less
PR interval	120–200 ms
QRS duration	100 ms or less
Corrected QT interval	440 ms or less in males
	460 ms or less in females

a negative S wave in lead V1 and a positive R wave in lead V6. The normal transition from leads V1 to V6 is marked by a progressive increase in R wave amplitude and a simultaneous decrease in S wave amplitude. QRS duration is usually 100 ms or less. Ventricular repolarization usually proceeds in the reverse direction to depolarization, i.e. apex to base and epicardium to endocardium, producing a deflection of similar polarity called the T wave. See Fig. 12.1 and Box 12.1.

- **PR interval.** The PR interval (Fig. 12.1 and Box 12.1) is measured from the start of the P wave to the start of the QRS complex. It is the time taken for electrical activity beginning in the sinus node to pass through to the ventricles.
- **ST segment.** The ST segment begins at the end of the QRS complex and, together with the T wave, represents ventricular repolarization.
- **QT interval.** The QT interval is measured from the start of the QRS complex to the end of the T wave and divided by the square root of the R–R interval to correct for the heart rate. It is the time taken for ventricular depolarization and repolarization; if prolonged, it may predispose to ventricular arrhythmias.
- **QRS.** In the frontal plane, the mean QRS axis ranges from −30° to +100°. Hence, the normal QRS pattern is very variable in the limb leads. **Left**

Kumar & Clark's Medical Management and Therapeutics

axis deviation is when the axis is more negative than −30° and right axis deviation is when the axis is more positive than +100°. Left axis deviation may be a normal variant or due to LV hypertrophy, left anterior hemiblock or inferior myocardial infarction. **Right axis deviation** may be a normal variant or due to right ventricular strain, left posterior hemiblock or lateral myocardial infarction.

Ambulatory ECG (Holter recordings)

These lightweight, battery-powered ECG recorders can be worn continuously for one or more days during routine activities. There is usually an internal clock and a manual symptom indicator that should be correlated to a patient's symptom diary. This allows the patient's symptoms to be correlated with any arrhythmias or changes in heart rate. Two leads are recorded and these are usually modifications of leads V1 and V5, which allow easy recognition of P waves and bundle branch blocks. The data is downloaded on to a computer and analysed, providing quantification of heart rate, premature atrial and ventricular complexes, and episodes of tachycardia and bradycardia. Holter monitoring is useful for detection of suspected arrhythmias, for the assessment of the efficacy of drug or ablation treatments and for risk stratification.

Patient-activated recorders

Some arrhythmias occur so infrequently that the diagnostic yield from Holter recorders is low. Hence, recorders that can be activated automatically by arrhythmias or manually by the patient are more useful. They can record at least 30 secs of information that can be retrieved subsequently. However, such devices are only useful in symptomatic arrhythmias that are of sufficient duration to allow their activation.

Implantable loop recorders

Asymptomatic arrhythmias or those causing significant incapacitation are best detected by loop recorders. These devices can be activated manually or automatically and record a 5-min loop that includes the rhythm prior to the recorder's activation. They are surgically implanted in a subcutaneous pocket and remain in situ for up to 18 months. Such devices are easy to implant with minimal risk and permit prolonged recording periods (up to 40 mins of prior ECG data when activated by a symptomatic patient) without the inconvenience of ECG cables. Following diagnosis of the arrhythmia or when the battery is drained, the device is easily explanted.

Electrophysiology study (EPS)

This is an invasive test used to detect suspected arrhythmias when the above techniques are equivocal. Electrode catheters are advanced, usually from the femoral veins, and placed at specific locations within the heart under fluoroscopic guidance. Intracardiac electrograms from each location are recorded and displayed simultaneously on a monitor, together with the surface ECG. Each electrode catheter can also be used to pace the heart from different locations. This permits the analysis of the electrical activation of the heart during both sinus rhythm and a tachyarrhythmia.

- **The four-wire study.** Electrode catheters are usually positioned high in the right atrium close to the sinus node, adjacent to the AV node and His bundle, along the coronary sinus and at the right ventricular apex. The coronary sinus runs in the AV groove and allows electrograms from the left atrium and ventricle to be recorded. Intracardiac electrograms are usually displayed at a sweep speed of 100 mm/second. A typical

Table 12.1 The basic electrophysiology study

Action	Measurements	Note
Sinus rhythm	Basic intervals (PA, AH, His duration, HV, QRS and corrected QT)	Is there pre-excitation or evidence for slowed conduction?
Single ventricular extra-stimulus testing	Retrograde AV node effective refractory period (AVNERP)	Is there VA conduction? If so, is it via the AV node and decremental, or an accessory pathway?
Incremental ventricular pacing	Retrograde Wenckebach cycle length (WCL)	
Single atrial extra-stimulus testing	Anterograde AVNERP	Is there AV conduction? If so, is it via the AV node and decremental, or an accessory pathway? Is there evidence for dual AV node physiology?
Incremental atrial pacing	Anterograde WCL	
Arrhythmia induction pacing from the atrium	Atrial effective refractory period (AERP) Coupling interval(s) for arrhythmia induction	Extra-stimulus testing with 2 or more extra-stimuli, burst pacing and 2 or more premature beats during sinus rhythm
Wellen's protocol	Ventricular effective refractory period (VERP) Coupling interval(s) for arrhythmia induction	Used to induce ventricular tachycardia. Ventricular extra-stimulus testing with up to 3 extra-stimuli

recording during sinus rhythm shows the earliest electrical activation in the high right atrium proceeding down the His bundle and proximal to distal along the coronary sinus. The earliest ventricular activation is usually at the QRS complex. The steps in a basic electrophysiology study are listed in Table 12.1.

- **Advanced mapping techniques.** Complex ablation procedures for atrial fibrillation and in the grown-up congenital heart disease population are lengthy and often guided by cardiac anatomy. Advanced mapping systems facilitate such procedures by minimizing radiation exposure and by providing three-dimensional representations of cardiac anatomy and electrical activation patterns. The anatomy (or geometry) of the cardiac chamber of interest can be created manually during the procedure, or a previously acquired contrast CT or MRI scan can be loaded into the mapping system. The scan image can then be segmented, leaving only the chamber of interest, on to which are superimposed real-time catheter movements and electrical activation patterns.

Kumar & Clark's Medical Management and Therapeutics

Pathophysiology of arrhythmias

● **Normal electrical activation.** The heart contains specialized conduction tissue that can generate rhythmic electrical pulses spontaneously. This is due to cyclical variations in the permeability of cell membranes to potassium, sodium and calcium ions. The activity of the specialized conduction tissue is modulated by the autonomic nervous system. Electrical pulses are rapidly conducted to the mass of cardiac myocytes, producing the mechanical events of each cardiac cycle. Usually, the cells of the sinus node generate electrical pulses most rapidly and are the physiological pacemaker. Cardiac myocyte activation can be divided into four stages (Fig. 12.2). Abnormalities during any of these stages can result in both **bradyarrhythmias** and **tachyarrhythmias**.

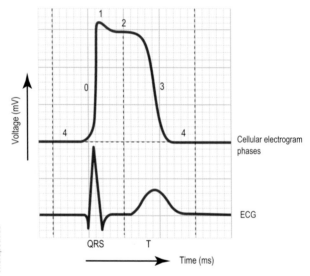

Phase	Event	Mechanism
0	Rapid depolarization	Sodium ion influx into myocyte
1		Sodium influx stops + efflux of potassium and chloride ion
2	Plateau	Calcium ion influx balanced by potassium ion efflux
3	Repolarization	Calcium influx stops and potassium ion efflux continues
4	Resting membrane potential	No net ionic movement

Fig. 12.2 The cardiac myocyte action potential.

- **Enhanced automaticity.** Any cardiac myocytes depolarizing faster than the sinus node can override it and cause arrhythmias. These foci of abnormal cells typically occur at the ostia of the caval or pulmonary veins, along the crista terminalis in the right atrium, within the coronary sinus, close to the AV node, around the insertions of both AV valves and within the ventricular outflow tracts.
- **Triggered activity.** Oscillations in the membrane potential during stage 3 or 4 of the action potential are called early and late after-depolarizations respectively. If they achieve the threshold potential, premature action potentials may be triggered, causing arrhythmias. Myocardial ischaemia, electrolyte disturbances, pacing, catecholamines and certain drugs are potential causes. Torsades de pointes from QT interval prolongation and arrhythmias due to digoxin toxicity are examples.
- **Re-entry.** This causes the majority of clinical tachyarrhythmias. It is due to the rotation of electrical activity around a region of conduction block that is either fixed, e.g. scar, or functional. The initiating event is usually an ectopic beat that is conducted around the region of conduction block in one direction only due to differences in conduction velocity and refractoriness. As long as the head of the rotating electrical wavefront meets excitable myocardium, a stable re-entry circuit is established.
- **Suppressed automaticity and conduction block.** If depolarization of the sinus node is slowed by either excessive vagal tone or drugs such as β-blockers, sinus bradycardia results. Bradyarrhythmias also occur if conduction through the AV node is slowed or blocked by excessive vagal tone, drugs or disease. Other parts of the specialized conduction system may assume the role of cardiac pacemaker, producing an escape rhythm.

MECHANISMS AND DIAGNOSIS OF BRADYARRHYTHMIAS

Sinus node-dependent arrhythmias

These include sinus bradycardia and sinus pauses with or without an escape rhythm.

Sinus bradycardia

Sinus bradycardia is a heart rate of < 60 bpm during sinus rhythm, with every P wave associated with a QRS complex. The causes of sinus bradycardia can be:

- **Cardiac,** e.g. sinus node ischaemia/infarction, sinus node and atrial fibrosis, myocarditis and cardiomyopathies
- **Systemic,** e.g. hypothermia, hypothyroidism, cholestatic jaundice, raised intracranial pressure, carotid sinus hypersensitivity and vasovagal syncope. Drugs include **β-blockers**, **calcium channel blockers**, **amiodarone**, **digoxin** and **disopyramide**.

Treatment of sinus bradycardia involves identifying and excluding specific causes, if possible. Specific measures are summarized in Box 12.2.

Sinus pauses

Sinus pauses can be due to either sinus node exit block or sinus arrest. Exit block is when an electrical impulse generated within the sinus node fails to conduct into the atria. Sinus arrest is when the sinus node fails to generate electrical impulses. In either case there is an absent P wave on the ECG; if the pause is prolonged, an escape rhythm may occur.

Kumar & Clark's Medical Management and Therapeutics

> **Box 12.2** Treatment of sinus bradycardia
>
> **Emergency**
> - IV atropine in 300–600 mcg boluses to a maximum of 3 mg
> - Adrenaline infusion from 2–10 mcg/min (alternative isoprenaline 0.5-10mcg/min)
> - Temporary pacing wire or transcutaneous pacing
>
> **Long-term therapy**
> - Stop relevant drugs
> - Permanent pacemaker implant in chronic sick sinus syndrome, carotid sinus hypersensitivity with pauses > 3 secs and cardio-inhibitory form of vasovagal syncope
> - Anticoagulation in tachycardia-bradycardia syndromes with atrial fibrillation

Sick sinus syndrome

Sick sinus syndrome encompasses sinus bradycardia, sinus pauses, permanent atrial fibrillation with bradycardia and tachycardia-bradycardia syndrome. The latter is a failure of stable sinus rhythm to establish following termination of a tachycardia such as atrial fibrillation and flutter, focal atrial tachycardia, junctional tachycardia and AV node re-entry tachycardia. Many patients also exhibit AV conduction abnormalities and bundle branch blocks.

Atrio-ventricular node-dependent arrhythmias

First-degree AV block

This is when every atrial electrical impulse is conducted slowly to the ventricles. Hence, each P wave is associated with a QRS complex but the PR interval is > 200 ms.

Second-degree block

This is when one or more, but not all, atrial electrical impulses fail to conduct to the ventricles. This encompasses both physiological and pathological variations in AV node conduction. The normal AV node exhibits the property of decrementation, which prevents excessive ventricular rates. Hence, increasingly premature atrial electrical impulses either are conducted to the ventricles more slowly or are blocked. This is due to the refractory properties of the AV node and is associated with changes in the PR intervals.

- **Wenckebach AV block (Mobitz type 1 block).** This is a benign form of second-degree block in which the PR interval progressively lengthens until an atrial electrical impulse fails to conduct to the ventricles (Fig. 12.3). However, successive PR intervals change in smaller increments, producing a progressive decrease in the RR intervals. The longest RR interval during Wenckebach periodicity incorporates the non-conducted P wave. Anatomically, this usually occurs at the level of the AV node. Patients are usually just monitored. If symptomatic, give **atropine** 0.5 mg IV every 2 mins, maximum dose 0.04 mg/kg.
- **Mobitz type 2 block.** Atrial electrical impulses failing to reach the ventricles despite a normal PR interval usually indicate a pathological process and may be associated with bundle branch block. Anatomically,

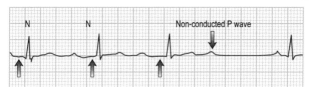

Fig. 12.3 Rhythm strip ECG showing **Wenckebach AV block** with progressive PR prolongation, as marked out by the arrows, followed by a non-conducted P wave.

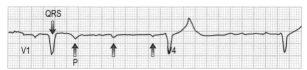

Fig. 12.4 Complete heart block. The P waves and QRS complexes are completely dissociated from each other, with different PP and RR intervals.

the block is usually at the infra-nodal level of the His bundle and the ratio of non-conducted to conducted P waves is variable. The risk of progression to heart block is greater than Wenckebach AV block, and cardiac pacing is usually indicated. Atropine is not used and may in fact worsen the block.

Third-degree or complete block (AV dissociation)

This is when no atrial electrical impulses are conducted to the ventricles. Hence, there is a continuously changing relationship between the P waves and QRS complexes (Fig. 12.4). Usually, there is a regular escape rhythm that arises below the level of block. A **narrow QRS complex** (< 125 ms) escape rhythm is from the His bundle and more stable than a **broad QRS complex** (> 125 ms), ventricular escape rhythm.

- Causes of third-degree block include ischaemic heart disease (e.g. acute myocardial infarction), post-cardiac operations/ablation, congenital abnormalities, autoimmune rheumatic disorders (e.g. SLE, rheumatoid arthritis, systemic sclerosis), infiltrative disorders (e.g. amyloid, sarcoid), haemochromatosis, infections and drugs.
- Treatment depends on aetiology. Recent-onset **narrow-complex AV block** may respond to **IV atropine** 600 mcg boluses but temporary pacing may be required. Chronic block will require permanent (dual chamber) pacing (p. 410). **Broad-complex AV block** presenting with a slow (15–40 bpm) rhythm, dizziness and blackouts (Stokes–Adams, p. 385) is treated with temporary, followed by permanent, pacing, which reduces the mortality. As ventricular arrhythmias are not uncommon, an **implantable cardioverter-defibrillator (ICD)** may be required.

Bundle branch blocks and hemiblocks

These are due to delayed conduction within the His–Purkinje system, producing QRS complex durations > 120 ms. Causes include ischaemic heart disease, idiopathic fibrosis of the conduction system,

Kumar & Clark's Medical Management and Therapeutics

cardiomyopathies, aortic stenosis, hypertensive heart disease, recurrent pulmonary emboli, cor pulmonale, congenital lesions, infective endocarditis and myotonic dystrophy.

- **Left bundle branch block (LBBB).** In LBBB depolarization of the left ventricle is delayed, giving a deep QS pattern in lead V1 and tall R waves in leads 1 and V6 (Fig. 12.5). This is usually associated with heart disease and causes a reverse split of the second heart sound. In some patients with poor LV function this can result in dyssynchronous ventricular contraction that requires biventricular pacing.
- **Right bundle branch block (RBBB).** In RBBB depolarization of the right ventricle is delayed, giving an RSR complex in lead V1 and deep S waves in leads 1 and V6. This may be a normal finding in 1% of young adults and in 5% of the elderly population.
- **Hemiblock and bifascicular blocks.** The left bundle has anterior and posterior divisions, also known as fascicles. Conduction block may also occur at this level, producing the **hemiblocks**. Left anterior hemiblock causes left axis deviation, and left posterior hemiblock causes right axis deviation. Either hemiblock together with an RBBB is called a **bifascicular block**. In this situation, conduction block within the remaining fascicle will produce complete heart block.

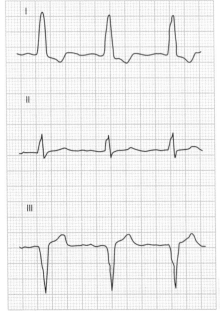

Fig. 12.5 Part of a 12-lead ECG showing typical **left bundle branch block** with a broad, negative QRS complex in lead V1.

MECHANISMS AND DIAGNOSIS OF TACHYARRHYTHMIAS

Atrial origin

Sinus node tachycardias

These are sinus rhythms with a heart rate > 100 bpm. **Causes** are cardiac or systemic. Cardiac causes include acute myocardial ischaemia, acute heart failure, sinus node re-entry or enhanced sinus node automaticity. Systemically, it is found normally in children, exercise and pregnancy. Anaemia, hypovolaemia, acute hypoxia, thyrotoxicosis, pyrexia, catecholamine excess and drugs also cause sinus tachycardia.

- Specific treatment is directed against the potential causes, together with rate-slowing drugs such as β-blockers and calcium channel blockers. Enhanced sinus node automaticity or sinus node re-entry may require catheter ablation with or without permanent pacemaker implantation.

Focal tachycardias

These are uncommon tachycardias, caused by atrial foci that exhibit enhanced automaticity, triggered activity or micro re-entry. Typical **causes** include myocardial infarction, myocarditis, digoxin toxicity, chronic lung diseases, alcohol, hypokalaemia and catecholamine release. Foci can occur anywhere within the atria and at the junctions with their respective veins. They are usually conducted to the ventricles with varying degrees of AV block. Automatic foci usually exhibit gradual acceleration and deceleration. They also cause incessant tachycardias with a subsequent tachycardia cardiomyopathy.

The morphology of the P waves during tachycardia is highly variable, depending on the site of the tachycardia focus. If the focus is close to the sinus node, typical P waves may be seen. P wave morphologies may give some indication as to the site of the tachycardia focus (Table 12.2).

- Treatment. Some focal atrial tachycardias respond to **adenosine** IV up to 0.25 mg/kg and are subsequently treated pharmacologically or by catheter ablation.

Table 12.2 P wave morphologies in different ECG leads for focal atrial tachycardias

Origin	I	aVL	aVR	II	III	aVF	V1	Comments
Cristal	+	+		+			Biphasic	Broad
Septal and CS os		+	+	−	−	−		
LAA and LUPV				+	++	+	+	
RUPV	Isoelectric			+	+	+	Biphasic/+	Narrow

The positive and negative signs refer to the polarities of the P waves during focal atrial tachycardias from different sites. CS, coconary sinus; LAA, left atrial appendage; LUPV and RUPV, left and right upper pulmonary vein. (Adapted from Josephson ME 2008.)

Kumar & Clark's Medical Management and Therapeutics

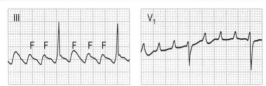

Fig. 12.6 Atrial flutter. Flutter waves are marked with an F with a frequency of 240/min. Every fourth flutter wave is transmitted to the ventricles with a ventricular rate of 60/min.

Flutters

These are **caused** by atrial macro re-entry circuits that rotate around anatomical structures and scars. They are associated with a slightly increased risk of embolic stroke and may compromise ventricular filling causing breathlessness.

Typical atrial flutter usually, but not always, has negative sawtooth-like flutter waves in the inferior ECG leads and positive flutter waves in lead V1 (Fig. 12.6). Frequently, typical atrial flutter is conducted with a 2-to-1 AV block, giving a heart rate of 150 bpm. The re-entry circuit is well characterized, and the zone of slow conduction critical to sustaining the circuit is the cavo-tricuspid isthmus.

- **Treatment.** Patients should be given **warfarin** and either rate control with **digoxin** and **β-blockers**, or **rhythm control**. Some patients also benefit from **DC cardioversion**. Catheter ablation of the cavo-tricuspid isthmus can successfully terminate and prevent recurrence of typical atrial flutter with minimal risk in 95% of patients. It is used for all patients with recurrent or haemodynamically significant atrial flutter.

Atrial fibrillation (AF)

AF is the commonest arrhythmia globally, with a prevalence of 0.5–1% of the general population and 5–10% of the population over 65 years. It is characterized by rapid (300–600 bpm), irregularly irregular contractions of the atria. The 12-lead ECG shows no regular atrial activity (Fig. 12.7) and the ventricles beat in an irregularly irregular fashion at rates of up to 150–200 bpm. The mechanisms underlying AF are thought to be a combination of triggering atrial ectopics usually originating within the pulmonary veins, and progressive electrical changes within the atrial myocardium (remodelling) that allow it to be sustained. AF is a consequence of a wide range of pathologies but it can exist independently in a structurally normal heart (lone AF).

Clinically, patients either are asymptomatic or complain of palpitations, breathlessness, dizziness and, less commonly, syncope. AF is a spectrum ranging from infrequent episodes (paroxysmal), to those requiring termination with drugs or DC cardioversion (persistent), to permanent AF.

Management of AF consists of either restoring rate and rhythm or, if this is not possible in the long term, controlling rate and preventing complications.

- Acute AF
  - *AF that is a complication of an acute illness*, e.g. a respiratory infection or alcohol toxicity, often reverts to sinus rhythm when the infection/cause is treated and resolves.

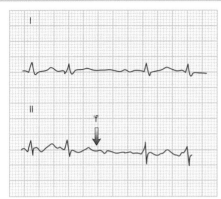

Fig. 12.7 A 12-lead ECG showing **atrial fibrillation**. There are no P waves but in leads V1 and V2 there is a rapid undulation of the baseline between the QRS complexes, demonstrating the fibrillatory activity. The RR intervals are continuously changing, resulting in an irregularly irregular pulse that is characteristic.

- *Acute symptomatic AF, if documented < 48-hour duration,* can be treated with synchronized DC cardioversion following immediate heparinization. This is successful in over 75% of cases but can recur.
- *If AF lasts for > 48 hours,* patients should be anticoagulated with **warfarin** (INR 2–3) for 3 weeks prior to cardioversion. The anticoagulation should be continued after successful cardioversion for at least 4 weeks, or longer if there are high risk factors for strokes. Alternatively, a transoesophageal echocardiogram (TOE) can be performed to rule out thrombosis in the left atrial appendage, obviating the need for anticoagulation prior to DC shock.
- *Chemical cardioversion* can alternatively be achieved by using an IV infusion of **flecainide** 2 mg/kg over 30 mins, maximum dose 150 mg or **amiodarone** IV infusion via a central venous catheter, initially 5 mg/kg over 20–120 mins with ECG monitoring. Patients again should be warfarinized prior to treatment
- *If cardioversion fails* (or the AF recurs), give **amiodarone** 300 mg over 1 hour before a further attempt at cardioversion. A second dose of **amiodarone** can be administered if necessary. Biphasic waveforms for cardioversion require less energy and have a higher efficacy than monophasic waves. The aims are as follows.
- Chronic AF
  - *Maintain sinus rhythm* following DC conversion with anti-arrhythmic drugs (class 1c, e.g. **flecainide**, **propafenone**; or class III, e.g. **amiodarone**, **sotalol** — see p. 411).
  - *Control rate* with a combination of **digoxin**, β-**blockers** or **verapamil** or **diltiazem**. The heart rate should be between 60 and 80 bpm at rest. **Anticoagulant therapy** should be continued. **Dabigatran** 220 mg oral daily, a direct thrombin inhibitor, is now being used instead of the more traditional warfarin (p. 245) as monitoring is not required.

Kumar & Clark's Medical Management and Therapeutics

- *If rate control is poor despite optimal medical therapy* patients should be considered for AV node ablation and pacemaker implantation ('**ablate and pace strategy**') but will require lifelong anticoagulation therapy.
- *Catheter ablation* should be offered to patients who remain symptomatic despite drug therapy with two different agents.
- *For paroxysmal AF* the pulmonary veins are electrically isolated, thereby eliminating the triggers. Success rates are between 80 and 85%.
- *In persistent AF* additional linear ablation is undertaken to compartmentalize the left atrium (catheter maze). This aims to prevent the formation of multiple re-entry circuits that sustain the AF. The success rate for permanent AF is 60–70% after one procedure. The ablation is a complex procedure, usually requiring an advanced mapping system, which can last up to 4 or 5 hours. The main risks include cardiac tamponade (1%), stroke (1–2%) and pulmonary vein stenosis (1%). Patients with structurally abnormal hearts and those over 65 years have an increased risk for embolic strokes (up to 5% per year) and should be anticoagulated with warfarin or **dabigatran**, even after ablation.

Atrio-ventricular junction origin

Atrio-ventricular node re-entry tachycardia (AVNRT)

This is one of the commonest causes of a paroxysmal supraventricular tachycardia, occurring in up to 60% of cases. It is more frequently found in females and most patients have structurally normal hearts.

- Clinical features. **Typical symptoms** include palpitations, dizziness, neck pulsations, chest discomfort and a polyuria that follows the termination of an episode. Syncope may occur in patients with impaired ventricular function and following termination from tachycardia-induced sinus arrest. AVNRT usually has an abrupt onset and termination, and can last from seconds to days. Patients usually have two functional and anatomically different pathways within the AV node — a fast conducting pathway and a slow pathway. The slow pathway repolarizes faster than the fast pathway. During sinus rhythm, antegrade conduction usually occurs via the fast pathway. If an atrial impulse occurs early, e.g. a premature beat when the fast pathway is refractory, antegrade conduction proceeds via the slow pathway in propagating the atrial impulses to the ventricles. Not all patients with dual AV node physiology develop AVNRT.
- Investigations. AVNRT can only occur if a stable micro re-entrant circuit can be established within the AV node between the fast and slow pathways. Usually, an atrial premature beat initiates the tachycardia. Less frequently, the initiation is from a ventricular premature beat.
  - *In typical AVNRT*, the antegrade limb of the circuit is the slow pathway, with retrograde conduction up the fast pathway. Consequently, the atria and ventricles are depolarized almost simultaneously. This produces a narrow complex tachycardia (QRS < 0.125 sec) with rates between 150 and 240 bpm. The P wave resulting from retrograde conduction up the fast pathway is usually fused with the QRS complex. Sometimes, its terminal portion may be seen as a small positive deflection at the end of the QRS complex in lead V1 (Fig. 12.8).

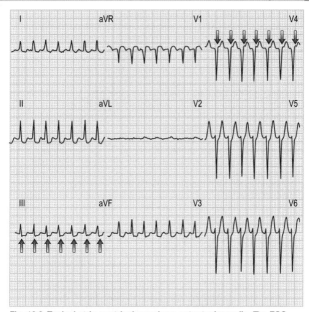

Fig. 12.8 Typical atrio-ventricular node re-entry tachycardia. The ECG shows a regular narrow-complex tachycardia with retrograde P waves that are fused with the QRS complexes and appear as small 'pseudo-R waves' in V1 and 'pseudo-S waves' in the inferior leads, as marked by the blue arrows. These deflections are absent in the sinus rhythm QRS complexes.

- *In atypical AVNRT,* the antegrade limb is the fast pathway. Hence, atrial depolarization follows that of the ventricles, producing a distinct retrograde P wave and a long RP tachycardia.
- **Treatment.** AVNRT can be terminated using vagal manœuvres, e.g. Valsalva manœuvre, and drugs, e.g. **IV adenosine**, **calcium channel blockers**, e.g. **verapamil**, and **β-blockers**, e.g. **propranolol**. Prophylaxis with **calcium channel blockers** and **β-blockers**, **flecainide** and **propafenone** is used, but symptomatic AVNRT should be referred for catheter ablation, which has a low complication rate and is curative in 95% of cases.

Junctional tachycardia
This is caused by an automatic focus in the AV node. The commonest cause of this is digoxin toxicity, which produces a tachycardia with a Wenckebach-type AV block. Other causes include acute myocardial infarction, cardiac surgery, chronic obstructive pulmonary disease, rheumatic fever and hypokalaemia. The ECG usually shows a narrow-complex tachycardia with retrograde P waves that may be fused with the QRS complex or occur either side of it.

- **Treatment** is directed at the underlying cause.

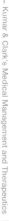

Kumar & Clark's Medical Management and Therapeutics

Accessory pathway-dependent tachycardias

Accessory pathways (APs) are myocardial bundles that electrically couple the atria and ventricles, at one or several points across the AV junction, in addition to the AV node and His–Purkinje system. Most APs do not exhibit decremental conduction and are therefore able to conduct rapidly between atria and ventricles. APs may conduct both antegradely and retrogradely, or only retrogradely. The former are seen in the Wolff–Parkinson–White syndrome and the latter are known as concealed APs. A rare form of AP is the atrio-fascicular or Mahaim connection between the right atrium and the right bundle branch. These APs usually conduct in the antegrade direction only and exhibit decrementation.

● Wolff–Parkinson–White syndrome (WPW) has a prevalence of 0.1–0.4% and typically presents during infancy or in the second and third decades. **Antegrade conduction** via the AP causes ventricular pre-excitation, characterized by a PR interval of < 0.12 secs and a slurred initiation to the QRS complex called a delta wave (Fig. 12.9). During sinus rhythm, the extent of pre-excitation is determined by the relative conductions through the AP and the AV node–His–Purkinje system. AP conductivity and location, as well as the effects of autonomic tone on AV nodal conduction, are significant factors. Several detailed ECG algorithms have been devised for identifying AP location. Orthodromic AV re-entry tachycardia (AVRT) is seen in 84% of cases of WPW, AF in 51%, antidromic AVRT in 10% and ventricular fibrillation in less than 1%.

  • *Orthodromic AVRT* is usually initiated by a premature ventricular or atrial beat establishing the macro re-entry circuit shown in Fig. 12.10a. The 12-lead ECG shows regular, narrow QRS complexes with retrograde P waves (Fig. 12.10b). However, functional delay in one of the bundle branches can produce broad QRS complexes. Orthodromic AVRT usually terminates with block in the AV node, although any limb of the circuit may be responsible. This is also the re-entry circuit seen with concealed AP tachycardias.

  • *Antidromic AVRT* has a re-entry circuit that is the reverse of that for orthodromic AVRT (Fig. 12.11a). The ventricles are fully pre-excited and the 12-lead ECG demonstrates regular, broad QRS complexes

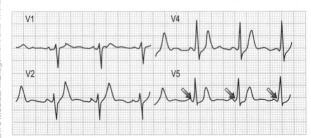

Fig. 12.9 Wolff–Parkinson–White syndrome. The ECG shows sinus rhythm with pre-excitation, as demonstrated by a short PR interval (marked in V5 by the blue lines) and a slurred upstroke to the QRS complex or 'delta wave' (marked in V5 by blue arrows).

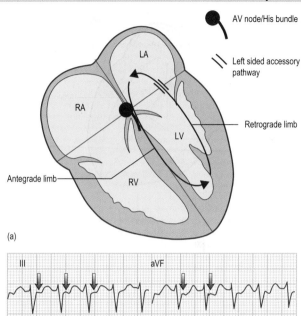

AV node/His bundle

Left sided accessory pathway

LA

RA

Retrograde limb

LV

Antegrade limb

RV

(a)

III   aVF

(b)

Fig. 12.10 (a) Orthodromic AV re-entry. This circuit involves four sequential anatomical components — the left (or right) atrium, the AV node and His–Purkinje system, the left (or right) ventricle and the accessory pathway. The ventricles are activated via the AV node and His–Purkinje system. The atria are activated retrogradely via the accessory pathway. RA, right atrium; LA, left atrium; RV, right ventricle; LV, left ventricle.

(b) Orthodromic AV re-entry tachycardia. The ECG complex shows a regular narrow-complex tachycardia with no pre-excitation. There are retrograde P waves that are shown in leads III and aVF by the blue arrows.

Kumar & Clark's Medical Management and Therapeutics

similar to those in ventricular tachycardia (Fig. 12.11b). Antidromic AVRT usually terminates with block in the AV node. Atrio-fascicular or Mahaim APs produce a characteristic antidromic AVRT with LBBB morphology and left axis deviation.

- *Atrial fibrillation in WPW* has the greatest risk of causing haemodynamic compromise and ventricular fibrillation. The initiation is thought to be secondary to orthodromic and conducted ventricular ectopics AVRT, and the 12-lead ECG demonstrates a variably pre-excited, rapid, irregularly irregular broad QRS complex tachycardia (Fig. 12.12). However, there may be occasional normal QRS complexes due to dominant anterograde conduction down the AV node–His–Purkinje system.

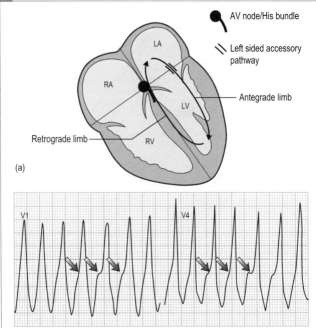

(a)

(b)

Fig. 12.11 (a) Antidromic AV re-entry. This circuit has four sequential anatomical components — the left (or right) atrium, the AV node and His–Purkinje system, the left (or right) ventricle and the accessory pathway. The ventricles are pre-excited via the accessory pathway. The atria are activated retrogradely via the AV node. RA, right atrium; LA, left atrium; RV, right ventricle; LV, left ventricle.

(b) Antidromic AV re-entry tachycardia. The ECG shows a regular broad-complex tachycardia with full pre-excitation. There are delta waves in each QRS complex that are marked in leads V1 and V4 by the blue arrows.

- **Treatment.** Haemodynamically unstable patients should be treated by DC cardioversion. Drug therapy is targeted at the AV node, accessory pathway or both (Box 12.3).
  - *Orthodromic AVRT* is usually terminated with IV AV nodal-blocking drugs such as **adenosine**, **verapamil** or **diltiazem**. If this fails, IV **procainamide** is administered with BP monitoring (Fig. 12.13). Chronic drug prophylaxis can be with either AV node-blocking drugs or those affecting the accessory pathway.
  - *Antidromic AVRT and pre-excited AF* are treated with **procainamide** as first-line therapy, since AV nodal-blocking drugs may

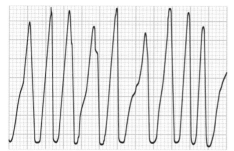

Fig. 12.12 Atrial fibrillation in Wolff–Parkinson–White syndrome. Note tachycardia with broad QRS complexes and fast and irregular ventricular rate.

Box 12.3 Sites of anti-arrhythmic drug action

AV node
- Digoxin
- Beta-blockers
- Adenosine
- Verapamil

Accessory pathway
- Quinidine
- Procainamide
- Disopyramide

Both
- Flecainide
- Propafenone
- Sotalol
- Amiodarone

(From Dhinoja and Lambiase 2005, with permission)

---

accelerate the tachycardia and cause ventricular fibrillation. Chronic drug prophylaxis is usually with **flecainide** and **propafenone**, which suppress conduction via the AP and AV node. Alternative drugs include **procainamide**, **quinidine** and **disopyramide**. **Amiodarone** is used only if other drugs are ineffective, due to its potential side-effects.

All patients with symptomatic WPW should be assessed for curative catheter ablation of the AP. This can be performed safely and has a success rate of 95%.

Long RP tachycardias

This is a special group of supraventricular tachycardias whose RP interval is > 50% of the RR interval (Fig. 12.14). The possible causes include focal atrial tachycardia, atypical AVNRT and orthodromic AVRT.

- Atypical AVNRT involves antegrade conduction via the fast pathway and retrograde conduction over the slow pathway. The retrograde P

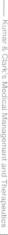

Kumar & Clark's Medical Management and Therapeutics

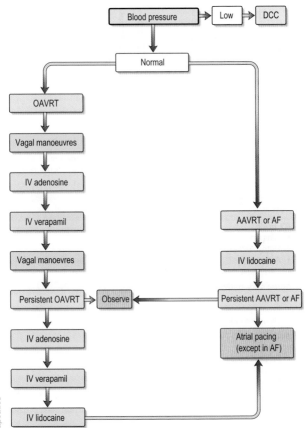

Fig. 12.13 Management strategy for tachycardias in Wolff–Parkinson–White syndrome.
AAVRT, antidromic AV re-entry tachycardia; AF, atrial fibrillation; DCC, DC cardioversion; OAVRT, orthodromic AV re-entry tachycardia (Modified from Dhinoja & Lambiase 2005, with permission).

waves are therefore clearly visible after their associated QRS complexes.

• **Orthodromic AVRT,** also known as permanent junctional reciprocating tachycardia (**PJRT**), a type of AVRT, usually involves a concealed posteroseptal accessory pathway. The latter usually conducts slowly and may have decremental properties. The tachycardia is often incessant, causing a tachycardia-mediated cardiomyopathy that resolves following successful ablation of the accessory pathway.

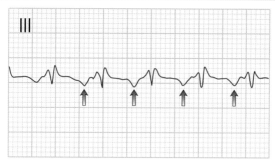

Fig. 12.14 Long RP tachycardia. The ECG shows a regular narrow-complex tachycardia. There is a long RP interval and the retrograde P waves are marked by the blue arrows in lead III. The cause in this patient was an atypical AVNRT.

Ventricular origin

Ventricular tachycardia (VT)

This tachyarrhythmia originates from the ventricles and is usually a broad-complex tachycardia (QRS > 140 msec) with rates between 150 and 200 bpm, which can cause haemodynamic compromise. In monomorphic VT the QRS complexes are identical, whereas they vary in polymorphic VT. There is frequently underlying heart disease, most commonly ischaemic heart disease with previous myocardial infarction. Other pathologies include cardiomyopathies, ion channel disorders and congenital heart disease. Rarely, VT occurs in structurally normal hearts.

Typical **symptoms** of VT include palpitations, chest pain, dizziness, syncope and breathlessness. In some patients the presentation is with sudden death.

- **Monomorphic VT** is usually a re-entrant tachyarrhythmia. It is initiated by a premature ventricular beat that establishes a macro re-entry circuit around a region of scarring. The re-entry wavefront may traverse the scar through several different channels, occasionally producing a variable RR interval. Table 12.3 shows the ECG features that distinguish VT from an aberrantly conducted supraventricular tachycardia (SVT) and a pre-excited tachycardia. Fig 12.15 shows the Resuscitation Council (UK) management for tachycardias in adults.
- **Bundle branch re-entry VT** (BBR VT) is a re-entrant tachyarrhythmia in which the circuit involves the His bundle, both bundle branches and interventricular septal myocardium. As with other macro re-entry circuits, a zone of slow conduction is necessary to sustain the tachycardia. This is the LBB in the common form of BBR VT, which is the retrograde limb and gives an LBBB pattern on the ECG. However, since antegrade conduction is via the His–Purkinje system, the QRS complexes are similar to those for an SVT with aberrant conduction. There is usually underlying heart disease, particularly dilated cardiomyopathy.
- **Idiopathic VT** occurs in structurally normal hearts and can arise from either ventricle. Patients usually present with palpitations or syncope and the prognosis is good. The QRS duration is relatively short at

Kumar & Clark's Medical Management and Therapeutics

Table 12.3 ECG features distinguishing ventricular tachycardia from supraventricular tachycardia with aberrant conduction

ECG criterion	VT	SVT with aberrant conduction
AV relationship	Usually dissociated	Usually associated
Capture and fusion beats	Present	Absent
QRS duration	> 140 msec with RBBB morphology > 160 msec with LBBB morphology	≤ 140 msec ≤ 160 msec
Mean frontal plane axis	−90 to ±180°	Similar to sinus rhythm
QRS transition across chest leads	Usually positive or negative concordance, i.e. no transition	Similar to sinus rhythm

LBBB/RBBB, left/right bundle branch block.

0.13–0.16 secs and VT may be misdiagnosed as SVT with aberrant conduction.

- *The left ventricular type* (also known as fascicular VT) is a re-entrant arrhythmia that responds to **verapamil**. The 12-lead ECG shows an RBBB monomorphic VT with left axis deviation.
- *The right ventricular type*, which is adenosine-sensitive, usually originates from the right ventricular outflow tract and is thought to be caused by triggered activity; it may, however, also arise from the LV outflow tract and aortic cusps. The 12-lead ECG usually shows LBBB with an inferior axis.
- Investigations
  - Patients should have transthoracic echocardiography.
  - Some require further investigations with contrast echocardiography, cardiac MR scan, ajmaline testing and signal-averaged ECG.
  - Certain patients may benefit from further risk stratification by VT stimulation testing. This especially applies to people with ischaemic heart disease and Brugada syndrome.
  - Idiopathic and bundle branch re-entry VTs are referred for electrophysiology studies and possible curative ablation.
- Treatment
  - Haemodynamically compromising VT requires **immediate** DC cardioversion.
  - **Drug therapy** is usually with **β-blockers** and **amiodarone**.
  - Fascicular VT is especially sensitive to **verapamil**.
  - All patients with impaired LV function should also have optimal heart failure drug therapy (p. 419).
  - Most other patients with symptomatic VT should have an **ICD fitted** (p. 410).

The only treatments to improve prognosis are β-blockers and ICDs.
N.B. In patients with LV impairment, **flecainide** and **propafenone** increase mortality and should not be used.

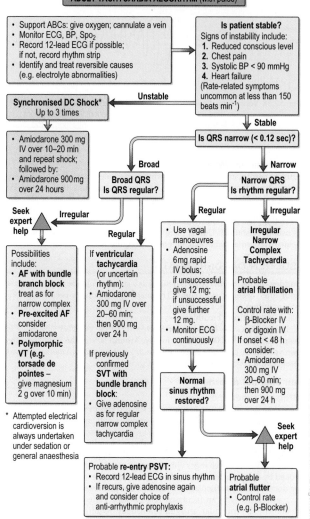

Fig. 12.15 Adult tachycardia algorithm (with pulse). (Reproduced with permission from the Resuscitation Council (http://www.resus.org.uk/siteindex.htm.)

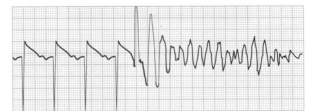

Fig. 12.16 Ventricular fibrillation. Four beats of sinus rhythm are followed by a ventricular ectopic beat that initiates ventricular fibrillation. The ST segment during sinus rhythm is elevated owing to acute myocardial infarction in this case.

Ventricular fibrillation (VF)

This is a cardiac arrest rhythm requiring immediate electrical defibrillation. There are advanced life support treatment algorithms that should be applied (p. 705). The underlying causes are similar to those of VT; the commonest is ischaemic heart disease with previous or acute myocardial infarction. The ECG shows disorganized electrical activity (Fig. 12.16) that is usually sustained. Unless there is an obvious reversible cause, such as acute myocardial ischaemia, all patients require ICD implantation.

SUDDEN CARDIAC DEATH

Sudden cardiac death (SCD) is defined as a sudden collapse within the first hour after onset of symptoms. The majority of patients become unconscious within seconds to minutes. This is sometimes preceded by chest pains, palpitations, breathlessness or generalized weakness.

In the USA, the incidence of SCD is 0.1–0.2% per year and SCD is responsible for 300000 deaths annually. Around 50% of the 700000 deaths per year from coronary heart disease are due to SCD (American Heart Association 2003, *Heart and Stroke Statistical Update*).

Ion channel disorders

Brugada syndrome

This is an inherited cause of idiopathic VF. It is commonest in young males from South-East Asia and classically presents with sudden death during sleep. Other symptoms include dizziness and syncope; some patients remain asymptomatic. In 20% of cases there is a sodium channel mutation (SCN5A) that causes characteristic coved ST segment elevation in ECG leads V1–V3. These changes either are present at baseline or may be provoked by drugs such as **flecainide** or **ajmaline**. In the absence of symptoms or documented ventricular arrhythmias, the presence of ECG changes is not associated with an increased risk of SCD. Patients with syncope or documented ventricular arrhythmias usually require ICD implantation, which improves prognosis.

Long QT syndrome (LQTS)

This is another cause of potentially lethal ventricular arrhythmias in structurally normal hearts and presents with sudden death or syncope. It is characterized by prolongation of the QT interval > 440 msec due to abnormal myocardial repolarization. The underlying causes may be ion channel

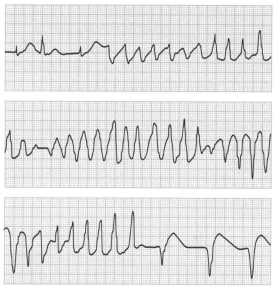

Fig. 12.17 Supraventricular rhythm with a long QT interval giving way to atypical ventricular tachycardia (torsades de pointes). The tachycardia is short-lived and is followed by a brief period of idioventricular rhythm.

mutations, certain drugs and electrolyte disturbances. The prevalence is around 1 in 4000, although it is probably under-diagnosed.

Two major forms of **inherited LQTS** have been described. They are the Romano–Ward and Jervell–Lange–Nielson (JLN) syndromes, which have ion channel mutations. These mutations affect currents generated by sodium or potassium ions. QT prolongation is the result of overloading cells with positive ions during repolarization. They each cause variations in T wave morphology. Some have a normal corrected QT interval (15%) but QT interval prolongation during exercise testing at faster heart rates. Ventricular arrhythmias are usually caused by adrenergic stimuli such as exercise, emotion and loud noises.

The classical VT in LQTS is **torsades de pointes**. This is a polymorphic VT in which the amplitude of the QRS complexes constantly changes around the isoelectric line (Fig. 12.17). This causes palpitations or syncope. Most episodes are self-terminating but SCD results from degeneration into VF.

● **Management.** All patients should undergo echocardiography to exclude any structural abnormality. Secondary causes of QT prolongation from drugs and electrolyte abnormalities should also be excluded (Box 12.4). All patients with confirmed congenital LQTs and family members should undergo genetic screening; mutations are only found in 50%. VT stimulation testing does not appear to be useful for risk stratification.

Box 12.4 Acquired causes of long QT syndrome

Electrolyte abnormalities
- Hypokalaemia, hypomagnesaemia, hypocalcaemia

Drugs
Anti-arrhythmics
- Amiodarone, disopyramide, dofetilide, flecainide, ibutilide, procainamide, propafenone, quinidine, sotalol

Antibiotics/antifungals
- Chloroquine, clarithromycin, erythromycin, fluoroquinolones, itraconazole, ketoconazole, trimethoprim

Antihistamines
- Terfenadine

Others
- Cisapride, domperidone, glibenclamide, tricyclic antidepressants (e.g. amitriptyline), phenothiazines (e.g. chlorpromazine)

- *Inherited LQTS.* The mainstay of treatment is β-blockers and ICD implantation, as well as avoiding competitive sports. Adrenergic effects on the heart may be further reduced by left cervico-thoracic sympathectomy.
- *Acquired LQTS.* This is treated by stopping causative drugs and correcting electrolyte disturbances. **IV magnesium sulphate** 8 mmol over 10–15 min is effective at terminating torsades de pointes. Temporary pacing may also prevent bradycardia and VT.

Cardiomyopathies

SCD is uncommon in hypertrophic cardiomyopathy but is the commonest cause of SCD in young adults (p. 408).

DRUG THERAPY

Anti-arrhythmic drugs are commonly used and work by affecting different components of the cardiac action potential. Consequently, they may precipitate arrhythmias and depress cardiac contractility. The Vaughan Williams classification describes them according to the effect on the action potential (Table 12.4). The use of individual drugs has been outlined in previous sections.

DEVICE THERAPY

Pacing

Pacemakers are commonly used in the treatment of symptomatic bradycardias. Symptoms include syncope, dizziness, breathlessness and reduced exercise capacity. Pacemakers can be either temporary or permanent systems. All pacing systems usually consist of a transvenous endocardial pacing wire and a pacing generator.

- *Temporary systems* usually require a single pacing wire that is introduced aseptically via the internal jugular, subclavian or femoral

Table 12.4 The Vaughan Williams classification of anti-arrhythmic drugs

Class	Examples	Effect on action potential	Ion channels or receptors affected	Used for	Other
I	Na channel blockade				
Ia	Disopyramide, procainamide, quinidine	Slow down phase 0 and lengthen action potential	Sodium channel blockade	Atrial tachycardias, AF, atrial flutter, VT	
Ib	Lidocaine, mexiletene	Slow down phase 0 and shorten action potential	Sodium channel blockade	VT	
Ic	Flecainide, propafenone	Slow down phase 0 and no effect on action potential duration	Sodium channel blockade	Atrial tachycardias, AF, atrial flutter, VT	Avoid in structurally abnormal hearts
II	Beta-blockers except sotalol	Suppress sinus and AV node conduction	Beta-adrenoceptor blockade	Atrial tachycardias, AF, atrial flutter, VT	
III	Amiodarone, dronedarone, sotalol	Lengthen action potential		Atrial tachycardias, AF, atrial flutter, VT	Suitable in structurally abnormal hearts
IV	Verapamil, diltiazem (calcium channel blocker)	Reduce plateau phase and slow AV node conduction	Calcium channel blockade	Atrial flutter, AF, AVNRT	Avoid in WPW syndrome
Other	Digoxin	Slow AV node conduction		Ventricular rate control in atrial flutter, AF, AVNRT	Avoid in WPW syndrome
	Adenosine	Short-acting AV node blockade		Terminating AVNRT, diagnosis of broad-complex tachycardia	Avoid in WPW syndrome and asthma

AF, atrial fibrillation; AVNRT, atrio-ventricular nodal re-entry tachycardia; VT, ventricular tachycardia; WPW, Wolff-Parkinson–White syndrome.

Table 12.5 International pacemaker nomenclature

I Chamber paced	II Chamber sensed	III Response to sensing
O: None	O: None	O: None
A: Atrium	A: Atrium	T: Triggered
V: Ventricle	V: Ventricle	I: Inhibited
D: Dual (A and V)	D: Dual (A and V)	D: Dual (T and I)

DDD and VVI are most commonly used.

veins and positioned within the right ventricle. The pacing generator is an external box. These systems should be left in situ for the least time possible, as there is a significant risk of infection.

- *Permanent systems* can have up to three wires that are usually introduced via the cephalic and/or subclavian veins. They can be positioned within the right atrium, right ventricle and, if indicated, tributaries of the coronary sinus for LV pacing. The pacing generator is a small box containing the pacing/sensing circuitry and a lithium iodine battery that lasts from 4 to 10 years. The system implant requires minor surgery to the pectoral region under local anaesthesia.

- Nomenclature. The basic function of a pacing system is described by a three-letter code that is recognized internationally. The first letter refers to the chamber(s) being paced, the second to the chamber(s) being sensed; the third describes the response to sensing (Table 12.5). **Commonly used pacing modes** include VVI, DDD and DDI.

- Indications. Symptomatic bradycardias can be caused by pathology within the specialized cardiac conduction system. The indications for permanent pacing are summarized in Box 12.5. Emergency temporary pacing is indicated in all haemodynamically unstable patients.

Ventricular mechanical dyssynchrony causes uncoordinated contraction of the different LV segments, thereby compromising ventricular function. This is often present in patients with a QRS duration of at least 130 ms and LBBB.

- Complications
  - *Pacemaker syndrome.* This is seen in patients with VVI pacemakers whose AV nodes conduct retrogradely to the atria. Consequently, every ventricular paced beat causes atrial contraction against a closed AV valve. This leads to dizziness, breathlessness, syncope, fullness in the neck and pounding sensations or fullness in the head. Reducing the pacing rate or implanting an atrial pacing wire restores AV synchrony and relieves symptoms.
  - *Pacemaker-mediated tachycardia.* This is seen with dual chamber pacing modes (VDD, DDD) when a ventricular paced beat is conducted retrogradely to the atria and is sensed by the atrial wire, triggering ventricular pacing again. This can be resolved by extending the post-ventricular atrial refractory period (PVARP) to prevent sensing of the retrograde P wave. Alternatively, the device could be reprogrammed to DDI mode, thereby preventing the ventricular pacing in response to the retrograde P wave.

> *Box 12.5* Indications for pacing
>
> - Sinus node disease (tachycardia-bradycardia syndrome)
> - AV block
>   - Mobitz type 2 (with or without symptoms)
>   - Complete (third-degree)
>   a) AV nodal or infranodal, symptomatic
>   b) AV nodal, asymptomatic with pauses > 3 sec or heart rate < 40 bpm
>   c) Infranodal, asymptomatic
>   d) Post-cardiac surgery (if not resolved by 5–7 days)
>   e) Post-AV node ablation
>   - Bifascicular block + intermittent
>   a) Second-degree block
>   b) Complete (third-degree) block
>   c) Alternating bundle branch block
>   - Trifascicular block + intermittent
>   a) Second-degree block
>   b) Complete (third-degree) block
> - Post-anterior myocardial infarction
>   - Mobitz type 2 block
>   - Complete (third-degree) block
>   - Transient Mobitz type 2 or complete block with bundle branch block
>   - Temporary pacing wire if new bifascicular block (right bundle branch block + left anterior or posterior hemiblock)
> - Post-inferior myocardial infarction
>   - Persistent, symptomatic bradycardia (rare)
>   - Temporary pacing wire if bradycardia-induced hypotension (unresponsive to atropine), ventricular tachycardia or heart failure
> - Sustained pause-dependent ventricular tachycardia
> - Some high-risk congenital long QT syndrome patients

- *Atrial tachycardias.* Any atrial tachycardia (commonly atrial flutter or fibrillation) can cause rapid ventricular pacing and consequent palpitations, dizziness, breathless or syncope. This is resolved by programming the pacemaker to switch pacing mode to VVI above a certain atrial rate or reprogramming to DDI mode (p. 412). Treatment (drugs and/or ablation) should be instituted for the atrial tachycardia.

Biventricular (cardiac resynchronization) pacing

This technique of pacing has been used in patients with severe heart failure to improve symptoms. It is offered to patients with New York Heart Association class 3 or 4 symptoms despite optimal medical therapy, an LV ejection fraction of 35% or less, an LV end-diastolic diameter of at least 55 mm and significant ventricular dyssynchrony.

Implantable cardioverter-defibrillators (ICDs)

These are specialized pacing devices that retain all of the functions of a standard pacemaker but, in addition, have the capacity to recognize and treat ventricular arrhythmias (VT, VF). The treatment modalities include

---

Box 12.6 Permanent indications for ICD implantation
(based on NICE guidelines)

Primary prevention
- Myocardial infarction > 4 weeks ago + LV ejection fraction
  < 35% + non-sustained VT on Holter + positive VT stimulation
  test
- Myocardial infarction > 4 weeks ago + LV ejection fraction
  < 30% + QRS duration ≥ 120 ms
- Familial cardiac conditions with a high risk of sudden death,
  including long QT and Brugada syndromes, HCM and
  arrhythmogenic right ventricular dysplasia (p. 458)
- Non-ischaemic dilated cardiomyopathy + syncope

Secondary prevention
- Survivors of cardiac arrest due to VT or VF
- Sustained VT causing syncope or significant haemodynamic
  compromise
- Sustained VT without syncope or cardiac arrest + LV election
  fraction < 35%

---

ventricular burst pacing at rates exceeding the VT rate (anti-tachycardia pacing, ATP) and shocks (up to 41 J).

The devices consist of endocardial pacing wires as for a standard pacemaker, except for the right ventricular wire. This has one or two shocking coils in addition to the pacing and sensing component. One coil is always inside the right ventricle, with the second in the superior vena cava, although the latter is not mandatory. As with standard pacemakers, ICDs can be single chamber (right ventricle), dual chamber (right atrium and ventricle) and biventricular (for cardiac resynchronization therapy). The ICD generator is larger but still easily implanted in the pectoral region like a standard pacemaker. In addition to the pacing/sensing circuitry there is a lithium silver vanadium oxide battery and capacitors to store charge for the shocks.

ICDs are implanted for both primary and secondary prevention of SCD and are the most effective treatment available at present. The indications are summarized in Box 12.6.

Inappropriate therapies and device failure

Atrial tachycardias may result in inappropriate anti-tachycardia pacing or shocks. The most common problems are due to rapidly conducted AF or atrial flutter. If the ventricular rate encroaches into either the VT or VF therapy zones, the ICD will deliver therapy and may restore sinus rhythm. This problem is prevented by starting an anti-arrhythmic drug such as sotalol or amiodarone to prevent the atrial tachycardia, or by using AV nodal-blocking drugs to prevent excessive ventricular rates. Furthermore, the ICD may be reprogrammed to activate the atrial tachycardia discriminators. Some patients may require an electrophysiology study with a view to ablating the atrial tachycardia.

In some patients, the ICD over-senses the ventricular activity, giving an erroneously fast ventricular rate that may cause inappropriate therapies. This can be due to high T wave voltages, atrial activity, skeletal muscle activity (myopotentials) and noise from electrical appliances, e.g. lead fractures or a loose set screw securing the shocking lead to the generator. Over-sensing of the T wave or atrial activity may be resolved by decreasing the ventricular lead's sensitivity without compromising VF detection. Alternatively, the shocking lead would require repositioning or replacement if fractured.

If the shocking lead becomes displaced or there is excessive fibrosis at the tip compromising electrical contact, the ventricular sensing will be compromised (under-sensing). The most serious consequence is a failure to detect VT or VF so that no therapy is delivered. This problem will usually necessitate a lead revision procedure.

Electrical storm

This is arbitrarily defined as at least three separate episodes of VT or VF within a 24-hour period requiring ICD therapy. Patients usually present with multiple anti-tachycardia pacing (ATP) episodes and/or shocks, which are painful and psychologically distressing.

Typical precipitants are listed in Box 12.7. Not infrequently, there is no obvious cause. The ICD is studied to confirm VT/VF and exclude atrial tachycardias. The treatment of storms is to identify and correct the precipitant and to provide symptomatic relief. If patients are receiving multiple shocks, they should be sedated and given opiates. If the VT can be treated by ATP rather than shocks, the ICD should be reprogrammed appropriately. Patients with a monomorphic VT should also be considered for catheter ablation. The mainstay of drug therapy is **β-blockade**, which may be IV initially, together with **amiodarone** or **mexiletene**. In Brugada syndrome, these drugs may exacerbate the storm and should be avoided if possible. Instead, patients should be started on an **isoprenaline infusion**, and **class Ia drugs** such as **quinidine** have been shown to be effective. If electrical storms fail to abate despite all treatment, general anaesthesia and intra-aortic balloon counterpulsation therapy may be effective.

Appropriate therapies

If patients are repeatedly receiving therapy from the ICD, particularly shocks, the device programming and medications should be reviewed. Recently, there have been reports demonstrating that ATP is very effective for termination of fast VT, where previously a shock would have been delivered. All patients should be assessed for acute heart failure and treated appropriately. As the heart failure progresses, many patients develop slower VTs that may fall outside the VT therapy zone. These are difficult problems to treat, since patients may already be on optimal

---

Box 12.7 Causes of electrical storm

- Electrolyte disturbances — usually from heart failure medications
- Thyrotoxicosis — if already on amiodarone
- Acute heart failure
- Fever
- Acute myocardial ischaemia
- Atrial tachycardia
- Idiopathic

— Kumar & Clark's Medical Management and Therapeutics

medical therapy and ICD reprogramming may lead to inappropriate therapy for sinus tachycardia. Catheter ablation of VT may be considered but remains a high-risk procedure in these patients.

HEART FAILURE

Heart failure results from any structural or functional cardiac disorder that impairs the ability of the heart to function as a 'pump' to support the physiological functions of the body. Its incidence increases with age, rising to > 10% in 65-year-olds. Mortality is 50% 5 years after the diagnosis, despite current therapy.

Causes

Systolic and diastolic ventricular dysfunction usually coexist to cause decreased cardiac output.

● Systolic ventricular dysfunction
  ● This is most commonly due to ischaemic heart disease or hypertension.
  ● The left ventricle is usually dilated and fails to contract forcefully.
● Diastolic ventricular dysfunction. Impaired diastolic ventricular filling is due to:
  ● impaired myocardial relaxation
  ● increased stiffness in the ventricular wall
  ● decreased LV compliance.

Pure diastolic dysfunction is increasingly being recognized, possibly accounting for 30% of patients with heart failure.

Pathophysiology

● Systolic dysfunction arises from a reduction in the number of functioning myocytes, a reduction in the function of each myocyte or an increase in the demand, e.g. anaemia, where an increase in cardiac output is required. It can also arise from or lead to ventricular dilatation and remodelling, e.g. following acute myocardial injury.
● Impaired myocardial relaxation leads to increased diastolic pressure and wall stress.
  ● This increase leads to neurohormonal activation of the renin–angiotensin–aldosterone axis causing sodium and water retention.
  ● B-type natriuretic peptide is released in response to atrial stretch, again causing salt and water retention.
  ● Aldosterone also causes an increase in interstitial fibrosis, reducing the ability of the ventricle to relax.
  ● Activation of the sympathetic system causes tachycardia, increased myocardial oxygen demand and increased peripheral vascular resistance.
  ● Microvascular constriction occurs due to endothelin-related vasoconstriction.
● In valvular disease, regurgitant valves lead to unnecessary repeated ejection of blood from the heart and stenosed valves demand an increased force of contraction to eject the same volume of blood.
● In hypertension, increased wall stress is a stimulus to myocyte hypertrophy and thus ventricular hypertrophy. Hypertrophied ventricles relax poorly and contribute to the diastolic component of heart failure.

Clinical syndromes of heart failure

Symptoms depend on how rapidly the heart decompensates, the age and co-morbidities of the patient, and the aetiology of the failure.

- Acute heart failure (acute pulmonary oedema or cardiogenic shock, p. 443). This is usually seen after an acute myocardial infarction, a rupture of the interventricular septum or an acute valvular regurgitation.
- Chronic heart failure develops more insidiously and is often punctuated by episodes of acute heart failure.
- Left heart failure is caused by ischaemic heart disease (IHD) (commonest), systemic hypertension, mitral and aortic valve disease, and cardiomyopathies.
- Right heart failure occurs with left heart failure, chronic lung disease (cor pulmonale), pulmonary embolism (PE), pulmonary hypertension, right to left shunts, isolated right ventricular cardiomyopathy and mitral valve disease with pulmonary hypertension.

Symptoms of heart failure

(See New York Heart Association classification, Table 12.6.)

- Fatigue.
- Exertional dyspnoea.
- Orthopnoea.
- Paroxysmal nocturnal dyspnoea (PND).

Signs of heart failure

- Cardiomegaly.
- Third or fourth heart sounds.
- Tachycardia (gallop rhythm).
- Bi-basal crackles.
- Pleural effusion (transudate).
- Peripheral oedema with or without ascites.
- Smooth, tender, enlarged (and sometimes pulsatile) liver.

Table 12.6 New York Heart Association (NYHA) classification of heart failure with therapy

NYHA class	Essential drugs to improve prognosis			Optional for symptoms	
I No limitation of physical activity	ACE inhibitors/ ARB if ACE-intolerant			Thiazide or loop diuretic	
II Slight limitation of physical activity		Beta-blockers			
III Marked limitation of physical activity			Aldosterone antagonist	Thiazide and loop diuretic	Digoxin
IV Inability to carry out physical activity					

ACE, angiotensin-converting enzyme; ARB, angiotensin receptor blocker.

Objective evidence, e.g. an echo, is required for diagnosis and management of the cause.

Diagnosis

- **ECG.** When a patient presents with symptoms suggestive of heart failure, a normal 12-lead ECG excludes almost all cases of heart failure. It has a sensitivity of around 90% and a positive predictive value of 20–30%.
- **CXR.** The cardio-thoracic ratio is increased; signs of pulmonary venous congestion, fluid overload or pleural effusions are present.
- **Natriuretic peptides.** A normal serum B-type natriuretic peptide (BNP) and NT-pro BNP in combination with a normal ECG excludes the vast majority of cases of heart failure. A serum BNP < 100 pg/mL excludes heart failure as a cause of breathlessness, while > 500 pg/mL makes heart failure very likely.
- **Other blood tests.** These include U&E, calcium, fasting blood glucose, liver biochemistry, fasting lipid profile, FBC, thyroid function tests, ESR and CRP, auto-antibodies, iron studies, selenium level, serum amyloid and viral screen (Coxsackie, enterovirus, HIV).
- **Transthoracic echocardiography (TTE).** Two-dimensional and Doppler echocardiography are the diagnostic and quantitative tests of choice in suspected heart failure.
  - Ventricular function can be measured in a variety of ways from the simple inner dimensions of the ventricles to the ejection fraction, relaxation, ventricular wall thickness and systolic thickening. An ejection fraction of < 0.45 is good evidence of systolic dysfunction.
  - Stress echocardiography is useful to detect ischaemia as a cause of reversible heart failure. It assesses the viability of dysfunctional myocardium; dobutamine infusion identifies the contractile reserve in stunned or hibernating myocardium (p. 424).
- **Nuclear cardiology.** Radionuclide angiography (RNA) provides accurate measurements of left (and to a lesser extent, right) ventricular function, cardiac volumes and regional wall motion.
  - *Single photon-emission computed tomography (SPECT)* can be used at rest or during stress (e.g. dobutamine infusion) with different radionuclides (e.g. ^{20}thallium or ^{99m}technetium) to detect ischaemia.
  - *Positron emission tomography (PET)* uses a marker of metabolism (^{18}FDG) and combines this with a measure of perfusion. It can detect glycolytic activity and therefore distinguishes viable, non-perfused muscle from non-viable, non-perfused muscle. It helps detect the reversibility of cardiac damage, in particular if revascularization may improve cardiac function by reawakening hibernating myocardium.
  - *Cardiac MRI (CMR)* allows accurate measurements of cardiac volumes, wall thickness and LV mass. The use of dobutamine (for contractile reserve) or gadolinium (for delayed enhancement) helps assess viability of myocardium.
  - *Cardiac catheterization* is used for the diagnosis of IHD (and suitability for revascularization). Measurement of pulmonary artery pressure, left atrial (wedge) pressure and LV end-diastolic pressure can be made.
  - *Holter (24-hour ambulatory ECG) monitoring* excludes the presence of asymptomatic non-sustained ventricular tachycardia where

ejection fraction is < 35% and the patient does not have symptoms of heart failure at rest. If VT is present, there is evidence to support the insertion of an ICD.

Management

Lifestyle

Patients and their family should be counselled and education given on healthy lifestyles, including weight/obesity control, exercise and diet.

- **Smoking.** The patient should stop.
- **Exercise.** Exertional breathlessness is not solely related to the lack of cardiac reserve but also to the lung function and skeletal muscle function of the patient. Patients should join cardiac rehabilitation programmes when their heart failure is stable. Bed rest is recommended for a short time because of its effect on reducing renin–angiotensin activation, when in acute heart failure.
- **Diet.** A healthy diet should be recommended to everyone. Salt intake should be reduced, with the patient avoiding foods rich in salt, and not adding salt during cooking or at the table. Fluid restriction is only necessary in severe heart failure. Alcohol acts as a diuretic but its effect on the myocardium is generally deleterious, with the possibility of developing alcoholic cardiomyopathy.
- **Weight loss.** Losing weight reduces disability by increasing mobility for the same effort. The direct cardiac effects include reduced systemic vascular resistance.

Pharmacological (Tables 12.6 and 12.7)

- Diuretics
  - *Loop diuretics.* These are effective for fluid retention. In general, the principle is to use the minimum effective dose. Where more diuresis is required, increases in doses can later be accompanied by another class of diuretic (thiazide or metolazone) or a twice-daily dose. The diuresis lasts several hours (≥ 6) and the drugs are best taken in the morning to avoid nocturia.

    Side-effects include hypotension, hyponatraemia, hypokalaemia and hypomagnesaemia (both of the latter can lead to QTc prolongation), renal impairment, hyperuricaemia and worsening control of diabetes mellitus.
  - *Thiazides.* With the exception of metolazone, these diuretics are not as effective as loop diuretics in producing a diuresis. However, they act synergistically in combination with loop diuretics and are therefore useful where further diuresis is required despite adequate doses of these drugs.

    Side-effects are similar, with hyponatraemia, hypokalaemia, hypomagnesaemia, hyperuricaemia and worsening control of diabetes mellitus.
- **ACE inhibitors.** These improve prognosis in terms of both mortality and reduced hospitalizations, as well as improving symptoms.
  - Initiating ACE inhibitors is a priority for any patient with heart failure but monitoring of serum U&E is essential before and after initiation of treatment and 5–7 days after every increase in dose. Deterioration in renal biochemistry is likely if there is underlying renal impairment but the benefits of ACE inhibition in these circumstances are likely to be greater, provided acute kidney injury can be avoided.

Table 12.7 Drugs available for the treatment of heart failure

	Starting dose (daily)	Maximum dose (daily)
Loop diuretics Furosemide	20–40 mg	250–500 mg
Bumetanide	0.5–1 mg	5–10 mg
Torasemide	5.0 mg	40 mg
Thiazide diuretics Bendroflumethiazide	2.5 mg	10 mg
Chlortalidone	25 mg	200 mg
Metolazone	2.5 mg	10 mg
Angiotensin-converting enzyme (ACE) inhibitors Captopril	6.25 mg 3 times daily	50 mg 3 times daily
Enalapril	2.5 mg	10–20 mg twice daily
Lisinopril	2.5–5.0 mg	30–35 mg
Perindopril	2 mg	4 mg
Ramipril	1.25 mg	10 mg
Angiotensin II receptor antagonists (ARBs) Candesartan	4 mg	32 mg
Valsartan	20 mg twice daily	160 mg twice daily
Beta-adrenoreceptor blocking drugs Carvedilol	3.125 mg twice daily	25-50 mg twice daily
Bisoprolol	1.25 mg	10 mg
Nebivolol	1.25 mg	10 mg
Aldosterone antagonists Spironolactone	12.5–25 mg	50–200 mg
Eplerenone	25 mg	50 mg
Cardiac glycoside Digoxin	Loading dose: 375–1500 mcg in divided doses over 24 hours	Maintenance dose: 62.5–500 mcg once daily with serum concentration $\geq$ 6 hrs post-dose of $\leq$ 2 ng/mL

- If creatinine rises to more than 50% of the baseline or to more than 200 µmol/L, stop all other nephrotoxic drugs and reduce the dose of ACE inhibitor. This may be an indicator of the presence of renal artery stenosis (p. 346). If the rise is more than 100% of baseline creatinine or above 350 µmol/L, stop the ACE inhibitor.
- A rise in serum potassium is common and is made worse by the concomitant use of potassium-sparing diuretics. Stop the ACE inhibitor when the serum K^+ is $\geq$ 6.0 mmol/L; a serum potassium $\geq$ 6.5 needs urgent treatment (p. 711).

- When starting, use a small dose to allow for the possibility of a hypotensive response. Doses can then be doubled at 2-weekly intervals until a target dose is reached or adverse side-effects occur. If symptomatic hypotension supervenes, reduce the dose to the previous step. Other drugs that cause hypotension should be stopped to allow the maximum tolerated dose of ACE inhibitor.
- ACE inhibitors also increase the levels of bradykinin; this may help to explain a beneficial effect of these drugs over angiotensin receptor blockers, which are more specific for renin–angiotensin. Unfortunately, it also explains the increased incidence of dry cough (15%) in patients receiving ACE inhibitors, which is bradykinin-mediated.
- ACE inhibitors are the most effective drugs for heart failure and should always be prescribed if possible.

- **Angiotensin receptor blockers (ARBs).** These offer a theoretical advantage over ACE inhibitors because they do not increase the bradykinin levels, as seen with ACE inhibitors, so there is no troublesome cough. As there is no additional benefit over ACE inhibitors, ARBs are only recommended as a substitute to ACE inhibitors when cough is intolerable.

- **Beta-adrenoreceptor blockers (β-blockers).** Large RCTs have found benefit in patients treated with these drugs, including a decrease in mortality and hospitalization. There are no data to recommend one drug over the other and their clinical use is similar. Trials have used them as additional drugs to baseline diuretics and ACE inhibitors; the best results are seen in those with NYHA class III–IV symptoms. Start at a low dose and titrate upwards. Patients may experience transient fatigue, increased fluid retention and hypotension, with symptomatic improvement only occurring after several weeks. Dose titration may be aided by increased diuretic use if fluid retention is a problem. Bradycardia may be due to heart block, and a 12-lead ECG before and after initiating therapy will reveal any AV blockade. First-degree heart block need not preclude the use of β-blockers but in higher degrees of heart block, β-blockers are not usually used.

- **Aldosterone antagonists**
  - *Spironolactone.* The addition of a low (sub-diuretic) 25 mg dose of spironolactone to ACE inhibitors, diuretics and β-blockers in cases of NYHA III–IV heart failure reduces mortality due to sudden death and due to heart failure. There is a significant risk of hyperkalaemia and renal dysfunction with this combination and monitoring is essential, starting before administration and continuing 5–7 days after commencing the drug. The trial evidence is based on a population with baseline creatinine ≤ 250 μmol/L, and if serum K^+ rises to a threshold of 5.5 mmol/L, the dose should be halved and stopped if it goes over this.

    Side-effects other than hyperkalaemia include gynaecomastia, which may be painful in up to 10% of patients taking the drug.
  - *Eplerenone* This is a more selective **aldosterone receptor antagonist**, which avoids the side-effect of gynaecomastia seen with spironolactone. It has been shown to be effective in patients with an ejection fraction ≤ 0.4 post myocardial infarction, with clinical signs of pulmonary congestion or radiographic evidence of this. It has not been

shown to be effective in chronic heart failure or heart failure due to non-infarction-related causes.

- **Digoxin.** Digoxin has a positive inotropic effect and has been shown to improve symptoms of heart failure and to reduce the frequency of hospital admission due to heart failure, but it has no effect on mortality. In addition to this, its negative chronotropic effect and potential nephrotoxic effects may prevent adequate therapy with other, more effective drugs. Digoxin is therefore mainly used in patients who require rate control for AF where β-blockade does not produce the desired rate reduction at rest. It is also used in treatment-resistant cases. The risk of toxicity increases with hypokalaemia and pre-existing renal dysfunction. There are numerous potential drug interactions and the manifestations of toxicity include anorexia and fatigue. These may lead on to AV block, VT, atrial tachycardia and accelerated junctional rhythm associated with AF. Chronic use is also associated with gynaecomastia and down-sloping ST segment depression on ECG. Co-prescription with maximal therapy with ACE inhibitors, β-adrenergic blockers, diuretics and spironolactone has been studied and may offer additional benefits in patients with NYHA class III–IV heart failure.

    Side-effects are hypotension, hyperkalaemia and renal impairment similar to those seen with ACE inhibitors.

- **Warfarin.** Although there is an excess of thromboembolic events in the heart failure population, risk stratification is difficult and the risks of warfarinization over a lifetime of heart failure is significant. In the presence of AF or a prior thromboembolic event and heart failure, long-term anticoagulation is beneficial. In addition, in the acute stages of ventricular thrombus or aneurysm, anticoagulation is indicated. There is little evidence otherwise to support its continuation and most protocols recommend cessation after 6 months' therapy.

- **Vasodilators.** Owing to the superiority of ACE inhibitors and ARBs, **nitrates** should only be used when the former classes are contraindicated. However, when used at a relatively high dose, they are effective in reducing mortality due to heart failure. Oral nitrates in combination with conventional therapy for heart failure can sometimes be helpful in symptomatic relief of breathlessness. Examples include isosorbide mononitrate 20–40 mg 3 times daily.

- **Aspirin.** Aspirin 75 mg is recommended where atherosclerotic disease and heart failure coexist.

- **Statins.** These are used in patients with ischaemic heart disease.

- **Ivabradine.** This inhibits the I_F channels in the sino-atrial node. It slows the heart rate and may be beneficial in heart failure.

- **Drugs to avoid or stop:**
    - *Calcium channel blockers,* such as diltiazem and verapamil, are negatively inotropic and promote fluid retention; they should be avoided if possible.
    - *Alpha-adrenergic blockers* similarly showed a lack of benefit in heart failure and may lead to an excess of heart failure in patients treated for hypertension.
    - *Class I anti-arrhythmic drugs* have been shown to increase the incidence of life-threatening arrhythmia in heart failure and also lower BP; they should be avoided.

- *NSAIDs,* including COX-II inhibitors, promote fluid retention and have been shown to increase the incidence of cardiac events.
- *Positive inotropes,* such as dobutamine, have been used in acute exacerbations of heart failure in order to support a low BP and increase cardiac output at the cost of increasing cardiac oxygen consumption and ventricular arrhythmia. They are therefore not recommended for routine use and should only be given if a more definitive treatment is awaited (e.g. reperfusion therapy) or if there is a clear exacerbation of heart failure.

Devices

The drug treatment of each patient should be optimized and all reversible ischaemia managed by revascularization.

- **Cardiac resynchronization therapy (CRT) (biventricular pacing).** An LBBB causes an interventricular conduction delay. This 'block' allows the septum to contract along with the right ventricle and the left ventricle, then contract as the septum is relaxing. This causes loss of a major contribution to ventricular function. To overcome this, pacing is required (p. 410).
- **ICDs.** Combining CRT with an ICD improves survival by preventing sudden death due to ventricular arrhythmia (p. 405).
- **Ventricular assist devices.** These are reserved for patients on maximal medical therapy but with severe intractable symptoms and awaiting transplant. These devices have a high incidence of infective and thrombotic side-effects but can provide some patients with support. They obviate the need for a transplant in some patients with reversible cardiomyopathies (e.g. peripartum cardiomyopathy and viral myocarditis).
- **Heart transplantation.** This is the treatment of choice for younger patients with severe intractable heart failure and a life expectancy of < 6 months. The median survival of recipients is 9 years. However, the demanding nature of follow-up and limited number of donors have meant that stringent selection criteria are applied to recipients in order to ensure the most effective use of the organs available to the people most likely to benefit. Absolute contraindications include life-threatening medical conditions likely to cause death within 5 years, age over 60 years, a history of non-concordance with drug therapy and severe mental ill health.

DIASTOLIC HEART FAILURE

The prevalence of this is unclear because of differing criteria for diagnosis and thus there is a lack of definitive trials showing a mortality benefit of any drug. The uncontentious criteria are symptoms of congestive heart failure and evidence of abnormal LV relaxation, filling, diastolic distensibility or diastolic stiffness with normal LV function on echocardiography. Diastolic heart failure has an estimated annual mortality of 5–8%. The cause and associated conditions, such as hypertension, ischaemia or diabetes or any other cause of LV hypertrophy, should be ascertained. Fluid retention may respond to cautious use of diuretics but high diastolic filling pressures are needed to maintain filling in stiff ventricles.

ACUTE HEART FAILURE

Acute heart failure (AHF) occurs with the rapid onset of symptoms and signs of heart failure secondary to abnormal cardiac function, causing

Kumar & Clark's Medical Management and Therapeutics

elevated cardiac filling pressures. This leads to severe dyspnoea as fluid accumulates in the interstitial and alveolar spaces of the lung (pulmonary oedema). AHF has a poor prognosis, with a 60-day mortality rate of nearly 10% and a rate of death or rehospitalization of 35% within 60 days. In patients with **acute pulmonary oedema** the in-hospital mortality rate is 12% and by 12 months this rises to 30%. Poor prognostic indicators include a high (≥ 16 mmHg) pulmonary capillary wedge pressure (PCWP), low serum sodium concentration, increased LV end-diastolic dimension on echo and low oxygen consumption.

The aetiology of AHF is similar to chronic heart failure.

- Patients with ischaemic heart disease present with an acute coronary syndrome or develop a complication of a myocardial infarct, e.g. papillary muscle rupture or ventricular septal defect requiring surgical intervention.
- Patients with valvular heart disease also present with AHF due to valvular regurgitation in endocarditis or prosthetic valve thrombosis. A thoracic aortic dissection may produce severe aortic regurgitation.
- Patients with hypertension present with episodes of flash pulmonary oedema despite preserved LV systolic function.
- In both acute and chronic kidney disease fluid overload and a reduced renal excretion will produce pulmonary oedema.
- Atrial fibrillation is frequently associated with AHF and may require emergency cardioversion.

Several clinical syndromes of AHF can be defined (Table 12.8). In a clinical environment both the Killip score (based on a cardio-respiratory clinical assessment) and the Forrester classification (based on right heart catheterization findings) are used to provide therapeutic and prognostic information.

Pathophysiology

The pathophysiology of AHF is similar to that of chronic heart failure with activation of the renin–angiotensin–aldosterone axis and sympathetic nervous system. In addition, prolonged ischaemia (e.g. in acute coronary syndromes) results in *myocardial stunning* that exacerbates myocardial dysfunction but may respond to inotropic support. If myocardial ischaemia persists, the myocardium may exhibit hibernation (persistently impaired function due to reduced coronary blood flow), which may recover with successful revascularization.

Diagnosis

- **CXR.** This is required to confirm the presence of pulmonary oedema. Typically, there will be distended upper lobe pulmonary veins with septal lines and diffuse shadowing in a perihilar distribution. The cardio-thoracic ratio will be increased if there is pre-existing heart failure. Other causes of breathlessness may be apparent on the CXR.
- **ECG.** This is needed to assess cardiac rhythm, potential acute coronary syndromes, myocarditis, cardiomyopathy, evidence of LV hypertrophy or RV strain.
- **TTE.** TTE in patients without a prior diagnosis of cardiac disease assesses valve function, chamber size and function, and pulmonary arterial pressures.
- **Routine blood tests.** These include FBC, U&E, glucose, LFTs, troponin and/or creatine kinase (CK-MB). Measure ABGs if there is severe heart

Table 12.8 Clinical presentation of acute heart failure

Range of presentations	Signs and symptoms	Criteria
Mild acute decompensated heart failure	Mild signs and symptoms of AHF	Does not fulfil criteria for cardiogenic shock, pulmonary oedema or hypertensive crisis
Hypertensive acute heart failure	Signs and symptoms of heart failure are accompanied by high BP	High BP, CXR evidence of pulmonary oedema, relatively preserved LV function
Pulmonary oedema	Severe respiratory distress, with basal lung crackles and orthopnoea	O_2 saturation < 90% on room air prior to treatment and CXR evidence of pulmonary oedema
Cardiogenic shock	Low BP, tachycardia, cool peripheries, pulmonary oedema, oliguria and/or altered mental state	Systolic BP < 90 mmHg, reduction of MAP (> 30 mmHg) ± oliguria (< 0.5 mL/kg/hour), pulse rate > 90 bpm
High-output failure	High heart rate with warm peripheries, pulmonary congestion, and sometimes low BP as in septic shock	High cardiac output, warm peripheries, tachycardia and pulmonary congestion
Right heart failure	Raised JVP, hepatomegaly, peripheral oedema, ascites and hypotension	

MAP, mean arterial pressure.
(Adapted from Nieminen et al 2005)

failure, and D-dimer if there is a high suspicion of PE and no history suggestive of sepsis.
- **Plasma BNP.** Levels > 100 pg/mL indicates heart failure.
- **Cardiac catheterization.** Contrast given during angiography exerts an additional fluid load and may worsen acute heart failure, but cardiogenic shock and AHF secondary to acute coronary syndromes can be improved by emergency revascularization; this can be facilitated by intra-aortic balloon pump (IABP) support if necessary.

Treatment
The goals of treatment in a patient with AHF include:
- short-term benefits:
  - the immediate relief of symptoms
  - stabilization of haemodynamics

- long-term benefits:
  - reduction in length of hospital stay and hospital readmissions
  - reduction in mortality from heart failure.

Patients with AHF should be managed in a high-care area with regular measurements of temperature, heart rate and BP, and cardiac monitoring. All patients require prophylactic anticoagulation with low molecular weight heparin (LMWH), e.g. **enoxaparin** 1 mg/kg SC daily or an antithrombin, e.g. dabigatram 220 mg daily.

Patients with haemodynamic compromise may require arterial lines (invasive BP monitoring and ABGs), central venous cannulation (IV medication, inotropic support, monitoring of CVP) and pulmonary artery cannulation (calculation of cardiac output/index/peripheral vasoconstriction/pulmonary wedge pressure).

- Initial therapy (Box 12.8) includes **oxygen**, **diuretics** and **vasodilator therapy** (Table 12.9) if the BP is maintained (systolic > 85 mmHg).
- Inotropic support (Table 12.10) with **dobutamine**, **phosphodiesterase inhibitors** or **levosimendan** (or nesiritide in the USA) can be added in patients who do not respond to the initial therapy (Fig. 12.18).

> ### Box 12.8 Treatment of acute heart failure
>
> - Oxygen 60% via face mask
> - Diuretic, e.g. furosemide 20–50 mg by slow IV injection, venodilates with reduction in preload and reduction in pulmonary congestion
> - Morphine 5–10 mg IV (depending on size of patient), with an antiemetic, e.g. metoclopramide 10 mg IV, relieves anxiety and causes systemic vasodilatation
> - Glyceryl trinitrate IV infusion 10–200 mcg/min venodilates and reduces preload

---

Table 12.9 Indications and dosing of IV vasodilators in acute heart failure

Vasodilator	Indication	Dosing	Main side-effects	Other
Nitroglycerine	Pulmonary congestion/ oedema BP > 90 mmHg	Start 10–20 mcg/min, increase up to 200 mcg/min	Hypotension, headache	Tolerance on continuous use
Isosorbide dinitrate	Pulmonary congestion/ oedema BP > 90 mmHg	Start with 1 mg/hour, increase up to 10 mg/hour	Hypotension, headache	Tolerance on continuous use
Nitroprusside	Hypertensive heart failure congestion/ oedema BP > 90 mmHg	Start with 0.3 mcg/kg/ min, increase up to 5 mcg/ kg/min	Hypotension, isocyanate toxicity	Light-sensitivity

(Dickstein et al 2008, with permission)

Table 12.10 Dosing of positive inotropic agents in acute heart failure

	Bolus	Infusion rate
Dobutamine	No	2–20 mcg/kg/min (β+)
Dopamine	No	< 3 mcg/kg/min: renal effect (δ+) 3–5 mcg/kg/min: inotropic (β+) > 5 mcg/kg/min: (β+), vasopressor (α+)
Milrinone	25–75 mcg/kg over 10–20 mins	0.375–0.75 mcg/kg/min
Enoximone	0.25–0.75 mg/kg	1.25–7.5 mcg/kg/min
Levosimendan*	12 mcg/kg over 10 mins (optional)†	0.1 mcg/kg/min, which can be decreased to 0.05 or increased to 0.2 mcg/kg/min
Noradrenaline (norepinephrine)	No	0.2–1.0 mcg/kg/min
Adrenaline (epinephrine)	Bolus: 1 mg can be given IV during resuscitation, repeated every 3–5 mins	0.05–0.5 mcg/kg/min

*This agent also has vasodilator properties.
†In hypotensive patients (systolic BP < 100 mmHg) initiation of therapy without a bolus is recommended.
(Dickstein et al 2008, with permission)

- Patients with profound hypotension may require inotropes and vasopressors to improve the haemodynamic status and alleviate symptoms but these agents have not been shown to improve mortality.
- Further therapy with non-invasive ventilation − CPAP/NIPPV (p. 542) − may be needed to improve oxygen saturation and reduction in the work of breathing. Mechanistic therapy may also be required (see below).
- New therapies include **relaxin**, a naturally occurring hormone, which has been used with success in heart failure.

Mechanical assist devices

Mechanical assist devices can be used in patients failing to respond to standard medical therapy but in whom there is either transient myocardial dysfunction with likelihood of recovery (e.g. post anterior myocardial infarction treated with coronary angioplasty) or as a bridge to cardiac surgery including transplantation.

Ventricular assist devices (VADs)

VADs are mechanical devices that replace or help the failing ventricles in delivering blood around the body. The left ventricular assist device (LVAD) receives blood from the left ventricle and delivers it to the aorta;

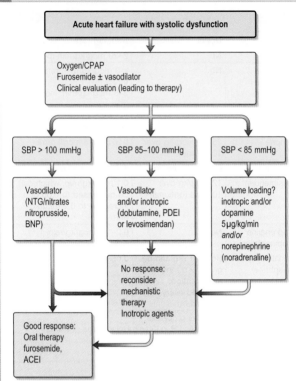

Fig. 12.18 Algorithm for the management of acute heart failure with systolic dysfunction.

ACEI, angiotensin-converting enzyme inhibitor; BNP, brain natriuretic peptide; CPAP, continuous positive airway pressure; NTG, nitroglycerine (glyceryl trinitrate); PDEI, phosphodiesterase inhibitor; SBP, systolic blood pressure (Nieminen et al 2005, with permission).

the right ventricular assist device (RVAD) receives blood from the right ventricle and delivers it to the pulmonary artery. The devices can be extra-corporeal (suitable for short-term support) or intracorporeal (suitable for long-term support as a bridge to transplantation or as destination therapy in patients with end-stage heart failure who are not candidates for trans-plantation). The main problems with VADs include thromboembolism, bleeding, infection and device malfunction.

CORONARY ARTERY DISEASE

Epidemiology

Cardiovascular disease (CVD) is the leading cause of death in many parts of the world.

Approximately 50% of CVD deaths are from coronary artery disease (CAD). CAD is the most common cause of death in men under the age of 75 and the second most common cause of death in women under the age of 75.

Risk factors

Several risk factors for developing CAD have been well established, through numerous large epidemiological studies. These can be divided into non-modifiable and modifiable risk factors.

- Non-modifiable risk factors
  - *Age.* This is a major risk factor for atherosclerosis. While fatty streaks can be found in teenagers, the volume of atheromatous plaques increases with age, and thus the risk of CAD. Using intravascular ultrasonography (IVUS) plaques are detectable in one-third of healthy people aged 20–29 who have no evidence of CAD on angiography.
  - *Gender.* Pre-menopausal women have a lower incidence of CAD than age-matched men. After the menopause the incidence of CAD in women approaches that of men, suggesting a potential protective role of oestrogen. However, there is no evidence that hormone replacement therapy reduces the risk and isolated oestrogen replacement can increase cardiovascular events.
  - *Family history.* The genetics of CAD are complex and polygenic. Having a first-degree relative who has developed CAD before the age of 50 in men and 55 years in women is an accepted risk factor for CAD.
- Modifiable risk factors
  - *Cigarette smoking.* Both smokers and those exposed to environmental smoke (passive smoking) are at an increased risk of CAD. Smoking acts synergistically with other risk factors. It is probably the most significant modifiable factor. The risk from smoking declines to almost normal after 10 years of abstention.
  - *Diabetes.* Type 1 and type 2 diabetes, an abnormal glucose tolerance test or a raised fasting glucose, are associated with an increased risk of CAD.
  - *Metabolic syndrome.* This consists of visceral obesity, dyslipidaemia, hyperglycaemia, insulin resistance and hypertension.
  - *Dyslipidaemia.* Raised levels of low-density lipoprotein (LDL) and reduced levels of high-density lipoprotein (HDL) are well-established risk factors. In addition, elevated triglyceride levels are an independent risk factor.
  - *Hypertension.* The level of hypertension (both systolic and diastolic) is associated with a linear increased risk of CAD. Hypertension is often asymptomatic and therefore clinically 'silent'. It should be measured regularly in patients above 55 years.
  - *Obesity.* The body mass index (BMI) is used to measure obesity and the risk of CAD is correlated with an increasing BMI. Patients should aim for a BMI of < 25. There has been an increasing recognition that

central obesity (due to visceral fat) is a risk factor for CAD. Central obesity is detected by a high waist to hip ratio and this is probably a more reliable marker of obesity than BMI.

- *Physical activity.* Lack of physical activity is now an established risk factor for CAD and a contributor to other risk factors, e.g. obesity and diabetes. Regular physical exercise (30 mins exercise of moderate intensity 5 or more days per week) protects against the development of CAD.
- *Alcohol.* A high intake of alcohol is associated with an increased risk of CAD. Moderate alcohol intake (2–4 U/day) may be associated with a reduced risk of CAD.
- *C-reactive protein (CRP).* There is evidence that a raised CRP is a risk factor, although there has been recent controversy. The exact mechanisms have not been fully elucidated. The high-sensitivity CRP (hs-CRP) assay has been shown to be useful in refining the level of risk in those already known to be at an increased risk of CAD.
- *Coagulation factors.* Factor VII polymorphisms, high serum fibrinogen and raised homocysteine levels have all been shown to be independent risk factors for CAD.
- *Diets.* Diets low in fresh fruit and vegetables, as well as low polyunsaturated fatty acids, are associated with increased risks.

DEFINITIONS AND SPECTRUM OF DISEASE

CAD causes a spectrum of disease from atherosclerotic plaques not limiting flow, to fibrotic, organized, flow-limiting atherosclerotic plaques.

- **Chronic stable angina** is due to flow-limiting lesions that restrict coronary blood flow.
- **Acute coronary syndromes (ACS)** occur when a plaque ruptures and a thrombus forms, which may result in myocardial necrosis (myocardial infarction). In order to diagnose an acute, evolving or recent myocardial infarction (MI), one of the following criteria must be fulfilled:
  - a typical rise and/or fall in markers of myocardial necrosis (preferably troponin) above the 99th centile of the upper limit of normal (p. 431) with at least one of the following:
    - a) ischaemic symptoms
    - b) development of pathological Q waves on the ECG
    - c) ECG changes indicative of new ischaemia (new ST–T changes or LBBB)
    - d) other imaging showing new loss of viable myocardium or new regional wall motion abnormality.
  - abnormal findings on ECG of an acute MI
  - For the definition of an MI following percutaneous coronary intervention (PCI) a cutoff of 3 times the 99th centile of the upper limit of normal is used.

This **definition** of MI is based on the European Society of Cardiology (ECS) and American College of Cardiology consensus statement from 2007. As a result, many more patients are now diagnosed as having had an MI, especially those who have had intervention.

- **STEMI, NSTEMI and unstable angina (UA).** MI is classified according to the ECG changes as either ST elevation myocardial infarction (STEMI) or non-ST elevation myocardial infarction (NSTEMI). This dictates subsequent management. UA differs from NSTEMI, in that there is no elevation in the serum markers. However, initially NSTEMI and UA may be indistinguishable; increased markers of necrosis may not be detectable for hours, as ischaemia needs to be severe enough in NSTEMI to cause sufficient myocardial damage to produce measurable quantities of markers, e.g. troponins, creatine kinase (CK-MB).

The new highly sensitive troponin assays have changed the above definitions and more patients are being diagnosed as having an M1.

Clinical features

- Ischaemic cardiac chest pain (angina) is most often described as a heavy central chest pain that classically radiates to the arm(s), neck and/or jaw.
- Angina may be atypical in nature (e.g. epigastric pain with inferior ischaemia) or may be asymptomatic, e.g. in diabetics. In diabetics shortness of breath on exertion may well be due to myocardial ischaemia.
- Unprovoked angina at rest lasting more than 20 mins or crescendo angina is typical of an ACS.
- The pain in ACS is often associated with autonomic symptoms (nausea, vomiting and sweating).
- The symptoms of gastro-oesophageal reflux may be indistinguishable from ischaemic pain.
- Examination may reveal no abnormalities but it is essential to rule out cardiac failure, cardiac dysfunction and other coexisting diagnoses.

Investigations

Twelve-lead ECG

This must be performed in any patient with suspected CAD.

- A baseline ECG is always helpful but it may be normal or only show minor changes.
- ECGs should be repeated every 10–15 mins in any patients with suspected ACS or if pain worsens or recurs.
- A right-sided lead (V_2R) should be recorded in patients with suspected right-sided infarcts.

Biochemical serum markers of myocardial damage

- **Troponins.** Troponins are the most commonly used markers of myocardial necrosis.
  - Either cardiac-specific troponin T or I is used; both are highly specific and sensitive for cardiac damage. They rise ~3–12 hours after an MI, peak at 24–48 hours and gradually decrease over a week. The new troponin assays are much quicker and more sensitive but some specificity is lost.
  - In patients with suspected ACS troponin should be measured on admission and 12 hours afterwards.
  - A raised troponin is a marker of myocardial ischaemia, of which there are many other causes (e.g. massive PE) and the troponin value should be used in conjunction with other findings to make a clinical diagnosis.
  - Troponins are useful for predicting prognosis (the increase in level is directly proportional to the risk of cardiac death), stratifying risk (p. 440) and guiding further management in ACS.

- Creatine kinase (CK-MB)
  - CK-MB is the proportion of the total CK released from the myocardium and therefore a marker of myocardial injury. It rises 3–12 hours after an MI, peaks around 24 hours and rapidly returns to normal in 48–72 hours.
  - CK-MB is less sensitive and specific than cardiac troponins and therefore tends not to be used as a first-line marker of myocardial damage.
  - CK-MB is often used for the diagnosis of MI caused by PCI.
- Other markers. Serum myoglobin rises early (2 hours) after an MI but is not cardiac-specific as it is also raised in end-stage renal disease. Heart-fatty acid binding protein (H-FABP) is another early marker of myocardial damage.

Imaging

- Coronary angiography. This is the gold standard for assessing the coronary arteries and identifying atherosclerotic lesions. Elective angiography is a very safe procedure with a combined risk of death, MI or stroke of < 0.1%. Indications include patients with a positive exercise test with angina, all NSTEMI ACS, patients who have had an MI revascularization with a positive stress test and those who have survived a sudden cardiac arrest. The timing will depend on the clinical scenario. Angiography allows identification of lesions that need revascularization (percutaneous or bypass graft surgery) and provides useful prognostic information.
- Additional tools. Additional tools, including IVUS and/or pressure wire, can be of great use in assessing functional implications and identifying the need for revascularization of coronary lesions.
- Transthoracic Echocardiography TTE. This is a non-invasive test and allows a full assessment of ventricular and valve structure and function. It also permits the identification of regional wall motion abnormalities due to myocardial ischaemia. Exercise or pharmacological (usually dobutamine) stress echo is useful and safe for the diagnosis and assessment of CAD. It highlights areas of ischaemia that are producing abnormal wall movement.
- CT. Electron beam CT (EBCT) scanners and 64 multi-detector CT (MDCT) can produce thin axial slices of the heart. The calcium score (i.e. the assessment of the degree of coronary calcification) can be calculated. This is of some prognostic use. A calcium score of '0' gives a 0.3% chance of having CAD whilst with a score of > 400, the chance of CAD is 61–90%. CT coronary angiography (CTCA) is used for diagnostic coronary angiography and involves the injection of an iodinated contrast agent. It has 85% sensitivity with 90% specificity. It is especially useful in defining coronary anomalies and is also valuable in excluding other causes of chest pain, e.g. aortic dissection, PE.
- Cardiovascular magnetic resonance (CMR). CMR can be used as a 'one-step' approach for assessing CAD. It is used for the assessment of ischaemia in patients with suspected coronary disease and to assess myocardial viability prior to revascularization in patients with impaired cardiac function.
  - *Coronary artery anatomy* and stenoses can be identified with ultrafast breath-hold or respiratory-gated sequences; at present this is predominantly a research tool.

- *Left ventricular function* and wall motion abnormalities are detected with cine imaging performed at rest and during dobutamine-induced stress (stress echocardiogram).
- *Myocardial perfusion* is assessed with gadolinium and first-pass imaging. Ischaemia is demonstrated with adenosine for coronary vasodilatation.
- *Myocardial viability* is determined by using gadolinium and 'delayed enhancement' images.

- **Nuclear imaging.** Radionucleotide myocardial perfusion imaging is useful for the diagnosis and functional assessment of CAD. Single photon emission computed tomography (SPECT) involves the injection of an isotope of either ^{99m}technetium-tetrofosmin or ^{201}thallium. Perfusion images are then obtained at rest and peak stress (exercise or pharmacological); comparison of these images in different views allows the identification of areas of ischaemia.

  - In patients with known CAD this technique can be used to assess the haemodynamic impact of known stenosis and thus guide revascularization.
  - It also provides useful prognostic information in these patients, as a normal scan is associated with a very low risk of coronary events.

MANAGEMENT OF ACUTE CORONARY SYNDROMES

Classification of ACS

When assessing any patient with a suspected ACS, remember '**time is muscle**'; these patients must be seen as a priority.

On the basis of history, examination and 12-lead ECG, patients can immediately be split into two groups to dictate subsequent management:

- **ST elevation (STEMI) or new-onset LBBB** (Figs 12.19 and 12.20). These patients need immediate reperfusion, preferably by PCI. However, if this is not available or a long delay is envisaged, then prompt thrombolytic therapy should be given.
- **Non-ST elevation (NSTEMI).** These patients are risk-stratified and referred for PCI according to this risk.

The **diagnosis** of STEMI, NSTEMI or troponin-negative ACS (unstable angina) becomes apparent when the troponin result becomes available. However, waiting for troponin results should never delay initial management, which is based on clinical findings and ECG (i.e. STEMI or NSTEMI). Sensitive and fast troponin assays are becoming more available.

Immediate medical management in A&E (Table 12.11)

All hospitals are expected to have a rapid triage for chest pain to ensure that all suspected ACS patients are seen without delay. There should be a multi-disciplinary team approach with defined guidelines (see Emergencies in medicine, Fig. 20.10). With all ACS patients:

- IV access should be gained and bloods sent for cardiac markers, biochemistry, lipid profile, FBC and clotting profile.
- **Oxygen** is no longer recommended (2008 British Thoracic Society guidelines), unless the patient is hypoxaemic.
- **Aspirin** 300 mg chewed, then 75–150 mg daily, should be given.

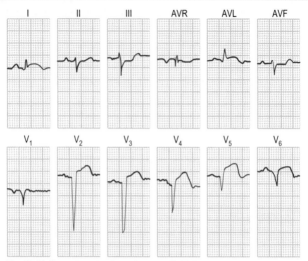

Fig. 12.19 An acute anterolateral myocardial infarction shown by a 12-lead ECG. Note the ST segment elevation in leads I, aVL and V2–V6. The T wave is inverted in leads I, aVL and V3–V6. Pathological Q waves are seen in leads V2–V6.

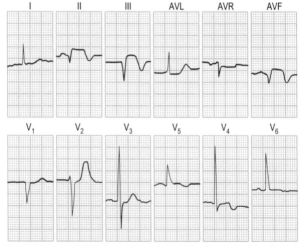

Fig. 12.20 An acute inferior wall myocardial infarction shown by a 12-lead ECG. Note the raised ST segment and Q waves in the inferior leads (III, III and aVF). The additional T wave inversion in V4 and V5 probably represents anterior wall ischaemia.

Table 12.11 Pharmacological therapy in acute coronary syndromes

Drug	Dose	Notes
Antiplatelet		
Aspirin	150–300 mg chewable or soluble aspirin, then 75–100 mg oral daily	Caution if active peptic ulceration
Clopidogrel	300 mg oral loading dose, then 75 mg oral daily	Caution — increased risk of bleeding, avoid if CABG planned
Prasugrel	60 mg loading dose then 10 mg if >60 kg or 5 mg if <60 kg daily	Used in combination with aspirin
Anti-thrombin		
Heparin	5000 U IV bolus, then 0.25 U/kg/hour	Measure anticoagulant effect with APTT at 6 hours
Low molecular weight heparins	e.g. Enoxaparin 1 mg/kg SC twice daily	
Fondaparinux	2.5 mg SC once daily	
Bivalirudin	750 mcg/kg IV bolus, then 0.75 mg/kg/hour	
Glycoprotein IIB/IIIA inhibitors		
Abciximab	0.25 mg/kg IV bolus, then 0.125 mcg/kg/min up to 10 mcg/min IV × 12 hours	Indicated if coronary intervention likely within 24 hours
Eptifibatide	180 mcg/kg IV bolus, then 2 mcg/kg/min IV × 72 hours	Indicated in high-risk patients managed without coronary intervention or during PCI
Tirofiban	0.4 mcg/kg/min for 30 mins, then 0.1 mcg/kg/min × 48–108 hours	Indicated in high-risk patients managed without coronary intervention or during PCI
Analgesia		
Diamorphine or morphine	2.5–5.0 mg IV 10 mg IV	Prescribe with antiemetic, e.g. metoclopramide 10 mg IV

Table 12.11 Continued		
Drug	**Dose**	**Notes**
Myocardial energy consumption reduction		
Atenolol	5 mg IV, repeated after 15 mins, then 25–50 mg oral daily	Avoid in asthma, heart failure, hypotension, bradyarrhythmias
Metoprolol	5 mg IV, repeated to a maximum of 15 mg, then 25–50 mg orally twice daily. In STEMI, wait 48 hours	Avoid in asthma, heart failure, hypotension, bradyarrhythmias
Coronary vasodilatation		
Glyceryl trinitrate	2–10 mg/hour IV/ buccal/sublingual	Maintain systolic BP > 90 mmHg
Plaque stabilization/ventricular remodelling		
HMG-CoA reductase inhibitors (statins)		
Simvastatin Pravastatin Atorvastatin	20–40 mg oral 20–40 mg oral 80 mg oral	Combine with dietary advice and modification
ACE inhibitors		
Ramipril Lisinopril	2.5–10 mg oral 5–10 mg oral	Monitor renal function

APTT, activated partial thromboplastin time; CABG, coronary artery bypass graft; PCI, percutaneous coronary intervention; STEMI, ST elevation myocardial infarction.

- **Sublingual glyceryl trinitrate (GTN)** 0.3–1 mg should be given for pain relief, repeated as necessary (provided BP is not compromised). This can be followed by an IV infusion of 1–10 mg/hour, which is titrated to pain whilst aiming to keep systolic BP > 100 mmHg.
- **IV diamorphine** (2.5–5 mg) or **morphine** 10 mg is used as analgesia, with **metoclopramide** 10 mg as an antiemetic.
- If there is **ongoing or continuous recurrent ischaemia** IV β-blockade with **metoprolol** is given in 5 mg boluses (up to a total of 15 mg), provided the patient is not in cardiogenic shock and/or hypotensive, and that there are no contraindications (e.g. asthma).
- Patients with a STEMI ideally should start β-blockers on the first day, provided they are definitely haemodynamically stable. If there is any doubt, wait until they are stable, to avoid the possibility of cardiac shock developing.
- All ACS patients should be transferred to a coronary care unit (CCU) for continuous monitoring and further specialist care.
- Patients with ACS should have **clopidogrel** 600 mg loading dose, unless PCI is not being considered, in which case the loading dose should be 300 mg; thereafter 75 mg daily is given in addition to aspirin. It has been shown to reduce mortality and the occurrence of major vascular events without an increase in the risk of bleeding in STEMI ACS. **Prasugrel** is an alternative.

- **N.B**. Proton pump inhibitors, particularly omeprazole, have now been shown not to reduce the antiplatelet effect of clopidogrel as they are inhibitors of cytochrome p450 (CYP2C19).
- In addition, urgent reperfusion (see below) is needed.

Reperfusion in STEMI ACS

Percutaneous coronary intervention (PCI)

PCI (if available on site or within 90 mins) is the treatment of choice in STEMI ACS. It should be used as soon as possible but within 90 mins of the patient arriving at hospital. It improves vessel patency and clinical outcome compared to thrombolytic therapy.

- Pre-procedure use of a glycoprotein (GP) IIb/IIIa inhibitor, e.g. abciximab, improves the outcome further; if nothing else, the bolus should always be given prior to angiography.
- Successful primary PCI for STEMI requires a dedicated service to be running within a hospital with a 'door to balloon' time of < 90 mins.
- Primary PCI should always be the first choice for patients with cardiogenic shock. However, it must be carried out within 24 hours or there is little benefit.
- **Drug-eluting stents**: coated stents lined with substances, e.g. sirolimus or paclitaxel, significantly reduce the incidence of coronary artery re-stenosis but late-stent thrombosis may be increased. Prolonged dual antiplatelet therapy (aspirin and clopidogrel) is therefore required with these stents for 1 year. Bare metal stents are currently used in STEMI, but there is increasing evidence that drug-eluting stents may confer a survival benefit.

Thrombolytic therapy

This still forms the mainstay of treatment of STEMI ACS in many countries. A 'door to needle' time of < 30 mins should be the minimum goal.

- There is clear benefit from thrombolysis for up to 12 hours after symptom onset. After 12 hours patients should be referred for PCI, as there is no clear benefit from thrombolysis in this group.
- Thrombolytic therapy should be administered to STEMI patients (PCI not being available) if they have:
  - no contraindications, e.g. history of a stroke, gastrointestinal bleeding, trauma, anticoagulant therapy
  - symptom onset within the last 12 hours *and either*
  - ≥ 1 mm (0.1 mV) ST elevation in at least two contiguous precordial leads or at least two adjacent limb leads *or*
  - new-onset LBBB.
- There is no good evidence to support the use of thrombolysis in patients with ST depression
- Rescue PCI is being performed (within 12 hours) in patients who fail to reperfuse.

Thrombolytic agents (Table 12.12)

- **Alteplase (tPA), reteplase and tenecteplase** all achieve faster reperfusion than streptokinase but need to be followed with a 24–48 hour-infusion of IV heparin therapy.
- However, there is evidence that 4–8 days on LMWH results in a reduction in reinfarction and mortality rates, irrespective of the thrombolytic agent given.

Table 12.12 Fibrinolytic regimes for ST elevation myocardial infarction (STEMI)

	Initial treatment (route is IV for all)	Need for heparin
Streptokinase	1.5 million U in 100 mL of 5% dextrose or 0.9% saline infusion over 30–60 mins	No
Alteplase (tPA)	0.15 mg bolus 0.75 mg/kg infusion over 30 mins *then* 0.5 mg/kg infusion over 60 mins Total dose must be < 100 mg	24–48 hours (or 4–8 days with LMWH), e.g. enoxaparin 1 mg/kg SC twice daily
Reteplase (rPA)	10 U bolus + 10 U bolus (30 mins apart)	24–48 hours (or LMWH as above)
Tenecteplase (TNK-tPA)	30 mg single bolus if < 60 kg 35 mg single bolus if 60 to < 70 kg 40 mg single bolus if 70 to < 80 kg 55 mg single bolus if 80 to < 90 kg 50 mg single bolus if ≥ 90 kg	24–48 hours (or LMWH as above)

LMWH, low molecular weight heparin.

- **Streptokinase** should not be given to a patient who has had streptokinase previously because of the risk of anaphylaxis and/or immune tolerance. Apart from its low cost, there is little to favour streptokinase as a first-choice thrombolytic agent.
- Pre-hospital thrombolysis can be given to patients with STEMI by trained paramedics.
- For anterior MI there is evidence that alteplase is superior to streptokinase.
- **Reteplase** and **tenecteplase** are often favoured due to their ease of administration (bolus doses, as opposed to infusions that have to be made up for alteplase or streptokinase).

If, after 60–90 mins, the ST elevation and/or pain have not resolved (or have recurred), the patient should be discussed immediately with a cardiologist, who should advise transfer with a view to rescue PCI (provided the patient is stable enough to transfer); if this is not possible, further thrombolytic therapy may be given.

It is not standard practice to use combined fibrinolytic regimes (e.g. reduced-dose thrombolysis and glycoprotein IIb/IIIa inhibitors). Although there is some evidence that they may reduce reinfarction, there is no benefit in terms of mortality reduction.

Patients can be transferred to CCU and given fibrinolysis, provided there is *no* delay. Otherwise, fibrinolysis should be started in A&E in a monitored bed. The transfer of a patient should *never* delay initiation of thrombolytic therapy.

After appropriate reperfusion therapy (either PCI or fibrinolysis), the patient should be monitored and managed on CCU.

NSTEMI ACS

- The ESC guidelines recommend that NSTEMI ACS patients undergoing immediate PCI receive either an LMWH (usually **enoxaparin** 1 mg/kg SC twice daily) or **bivalirudin** (a thrombin-specific anticoagulant) IV bolus 0.75 mg/kg; the actual clotting time (ACT) should be checked 5 mins after this, and if < 225, a second bolus of 0.3 mg/kg should be given (provided glomerular filtration rate (GFR) is > 30 mL/min), followed by an infusion of 1.75 mg/kg/hour.
- In patients not undergoing immediate PCI, the ESC guidelines now recommend the pure factor Xa inhibitors; **fondaparinux** 2.5 mg SC once daily should be used as the first-choice anticoagulant, as it is at least as effective as LMWH and is associated with fewer adverse bleeding episodes. If fondaparinux is not available, then an LMWH (usually **enoxaparin** 1 mg/kg SC twice daily) may be used.

Risk stratification, GP IIb/IIIa antagonists and revascularization in NSTEMI ACS

Patients with a NSTEMI ACS who have severe ongoing ischaemia (continuing chest pain and ischaemic ECG changes), haemodynamic instability or major arrhythmias, despite full medical therapy (as outlined earlier), are at very high risk and need immediate referral for angiography and PCI. These patients should be discussed with a cardiologist, who will often advise starting a **GP IIb/IIIa antagonist**, e.g. **abciximab** IV 250 mg/kg over 1 min, then IV infusion 125 ng/kg/min 10–60 mins before PCI; this is usually continued for 12 hours post PCI. For patients not going immediately to the laboratory for PCI, either **tirofiban** or **eptifibatide** given as infusions is usually the IIb/IIIa antagonist of choice (see below for dose schemes).

All other patients must be 'risk-stratified' using the results of their serum troponin level 12 hours post admission. There is a clear increase in risk of mortality with increasing troponin levels. Either the TIMI (Table 12.13) or the GRACE risk score can be used. A TIMI score of > 4 (or a GRACE risk score of > 140) is classified as high-risk.

- **Low-risk patients.** Patients who have no troponin rise 12 hours post admission, remain pain free and have minor or no ECG changes can be considered as low-risk. In this group SC LMWH and GTN infusions should be discontinued, and patients should be fully mobilized and have a pre-discharge exercise stress test. Patients with ischaemia at a very low workload should be discussed with a cardiologist prior to discharge, as they usually need either an early outpatient angiogram or possible retention for further assessment. All other patients can be managed as outpatients.
- Intermediate- and high-risk patients
  - **Angiography** should be performed in all of this group, with a view to PCI. Provided patients are stable, this can be done after 48 hours of admission (whilst they are still inpatients).
  - Treatment with a **GP IIb/IIIa antagonist** is beneficial in this group, with the benefit being greatest in diabetics with NSTEMI.

Table 12.13a TIMI risk score in acute coronary syndrome (NSTEMI/UA)

Risk factor	Score
Age > 65	1
≥ 3 risk factors for CAD	1
Known CAD (stenosis > 50%)	1
Aspirin use in last 7 days	1
Recent (≤ 24 hours) severe angina	1
Raised cardiac markers	1
ST deviation ≥ 0.5 mm	1
Elevated cardiac markers (CK-MB or troponin)	1

CAD, coronary artery disease; CK-MB, creatine kinase; NSTEMI, non-ST elevation myocardial infarction; UA, unstable angina.

Table 12.13b Risk of cardiac events (%) by 14 days in TIMI IIb

Total score	Death or MI (%)	Death, MI or urgent revascularization (%)
0/1	3	4.75
2	3	8.3
3	5	13.2
4	7	19.9
5	12	26.2
6/7	19	40.9

- Generally, **abciximab** is used if PCI is planned within 24 hours; otherwise use either **tirofiban** IV infusion 400 ng/kg/min for 30 mins, then 100 ng/kg/min for at least 48 hours (continue during and for 12–24 hours after PCI; max. duration 108 hours) or **eptifibatide** IV injection 180 mcg/kg, then IV infusion 2 mcg/kg/min for 72 hours (up to 96 hours if PCI is performed during treatment). GP IIb/IIIa antagonists can be safely co-prescribed with **enoxaparin** (an LMWH) and **clopidogrel**.
- Patients with **refractory ischaemia** (ongoing chest pain and/or persistent ischaemic ECG changes), despite full medical therapy, should be sent for urgent PCI after being started on a IIb/IIIa antagonist (e.g. **abciximab**).
- In the **stable group** of patients (pain-free and no ongoing dynamic ischaemic ECG changes), the decision as to whether GP IIb/IIIa antagonists should be started immediately and kept running until the time of angiography depends on local policies and should be discussed with a cardiologist. Evidence suggests that all patients having PCI benefit from IIb/IIIa antagonists. If the patient is not already on a GP IIb/IIIa antagonist, one is usually started in the catheter laboratory, just prior to the procedure, and continued for 12–24 hours afterwards.

- There is no benefit in the use of GP IIb/IIIa antagonists in patients who are going to be treated with medical therapy only and/or are not candidates for angiography.

Other therapies used in ACS

- Glucose-insulin-potassium (GIK) infusions. These are not given routinely but there is some evidence that they are beneficial in some ACS patients.
- IV magnesium. There is no evidence that routine use of this is of any benefit in ACS patients.

Secondary prevention and medical treatment

- Lifestyle advice and rehabilitation should ensure that all patients:
  - stop smoking and be referred to a smoking cessation clinic if necessary
  - start a low-cholesterol diet
  - lose weight (with the aim of reaching their optimal weight)
  - follow an appropriate exercise programme to improve their physical fitness.
- Education and advice regarding when patients can resume various activities (e.g. work, driving and sexual intercourse) should also be provided. Specialist cardiac rehabilitation nurses usually do this and offer a rehabilitation course. All diabetics should be referred to a clinic/diabetic nurse to ensure that their diabetes is kept under adequate control.

Pharmacological treatment

All ACS patients should be prescribed (and be discharged on) all of the following medications:

- **Aspirin.** Dosage is 75 mg once daily.
- **ACE inhibitors.** There is good evidence that all ACS patients benefit from an ACE inhibitor and that those with LV dysfunction benefit the most. An ACE inhibitor should be prescribed at the earliest safe opportunity (within the first 24 hours if possible) in all patients, provided they are not hypotensive and/or do not have significant renal dysfunction. Start with a low dose (e.g. **ramipril** 2.5 mg in the evening) and gradually titrate the dose upwards, aiming for the target dose (e.g. **ramipril** 10 mg once daily). **Angiotensin II receptor antagonists** (ARBs, e.g. **valsartan**) 160 mg twice daily is used in patients intolerant of ACE inhibitors.
- **Beta-blockers.** These reduce heart rate and thus myocardial oxygen demand, and should be given to all ACS patients once they are haemodynamically stable (provided there are no contraindications). Aim for a resting heart rate of < 60 bpm with either **atenolol** 25–100 mg once daily or **metoprolol** 25–100 mg 3 times daily.
- **Statins (HMG-CoA reductase inhibitors).** All patients should be started on a statin within the first 24 hours of hospital admission, irrespective of their lipid profile, e.g. **atorvastatin** 80 mg daily (p. 617). There is increasing evidence that, in addition to their beneficial lipid-lowering effect, statins also have other beneficial effects in ACS, such as a plaque stabilization. In the first 10 days intensive treatment aims for an LDL-C of < 1.8 mmol/L (70 mg/dL). After this, the dose may be lowered to aim for an LDL-C of < 3 mmol/L (114 mg/dL). After discharge from

Kumar & Clark's Medical Management and Therapeutics

hospital, patients should be continued indefinitely on their statins; generally, the lower the cholesterol, the better the outcome. A serum cholesterol of < 5 mmol/L (190 mg/dL) (LDL-C < 3 mmol/L (114 mg/dL)) or a reduction by 30%, whichever is greater, should be achieved.

Full fasting lipid profiles should be obtained in all patients with CAD, to include LDL-C, HDL-C and triglycerides. Diet must be modified (p. 617), as this will improve the lipid profile in addition to medical therapy, e.g. **bezafibrate** 200 mg 3 times daily, used in addition to a statin in patients with a low HDL-C. Patients who have any of the following will need further assessment, treatment and family screening, if necessary, in the lipid clinic:

- no response to statin therapy
- a markedly elevated LDL-C
- a markedly elevated serum triglyceride
- an unusual lipid profile.

In addition to the four agents listed above, all ACS patients who have had an MI (STEMI or NSTEMI) should be given:

- **Clopidogrel.** In patients with a STEMI, clopidogrel should be continued at 75 mg orally once daily for at least 4 weeks (COMMIT trial). However, there may be a benefit with longer-term treatment (CURE trial) and the ESC guidelines recommend use of clopidogrel for 12 months. In NSTEMI clopidogrel 75 mg once daily should be continued, in addition to aspirin, for at least 12 months.
- **Prasugrel.** This drug (10 mg daily) is being used instead of clopidogrel; it has a more rapid action and greater platelet inhibition.

The following may also be of use in ACS patients:

- **Oral nitrates.** These can be used if additional anti-anginal medications are needed. They do not improve prognosis.
- **Calcium channel blockers.** These can be used as an alternative agent in patients who cannot tolerate β-blockers and need anti-anginal therapy. Non-dihydropyridine calcium antagonists are used, e.g. **diltiazem** 60 mg 3 times daily, up to max. dose of 360 mg daily, or **verapamil** slow-release 120–480 mg daily. Avoid short-acting calcium antagonists, e.g. **nifedipine**, as they may increase mortality.

The following should be given in particular circumstances:

- **Oral anticoagulants.** There is no proven benefit for warfarin therapy in post-MI patients unless they have specific indications. The **absolute cardiac indications for warfarin** include atrial fibrillation, LV dysfunction with a documented embolic event, LV aneurysm and documented LV thrombus. Relative cardiac indications include severe LV dysfunction and an extensive anterior wall motion abnormality. Oral antithrombin agents, e.g. dabigatran may well replace warfarin.
- **Eplerenone.** 25 mg once daily, an aldosterone antagonist, should be given to all who have post-M1 heart failure.

Pre-discharge risk stratification and follow-up

All STEMI patients who have received successful fibrinolysis should proceed to a coronary angiogram. Those with a low risk, or if coronary angiography is not immediately available, should have a submaximal (modified Bruce) pre-discharge exercise test for risk stratification and an early outpatient (usually 6 weeks post discharge) symptom-limited (full Bruce) exercise test. Alternative non-invasive imaging (e.g. dobutamine stress echocardiography) should be used when exercise testing is contraindicated. Patients who have had successful PCI do not need routine exercise tests prior to discharge. Exercise testing is now less often performed, being replaced by a functional imaging study.

All ACS patients should be seen 4–6 weeks post discharge in the outpatient clinic to ensure that they are receiving appropriate secondary prevention, to up-titrate drug doses as necessary, to review symptoms and investigations, and to assess any need for further investigation and/or revascularization.

MANAGEMENT OF COMPLICATIONS OF ACS

Refractory ischaemia

Any patient who develops recurrent ischaemia should be on or restarted on full medical therapy (heparin, nitrate and β-blocker) and moved to a monitored bed on CCU. If, despite full medical therapy, patients continue to have refractory ischaemia, they need urgent PCI.

Cardiogenic shock

Cardiogenic shock is associated with a very high mortality (70–80%). It is defined as an inadequate circulation (due to reduced cardiac output and hypotension) to meet the peripheral metabolic needs (usually manifested by oliguria or anuria and/or mental status changes). It is characterized by a low systolic pressure (usually < 90 mmHg) and adequate or high central filling pressure (pulmonary capillary wedge pressure ≥ 12 mmHg).

- Correctable causes for hypotension (inadequate filling, drugs (notably nitrate infusions), arrhythmias and electrolyte disturbances) need to be excluded.
- Patients need continuous invasive monitoring and high-dependency nursing care (**at least a level 2 critical care bed**).
- Central venous and arterial lines should be inserted. A pulmonary artery catheter is only occasionally necessary.
- Urgent bedside echo is essential to assess ventricular function and rule out other structural causes of hypotension.
- Serial ECGs should be performed.
- Give oxygen via a face mask (35–55%).
- Aim for a pulmonary wedge (filling) pressure of > 15 mmHg. If the patient remains hypotensive despite an adequate filling pressure, start **dobutamine** 5–10 mcg/kg and titrate this to aim for a systolic pressure of at least 90 mmHg.
- Patients with cardiogenic shock often require intra-aortic balloon pumping (IABP) urgently if they do not respond to dopamine therapy.

Patients with cardiogenic shock as a result of ischaemia need urgent angiography and percutaneous revascularization. This must be done urgently (**N.B.** Referring patients after 24 hours is too late!). Thrombolytic therapy should only be given when PCI is not available. Patients with cardiogenic shock due to other mechanical causes (e.g. ventricular septal defect) require surgery.

Right ventricular infarction

The treatment of cardiogenic shock due to right ventricular infarction is quite different from that due to LV infarction. Patients with RV infarction are dependent on high filling pressures and IV fluid loading is needed to optimize cardiac output. Avoid vasodilator drugs if possible.

Mechanical complications post MI

- **Mitral regurgitation.** Acute mitral regurgitation can be due to either papillary muscle ischaemia/rupture or mitral annulus dilatation. Papillary muscle ischaemia/rupture usually presents as acute haemodynamic deterioration with acute pulmonary oedema. On auscultation a pan-systolic murmur may be present. An echocardiogram will confirm the diagnosis and allows a full anatomical and functional assessment. Supportive therapy is required, including insertion of an IABP as a bridge to urgent mechanical therapy (PCI for ischaemic papillary dysfunction and valve replacement for papillary rupture).
- **Ventricular septal defect (VSD).** This usually occurs within the first 24 hours post thrombolysis and in patients who have not received thrombolysis either on day 1 or days 3–5. VSDs usually present with acute pulmonary oedema and haemodynamic deterioration; chest pain may be a feature. There is usually a loud pan-systolic murmur on examination. An echocardiogram shows the size and location of the defect. Supportive therapy is required, including insertion of an IABP as a bridge to surgical repair.
- **Free wall rupture.** This usually presents as either a cardiac arrest or acute haemodynamic compromise. Patients very rarely survive the initial insult. If they do, then pericardiocentesis (to relieve tamponade) and IABP insertion may act as a bridge to surgical repair, which is the only definitive treatment.

Heart failure

This is a poor prognostic feature post MI. Acute heart failure should be followed up and treated by the heart failure team (p. 419). An echocardiogram allows assessment of ventricular function and identification of other potentially treatable contributing causes (e.g. VSD). Any reversible causes, such as arrhythmia, ischaemia and drug therapy, need treatment. Any patients with an ejection fraction of < 35% is at high risk of SCD and must be discussed with a cardiologist (ideally, an electrophysiologist) prior to discharge, as they will benefit from insertion of an ICD, which can detect and treat dangerous ventricular arrhythmias.

Arrhythmias and bradycardias

Any arrhythmia that results in haemodynamic compromise needs urgent aggressive therapy; DC cardioversion should be used if necessary. Any contributing factors to an arrhythmia should be treated if possible (e.g. electrolyte disturbances). Reperfusion arrhythmias, such as ventricular ectopics, non-sustained ventricular tachycardia and accelerated idioventricular rhythm, are common and do not routinely need treatment.

- **Supraventricular tachycardias (SVT).** AF is common post MI and occurs in up to 20% of patients. Cardioversion is possible but relapse is frequent. Rate control with **digoxin**, **β-blockers** and prevention of thrombotic complications with **warfarin** are often required. Other SVTs should be treated (p. 403).
- **Ventricular tachycardia (VT)**
  - *Non-sustained VT* (three or more beats of VT, <30 secs in total) is common in the first 24 hours post MI and carries no adverse risk or need for treatment. If non-sustained VT occurs later than 24 hours post MI it carries a risk and should be treated (p. 406).

- *Sustained VT* occurring in post-MI patients is associated with an increased mortality. It must be treated with urgent synchronized DC cardioversion if there is haemodynamic compromise; this should be followed by prophylactic drug therapy (p. 406). If the patient is initially stable, an IV β-blocker may be tried but this should be discussed with an electrophysiologist first.
- *Recurrent VT* in patients who have had revascularization needs further investigation by an electrophysiologist with possible insertion of an implantable defibrillator.
- Bradycardias and heart block. These are common post MI, especially with an inferior MI. If sinus bradycardia is associated with hypotension, it can be treated with IV **atropine** 0.3–0.5 mg up to a total of 1.5–2.0 mg.
  - *First-degree heart block* requires no treatment.
  - *Type I second-degree heart block* needs no treatment unless there is haemodynamic compromise, in which case **atropine** should be used first, and failing this, pacing.
  - *Type II second-degree (Mobitz II) and third-degree (complete) heart block* need pacing if there is haemodynamic compromise or a broad escape rhythm.

If the patient is haemodynamically stable, then close monitoring on CCU is appropriate. In patients with an inferior STEMI, reperfusion should not be delayed, unless the patient is haemodynamically compromised, as heart block usually resolves with successful reperfusion. If pacing is required, then temporary transvenous pacing is used. However, those with persistent Mobitz II or complete AV block after 10 days are likely to need a permanent pacemaker inserted; this is usually the case with anterior infarcts.

Pericarditis and Dressler's syndrome

- Pericarditis is common post MI; it is necessary to rule out ischaemia before making the diagnosis. Treatment is with high-dose **aspirin** 600 mg every 4 hours. There is no good evidence to support the use of oral steroids. Patients on oral anticoagulants may develop haemorrhagic effusions that necessitate drainage.
- Dressler's syndrome is a form of autoimmune pericarditis that occurs 2–10 weeks post infarct. Treatment is with high-dose **aspirin** 600 mg every 4 hours.
- NSAIDs are best avoided in patients up to 4 weeks post MI, as they may impair infarct healing; after this they can be used.

MANAGEMENT OF CHRONIC STABLE ANGINA

Risk stratification and investigation

These patients are usually referred to a rapid-access chest pain clinic or an outpatient clinic; they may occasionally present in A&E. Based on age, sex, history and a 12 lead ECG, a diagnosis of angina can be made, and the patient treated for angina. An exercise ECG is now not recommended (NICE guidelines) if the likelihood of coronary artery disease (CAD) is more than 90%. If there is doubt, CT calcium scoring (p. 432) can be helpful. If the score is 1–400, CT coronary angiography should be performed. If the angiogram shows CAD, treat as angina; if there is doubt perform functional tests. These tests include myocardial perfusion scintigraphy with single photon emission computed tomography (MAS with SPECT), stress echocardiography or contrast enhanced MR, depending on availability of the tests. Exercise ECGs are still being performed.

ECG exercise test

This is useful in patients with suspected chronic stable angina for risk stratification. It is however being superseded in many hospitals by non invasive imaging (see above).

- In properly selected patients it has a 75% specificity and 68% sensitivity.
- A **Bruce** or **modified Bruce** protocol is used. The patient walks on a treadmill with increasing speed and incline; BP, heart rate symptoms and ECG are monitored during and after the test. A positive test is indicated by an inability to exercise > 2 mins, new ST depressions of > 1 mm in multiple leads, hypotension, heart failure or sustained ventricular arrhythmias, and a post-exercise interval of > 5 mins for ischaemic ST changes to return to normal.
- Patients with suspected **ACS** should *not* be subjected to exercise testing, e.g. an acute MI in the previous 2 days or unstable angina.
- Other *contraindications* include severe aortic stenosis, severe heart failure, acute PE, pericarditis, myocarditis, aortic dissection, physical immobility and a pacemaker.
- Exercise testing is not as helpful in young and middle-aged women or patients with LBBB, and alternative non-invasive investigations, e.g. stress echocardiography, should be used.

If an exercise ECG is contraindicated, then an alternative form of non-invasive imaging should be used, e.g. radionucleotide myocardial perfusion imaging or stress echocardiography.

Coronary angiography

If patients have a positive exercise test, coronary angiography is helpful in the following conditions:

- **severe stable angina** (i.e. marked limitation of ordinary activity, e.g. climbing one flight of stairs at a normal pace), especially if symptoms are inadequately responding to medical therapy
- **chronic stable angina** (i.e. slight or no limitation of ordinary activity) and a history of MI or ischaemia at a low workload
- **chronic stable angina in patients with bundle branch block** with readily inducible ischaemia demonstrated by non-invasive imaging
- patients with **stable angina being considered for major vascular surgery**
- patients with **serious ventricular arrhythmias**, e.g. survivors of cardiac arrest
- patients who have been **revascularized (PCI or coronary artery bypass graft (CABG))** with recurrent angina
- when it is essential to **establish a diagnosis** for occupational reasons.

Revascularization

- Left main stem stenosis or proximal triple vessel disease. These patients are generally referred for CABG surgery first. If they are not fit for surgery (e.g. due to severe co-morbidity) or refuse it, then PCI is the second choice. There is a proven benefit in terms of reduced mortality and MI rate from revascularization in patients with either of these patterns of disease.

- Other patterns of disease. These patients should be referred for PCI. Revascularization in this group of patients is an excellent treatment for symptomatic angina but provides no benefit in terms of either mortality or reduced MI rate. Diabetic patients with multi-vessel disease tend to do better with surgery than with PCI.

Secondary prevention and medical treatment

All patients should follow lifestyle advice (p. 441) and should be on aspirin 75 mg, a statin, an ACE inhibitor and a β-blocker (p. 441). All should be given a **GTN spray** to use as required. In addition, the following may be used as **second-line anti-anginal treatments**:

- Nitrates. Long-acting nitrates provide good symptomatic relief (e.g. **isosorbide mononitrate** up to 120 mg daily, in divided doses). Slow-release GTN patches are also available. Tolerance can be a problem with nitrates.
- Calcium channel blockers. Due to its rate-slowing properties **diltiazem** 60 mg daily up to total maximum dose of 360 mg can be used when β-blockers are contraindicated. It should only be co-prescribed with a β-blocker under close supervision. In patients on a β-blocker who need additional anti-anginal therapy, a dihydropyridine group such as long-acting **nifedipine,** e.g. 30–90 mg daily, or **amlodipine** 5–10 mg daily can be used, as these do not slow the heart rate.
- Nicorandil. This is good at relieving angina and has been shown to provide a reduced event rate in clinical trials. Give 10–30 mg orally × 2 daily.
- Ivabradine. This is an I_f channel inhibitor that reduces heart rate and has been developed as an anti-anginal drug. The usual dose is 2.5–7.5 mg orally twice daily. Reversible visual symptoms are reported at the higher dose. **Ivabradine** should not be co-prescribed with **β-blockers** or **diltiazem**.
- Ranolazine. This drug interacts with sodium channels but can cause QT interval prolongation. It is used if other drugs do not help.
- Eplerenone. This aldosterone antagonist is given 25 mg/day to patients post MI with clinical evidence of heart failure and reduced ejection fraction (monitor serum K^+ levels).

VALVULAR HEART DISEASE

Valvular heart disease is common in developing countries and in some cases can be life-threatening, but interventions can allow a normal life expectancy. The diagnosis of the cause of a murmur starts with clinical suspicion and clinical examination. In general, diastolic murmurs are never innocent, whereas asymptomatic ejection systolic murmurs often represent flow murmurs. Echocardiography usually confirms the diagnosis.

MITRAL REGURGITATION

Mitral regurgitation is common and may be a benign condition. It is secondary to intrinsic mitral valve disease or LV dilatation of any cause. Causes therefore include mitral valve prolapse, rheumatic heart disease, infective endocarditis and collagen vascular diseases, which primarily affect the valve, and ischaemic heart disease and dilated cardiomyopathy, which allow the mitral valve annulus to dilate. In addition to these chronic conditions, the mitral valve is susceptible to acute ischaemic, traumatic or infective injury with papillary muscle dysfunction, chordal rupture or valve leaflet destruction causing sudden valve failure.

Pathophysiology

- **Acute mitral regurgitation** involves destruction of part of the valve apparatus. A sudden severe valve failure in this high-pressure system leads to acute decompensation with excessive stress on the left atrium, coupled with a sudden loss in cardiac output, which leads to pulmonary oedema and cardiogenic shock. Often classical clinical signs may be absent and the diagnosis is made by echocardiography in a patient who presents with acute heart failure.
- **Chronic mitral regurgitation**, in contrast, allows partial or complete compensation with gradual ventricular hypertrophy and dilatation of the left atrium. Afterload is not affected but cardiac output may be reduced by the flow of blood into the left atrium. The ventricle assumes a hyperdynamic action, which can remain stable, deteriorate with progressive dilatation and systolic dysfunction only developing over a period of years.

Clinical features

- Symptoms of mitral regurgitation occur late in the disease and comprise fatigue and breathlessness.
- Examination findings include a forceful, displaced apex beat with a pan-systolic murmur that does not vary in intensity throughout its duration. Radiation is typically to the axilla but it may be to the base. The presence of a third heart sound indicates volume overload.

Diagnosis

- **ECG** may reveal concurrent AF or bifid, M-shaped P waves that are related to the presence of left atrial dilatation and delay of atrial contraction.
- **TTE** can reveal the degree of LV dilatation and whether there is related systolic dysfunction. An echocardiographic diagnosis of severe mitral regurgitation requires the presence of left atrial enlargement and LV dilatation. In asymptomatic patients, echocardiography is repeated annually to assess LV internal dilatation, as progressive enlargement is an indication for valve surgery. The aetiology may also be revealed by echocardiography with careful examination of the valve leaflets for valve tip thickening indicating rheumatic disease, evidence of prolapse, chordal or papillary muscle rupture or vegetations.
- **TOE** is helpful when transthoracic imaging is not clear and for pre- or intra-operative assessment when detailed images are required to plan the surgical intervention.
- **Cardiac catheterization** is commonly used for assessment of right and left heart pressures and to exclude the presence of concurrent CAD before planning surgical intervention. However, it can also be used as an additional tool to assess the degree of regurgitation.

Management

- **Acute mitral regurgitation.** In acute severe mitral regurgitation, **surgical intervention** is urgent. Other measures should be aimed at optimizing the patient for anaesthesia and avoiding organ hypoperfusion. If BP is normal, vasodilatation can aid forward cardiac output and reduce pulmonary congestion via the regurgitating valve. This can be achieved by the use of IV **sodium nitroprusside**. If BP falls, an alternative to nitroprusside alone is a combination with **dobutamine** or intra-aortic balloon counterpulsation.

- Chronic mitral regurgitation. If mitral regurgitation has resulted from LV dilatation (functional mitral regurgitation), treatment with **ACE inhibitors** and/or β-**blockers** is recommended. There is no indication for these drugs where LV function is normal.

Timing of **surgery** in intrinsic valve disease is complicated by the difficulty in assessing LV function owing to the ejection into the left atrium, which tends to over-estimate residual LV function. Operation is performed before LV ejection falls below 0.3 and the LV end-systolic dimension ≤ 55 mm in symptomatic patients. In asymptomatic patients the absolute indication for surgery is an ejection fraction of 0.3–0.6 and LV end-systolic dimension of ≥ 40 mm. Mitral valve replacement with a prosthetic valve tends to disrupt the papillary muscles, which contribute to overall LV function, and therefore mitral valve repair is generally preferred, as it can preserve more LV function and offers an option where there is particularly poor LV function.

Patients with mitral regurgitation should be followed yearly to monitor LV function and size; surgery should be performed before there is irreversible myocyte damage.

MITRAL STENOSIS

Mitral stenosis is almost always rheumatic in origin.

Pathophysiology

Obstruction to left atrial emptying leads to progressive hypertrophy and dilatation of the left atrium and this increases the atrial pressure further, leading to increased pulmonary venous pressure and eventually pulmonary hypertension. Chronic elevation in pulmonary venous pressure in mitral stenosis can lead to pulmonary oedema but the adaptive process is more gradual in the context of lower atrial pressure when compared to the ventricular pressure seen in mitral regurgitation. Thus the pulmonary veins reduce compliance and permeability, and the pulmonary arteries bear the brunt, leading to pulmonary arterial hypertension. Atrial hypertrophy and dilatation lead to AF, which is common in mitral stenosis, increasing the risk of thromboembolic disease.

Clinical features

Mitral stenosis is a slowly progressive disease. Symptoms of breathlessness, irregular palpitations, haemoptysis and embolic complications predominate.

The pulse may have a low volume and be irregularly irregular with AF. A malar flush may be present, and giant systolic 'v' waves in the jugular veins are almost always seen due to associated tricuspid regurgitation. Chest examination may reveal right ventricular heave, a palpable pulmonary second heart sound and usually an undisplaced apex beat.

Auscultation reveals a loud first heart sound, a low-pitched mid-diastolic murmur with pre-systolic accentuation and an opening snap heard in early diastole.

Diagnosis

- ECG may reveal AF or a bifid P wave due to atrial hypertrophy. There may be associated ECG evidence of right ventricular hypertrophy with a dominant R1 in V1.
- TTE assesses the severity of stenosis and the degree of associated pulmonary hypertension. More detailed anatomical assessment is required when assessing for suitability of surgery or percutaneous valvotomy, and TOE should be performed in these circumstances.
- CMR accurately defines the valve structure.

Management

- Mitral stenosis progresses slowly and medical therapy is used before serious adverse events warrant surgical intervention. However, medical therapy has not been shown to affect outcome.
- Exercise-induced tachycardia can lead to decompensation; in patients with mild symptoms, β-blockers or rate-limiting calcium antagonists can be used.
- Intermittent pulmonary oedema is controlled by diuretics.
- AF is common, although not invariable, in mitral stenosis. This poses the dual threat of uncontrolled rate and emboli. The former can be controlled with β-blockade or calcium antagonists.
- Digoxin may also be used but is not as helpful for controlling exercise-induced tachycardia.
- Anticoagulation is initially with heparin; warfarin is then required, whether AF is paroxysmal or permanent. Anti-thrombin agents are now being used.

When symptoms worsen (NYHA class III–IV) and the echo appearance is consistent with severe mitral stenosis (valve area < 1 cm^2), mechanical intervention should be considered. Patients may be suitable for percutaneous mitral valvuloplasty and this should always be discussed with a cardiologist. Alternatively, surgery with mitral valvuloplasty or mitral valve replacement can be performed. Pre-operative assessment of the coronary anatomy by angiography is required for the majority of patients in order to exclude underlying CAD.

AORTIC STENOSIS

Untreated symptomatic aortic stenosis has a poor prognosis, with median survival being in the order of 2–3 years, but surgery is highly successful and can restore the recipient to a normal life expectancy.

Pathophysiology

- The commonest causes of aortic stenosis are calcific atherosclerotic-like degeneration, a congenital bicuspid valve and rheumatic heart disease. Presentation normally around 60–70 years old.
- Progressive narrowing of the aortic valve leads to increasing gradients across the valve as the heart compensates for the restriction to flow.
- The increased pressure is generated by a hypertrophied ventricle, and the narrowed jet that is ejected into the aorta at high velocity often leads to post-stenotic arch dilatation.
- Progressive LV hypertrophy leads to relative myocardial ischaemia and fibrosis, which in turn eventually causes dilatation, systolic dysfunction and heart failure.
- The thickened ventricle also leads to arrhythmias, and sudden changes to peripheral vascular resistance may lead to syncope or sudden death.

The hypertrophic response in individuals varies and those with an inadequate response tend to develop heart failure earlier.

● There is a predisposition to develop an acquired von Willebrand syndrome with platelet dysfunction and a bleeding diathesis that correlates with the severity of stenosis.

Clinical features

Exertional chest pain can result from a mismatch between myocardial perfusion and hypertrophy or from coexisting CAD. Syncope is generally exertional and can be heralded by episodes of exertional pre-syncope. LV dysfunction, which tends to be predominantly diastolic in nature, can lead to breathlessness. The onset of systolic dysfunction and LV dilatation carries a particularly poor prognosis. In such circumstances, the pressure generated within the ventricle may be reduced, leading to an underestimate of the valve stenosis if measured by gradient across the valve.

Examination reveals a slow-rising pulse, a narrow pulse pressure (generally caused by low systolic pressure and maintained diastolic pressure) and a pressure-overloaded apex beat. There is typically a crescendo–decrescendo ejection systolic murmur, which radiates to the carotid arteries.

Diagnosis

● ECG typically reveals evidence of LV hypertrophy, with lateral lead ST depression due to strain. Exercise testing is *contraindicated* in symptomatic aortic stenosis. However, in patients who are asymptomatic but are planning to exercise, a failure of BP to rise ≥ 20 mmHg can indicate that the patient ought to avoid that level of exercise and may benefit from intervention.

● Echocardiography is required to confirm the diagnosis and can be used to grade severity of stenosis, but it correlates poorly with prognosis compared to symptoms.

● CMR — see below.

Management

● Medical management. The aim is to control cardiovascular risk factors (p. 441). Treatment of hypertension can be difficult, as vasodilators can worsen the gradient across the valve.

● Surgical management. Surgery is the definitive treatment. Pre-operative assessment of the coronary anatomy by angiography is required for the majority of patients in order to exclude underlying CAD. Patients should be operated on before symptoms and with good LV systolic function.

● Percutaneous aortic valve replacement (PAVR). This treatment is generally reserved for patients with severe co-morbidities that make surgical aortic valve replacement too high-risk. The short-term results are excellent but the long-term results are as yet unclear. These patients are assessed and treated as appropriate by a multi-disciplinary team, including an interventional cardiologist, cardiac surgeon and cardiac anaesthetist at a tertiary centre.

AORTIC REGURGITATION

Aortic regurgitation can present acutely or follow a chronic course. The relative paucity of symptoms early in the disease continues until there is advanced disease, in which case LV dysfunction may be irreversibly impaired. Exercise tolerance and serial estimations of valvular and ventricular function should be made by echo.

Pathophysiology

- Acute severe aortic regurgitation loads the ventricle beyond its capacity to dilate and leads to sudden increases in LV wall stress and subsequently left atrial pressure and pulmonary venous pressure. This may cause pulmonary oedema. If diastolic pressure in the ventricle is equal to that in the coronary arteries, the driving pressure gradient to perfuse the sub-endocardium ceases and this leads to ischaemia, reducing ventricular function further.

- Chronic aortic regurgitation leads to progressive LV dilatation and hypertrophy. The need for a greater volume of blood to be ejected into the aorta with each beat increases the afterload and with it the stimulus to hypertrophy due to pressure increase.

Clinical features

- Acute aortic regurgitation. Patients may present with sudden breathlessness, chest pain and cardiogenic shock. Tachycardia is common. The murmur can be shorter in acute severe aortic regurgitation, as there is rapid pressure equalization between ventricle and aorta in diastole. The diagnosis is a priority, as is exclusion of aortic dissection, even if the patient does not complain of chest pain.

- Chronic aortic regurgitation. There is a wide difference between systolic and diastolic BP (pulse pressure). The arterial pulse is bounding and collapsing. The apex beat is typically displaced owing to LV dilatation and it may feel hyperdynamic. The murmur of aortic regurgitation is diastolic and decrescendo in nature, occurring immediately after the second heart sound. A systolic flow murmur is commonly heard due to the need for increased forward flow through the aortic valve to compensate for the regurgitation.

Diagnosis

- ECG may show evidence of LV hypertrophy.
- TTE can be used to assess the cause of the valve lesion, as well as the severity of the regurgitation and LV dilatation and function. All these measurements are prognostically useful and can aid with decisions regarding progression and treatment.
- TOE, cardiac catheterization and CMR should be used if there is LV impairment or the patient has developed symptoms.

Management

Due to increased afterload, therapy with vasodilators such as **nitroprusside** and **hydralazine** may improve haemodynamic function. ACE inhibitors are less effective in this context. **Surgery** with mechanical prostheses or tissue valve replacement is performed before symptoms occur when the myocardium is failing (i.e. LV ejection fraction < 50%). A repair of the aortic valve may occasionally be surgically possible.

TRICUSPID REGURGITATION

There is almost always a minor degree of tricuspid regurgitation on echocardiography.

- Significant tricuspid regurgitation is usually secondary to right ventricular dilation of any cause, e.g. cor pulmonale.
- Rarely, it can be organic, e.g. rheumatic heart disease.

- It is usually detected clinically by giant 'v' waves in the JVP, a pulsatile, palpable liver and a blowing pan-systolic murmur best heard on inspiration. Management is that of right heart failure. The occasional organic disease might require surgical replacement.

Special considerations for valvular heart disease

Pregnancy

An increase in blood volume of 30% carries a number of potential problems and risk to the mother and fetus during pregnancy. Cardiac conditions during pregnancy, whether new or old, are managed by multi-disciplinary specialists. Conditions requiring anticoagulation, such as mechanical prosthetic valves, pose a problem, as **warfarin** is teratogenic in the first trimester and increases the bleeding risk during birth. The commonest strategy is therefore to plan pregnancy with anticoagulation using **LMWH** until the second trimester, when warfarin may be reinstated. At the onset of the third trimester, LMWH is restarted until birth, when warfarin is again restarted. This depends on the relative risk of thrombotic complications in each condition and requires expert consultation.

- Peripartum cardiomyopathy — see p. 459.
- Mitral stenosis is rare in women of childbearing age. However, it is commonly silent until pregnancy leads to a presentation with symptoms, normally around 20–24 weeks' gestation. Symptoms should be dealt with medically where possible. Diuretics may control volume overload and β-blockers may be required to control resting heart rate. If there is persistent haemodynamic compromise and the fetus is too young to deliver electively, emergency mitral balloon valvotomy can be performed. Women of this age are less likely to have valve calcification, a factor that facilitates the procedure.
- Cyanotic heart disease, combined with pulmonary hypertension (Eisenmenger syndrome), poses a prohibitive risk to mother and baby in pregnancy, with a maternal mortality of around 50%, a risk of spontaneous abortion of 20–40% and perinatal mortality of 8–28%. This risk means that it is considered in the best interests of the patient to have a therapeutic termination. Where pulmonary hypertension has not been established and symptom levels are low, pregnancy increases the risk of heart failure but this may be carefully managed by a combination of good fluid management and bed rest where necessary.

CARDIOMYOPATHY

The classification of cardiomyopathy into dilated, restrictive and hypertrophic has become blurred, as genetic screening reveals common roots between some hypertrophic and dilated cardiomyopathies. Moreover, the management of heart failure due to these conditions depends more on the physiology of the heart at that time rather than the original defect. As a rule, cardiac MR is very useful in the assessment of these patients.

Genetic screening offers help in the risk stratification of sudden death and the possibility of a more accurate estimation of prognosis, both in the index patient and in relatives.

- Primary cardiomyopathies include the genetic disorders, e.g. hypertrophic mitochondrial myopathies, as well as acquired, e.g. myocarditis.
- Secondary cardiomyopathies due to infiltrative disease (e.g. amyloidosis, Gaucher's disease, glycogen storage disease), adenomatosis, due to

Kumar & Clark's Medical Management and Therapeutics

toxic compounds (e.g. alcohol), and autoimmune rheumatic disorders (e.g. SLE), are potentially reversible with treatment of the underlying disorder. Cardiomyopathies due to cytotoxic agents are dose-related.

DILATED CARDIOMYOPATHY

In dilated cardiomyopathy there is dilatation of the left (and occasionally the right) ventricle, leading to impaired contraction. It has a prevalence of approximately 40 per 100 000 in Europe and North America.

Pathophysiology

As in other causes of systolic heart failure, the disturbances in haemodynamics are due to an ineffective cardiac pump, which leads to alterations in neurohumoral regulation and inappropriate fluid retention. Any disorder that affects the myocardium — either idiopathic, genetic (up to 25%) or secondary due to, for example, alcohol, autoimmune rheumatic disorders, nutritional deficiencies, storage diseases or cytotoxic agents — can lead to a dilated cardiomyopathy.

Clinical features

- Breathlessness, oedema and arrhythmia are the main clinical features, similar to chronic heart failure.
- Murmurs of tricuspid or mitral regurgitation can be heard due to the dilatation affecting the valves.
- Ventricular and atrial arrhythmias are common and can cause sudden death.

Diagnosis

This depends on the exclusion of ischaemic heart disease and other secondary causes.

- Echocardiography or radionuclide scanning shows dilated, poorly functioning ventricles.
- Doppler echo is useful to rule out other forms of cardiomyopathy.
- CMR excludes other causes of LV dysfunction or myocardial fibrosis. It is also useful for identifying myocardial thrombus.

Management

The treatment and complications of the condition mirror those of chronic systolic heart failure of any cause.

- The risk of sudden arrhythmic death is reduced by effective medical treatment for cardiac failure, including **β-blockers** and **angiotensin receptor antagonists** (ARBs).
- ICDs and pacemakers may also be necessary and discussion with an electrophysiologist is often helpful.
- The efficacy of immunosuppressive agents is not proven.
- Anticoagulants are not used unless there is a history of AF or thromboembolic events.
- If medical treatment fails, cardiac transplantation is required, as long as a cardiac biopsy does not show a lesion such as amyloid.

HYPERTROPHIC CARDIOMYOPATHY

Hypertrophic cardiomyopathy (HCM) is common in the general population, with an incidence of 1 : 500, and represents a common cause of SCD in young adults, although the annual risk of SCD is low (~1%). Increased surveillance and use of genetic screening have revealed a wide heterogeneity in the cardiac morphological characteristics and prognosis of this condition, even with similar genetic mutations. Thus some patients may have the disease-causing mutation without obvious hypertrophy but their histology shows the classical features of HCM.

Pathophysiology

- **Hypertrophied ventricle.** The hypertrophied ventricle is less able to relax and is relatively stiff due to its thickness and to the arrangement of cardiac myocytes that do not align and typically have an appearance of disarray on histological examination.
- **Obstructive disease.** A hypertrophied septum causes a partial blockage to LV outflow, leading to an acceleration of blood across the septum. This causes a Venturi effect — a reduction in the pressure of the blood passing through the narrowing due to its acceleration in order to maintain the same flow rate. As the adjacent structures (anterior mitral valve leaflet and septum) are relatively mobile, the reduction in pressure draws them closer together, worsening the obstruction. The anterior movement of the mitral valve and partial vacuum over the anterior mitral valve leaflet can lead to a functional mitral valve prolapse and regurgitation. Obstruction also takes place at a mid-cavity level due to excessive hypertrophy around this area. Obstruction occurs at rest but stress-inducible gradients, e.g. exercise, can occur where there is little or no resting obstruction. Exercise that increases the heart rate reduces the length of diastole and the thickened, stiff ventricle is less able to fill, leading to increased obstruction.
- **Genetics.** The genetic basis of HCM is complex, with new mutations of genes encoding for components of the cardiac sarcomere, a lack of concordance in the mutations between different families, and individual patient responses to stress and environment. The mode of inheritance is autosomal dominant. The electrophysiological abnormalities that may be a cause of sudden death are dependent on specific mutations.

Clinical features

The clinical course can be entirely benign, with 25% of patients with confirmed HCM surviving to a normal life expectancy. The age of presentation is highly variable, the increasing use of echocardiography revealing new cases in all age groups. Symptoms can occur at any age and those who present at a young age with symptoms have a particularly poor prognosis.

- **Breathlessness**
  - *In non-obstructive cases*, breathlessness is mainly due to diastolic dysfunction, which results from ventricular hypertrophy and ischaemia. Breathlessness is generally exertional and can precede any systolic dysfunction on echocardiography. The addition of AF and mitral regurgitation can contribute to the initial defect.
  - *In obstructive cases*, there is systolic impairment, which will respond to measures designed to alleviate obstruction (p. 457).
- **Chest pain.** Typical dull, central, exertional ischaemic chest pain can result from inadequate increase in perfusion through a thickened myocardium, from abnormal coronary arterioles and from coexisting atherosclerotic disease of the coronary arteries.
- **Syncope or pre-syncope.** This occurs typically with exertion.
- **SCD.** Risk factors are shown in Box 12.9.
- **Thromboembolic disease.** There is a higher than normal risk of thromboembolic events relating to the increased incidence of AF. However,

> **Box 12.9** Risk factors for sudden cardiac death in hypertrophic cardiomyopathy
>
> **Major**
> - Prior cardiac arrest
> - Spontaneous VT
> - Family history of SCD
> - Unexplained syncope
> - LV thickness ≥ 30 mm
> - Inadequate BP rise on exercise
> - Non-sustained VT on Holter
>
> **Minor**
> - AF
> - Myocardial ischaemia with normal coronary circulation
> - LV outflow tract obstruction
> - High-risk genetic mutation
> - Patients likely to perform intense exertion

routine anticoagulation is not recommended unless there is AF or a previous thromboembolic event.

Diagnosis

The heterogeneity of this condition and the possibility of confounding co-morbid conditions make clinical diagnosis more difficult. Where there is hypertension and concentric hypertrophy or borderline hypertrophy, genetic testing may be required to make the diagnosis.

- **ECG** markers of LV hypertrophy are usually present, with large-voltage QRS complexes and symmetrical T wave inversion in the distribution of hypertrophy.
- **Echocardiography** will show hypertrophy that is typically asymmetric but can be in any distribution or even concentric. The inner LV dimensions are normal or small. Establishing the degree of left ventricular hypertrophy (LVH) that constitutes a diagnosis of HCM is difficult due to overlap with normal variants and athletic hearts. LVH of ≥ 15 mm is more likely to be due to HCM. Systolic anterior motion of the mitral valve due to sub-aortic obstruction and asymmetric septal hypertrophy are the classic features but depend on predominantly septal hypertrophy. Anterior mitral valve leaflet thickening, presumably due to collision with the ventricular septum or markedly increased flow, is often seen. The presence of mitral valve prolapse with or without regurgitation should be noted. Obstruction is a dynamic process and is often not present at rest. However, a sub-aortic gradient of ≥ 30 mmHg is considered physiologically and prognostically significant. Exercise is the most reliable provocation for stress-induced obstruction and this can be used with echo to test for dynamic obstructions.
- **Cardiac MR** can detect both the hypertrophy and abnormal myocardial fibrosis, and is very useful in the assessment of any form of heart muscle disease.
- **Cardiac catheterization** is used when chest pain is a feature, or when gradients are difficult to measure by echocardiography. It can provide diagnostic information about coronary anatomy, can establish the

presence or absence of co-existing atherosclerotic disease, and can directly measure pressure within the left ventricle.

● Genetic testing to find the mutation in a particular case can be expensive and laborious because there are numerous genetic mutations. However, once the mutation is found, this can be used as a screening test for relatives. Once a genetic diagnosis has been made in a relative, decisions regarding follow-up can be made, particularly in cases where no echo abnormalities are present.

Management

● **Asymptomatic patients.** There is no evidence to support pharmacological intervention in asymptomatic patients with or without outflow tract gradients or LV hypertrophy. Where there is a high risk of SCD, device implantation is recommended (p. 410).

● **Beta-adrenergic antagonists.** There is little evidence to support the use of β-blockers, except in the context of symptomatic benefit. **Propranolol**, **atenolol**, **metoprolol** and **nadolol** have been used in order to relieve symptoms of breathlessness or chest pain in patients who suffer exercise-induced obstruction. They have the theoretical advantage of vasoconstriction, which could reduce the gradient between the ventricle and aorta and minimize the Venturi effect while prolonging diastole and reducing the force of myocardial contraction. Any benefit can be monitored by exercise testing, as subjective improvements in symptoms can be unreliable.

● **Calcium channel blockers. Verapamil** shares the negative inotropic effects of β-blockers but is a vasodilator and therefore can worsen the gradient across the obstruction if any exists. For this reason, it is a second-line drug and should be avoided in severely symptomatic patients. It can be a useful alternative in patients with milder symptoms where β-blockade is unsuccessful or unfeasible due to contraindications, e.g. asthma.

● **Diuretics.** Diuretics can be used but in low dose, as fluid retention maintains high filling pressures, which are required in cases of diastolic dysfunction.

● **Disopyramide.** This class 1a anti-arrhythmic agent also has negatively inotropic effects and antimuscarinic effects. The effect on inotropy can be harnessed in patients who suffer severe symptoms with resting obstruction but the reflex tachycardia often requires control with a combination of a low-dose β-adrenergic antagonist.

● **End-stage HCM.** Vasodilators are generally contraindicated in HCM, but in a small proportion of patients HCM evolves into a condition similar to dilated cardiomyopathy with systolic dysfunction and wall thinning. In this circumstance, patients can be treated with ACE inhibition/ARBs and diuretics.

● **Transplant.** HCM may cause end-stage heart failure at a relatively early age compared to patients with ischaemic heart disease. Patients with HCM also tend to have single organ involvement and this makes them attractive candidates for cardiac transplant.

● **Ventricular septal myectomy and alcohol-induced septal ablation.** Ventricular septal myectomy and alcohol-induced septal ablation are recommended for patients with symptoms attributable to a severe outflow tract gradient. Septal ablation by catheter has an advantage in that it is less invasive but produces results similar to those of surgical

Kumar & Clark's Medical Management and Therapeutics

myectomy. A higher proportion of patients who receive catheter ablation require a permanent pacemaker.

● ICD. Where no risk factors for SCD are present, patients have an excellent prognosis. However, each of the risk factors above constitutes a relatively weak predictor of adverse events and there is therefore some difficulty in deciding who merits implantation of an ICD. There is little evidence to support pharmacological prevention of malignant arrhythmia.

ARRHYTHMOGENIC RIGHT VENTRICULAR CARDIOMYOPATHY

Arrhythmogenic right ventricular cardiomyopathy (ARVC) is an uncommon (1/5000 people) inherited condition that predominantly affects the right ventricle, with fatty or fibro-fatty replacement of myocytes leading to segmental or global dilatation. LV involvement has been reported in up to 75% of cases. The fibro-fatty replacement causes ventricular arrhythmia and risk of sudden death in its early stages, and right ventricular or biventricular failure in its later stages.

Autosomal dominant ARVC has been mapped to eight chromosomal loci within mutations in four genes — cardiac ryanodine receptor RyR2 (also responsible for familial catecholaminergic polymorphic ventricular tachycardia, CPVT), desmoplakin, plakophilin-2, and mutations altering the regulatory sequences of the transforming growth factor-β gene.

There are two recessive forms — **Naxos disease** (associated with palmoplantar keratoderma and woolly hair), due to a mutation in junctional plakoglobin, and **Carvajal syndrome**, due to a mutation in desmoplakin.

Clinical features

● Most patients are asymptomatic.
● Symptomatic ventricular arrhythmias or syncope or sudden death occur. Occasionally, presentation is with symptoms and signs of right heart failure, although this is more common in the later stages of the disease. Some patients maybe detected through family screening.

Investigations

● ECG is usually normal but may demonstrate T wave inversion in the precordial leads related to the right ventricle (V1–V3). Small-amplitude potentials occurring at the end of the QRS complex (epsilon waves) may be present and incomplete or complete RBBB is sometimes seen. Signal-averaged ECG may indicate the presence of late potentials, the delayed depolarization of individual muscle cells. Twenty-four-hour Holter monitoring may demonstrate frequent extrasystoles of right ventricular origin or runs of non-sustained ventricular tachycardia.
● Echocardiography is frequently normal but with more advanced cases may demonstrate right ventricular dilatation and aneurysm formation; there may be LV dilatation.
● Cardiac MR can more accurately assess the right ventricle and in some cases can demonstrate fibro-fatty infiltration.
● Genetic testing may soon be the diagnostic gold standard.
● Endomyocardial biopsy shows reduced levels of plakoglobin on immunofluorescence (90% sensitive; 80% specific).

Treatment

Beta-blockers are first-line treatment for patients with non-life-threatening arrhythmias. **Amiodarone** or **sotalol** is used for symptomatic arrhythmias, but for refractory or life-threatening arrhythmias an ICD is required. Occasionally, cardiac transplantation is indicated for either intractable arrhythmia or cardiac failure.

RESTRICTIVE CARDIOMYOPATHY

Idiopathic familial restrictive cardiomyopathy is rare but may be part of a clinical spectrum of cardiac troponin gene mutations, a different physiological manifestation of HCM with the same autosomal dominant inheritance.

Secondary restrictive cardiomyopathy may be due to amyloidosis, sarcoidosis, haemochromatosis, Fabry's disease, tropical endomyocardial fibrosis and hypereosinophilic endomyocardial fibrosis.

Pathophysiology

Restrictive physiology results from a loss of ventricular wall compliance and diastolic filling. The stiffened ventricles require increased atrial force of contraction to fill and this leads to progressive atrial hypertrophy and dilatation, which is usually severe. The ventricular wall thickness and the internal dimensions remain normal. However, the right ventricular pressure increases and may be as high as 60 mmHg.

Clinical features

Symptoms are of biventricular failure and include a reduction in effort tolerance due to breathlessness and peripheral oedema. Patients may exhibit signs of the underlying condition.

Diagnosis

The differential diagnosis is constrictive pericarditis.

- CXR may be normal or may show pulmonary venous congestion.
- ECG may show P-wave changes consistent with bi-atrial enlargement and interventricular conduction defects due to the disease process infiltrating the myocardium.
- Echocardiography may show a brightened myocardium and also a pericardial effusion in amyloidosis. There will be severe bi-atrial enlargement and little or no respiratory variation in septal movement or in mitral or tricuspid inflow. Cardiac catheterization may be required to distinguish between restrictive and constrictive physiologies.

Where there is a clinical suspicion of infiltrative cardiomyopathy (e.g. hypercalcaemia in sarcoidosis) and there is no alternative diagnostic test, **myocardial biopsy** may be necessary as confirmation.

Management

Treatment of any underlying cause may reverse the defect, especially in Fabry's disease, sarcoidosis and haemochromatosis. Unfortunately, other causes are not amenable to therapy and medial treatment aimed at symptomatic relief may be the only option, with end-stage disease being eligible for cardiac transplantation.

PERIPARTUM CARDIOMYOPATHY

Peripartum cardiomyopathy is a dilated cardiomyopathy with an unknown pathophysiology. The definition involves exclusion of pre-existing cardiomyopathy and a time period of incidence of 1 month before delivery to 5 months post delivery. There can be a full spectrum of disease severity, from mild to fatal. Presentations include arrhythmia, peripheral and pulmonary oedema, emboli and shock. Fortunately, spontaneous resolution

Kumar & Clark's Medical Management and Therapeutics

is likely, provided adequate support can be given in the acute phase; this includes appropriate treatment for heart failure with diuretics, vasodilators and β-blockade if required. If medical therapy is insufficient, LVADs are particularly appropriate as a means of avoiding cardiac transplantation until resolution of heart failure. Mothers should be advised that recurrence in subsequent pregnancies is common.

PERICARDIAL DISEASE

CONSTRICTIVE PERICARDITIS

The cause of constrictive pericarditis is usually post-tuberculous pericarditis but other causes include post-cardiac surgery and radiation therapy.

Pathophysiology

The pericardium is a partly compliant sac of fibrous tissue; progressive inflammation leads to loss of compliance and encasement of the heart within this sac. The right ventricle is relatively collapsible compared to the more muscular left ventricle and therefore loses its chance to distend in diastole where there is competition for limited space with the left ventricle. Thus right-sided atrial and systemic venous pressure is increased. During inspiration, intrathoracic pressure decreases, which would normally lead to increased venous return and cardiac output. However, where there is constriction, the atrial pressures are increased, and when pulmonary venous pressure is reduced by inspiration, venous return to the left atrium is also reduced. This lowers cardiac output and produces an exaggerated reduction in systolic BP (≥ 10 mmHg) with inspiration (pulsus paradoxus).

Clinical features

The predominance of right heart failure symptoms points to the diagnosis. Breathlessness, pleural effusions, peripheral oedema, ascites and hepatic congestion are all common. The JVP is raised, and a further rise with inspiration is due to the inability of the right ventricle to fill and increased venous return due to inspiration.

Diagnosis

A history of previous TB, surgery or radiation may be present.
- **CXR** reveals pericardial calcification in a proportion of cases, and apical pulmonary calcification may signify previous TB.
- **ECG** may show small QRS voltages.
- **Echocardiography** will reveal the impaired diastolic relaxation and exaggerated responses to respiration, with mitral and tricuspid inflow varying by $\geq 25\%$. Pericardial thickening and effusions may also be seen.
- **CT** provides a more sensitive means of visualizing pericardial thickening and calcification.

Management

Pericardiotomy is the definitive management and, in the presence of pure pericardial disease, is highly effective. However, if there is concurrent ventricular dysfunction, the improvement is less impressive. Oedema can be palliated with diuretics.

AORTIC DISSECTION

This occurs when a tear forms in the intima of the arterial wall, which causes blood to separate the intima from the media, creating a false lumen.

This can extend proximally to involve the aortic root and therefore the coronary sinuses and aortic valve, or distally to involve any major vascular bed. It can be acute or chronic and, if untreated, carries a high mortality.

Risk factors

Any condition that weakens the aortic wall either by direct strain (e.g. hypertension) or structural changes (e.g. connective tissue diseases, inflammation or infection) may predispose to aortic dissection. Hypertension, bicuspid aortic valve and Marfan syndrome are the most common risk factors. Dissections are classified into those affecting the ascending aorta (type A) and those involving the descending aorta (type B).

Clinical features

The pain of aortic dissection is characteristically of sudden onset and severe, often described as tearing and commonly radiating through to the back. Dissection can present in many other ways including inferior STEMI, cardiovascular collapse, pulmonary oedema and neurological events.

On examination the patient may have neurological signs due to loss of blood supply to the spinal cord, aortic regurgitation, pulmonary oedema, a pulse and/or BP deficit, labile BP or tamponade and loss of peripheral pulses. Measurement of BP in both arms is mandatory.

Investigations

- ECG may show inferior ST elevation, indicating an inferior MI, if the dissection has involved the ostium of the right coronary artery.
- CXR shows widened mediastinum only in a traumatic dissection.
- TTE may be useful to look for aortic regurgitation and may occasionally be diagnostic. This should not delay a definitive investigation. Any patient with a suspected aortic dissection *must* have a definitive investigation.
- Definitive investigation should be chosen depending on what is available locally and how stable the patient is.
  - *TOE* has a high sensitivity and specificity. It can be done at the bedside by an experienced operator and is the first-line investigation, where available.
  - *CMR* is the gold standard imaging modality of choice and is being used more and more to establish the cause of acute central chest pain.
  - *CT scan* with contrast is used if MRI is unavailable.

Management

- BP should be continuously monitored via an arterial line.
- Systolic pressure should be kept at about 100 mmHg. This is usually achieved using an IV infusion of short-acting β-blocker, **esmolol** 50–200 mcg/kg/min, or **labetalol** 2 mg/min, which has α- as well as β-blocking effects.
- An alternative agent is IV **sodium nitroprusside** 0.25–0.5 mcg/kg/min, which *must* be used with the β-blocker, as the sympathetic stimulation increases LV contraction, leading to aortic shear stress.

Patients should be referred to a cardio-thoracic centre for guidance concerning further management.

- Type A dissections need *urgent* surgical repair with a composite graft to prevent aortic rupture and pericardial tamponade and to relieve aortic regurgitation.
- Type B dissections can often be managed medically, provided there is no progression/deterioration or involvement of other arteries, e.g.

coeliac or renal. There is a consensus that the prevention of life-threatening complications of type B dissection is an indication for surgery; these include persistent or recurrent chest pain, aortic expansion, pericardial haematoma and/or mediastinal haematoma. Treatment of other complications of type B dissections can often now be done by stenting.

After discharge, patients need tight control of their BP, regular imaging (MRI, CT or TOE) and outpatient clinic follow-up.

HYPERTENSION

Definition

Hypertension is elevated BP (> 140/90 mmHg). Elevated BP is a significant determinant in the cause of cerebrovascular, ischaemic heart and peripheral vascular disease.

Hypertension is very common in the developed world and with advancing age the prevalence of hypertension increases. The prevalence of hypertension has been estimated to be 42% in people aged 35–64 years. Hypertension rates are much higher in black people of African descent.

The **classification** of blood pressures is outlined in Table 12.14. A category of pre-hypertension has been introduced, as these patients are at risk of cardiovascular disease and require follow-up.

The risk of mortality or morbidity rises progressively with increasing systolic and diastolic pressures. All adults should have their BP measured every 5 years until the age of 80 years. Measurements taken after 5 mins sitting are usually sufficient. The cuff should be deflated at 2 mm/s and the BP measured to the nearest 2 mmHg. Two consistent BP measurements are needed to estimate the BP level. **Ambulatory BP** monitoring is useful in patients with fluctuating BP and also for monitoring therapy.

Causes

The majority (80–90%) of hypertensive patients have essential hypertension; the remainder have secondary hypertension, which is the result of a specific and potentially treatable condition.

Table 12.14 Joint National Committee 7 (JN7) classification of BP levels

Category	Systolic BP (mmHg)	Diastolic BP (mmHg)
Normal	< 120	< 80
Pre-hypertension	120–139	80–89
Hypertension		
Stage 1	140–159	90–99
Stage 2	> 160	> 100
Isolated systolic hypertension	> 160	< 90

(National Institutes of Health 2003, with permission)

- **Secondary causes** include renal parenchymal disease, reno-vascular disease, phaeochromocytoma, Cushing's syndrome, primary aldosteronism and coarctation of the aorta. It is impracticable and unnecessary to screen all hypertensive patients for secondary causes. The highest chances of detecting such causes are in:
  - subjects under 35 years, especially those without a family history of hypertension
  - those with accelerated (malignant) hypertension and those with evidence of renal disease (e.g. proteinuria, unequal renal sizes)
  - those with hypokalaemia before diuretic therapy
  - those resistant to conventional antihypertensive therapy (e.g. more than three drugs)
  - those with unusual symptoms (e.g. sweating attacks or weakness).
- **Essential hypertension** has a multi-factorial aetiology. This includes genetic, fetal, humoral and environmental factors, as well as evidence of insulin resistance (see metabolic syndrome, p. 429). The most significant environmental factors include obesity, alcohol intake, sodium intake and stress.
- **Malignant hypertension** is seen when BP rises rapidly and also with severe hypertension (diastolic BP > 120 mmHg). The characteristic histological change is fibrinoid necrosis of the arterial vessel wall. If the condition is left untreated, it will lead to death from progressive renal failure, heart failure, aortic dissection or stroke. There is a high risk of cerebral oedema and haemorrhage with encephalopathy. In the retina there are flame-shaped haemorrhages, cotton wool spots, hard exudates and papilloedema. Without effective treatment there is a 1-year survival of < 20%.

Investigations

- ECG — for LV hypertrophy.
- Echo — for LV function.
- Urine dipstick — for protein and blood.
- Fasting bloods — for lipids and glucose.
- Serum urea, creatinine, calculated GFR (cGFR) and electrolytes.

If urea or creatinine is elevated or cGFR reduced, then more investigations will be indicated, e.g. visualization of renal tract by US/renal isotope scan.

Treatment

In patients with **pre-hypertension** and **stage 1 hypertension**, there should be an initial 3–6-month period of assessment with repeated BP measurement, in association with advice and non-pharmacological measures. The British Hypertension Society suggests the following:

- weight reduction — BMI should be < 25
- low-fat and low-saturated fat diet
- low-sodium diet (< 6 g sodium chloride per day)
- limited alcohol consumption (< 21 U/week for men, < 14 U for women)
- dynamic exercise (e.g. walking 30 mins 5 times weekly)
- increased fruit and vegetable consumption
- stopping smoking.

Patients should be encouraged to check their BP regularly at home with a self-monitoring device.

Drug therapy

The **indications for initiating antihypertensive therapy** include:

- sustained systolic BP > 160 mmHg
- sustained diastolic BP > 100 mmHg
- sustained systolic BP between 140 and 159 mmHg or sustained diastolic BP between 90 and 99 mmHg, in patients who have evidence of target organ damage or a 10-year cardiovascular risk > 20% on a risk prediction chart.

In patients with diabetes mellitus, initiation of therapy should occur in the presence of:

- sustained systolic BP >140 mmHg
- diastolic BP > 90 mmHg.

Treatment goals

- In non-diabetic hypertensive patients BP should be < 140/85 mmHg.
- In diabetic patients hypertensive patients BP should be < 130/80 mmHg.
- Most require a combination of antihypertensive drugs to achieve the recommended targets, as well as **statins** and **aspirin** to reduce overall cardiovascular risk.
- Glycaemic control should be optimized in diabetics with HbA_{1C} of < 7%.

Specific treatments

The decision to commence specific drug therapy should usually be made after a period of assessment of up to 6 months, with repeated measurements of BP and the institution of non-pharmacological therapy. The aim of treatment is to reduce the risk of complications of hypertension.

Initial management of hypertension

In many patients initial therapy should be with a thiazide diuretic, although this has been questioned. Some recommend that the young hypertensive should start on an ACE inhibitor as first-line therapy. In the ALLHAT study **chlortalidone** 12.5 mg a day, rising to 25 mg daily, was used. **Bendroflumethiazide** 2.5 mg daily is also widely used. Patients over 55 years (and/or black) do not respond to diuretics and in this group, as well as in patients who have had an inadequate response to thiazide monotherapy, an ACE inhibitor is used. Angiotensin II receptor blockers (ARBs) are used in patients who cannot tolerate an ACE inhibitor. If this treatment fails to control BP adequately, a calcium channel blocker should be added in a stepwise manner until control is achieved. The use of β-blockers is not now recommended for routine initial treatment of uncomplicated hypertension.

Most patients require more than one drug to control their BP adequately, and other agents, such as directly acting vasodilators and adrenoreceptor-blocking drugs, are sometimes required in the resistant patient.

The recommended regimens for the treatment of hypertension are complex and depend on age, race and the patient's response. Most of the available evidence suggests that the attained BP, rather than the drug used, is of primary importance for effective therapy.

The available drugs are described below.

Diuretics
- Thiazide and thiazide-related diuretics
  - **Bendroflumethiazide** 2.5 mg daily.
  - **Chlortalidone** 12.5–25 mg daily.
  - **Indapamide** 2.5 mg daily.

Mode of action: a natriuresis is caused, thus reducing intravascular volume. Thiazides and related diuretics block sodium reabsorption in the distal convoluted tubule by inhibiting the Na/Cl co-transporter.

These are effective agents in the treatment of hypertension. Accumulated data suggest that they are safe and benefit the patient by reducing the risk of complications of hypertension. Thiazide diuretics may be more effective than α-adrenergic antagonists in the treatment of hypertension, and may lessen the risk of cardiovascular disease and stroke in patients with hypertension and at least one coronary heart disease risk factor. These relatively inexpensive agents have been shown to be effective for BP control and reduction in end points such as fatal and non-fatal MI.

Lower doses appear as effective as higher doses in reduction of BP. They act within 1–2 hours of oral administration and most have a duration of up to 24 hours. These drugs should not be used in pregnancy. The main concern regarding these drugs is their potential **adverse effects,** which tend to occur with higher doses and include raised serum cholesterol, impaired glucose tolerance, hyperuricaemia, hypokalaemia, hypomagnesaemia and hyponatraemia. Other side-effects include weakness, muscular cramps and erectile dysfunction.

- Loop diuretics
  - **Furosemide** 20–40 mg daily oral.
  - **Bumetanide** 1–2 mg daily oral.

Mode of action: loop diuretics block sodium reabsorption in the thick ascending loop of Henle through the inhibition of the Na/K/2 Cl co-transporter. They are not usually used for hypertension except in patients with renal impairment. **Side-effects** include electrolyte disturbances such as hypokalaemia, hyponatraemia and hypomagnesaemia but these are rare when these drugs are used for hypertension.

Potassium-sparing diuretics
- **Amiloride** 5–10 mg daily.
- **Triamterene** 50 mg orally.

These drugs are used in combination with a thiazide diuretic if hypokalaemia develops. They are not usually necessary in the treatment of hypertension and have no hypotensive effect on their own.

- **Spironolactone** 50–200 mg (only used in hypertension due to primary hyperaldosteronism).

Angiotensin-converting enzyme (ACE) inhibitors
- **Perindopril** 4 mg daily.
- **Enalapril** 5–20 mg daily.
- **Ramipril** 1.25–5 mg daily.
- **Fosinopril** 10–40 mg daily.
- **Lisinopril** 10–20 mg daily.
- **Quinapril** 20–40 mg daily.

These are now often used as first-line therapy in all patients. ACE inhibitors have beneficial effects in patients with coexisting heart failure. One study suggested that ramipril might significantly reduce MI and stroke in patients with heart failure or low ejection fraction.

Mode of action: these drugs block the conversion of angiotensin I to angiotensin II, which is a potent vasoconstrictor. They also block the degradation of bradykinin, which is a potent vasodilator. They lead to arterial and venous vasodilatation and natriuresis.

They are particularly useful in diabetics with nephropathy, where they have been shown to slow renal disease progression, and in patients with either symptomatic or asymptomatic LV dysfunction, as they improve survival.

The main **side-effects** include significant first-dose hypotension (particularly if the patient is on a diuretic) and deterioration of renal function in those with bilateral reno-vascular disease. Patients often describe a dry cough (20%), which can occur at higher doses. This is thought to be due to bradykinin degradation. Hyperkalaemia occurs. ACE inhibitors should be avoided in pregnancy and in patients who are breast feeding.

Angiotensin II receptor antagonists (angiotensin receptor blockers, ARBs)

- **Losartan** 50–100 mg daily.
- **Candesartan** 8–32 mg daily.
- **Valsartan** 80–160 mg daily.
- **Irbesartan** 75–300 mg daily.

This group of drugs is also now used as first-line therapy. **Mode of action**: they selectively block the receptors for angiotensin II and lead to decreased peripheral vascular resistance. The actions are similar to ACE inhibitors but they do not cause a dry cough, as they do not affect bradykinin degradation. They are effective in a diverse range of patients. They are also used in patients with heart failure and in diabetics who are unable to tolerate ACE inhibitors.

Side-effects occur occasionally and include angio-oedema, allergic reaction and rash. Avoid in pregnancy and breast feeding. These drugs should be used cautiously in patients with renal artery stenosis.

Calcium channel blockers

- **Amlodipine** 5–10 mg daily.
- **Verapamil** 80–480 mg 3 times daily.
- **Nifedipine** 10–20 mg 3 times daily.
- **Diltiazem** 60–180 mg twice daily).

Mode of action: these agents selectively block the slow inward calcium channels in vascular smooth muscle walls and hence reduce BP by arteriolar dilatation; some of them also reduce the force of cardiac contraction. They are useful in patients with coexisting ischaemic heart disease.

Calcium channel blockers are effective in treating hypertension and include benzothiazepines (**diltiazem**), diphenylalkylamines (**verapamil**) and dihydropyridines (**amlodipine**, **nifedipine**). In the mid-1990s concerns arose regarding the use of short-acting dihydropyridine calcium channel blockers and an increase in the number of ischaemic cardiac events. None the less, long-acting agents are safe in the management of hypertension.

The major **side-effects** are often seen with the short-acting agents and include headache, sweating, swelling of the ankles, palpitations and flushing. **Verapamil** can also be associated with nausea and constipation. The short-acting agents, such as **nifedipine** 10–20 mg 3 times daily, are being replaced by once-a-day preparations including **amlodipine** 5–10 mg daily. All are metabolized in the liver and doses should be adjusted for patients with cirrhosis. Some of these drugs also inhibit hepatically cleared medications, e.g. **ciclosporin**. They have no effect on electrolytes, lipid profiles or glucose metabolism. **Verapamil** and **diltiazem** can worsen heart failure and cause cardiac arrhythmias; they have negative inotropic and chronotropic effects.

Beta-adrenoceptor-blocking drugs (β-blockers)

- **Propranolol** 80 mg twice daily.
- **Atenolol** 25–50 mg daily.
- **Bisoprolol** 5–20 mg daily.
- **Metoprolol** 25–200 mg twice daily.

Mode of action: these agents exert their action by reducing the effects of the sympathetic nervous system and the renin–angiotensin system. They reduce the force of cardiac contraction and lower the increase between resting and exercise-induced heart rate. Some agents depress renin secretion. The exact mode of action of β-blockers in lowering BP is unclear. They reduce BP but are not as effective as other antihypertensives in reducing the incidence of stroke, MI and cardiovascular mortality, especially in the elderly.

Atenolol is relatively cardio-selective, i.e. it has less effect on the B2 receptors (non-cardiac) and it is less lipid-soluble and consequently less likely to produce side-effects originating from the CNS. Atenolol reduces brachial artery pressure but not aortic pressure, which is more significant in the causation of strokes and heart attacks.

The main **side-effects** include high-degree AV block, heart failure, glucose intolerance, bronchospasm, Raynaud's phenomenon, fatigue, nightmares, hallucinations and erectile dysfunction.

Renin inhibitors

- **Aliskerin** 150 mg once daily, increased if necessary to 300 mg daily.

Mode of action: this is the first orally active renin inhibitor that directly inhibits plasma renin activity; it reduces the negative feedback by which angiotensin II inhibits renin release. It has been used in combination with ACE inhibitors and ARBs, with a significant reduction in BP. **Side-effects** are few but hypokalaemia occurs.

Alpha-adrenoreceptor-blocking drugs

- **Doxazosin** 1–4 mg daily.
- **Indoramin** 25–200 mg twice daily.

Mode of action: these agents cause post-synaptic α-blockade with resultant vasodilatation and BP reduction. Long-acting examples such as doxazosin are used in combination with other antihypertensives. The updated results of the ALLHAT study suggested that α-adrenergic antagonists may be less efficacious than diuretics, calcium channel blockers and ACE inhibitors in reducing primary end points of cardiovascular disease when used as monotherapy.

The main **side-effect** of these agents is a first-dose effect, which results from a greater reduction in BP with the first dose than with subsequent doses. They can also cause syncope, orthostatic hypotension, dizziness, headache and drowsiness, and occasionally blood dyscrasias and liver dysfunction.

Agents with α- and β-blocking effect

- **Labetalol** 100–400 mg twice daily.
- **Carvedilol** 12.5–25 mg daily.

Mode of action: these agents have both α- and β-blocking activity. They antagonize the effects of catecholamines at β-receptors and peripheral αI receptors. Labetalol is not routinely used, except in pregnancy-induced hypertension. The main **side-effects** of labetalol include hepatocellular damage, postural hypotension, a positive ANA test, a lupus-like syndrome and tremors. Carvedilol has a similar side-effect profile to other β-adrenergic antagonists but is not commonly used in hypertension.

Centrally acting adrenergic agents
● **Methyldopa** 250–2000 mg twice daily.
● **Clonidine** 0.1–1.2 mg twice daily.
Mode of action: these agents stimulate the central pre-synaptic αII receptors and cause a decrease in peripheral sympathetic tone, which reduces systemic vascular resistance. They also cause a modest reduction in cardiac output and heart rate. Clonidine provides all the benefits of methyldopa without the rare autoimmune reactions. Methyldopa is still widely used despite central and potentially serious hepatic and blood **side-effects**. Common side-effects also include bradycardia, drowsiness, dry mouth, orthostatic hypotension, galactorrhoea and erectile dysfunction.

Direct-acting vasodilators
● **Hydralazine** up to 100 mg daily.
● **Minoxidil** up to 50 mg daily.
These agents are potent vasodilators that are reserved for patients resistant to other forms of treatment or for specific circumstances, such as the use of **hydralazine** in pregnancy.

   Mode of action: minoxidil causes direct arterial vasodilatation via hyperpolarization and relaxation of smooth muscle by stimulating an adenosine triphosphate-dependent K channel. The mechanism of action of hydralazine is unknown.

   These drugs can be used alone for a short time; however, their sustained antihypertensive action is limited by reflex sodium and fluid retention, with sympathetic hyperactivity producing tachycardia. Consequently, they are often used in combination with a diuretic or a β-blocker in order to reduce these unwanted **side-effects**. These drugs should be avoided in patients with ischaemic heart disease because of the reflex sympathetic hyperactivity. **Hydralazine** can be associated with headache, nausea, tachycardia, fluid retention and an SLE-like syndrome that may affect up to 10% of patients. Patients who are at risk of developing this side-effect include those receiving large doses (> 400 mg/day), those with impaired cardiac or renal function, and those with the slow acetylation phenotype. Hydralazine should be discontinued if there is clinical evidence of the development of a lupus-like syndrome and an ANA-positive test. The syndrome usually resolves with the removal of the drug. **Minoxidil** can cause severe oedema, excessive hair growth, coarse facial features and pericardial effusions.

Parenteral antihypertensives
● **Glyceryl trinitrate** (GTN) onset 1–2 mins, dose 1–10 mL/hour (50 mg/ 50 mL).
● **Labetalol** onset 5–10 mins, dose 20–80 mg every 10 mins.
● **Esmolol** onset 1–5 mins, dose 500 mcg/kg/min for 1st min, then 50– 300 mcg/kg/min.
These drugs are indicated in the immediate reduction of BP in patients with hypertensive emergencies, e.g. aortic dissection. They are also

indicated for patients with peri-operative hypertensive problems and those in need of emergency surgery. An accurate baseline BP should be obtained before initiating therapy. This is best achieved by admission to ICU for close intra-arterial monitoring. These drugs are not necessary for malignant hypertension.

GTN can be given as a continuous infusion and is the preferred agent in patients with moderate hypertension in the setting of acute coronary ischaemia or post-coronary bypass surgery. GTN reduces preload more than afterload and should be used with caution or avoided in patients who have inferior MI with right ventricular infarction.

Labetalol is the drug of choice in hypertensive emergencies that occur in pregnancy. When given intravenously, the β-adrenergic antagonist effect is greater than the α-adrenergic effect. As the half-life is 5–8 hours, intermittent IV bolus doses may be preferable to continuous IV infusion. IV infusion can be discontinued before an oral preparation is given.

Esmolol is a short-acting cardioselective β-adrenergic antagonist that can be used when β-blocker intolerance is a concern. It is useful in the treatment of aortic dissection.

Management of hypertension in special situations

Malignant hypertension/hypertensive crisis

Patients with severe hypertension (diastolic pressure > 140 mmHg), malignant hypertension (grade 3 or 4 retinopathy) or hypertensive encephalopathy should be admitted to hospital for initiation of therapy.

It is unwise to reduce the BP too quickly, as this can lead to cerebral infarction, blindness and myocardial ischaemia. The aim is to reduce the diastolic BP to 100–110 mmHg over 24–48 hours. This is achieved by oral medication such as **atenolol** 25 mg or **amlodipine** 5 mg. The BP can be normalized over the next 2–3 days, usually by adding an ACE inhibitor or ARB. Parenteral hypotensive therapy is rarely necessary; **sodium nitroprusside** (p. 461) is used, usually in dissection, if there is no response to oral therapy.

Management of hypertension in pregnancy

Treatment of hypertension should begin if the diastolic BP is > 100 mmHg. Non-pharmacological methods, such as weight reduction and vigorous exercise, are not recommended during pregnancy.

First-line therapy with **methyldopa** 250 mg 2–3 times daily is generally recommended because of its proven safety.

Hypertension can also be treated with **hydralazine** 25 mg twice daily or **labetalol** 100 mg twice daily and these drugs can be used parenterally in emergencies. ACE inhibitors are contraindicated in pregnancy.

When a patient has clinical evidence of pre-eclampsia or eclampsia, then the specialist help of an obstetrician should be sought.

The elderly hypertensive patient

Older patients often have other medical problems; however, benefit from BP reduction can be seen up to 80 years of age with BP levels over 160/90 mmHg. If antihypertensives are already being given, these should be continued despite the age of the patient.

Drugs should be increased slowly to avoid adverse effects and hypotension. Diuretics as initial therapy have been shown to reduce the BP and the incidence of stroke, fatal MI and overall mortality in this group of patients.

Older patients have an increased vascular resistance, decreased plasma renin activity and greater LVH than younger patients. Calcium channel blockers reduce vascular resistance and are very useful in the older patient. ACE inhibitors and ARBs may be effective agents in the elderly.

Long-term studies have shown the safety and effectiveness of β-blockers, particularly after MI. Agents that could cause postural hypotension should be avoided. Central α-adrenergic antagonists are effective in older patients but can cause drowsiness.

Isolated systolic hypertension with blood pressures > 160 mmHg are often seen in the elderly and should be lowered in the over-60s, even with a normal diastolic pressure. A thiazide diuretic or a calcium channel blocker (e.g. **amlodipine**) with the addition of an ACE inhibitor if necessary, is effective.

The diabetic hypertensive patient

Control of BP has been shown to slow down loss of renal function. ACE inhibitors should be used as first-line therapy. They have been shown to reduce proteinuria and to slow progressive loss of renal function independent of their antihypertensive effects.

ACE inhibitors may also be beneficial in reducing the rates of death, MI and stroke in diabetics who have cardiovascular risk factors but lack LV dysfunction. ARBs are used in patients with intolerance to ACE inhibitors.

Further reading

Battacharyya S, Shapira AH, Mikhailidis DP, Davar J: Drug induced fibrotic valvular heart disease, *Lancet* 374:577–585, 2009.

Braunwald E: Biomarkers in heart failure, *N Engl J Med* 358:2148–2158, 2008.

Carlberg B: Time to lower treatment blood pressure targets for hypertension, *Lancet* 374:503–504, 2009.

Chandrashekhar Y, Westaby S, Nerula J: Mitral stenosis, *Lancet* 374:1271–1283, 2009.

Dhinoja N, Lambiase P: A broad complex tachycardia, *Br J Hosp Med* 66:M85–M87, 2005.

Dickstein K, Cohen-Solal A, Filippatos G, et al: ESC guidelines for the diagnosis and treatment of acute and chronic heart failure 2008 of the European Society of Cardiology. Developed in collaboration with the Heart Failure Association of the ESC (HFA) and endorsed by the European Society of Intensive Care Medicine (ESICM), *Eur J Heart Fail* 10(10):93393–93398, 2008.

Ernst ME, Moser M: Use of diuretics in patients with hypertension, *New Engl J Med* 361:2153–2164, 2009.

Grove EL, Storey RF: The right oral antithrombotics in acute coronary syndromes, *Lancet* 374:1947–1948, 2009.

Jackson CE, Solomon SD, Gerstein HC, et al: Albuminuria in chronic heart failure: prevalence and prognostic importance, *Lancet* 374:543–550, 2009.

Jefferies JL, Towbin JA: Dilated cardiomyopathy, *Lancet* 375:752–762, 2010.

Josephson ME: *Clinical cardiac electrophysiology, techniques and interpretations*, ed 4, Philadelphia, 2008, Lippincott Williams & Wilkins.

Morrow DA: Clinical application of sensitive troponin assays, *New Engl J Med* 361:913–915, 2009.

Moss AJ, Jackson WJ, Cannon DS, et al: Cardiac resynchronisation therapy for the prevention of heart failure events, *New Engl J Med* 361:1328–1329, 2009.

National Institutes of Health: The seventh report of the Joint National Committee on Prevention, Detection, Evaluation, and Treatment of High Blood Pressure, *Hypertension* 42:1206, 2003.

Pfisterer M, Zellweger MJ, Gersh B: Management of stable coronary artery disease, *Lancet* 375:763–772, 2010.

Sibbing D, Kastrati A: Risk of combining PPIs with thienopyridines: fact or fiction? *Lancet* 374:952–954, 2009.

Sun JCJ, et al: Anti-thrombotic management of patients with prosthetic heart valves: current evidence and future trends, *Lancet* 374:565–576, 2009.

Xavier D, Pais P, Devereaux PJ, et al: Treatment and outcome of acute coronary syndromes in India (CREATE), *Lancet* 371:1435–1442, 2008.

Further information

www.acc.org/clinical/statements.htm
American College of Cardiology (ACC) and American Heart Association (AHA) joint guidelines

www.bhsoc.org/
British Hypertension Society

www.escardio.org/knowledge/guidelines/
European Society of Cardiology (ESC) guidelines

www.nhlbi.nih.gov/guidelines
National Heart, Lung and Blood Institute Clinical Practice Guidelines

www.nice.org.uk/CG034
NICE Clinical Guideline on Hypertension

Respiratory disease 13

CHAPTER CONTENTS

APPROACH TO THE PATIENT

- A **productive cough** is a feature of chronic obstructive pulmonary disease (COPD) or bronchiectasis (large volumes). Yellow sputum does not always indicate infection, as eosinophils in the sputum can give the same appearance, e.g. in asthma. Green sputum usually implies infection.
- **Haemoptysis** (blood-stained sputum) varies from small streaks of blood to massive bleeding.
  - Mild haemoptysis is usually caused by an acute infection, e.g. exacerbations of COPD, but it should not be attributed to this without investigation.
  - Other common causes are pulmonary infarction, bronchial carcinoma and TB.
  - In lobar pneumonia, the sputum is usually rusty in appearance rather than frankly blood-stained.
  - Pink, frothy sputum is seen in pulmonary oedema.
  - In bronchiectasis, the blood is often mixed with purulent sputum.
  - Massive haemoptyses (> 200 mL of blood in 24 hours) are usually due to bronchiectasis or TB.

Haemoptysis should always be investigated. Often, the diagnosis can be made from a CXR, but a normal CXR does not exclude disease. Bronchoscopy is only diagnostic in about 5% of patients with haemoptysis and a normal CXR.

For **management of a massive haemoptysis**, see Box 13.1.

Treatment of cough is the treatment of the underlying cause and often symptomatic. Anti-tussives include **codeine linctus** 5–10 mL 3–4 times daily or **pholcodine** 5 mL 3–4 times daily. There is no evidence that expectorants work but **simple linctus** 5 mL 3–4 times daily is comforting.

Shortness of breath

Most people get breathless on exertion; exercise tolerance should be documented. Breathlessness can be of sudden onset, e.g. in acute left ventricular

> **Box 13.1** Management of massive haemoptysis
>
> As little as 250 mL can fill the bronchial tree and be life-threatening. This is uncommon but frightening for everyone involved.
> - Monitor oxygen saturation with oximetry, BP and pulse rate
> - Exclude coagulation defects
> - Perform a CXR
> - Endotracheal intubation and suction may be required
> - Urgent bronchoscopy is needed
> - A double lumen endotracheal tube can be inserted by an anaesthetist to protect the unaffected lung
> - Bronchial artery embolization is highly effective if the bleeding vessel can be identified and bleeding continues

failure, or more progressive, as in COPD. It may vary at different times of the day, e.g. in asthma it is usually worse in the morning.

Breathlessness on lying flat occurs in, for example, pulmonary oedema (p. 425). Breathlessness with a wheeze occurring on exposure to an allergen is seen in asthma (e.g. horse riding). It can occur many hours after exposure to an allergen (p. 520) in, for example, hypersensitivity pneumonitis.

Inhalation of foreign bodies can cause choking and acute shortage of breath. Treatment is with the Heimlich manoeuvre. See Emergencies in Medicine p. 714.

Chest pain

Chest pain in respiratory disease is usually pleuritic. Pain can be due to other causes, e.g. localized pain in costochondritis. Shoulder tip pain suggests irritation of the diaphragmatic pleura. Retrosternal soreness occurs with tracheitis but also in other conditions, e.g. oesophagitis, when it is usually burning. Chest pain should always be differentiated from cardiac pain, which is usually a central crushing chest pain radiating to the jaw, neck and left arm (p. 431).

Respiratory investigations

These are discussed under specific diseases.

CHRONIC OBSTRUCTIVE PULMONARY DISEASE

Chronic obstructive pulmonary disease (COPD) is a slowly progressive condition predominantly caused by smoking and is the sixth commonest cause of death worldwide; its incidence is increasing. It is characterized by airflow limitation, which is not fully reversible. The lungs have an abnormal inflammatory response to inhaled particles or gases, resulting in airflow limitation. The GOLD (Global Initiative for Chronic Obstructive Lung Disease, WHO) criteria for the diagnosis of lung disease are shown in Table 13.1.

Table 13.1 COPD — Global Initiative in Obstructive Lung Disease (GOLD) criteria

Stage of COPD		Function	Symptoms of breathlessness
I	Mild	$FEV_1/FVC < 70\%$ $FEV_1 \geq 80\%$ predicted	None or mild
II	Moderate	$FEV_1/FVC < 70\%$ $FEV_1 \leq 50\%$ and $\leq 80\%$ of predicted	On exertion
III	Severe	$FEV_1/FVC < 70\%$ $FEV_1 \leq 30\%$ and $\leq 50\%$ of predicted	On minimal exertion, e.g. dressing
IV	Very severe	$FEV_1/FVC < 70\%$ $FEV_1 < 30\%$ predicted or $FEV_1 < 50\%$ predicted plus respiratory failure	At rest

FEV_1, forced expiratory volume in 1 sec; FVC, forced vital capacity.
(Modified from the Global Strategy for the Diagnosis, Management and Prevention of COPD, 2006. www.goldcopd.com)

Causes

Tobacco smoking, indoor air pollution from biomass fuel and environmental pollution are the major causes for COPD in the world, although only 10–20% of heavy smokers develop COPD.

Pathogenesis

- Inflammation, infection, scarring, loss of elasticity and increased secretion of mucus (which blocks airways) all play a role. There is also an imbalance of protease and antiprotease activity (α_1-antitrypsin being the major antiprotease).
- Small airways are particularly affected early in the process (obstructive bronchiolitis).
- If airway narrowing is combined with emphysema (loss of elastic recoil of the lung with collapse of small airways during expiration), airflow limitation is even more severe.
- **Microscopically**, there is infiltration of the walls of bronchi and bronchioles by acute and chronic inflammatory cells, with ulceration of epithelial layers leading to squamous metaplasia, scarring and thickening of walls.
- **Systemic** sequelae including skeletal muscle dysfunction (see below).

Thus, the characteristic physiological effects include airflow limitation and abnormal alveolar gas exchange, leading to cor pulmonale (pulmonary vascular disease).

Clinical features

COPD is suspected on the basis of chronic progressive symptoms, usually with a smoking history of more than 20 pack years (1 pack year = 20 cigarettes per day for 1 year). It is supported by objective evidence of airflow

Kumar & Clark's Medical Management and Therapeutics

limitation (or obstruction), usually with spirometry, which does not return to normal with treatment.

- Patients are usually over the age of 35, have a risk factor and present with one or more of exertional breathlessness, chronic cough, regular sputum production, frequent winter 'exacerbations/bronchitis' or wheeze.
- Effort intolerance, ankle swelling and fatigue also occur.
- Chest pain and haemoptysis are uncommon and an alternative diagnosis should be looked for.
- Extrapulmonary features occur, e.g. osteoporosis, depression and metabolic problems leading to weight loss, loss of muscle mass and weakness.

Signs

- In mild COPD, signs are absent, except for a wheeze.
- In more severe COPD, tachypnoea, prolonged expiration, pursed lip breathing, use of accessory muscles and intercostal in-drawing on inspiration are seen. Hypercapnic patients will be vasodilated with a bounding pulse and a coarse flapping tremor of the outstretched hands. Severe hypercapnia causes confusion and progressive drowsiness. Clubbing is *not* a sign of COPD and should alert the physician to the possibility of bronchiectasis or lung cancer.
- In advanced COPD, patients develop cor pulmonale.

Pulmonary hypertension/cor pulmonale

Pulmonary hypertension/cor pulmonale (p. 520) is defined as heart disease secondary to disease of the lung. It occurs in hypoxic patients with COPD. Pulmonary hypertension can be present for years without causing symptoms.

Cor pulmonale is enlargement of the right ventricle secondary to increased afterload due to primary lung disease in patients who have no other cause of ventricular dysfunction. Symptoms include worsening exertional dyspnoea, fatigue and chest pain. On examination JVP is raised and there is a right ventricular parasternal heave, a loud pulmonary component of the second heart sound, fluid retention and peripheral oedema.

Diagnosis and investigations

The diagnosis of COPD is usually clinical, supported by the presence of airflow obstruction on spirometry.

Lung function tests

- **Spirometry** shows evidence of airflow obstruction, with a reduced forced expiratory volume in 1 second (FEV_1) of < 80%, a reduced FEV_1 to forced vital capacity (FVC) ratio of < 70% and a reduced peak expiratory flow rate (PEFR). In COPD reversibility is less than in asthmatic patients (usually a change in FEV_1 of < 15%). Clinically significant COPD is not present if the FEV_1 and FEV_1/FVC ratio return to normal following treatment. FEV_1 determines severity (Table 13.1) and can also be used to monitor the course of the disease and response to therapy. In addition, FEV_1 can be used to test reversibility and is a predictor of mortality. Five-year survival is about 50% when FEV_1 falls to < 1 L.
- **Serial home PEF** measurements can be useful to exclude asthma. Reversibility to bronchodilators is also helpful in distinguishing patients who have asthma and to aid further management.

Other tests

- **Haemoglobin level and packed cell volume (PCV)** can be elevated as a result of persistent hypoxaemia causing secondary polycythaemia.
- **Arterial blood gases (ABGs)** determine the degree of hypoxia and hypercapnia. A baseline should always be taken for assessment of patients in acute exacerbations and will help in assessing the need for long-term oxygen therapy (LTOT).
- **Pulse oximetry** measures oxyhaemoglobin concentration but remember that it does *not* give information about the CO_2 ($Paco_2$ or arterial carbon dioxide tension) and hence alveolar ventilation.
- **CXR** can be normal or show hyper-expanded lung fields with low flattened diaphragms and the presence of bullae.
- **Sputum culture** is usually unnecessary.
- **ECG** is not necessary in routine assessment of COPD but can show advanced cor pulmonale; it is insensitive.
- **Alpha$_1$-antitrypsin level and phenotype** may be helpful (young non-smokers, lower lobe emphysema, a family history of chest problems). The normal range for α_1-antitrypsin is 2–4 g/L.

Management

With the exception of smoking cessation, the aims of COPD treatment are symptomatic relief and the prevention of exacerbations and complications. No existing medication has been shown to **modify decline** in lung function.

Smoking cessation

This is vital at any age or stage of the disease. An aggressive smoking cessation programme has been shown to reduce the age-related decline in FEV_1, significantly in middle-aged smokers with mild airways obstruction, and also lead to a decrease in cardiovascular and lung cancer mortality. Smokers should be told to stop and an agreed target date set. **Nicotine replacement therapy (NRT)** or **bupropion** is given, unless contraindicated, in addition to a support programme to improve the chances of success.

- **NRT** aims to replace nicotine and thus reduce the craving for a cigarette. **Chewing gum** 2 mg and 4 mg, **transdermal patches** 16-hour and 24-hour in varying doses, **nasal spray** 0.5 mg per spray, inhalational 10 mg **inhalation cartridge**, **sublingual tablets** 2 mg and **lozenges** 1, 2 and 4 mg are available. Nicotine patches should be limited to 3 months' usage. NRT should be stopped if the patient restarts smoking. **Common side-effects** are localized reactions, such as skin irritation with patches, and minor sleep disturbances. **Contradictions** include vascular disease and allergy to the drug; NRT should not be used in pregnancy or breast feeding.
- **Bupropion** sustained release is a weak, selective inhibitor of the neuronal re-uptake of dopamine and noradrenaline (norepinephrine). The exact mechanism by which it aids smoking cessation is unclear. The dose is 150 mg once a day for 1 week prior to stopping smoking and then 300 mg a day for a further 6–8 weeks, provided the patient abstains from further cigarettes. **Side-effects** include seizures in about 1 in 1000 patients. Avoid in patients with a previous history of seizures, or a concomitant administration of other medication that lowers the seizure threshold. Other side-effects include hypersensitivity reactions (0.1%), insomnia and dry mouth.

- **Combination therapy** with NRT or bupropion has so far shown no significant benefit.
- **Varenicline** is an oral partial agonist on the $\alpha_4\beta_2$ subtype of nicotinic acetylcholine receptor. A 12-week course increases the chances of stopping smoking four-fold; its main side-effect is nausea but severe depression has been recorded.

Drug therapy

This is used both for the short-term management of exacerbations and for the long-term relief of symptoms in patients with an $FEV_1 < 80\%$ predicted.

Bronchodilator therapy

Inhaler therapy remains the mainstay of treatment, despite the fact that COPD is characterized by irreversible airway obstruction. It causes relaxation of the smooth muscle and thus decreases airway resistance. Patients with mild COPD feel less breathless.

- **Inhaler technique.** Patients should be taught a good technique for using inhalers; this should be rechecked regularly. COPD patients may have problems in effective coordination and find it hard to use simple **metered-dose inhalers (MDIs)**. This can be improved by offering different types of inhaler and/or a spacer.
- **Beta$_2$-adrenoceptor agonists** act directly on the smooth muscle, have a relatively rapid onset of action and can therefore be used for symptomatic relief and prior to exercise. They can be used on an 'as required' or a 'regular' basis.
  - *Short-acting β_2-adrenoceptor agonists.* **Salbutamol** is usually given by pressurized aerosol inhalation 100–200 mcg (1–2 puffs) up to 4–6 times a day. **Terbutaline** is prescribed at a dose of 250–500 mcg (1–2 puffs) up to 3–4 times a day.
  - *Long-acting β_2-adrenoceptor agonists.* These are used in more severe airway limitation (moderate and severe COPD). They include **salmeterol** 50–100 mcg (2–4 puffs) twice a day and **formoterol** 12 mcg inhaled twice a day (depending on formulation and severity).

  Side-effects include fine tremor, nervous tension, tachycardia, arrhythmias and hypokalaemia.
- **Antimuscarinic agents** are used for achieving greater and more prolonged bronchodilatation.
  - *Short-acting antimuscarinics.* These cause bronchodilatation by blocking the bronchoconstrictor effects of cholinergic nerves. They have a longer onset of action and a more prolonged and greater bronchodilatory effect than β_2 agonists, and are associated with less toxicity. **Ipratropium bromide** is given by aerosol inhalation at a dose of 20–40 mcg 3–4 times a day or by nebulized solution 250–500 mcg 3–4 times a day.
  - *Long-acting antimuscarinics.* Inhaled **tiotropium** 18 mcg once daily improves the duration of bronchodilatation and the frequency of acute exacerbations in patients with moderate to severe COPD.

    Side-effects include dry mouth, nausea, constipation, bladder outlet obstruction, exacerbation of acute-angle glaucoma and headache.

  In **mild disease** short-acting β_2 agonists or short-acting antimuscarinic bronchodilators should be prescribed as required. Their effects are additive and once airflow becomes more severe a regular antimuscarinic can be added to a β agonist. Some patients prefer to use just one combined inhaler **ipratropium bromide 20 mcg and salbutamol 100 mcg**/metered dose 2 puffs 4 times a day.

Patients who remain symptomatic despite being treated with a combination of two short-acting bronchodilators or patients who have two or more exacerbations a year should be prescribed a long-acting bronchodilator and an inhaled corticosteroid should be added (see below).

Objective evidence of improvement in peak flow or FEV_1 may be small and the decision on whether to continue or stop therapy should be based on the patient's reported symptoms.

Corticosteroids

Corticosteroids are given to patients in the community with increasing shortness of breath that interferes with daily activities. Inhaled corticosteroids are usually reserved for stable COPD, but if already prescribed, should be continued throughout exacerbations.

- **Oral corticosteroids** The use of corticosteroids in patients with COPD remains contentious but a subgroup of patients respond to these drugs with improvement of lung function. Therefore in symptomatic patients a trial of **prednisolone** of 30 mg a day for 2 weeks can be given, with spirometry measurements before and after the treatment period. If patients show a response (FEV_1 increases > 15%), prednisolone should be stopped and an inhaled steroid such as **beclometasone** 400 mcg twice daily started. Regular oral corticosteroids are not recommended, but in advanced COPD, patients may require a maintenance dose when steroids cannot be withdrawn after an exacerbation.
- **Inhaled corticosteroids.** An inhaled corticosteroid should be given, in addition to a bronchodilator, in patients with an FEV_1 < 50% or with two or more exacerbations a year requiring treatment with antibiotics or oral corticosteroids. In addition, a trial of high-dose inhaled corticosteroid for 3 weeks in patients with moderate airflow obstruction can distinguish those patients who actually have a diagnosis of asthma and not COPD. There are a number of **different formulations and inhalers** available. The dose varies from 200 mcg to 800 mcg a day.

There are many **side-effects** associated with corticosteroids (see Box 15.2, p. 585). Inhaled steroids cause considerably fewer systemic side-effects, although at high doses adverse effects have been reported.

Combination therapy

Corticosteroids activate the $β_2$ receptor gene, increasing receptor numbers and decreasing desensitization, whilst long-acting $β_2$ agonists may amplify the anti-inflammatory effects of corticosteroids.

- Corticosteroids are used in combination with $β_2$ agonists for maintenance therapy in moderate to severe COPD, as they provide synergistic benefit for patients. They produce better control of symptoms, improved lung function and reduced exacerbation rates, with no greater risk of side-effects.
- Combinations include **fluticasone propionate** 50–500 mcg per metered dose and **salmeterol** 25–50 mcg per metered dose, or **budesonide** 100–400 mcg per metered dose and **formoterol** 6–12 mcg per metered dose. Patients usually require 1–2 puffs twice a day.

- **Other combinations** of treatment can be used if monotherapy does not control symptoms:
  - β_2 agonists and antimuscarinics
  - β_2 agonists and oral theophylline
  - antimuscarinics and oral theophylline.

Clinical effectiveness should be judged by improvements in symptoms, activities of daily living, exercise capacity and lung function. If there is no benefit after 4 weeks, therapy should be discontinued.

Antibiotics

See p. 482.

Oxygen therapy

- **Long-term oxygen therapy (LTOT)** benefits patients with progressive COPD who are hypoxic with a $Pao_2 < 8$ kPa (59 mmHg) *and* signs of cor pulmonale, such as peripheral oedema. These patients have a poor prognosis and, if left untreated, 5-year survival is < 50%.
- LTOT can also be used for exercise-induced hypoxia and to relieve acute shortness of breath. Oxygen therapy should always be used in a controlled manner, as some patients' respiratory drive depends on their degree of hypoxia (p. 483).
- **Continuous administration** of oxygen is given at 2 L/min, maintaining oxygen saturations > 90% for more than 15 hours a day. A fall in pulmonary artery pressure was achieved if oxygen was given for > 15 hours, but substantial improvements in mortality were achieved only if oxygen was administered for 19 hours daily.

The following patients should be assessed for oxygen therapy:

- those with severe airflow obstruction ($FEV_1 < 30\%$ predicted) or moderate airflow obstruction (30–49% predicted)
- cyanotic patients, polycythaemic patients and those with peripheral oedema, signs of right-sided heart failure, or oxygen saturations < 92% when breathing air.

Patients fulfil the **criteria for LTOT** when they have:

- a $Pao_2 < 7.3$ kPa (55 mmHg) when stable and breathing air; measurements should be taken on two occasions at least 3 weeks apart after appropriate bronchodilator therapy
- a Pao_2 7.3–8 kPa (55–59 mmHg) with polycythaemia, nocturnal hypoxaemia, peripheral oedema or evidence of pulmonary hypertension
- a carboxyhaemoglobin of < 3% (i.e. patients who have stopped smoking).

Guidelines for domiciliary oxygen are shown in Box 13.2.

Patients requiring LTOT will need an oxygen concentrator and education regarding its use. They should use the oxygen for at least 15 hours per day or, if possible, 20 hours per day. Once established, they should be reviewed at least once a year by a practitioner familiar with LTOT. They should be warned about the risks of explosion and fire if they continue to smoke. Short-burst oxygen should be reserved for patients with episodes of severe breathlessness that is not relieved by other treatment.

An **oxygen alert card** stating the oxygen saturation should be given to all patients who have had hypercapnic respiratory failure.

Non-invasive ventilation (NIV)

This is mainly used for exacerbations of COPD — see p. 485. The ventilators are small and can be used at home. Patients should be considered for

> **Box 13.2** Guidelines for domiciliary oxygen (Royal College of Physicians, 1999)
>
> - Chronic obstructive pulmonary disease with Pa_{O_2} < 7.3 kPa when breathing air during a period of clinical stability
> - Chronic obstructive pulmonary disease with Pa_{O_2} 7.3–8 kPa in the presence of secondary polycythaemia, nocturnal hypoxaemia, peripheral oedema or evidence of pulmonary hypertension
> - Severe chronic asthma with Pa_{CO_2} < 7.3 kPa or persistent disabling breathlessness
> - Diffuse lung disease with Pa_{O_2} < 8 kPa and in patients with Pa_{O_2} > 8 kPa with disabling dyspnoea
> - Cystic fibrosis when Pa_{O_2} < 7.3 kPa or if Pa_{O_2} 7.3–8 kPa in the presence of secondary polycythaemia, nocturnal hypoxaemia, pulmonary hypertension or peripheral oedema
> - Pulmonary hypertension without parenchymal lung involvement when Pa_{O_2} < 8 kPa
> - Neuromuscular or skeletal disorders, after specialist assessment
> - Obstructive sleep apnoea despite continuous positive airways pressure therapy, after specialist assessment
> - Pulmonary malignancy or other terminal disease with disabling dyspnoea
> - Heart failure with daytime Pa_{O_2} < 7.3 kPa (on air) or with nocturnal hypoxaemia

home NIV if, despite maximal treatment, they have hypercapnic respiratory failure and have required ventilatory support during an exacerbation, or are acidotic or hypercapnic on LTOT.

Diuretic therapy (p. 420)

This is necessary for all oedematous patients. Patients should be weighed daily.

Other agents

- Oral mucolytic drugs. Mucolytics increase the expectoration of sputum by reducing its viscosity. Regular use of mucolytics for at least 2 months can reduce the number of exacerbations of COPD and days of illness. They should be used in patients with a chronic productive cough but only continued if there is continual symptomatic improvement.
  - **Carbocisteine** 2.25 g a day in divided doses, then 1.5 g daily in divided doses. **Erdosteine** 300 mg twice daily is also used.
  - **Mecysteine hydrochloride** 200 mg 4 times a day for 2 days, followed by 200 mg 3 times a day for 6 weeks, then 200 mg twice daily.
- Anti-oxidants. **N-acetylcysteine** has both anti-oxidant and mucolytic properties, and has been shown to reduce frequency of exacerbations. However, it and other anti-oxidants, such as α-tocopherol and β-carotene supplements, are currently not recommended.

- **Anti-tussives.** Regular use of anti-tussive medication is not recommended in COPD, as there is insufficient evidence for its benefit, and although cough is a problematic symptom, it has a protective role.
- **Antibiotics**
  - There is no evidence for the use of prophylactic antibiotics.
  - Give antibiotics in acute exacerbations, as they shorten exacerbations and may prevent hospital admission.
  - Give the patient a supply of antibiotics to keep at home, to start when sputum turns yellow or green.
  - **Amoxicillin** 500 mg 3 times daily is still effective, although resistance to *H. influenzae* occurs in 10–20%. Resistance is less frequent to **cefaclor** 500 mg 8-hourly or **cefixime** 400 mg once daily; **co-amoxiclav** is an alternative.
    Long-term treatment with antibiotics was thought to be of little value but eradication of infection and keeping the lower respiratory tract free of bacteria may help prevent deterioration in lung function.
- **Vaccination/antiviral therapy**
  - *Polyvalent pneumococcal polysaccharide vaccine* usually provides lifelong immunity after a single dose.
  - *Annual influenza vaccination* should be given, unless patients have a hypersensitivity to eggs.
  - *Antiviral agents* include **zanamivir** inhalation of 10 mg twice daily for 5 days and **oseltamivir** 75 mg 12-hourly for 5 days. They are recommended for the treatment of 'at-risk' adults who can start therapy within 48 hours of presenting with an influenza-like illness. For **side-effects**, see p. 91.
- **Antidepressants.** These may be helpful in COPD, as mood disturbances such as anxiety and depression are common.
- **Alpha$_1$-protease inhibitor augmentation therapy.** Young patients with severe hereditary α_1-antitrypsin deficiency with serum levels < 0.31 g/L and abnormal lung function are candidates for α_1-antitrypsin replacement therapy. There is limited evidence for its benefit in modifying the disease in the long term.

Non-pharmacological interventions

- **Physiotherapy.** Physiotherapy is helpful for patients with excessive sputum. Patients should be encouraged to cough to remove sputum and taught the active cycle of breathing techniques and how to use positive expiratory pressure masks.
- **Nutrition.** Weight loss is common in patients with COPD and there is an association between low BMI and increased mortality. Patients with a low BMI should be referred for dietary advice and nutritional supplements. Overweight patients should also be offered dietary advice, as obesity puts additional strain on the cardio-respiratory system.
- **Pulmonary rehabilitation.** Patients with moderate to severe COPD on optimal medical treatment should be put on a pulmonary rehabilitation programme. The aim is to prevent or reverse the deconditioning that occurs in patients with COPD due to lack of exercise and immobility caused by symptoms. The rehabilitation programme is provided by a multi-disciplinary team and includes physical training, disease education, nutritional advice, and psychological, social and behavioural intervention.

Surgery

Surgical treatment for COPD is associated with a high morbidity and mortality, and patients must be carefully selected and be receiving optimal medical management prior to surgery. Bullectomy, lung volume reduction surgery and lung transplantation are used in severe disease.

Acute exacerbations of COPD (type II respiratory failure)

An acute exacerbation is defined as 'a sustained worsening of the patient's symptoms from his or her usual stable state that is beyond normal day-to-day variations, and is acute in onset'.

Exacerbations of COPD are among the commonest acute respiratory problems presenting to primary or secondary care.

- They are usually caused by infection, although only 50% of patients will have a positive sputum culture. The commonest organisms are *H. influenzae*, *Strep. pneumoniae* and *Moraxella catarrhalis*.
- Viruses, including rhinovirus, influenza (including H1N1 swine flu variant), coronavirus, adenovirus and respiratory syncytial virus, account for up to 30% of cases.
- Pollutants may also precipitate an exacerbation.
- Some patients with mild exacerbations can be treated at home, but factors such as acute confusion, a decreased level of consciousness, significant co-morbidities, severe breathlessness and acidosis require **hospital admission**.

Investigations

- **CXR** for signs of infection or other pathologies, e.g. pneumothorax or pulmonary oedema.
- **Baseline ABGs** on room air (or a known inspired oxygen concentration) to look for hypoxia or hypercapnia.
- **Purulent sputum** for culture.
- **ECG** to look for a cardiac cause for the deterioration.
- **Blood cultures** if the patient is pyrexial.
- **Routine bloods** for FBC and U&E.

Treatment

The treatment of respiratory failure in COPD is shown in Fig. 13.1. General care includes prophylaxis against deep vein thrombosis, optimizing fluid status and ensuring adequate nutrition.

- **Controlled oxygen.** A fixed performance mask can deliver 24%, 28% and 35% oxygen. It is given to correct hypoxia and maintain oxygen saturations > 90%. In a minority of patients respiratory drive is hypoxic and high oxygen concentrations can result in increasing levels of carbon dioxide, decreasing consciousness, and respiratory acidosis and arrest. Pulse oximetry should always be available to measure oxygen saturations. An ABG is performed on arrival in hospital to monitor CO_2 levels. Oxygen concentrations should never be reduced in patients who are hypoxic, even if CO_2 levels are high.
- **Bronchodilators (p. 478).** There is no benefit in delivering bronchodilators via a nebulizer over an inhaler in acute exacerbations of COPD. Bronchodilators are, however, given via a **nebulizer** with a face mask or mouth piece delivering higher doses if patients are too breathless to coordinate the use of an inhaler/spacer. If the patient is hypercapnic, the nebulizer should be driven with air and not oxygen. Oxygen can be given at the same time via nasal cannulae.

- Inhaled β_2 short-acting adrenergic agonists (p. 478). The frequency and dose of inhaled β_2-agonists can be increased in an acute exacerbation. They reach peak activity between 10 and 30 mins, and remain effective for about 4–6 hours. **Salbutamol** (via inhaler or nebulizer) is the most commonly used. *Nebulizers* are given at a dose of 2.5–5 mg, usually 4 times daily, although this can be increased provided side-effects are tolerated. Currently, there is no evidence to support the use of IV β_2-agonists in acute exacerbations of COPD.

- Inhaled short-acting antimuscarinics. These agents are often used **in combination with inhaled β_2-agonists** in acute exacerbations of COPD and are associated with fewer side-effects. They have a less rapid onset of action but a longer duration of action. They can be delivered via an inhaler as **ipratropium bromide** 20–40 mcg, or via a nebulizer **ipratropium bromide** 500 mcg, **salbutamol** 2.5 mg/2.5 mL vial, 1 vial 4 times a day.

- Systemic corticosteroids. These drugs reduce the increased airway inflammation in patients with acute exacerbations of COPD. Short courses of corticosteroids have been shown to reduce FEV_1, improve hypoxia and shorten duration of hospital stay compared to placebo. All patients admitted to hospital with an acute exacerbation should receive a course of **oral corticosteroids** 30 mg for 7–14 days, in addition to other therapies, provided there are no contraindications. The first dose of corticosteroids can be given intravenously as **hydrocortisone** or **methyl-prednisolone**. If patients do receive a prolonged course of corticosteroids, the dose should be gradually tapered down.

- Antibiotics (p. 482). There is some evidence for a small but significant benefit with antibiotics in acute exacerbations of COPD, especially in those with more severe disease. The use of antibiotics is recommended in patients with a history of increased purulence or production of sputum or in those with consolidation on CXR or clinical signs of pneumonia. Initially, treatment is empirical, with an **aminopenicillin**, a **macrolide** or a **tetracycline**, and then changed when culture results and sensitivities become available. Antibiotic use should be guided by local policy. Commonly used antibiotics include **amoxicillin** 250–500 mg 3 times daily (15% of *Haemophilus* strains may be resistant), **doxycycline** 200 mg then 100 mg daily, or **erythromycin** 250–500 mg every 6 hours or 0.5–1 g every 12 hours. **Ampicillin** can be used instead of amoxicillin.

- Methylxanthines. The use of methylxanthines such as **theophylline** (p. 501) remains controversial, as there is currently no clear evidence of benefit in acute exacerbations of COPD. IV theophylline should only be used in patients refractory to nebulized bronchodilators, and levels should be monitored within 24 hours of treatment and regularly after this period. Patients already taking oral methylxanthines should continue on this medication during an exacerbation and should *not* receive additional IV methylxanthines. IV methylxanthines are usually prescribed as **aminophylline loading dose** 5 mg/kg (250–500 mg) over at least 20 mins, followed by 0.5 mg/kg/hour over 24 hours adjusted according to plasma levels. Patients should be closely monitored throughout.

- Respiratory stimulants. These (e.g. **Doxapram** 1.5–4.0 mg/min) are only recommended for use when NIV is unavailable or considered inappropriate.

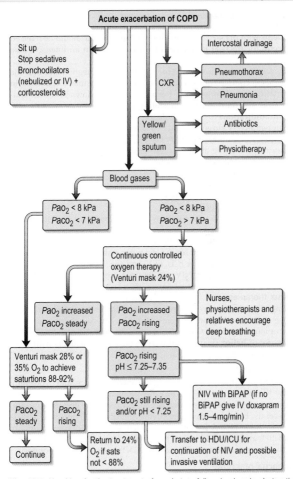

Fig. 13.1 Algorithm for the treatment of respiratory failure in chronic obstructive pulmonary disease. BiPAP, bilevel positive airways pressure; CPAP, continuous positive airways pressure; LVF, left ventricular failure; NIV, non-invasive ventilation (Calvaley & Walter 2008, with permission).

● Non-invasive ventilation (NIV)

This is the treatment of choice in patients with exacerbations of COPD who, despite maximal medical therapy and controlled oxygen therapy, have a persistent respiratory acidosis (pH 7.25–7.35, [H+] 45–56 nmol/L).

A tight-fitting facial mask delivers bi-level positive airway pressure ventilatory support (BiPAP). Continuous positive airway pressure

(CPAP, p. 542) is also used. NIV can avoid the need for endotracheal intubation.

- Patients with pH < 7.25 respond less well to NIV and should be referred directly for tracheal intubation or a trial of NIV in an intensive care setting.
- NIV results in a reduced need for endotracheal intubation and thus the associated complications. There is improved acidaemia, a reduction in mortality and a shortening of hospital stay. NIV allows better communication, and nutrition and physiotherapy to continue as normal.
- **Contraindications** to NIV include impaired consciousness, recent facial or upper airway surgery, facial abnormalities such as burns or trauma, undrained pneumothorax, hypoxaemia, cardiovascular instability, inability to protect the airway, recent gastrointestinal surgery, vomiting and copious respiratory secretions.
- Endotracheal intubation

Endotracheal intubation and mechanical ventilation are used in patients with acidaemia or with persistent or worsening hypoxia despite NIV, and when NIV is contraindicated.

- **Mortality** in patients with COPD who are intubated for an exacerbation is about 20%.
- Assessment for suitability for intubation and ventilation includes functional status, requirement for oxygen when stable, BMI, co-morbidities, previous admissions to the ICU, FEV_1 and age. Weaning from a ventilator can be difficult and NIV can be used post extubation to shorten weaning time.
- Other therapies

Although there is no proven benefit, chest physiotherapy, particularly with the use of positive expiratory pressure masks, can be helpful in patients with copious secretions. Currently, there is no evidence showing benefit for the use of **heliox** (helium and oxygen mixture) in patients with exacerbations of COPD.

Prognosis of COPD

The predictors of a poor prognosis are increasing age and worsening airflow limitation, i.e. a fall in FEV_1. A predictive index (BODE = **b**ody mass index, degree of airflow **o**bstruction, **d**yspnoea and **e**xercise capacity) has recently been modified, improving prediction of outcome, and is shown in Table 13.2. A patient with a BODE index of 0–2 has a mortality rate of 10% and with 7–10 it rises to 80% at 4 years. A simpler index using **a**ge, **d**yspnoea and airflow **o**bstruction (ADO) gives a similar prognosis.

Discharge planning

- Prior to discharge patients should have adequate and stable gas exchange (oxygen saturations and ABGs) on optimal maintenance bronchodilator therapy.
- They should understand what medication to take, including oxygen therapy if required.
- Spirometry should be measured prior to discharge as a baseline for further measurements.
- A follow-up appointment should be made for 4–6 weeks, especially for those with respiratory failure who may require assessment for LTOT.
- Ensure that there is adequate support at home.

Table 13.2 Assignment of points for the updated BODE index

	0 points	1 point	2 points	3 points	4 points	7 points	9 points
BMI (kg/m^2)	> 21	≤ 21	–	–	–	–	–
FEV$_1$ (% predicted)	≥ 65%	≥ 36–64%	≤ 35%	–	–	–	–
Dyspnoea (MRC scale)	0–1	2	3	4	–	–	–
6-min walk distance (m)	≥ 350	–	–	–	≥ 250–349	≥ 150–249	< 150

BMI, body mass index; FEV$_1$, forced expiratory volume in 1 s; MRC = Medical Research Council.
Dyspnoea (MRC) scale ranges from 0–4, with 4 indicating that the patient is breathless when dressing (Schünemann 2009, with permission).

OBSTRUCTIVE SLEEP APNOEA/ HYPOPNOEA SYNDROME

- Obstructive sleep apnoea/hypopnoea syndrome (OSAHS) affects 1–2% of the population and is commonly seen in overweight, middle-aged men.
- It is a syndrome caused by abnormal size and/or collapsibility of the pharynx during sleep, which disrupts sleep and causes symptoms.
- During sleep, activity of the respiratory muscles is reduced and in OSAHS this results in collapse of the upper airways intermittently and repeatedly. If there is complete collapse, there is total obstruction of the airway and no respiratory flow (apnoea); partial collapse may cause snoring; and if there is critical collapse, there is reduced flow (hypopnoea).
- Apnoea results in hypoxia and increasingly strenuous respiratory efforts until the patient overcomes the resistance and there is termination of the apnoea and resumption of breathing.
- The patient wakes up as a result of the combination of this increased respiratory effort and central hypoxic stimulation. Patients may wake up hundreds of times per night, resulting in reduced rapid eye movement (REM) sleep and sleep deprivation. Patients are usually unaware of these night-time awakenings.

    Factors predisposing to OSAH include increasing age, male gender, obesity, sedative drugs, smoking and alcohol consumption.

- **Differential diagnosis. Central sleep apnoea** is due to impairment of central ventilatory control secondary to brainstem pathology. It occurs at the onset of sleep and is seen in non-obese patients with no history of snoring.

Diagnosis

Symptoms

These include excessive daytime somnolence (90%), impaired concentration and loud snoring (95%). Patients may fall asleep at work, whilst driving or in mid-conversation.

If patients present with typical symptoms, they should be asked to complete an **Epworth Sleepiness Scale (ESS)**. The maximum score is 24, normal range is < 11, mild daytime sleepiness 11–14, moderate subjective daytime sleepiness 15–18 and severe daytime sleepiness > 18. Patients and their partners should fill out the Epworth Sleepiness Scale independently, as patients often under-estimate the severity of their symptoms because onset is often gradual and there may be concerns over driving.

Examination

Examination includes a recording of weight, height, neck circumference and BP. Mandible size should be noted. There should be a full examination of the nose, oral cavity and upper airways, and a complete respiratory, cardiovascular and neurological assessment.

Complications

OSAHS has been associated with hypertension, hypothyroidism, diabetes and lipid abnormalities, and there is increasing evidence of an association with increased cerebrovascular events. Patients with OSAHS may decompensate with hypercapnic respiratory failure or cor pulmonale, especially if there is co-existent COPD.

Referrals

Patients with an abnormal Epworth Sleepiness Scale; those with symptoms suggestive of OSAHS with sleepiness in dangerous situations, such as driving or operating hazardous equipment, even if the ESS is normal; and those with likely OSAHS and COPD should be referred to a specialist sleep centre.

Investigations

Sleep studies

The primary aims of sleep studies are to assess sleep fragmentation, to establish whether a respiratory problem is responsible and to decide if upper airway obstruction is the primary cause.

- **Oximetry** is cheap and widely available. It can be used to measure the number of oxygen desaturations per hour or the time spent below an agreed SpO_2 level during the study. Oximetry has a role in initial assessment but limited sleep studies or polysomnography are usually required for diagnosis of OSAHS.
- **Polysomnography** records sleep and breathing patterns simultaneously. Full polysomnography monitors sleep stage, oxygen saturation, respiratory effort, airflow, thoraco-abdominal movement, snoring, ECG, body position and limb movements. This is an expensive technique, as the patient needs to spend the night in a sleep centre and a technician must be available throughout. Full polysomnography is not necessary for diagnosis in most cases.
- **Limited sleep studies** can measure thoraco-abdominal movement, oximetry, flow and heart rate. The limited sleep studies can be performed at home, although there is reduced sensitivity and specificity, compared to full polysomnography.

Treatment

Treatment depends on the severity of disease, underlying medical conditions and patient compliance. Management should consist firstly of correction of treatable and potentially reversible factors.

- **Who to treat.** Patients who have a sleep study showing a > 4% oxygen saturation dip more than 10 times an hour should be referred for treatment. Treatment is also necessary in those with mild OSAHS who are symptomatic or have complications.

Behavioural interventions

Weight loss can reduce symptoms, as can smoking cessation and avoidance of alcohol, sedatives and sleeping tablets. Some patients may benefit from sleeping on their side. Keeping the nose as clear as possible, with the use of nasal decongestants if required, may improve symptoms.

Treatment of underlying conditions such as hypothyroidism may greatly improve symptoms of OSAHS.

The above measures may alleviate symptoms in patients who snore or have mild OSAHS. However, in those with more severe disease, additional treatment, as well as behavioural change, is likely to be required and should not be delayed.

Non-surgical interventions

- **NIV**
  - *CPAP.* This involves wearing a tight-fitting mask during sleep, which delivers pressure via air tubing from a flow generator in the

region of 5–10 mmHg. The pressure splints open the pharynx and prevents collapse, allowing unobstructed breathing and an undisturbed night. Nasal CPAP is currently the treatment of choice. There are machines available that automatically 'hunt' the pressure required to overcome the collapse of the airway. Supplemental oxygen can be delivered via the machine if oxygen saturations are low, such as in COPD patients. Treatment with CPAP improves symptoms and may improve BP. Once patients are established on CPAP, they are likely to require it for life. However, compliance is poor because of the discomfort and noise. Other **side-effects** include rhinitis, nasal congestion, nasal bridge abrasions, claustrophobia and abdominal bloating.

- *Intra-oral devices.* Mandibular advancement devices may be worn at night; by holding the lower jaw forward, they increase the space behind the tongue and thus pharyngeal volume. This improves airflow. Alternatives include tongue-retaining devices, which hold the tongue forward. These devices need to be made individually and are useful in patients with mild OSAHS and for snorers.
- Pharmacological treatment
  - *Supplementary oxygen* may benefit a small subset of patients, especially those living at altitude.
  - *Modafinil* 200–400 mg daily (100 mg in the elderly) in the morning is a wake-promoting drug that is a potential adjunctive therapy. There are, however, ongoing debates regarding its efficacy.

Surgery

The aims of surgery are to increase the calibre of the pharynx and thus reduce pharyngeal resistance during sleep.

- **Uvulopalatopharyngoplasty** involves resection of the uvula, redundant retro-lingual soft tissue and palatine tonsillar tissue if present. The outcome is difficult to predict and it is not uniformly successful. **Side-effects** include post-operative pain, changes in voice and nasal regurgitation of food. In addition, patients are more likely to have difficulty with CPAP following surgery.
- **Tonsillectomy** may help patients with large tonsils.
- **Tracheostomy** is only used in patients with life-threatening apnoea in whom all other treatments have failed. It works by bypassing the obstruction.

Mandibular advancement, suprahyoid tensing, weight reduction surgery and nasal surgery have been used but there is insufficient evidence to recommend these treatments.

Driving

It is the doctor's responsibility to inform the patient of the risks associated with continued driving, even if the diagnosis is clinically suspected but not yet formally diagnosed. Once a diagnosis is made, patients must be told verbally and in writing that it is their responsibility to inform the authorities.

CYSTIC FIBROSIS

Cystic fibrosis (CF) is a common recessively inherited disease with an incidence of 1 in 2500 and a calculated carrier frequency of 1 in 25 in the UK. It is more common in the Caucasian population.

Genetics

- CF is caused by a genetic mutation in the cystic fibrosis gene, which codes for a protein known as the cystic fibrosis transmembrane regulator (CFTR) protein. The gene is situated on the long arm of chromosome 7 (7q21.3→7q22.1).
- The commonest mutation in the European population is δF508, which is found in about 70% of affected cases and causes defective synthesis, defective maturation, blocked activation or defective function of the CFTR protein.

Pathophysiology

- The CFTR protein is essential for regulation and transport of electrolytes across the epithelial cell and intracellular membranes. In the presence of a mutant CFTR protein, chloride channels in the epithelial cells fail to open in response to elevated cyclic adenosine monophosphate (cAMP), leading to a decreased excretion of chloride ions and an increased reabsorption of sodium. As a result, less water is secreted into the airways, making the secretions more tenacious and viscous, more difficult to expectorate, and prone to infection. There is a continuous cycle of infection and inflammation, resulting in severe airway damage, bronchiectasis and loss of respiratory function.
- In the sweat ducts a similar process results in increased concentrations of sweat sodium and chloride, which is useful for diagnosis. Other organs involved include the pancreas, liver, biliary tree and gut.

Clinical features

Respiratory

The commonest presentation is with recurrent respiratory infections. A cough productive of purulent sputum in childhood eventually results in bronchiectasis and chronic airway obstruction. Increased breathlessness occurs as the disease develops. Other pulmonary complications include haemoptysis, pneumothorax and allergic bronchopulmonary aspergillosis. Eventually, cor pulmonale and respiratory failure develop. Nasal polyps and purulent sinusitis occur. **Physical signs** include clubbing, cyanosis, wheeze and scattered coarse crackles.

- **Infection** is a major problem. The bacteria are described in the treatment section. Colonization with *Burkholderia cepacia* is an increasing problem. It is multi-resistant and is spread by patient-to-patient contact, resulting in clinic segregation and the end of 'CF holidays'.
- Clinically, one-third of patients have no change in symptoms or lung function, in one-third there is deterioration of lung function, and in one-third there is rapid deterioration resulting in death, even in patients with previous mild disease. The latter is known as 'cepacia syndrome'.
- **Viral infections** also occur.

Gastrointestinal

About 85% of patients have pancreatic insufficiency from birth, resulting in malabsorption of fat and protein, and causing steatorrhoea and malnutrition. Infants and children may present with failure to thrive, diarrhoea or acute pancreatitis. Bowel obstruction secondary to meconium ileus (10%) can occur soon after birth; if it occurs later in life, it is known as 'meconium ileus equivalent' or 'distal intestinal obstructive syndrome'

Kumar & Clark's Medical Management and Therapeutics

(DIOS). These patients present with volvulus or rectal prolapse. Biliary obstruction may result in cholecystitis, while chronic liver disease and cirrhosis can lead to portal hypertension, varices and splenomegaly. There is an increased prevalence of gallstones (especially cholesterol), reflux oesophagitis, peptic ulceration and gastrointestinal malignancy in CF.

Endocrine

There is gradual loss of pancreatic islet cells with the development of diabetes mellitus in about 11% of adult patients with CF. Diabetic ketoacidosis is rare. Male patients are infertile as a result of failure of the vas deferens and epididymis to develop. Female patients are able to conceive but their fertility may be reduced secondary to thickened cervical mucus.

Other

Puberty and skeletal maturity are delayed in many CF patients. Growth retardation, demineralization and osteoarthropathy may occur. Patients on long-term steroids may develop osteoporosis (p. 585).

Diagnosis and investigations

- Positive family history.
- **Sweat test.** This is the gold standard test for diagnosis of CF and must be performed in an experienced laboratory. Sweat is collected with pilocarpine iontophoresis; chloride levels with CF are > 60 mmol/L. The test can be repeated the day after receiving fludrocortisone 3 mg/m^2 for 2 days, when the sweat electrolyte concentration fails to suppress into the normal range in CF patients.
- **Nasal potential difference.** Normal values are −10 to −30 mV; in CF they are −34 to −60 mV. The test is performed in specialist centres.
- **Genotyping.** The diagnosis can be confirmed if two abnormal mutations (see above) are found.
- **Radiology.** A CXR or CT showing enlarged lung volumes and evidence of bronchiectasis supports a diagnosis of CF.
- **Pancreatic insufficiency.** This is demonstrated by a low stool elastase, abnormal pancreatic stimulation tests or fat malabsorption.

Treatment

The main aims of therapy should be to reduce exacerbations and hospitalization, enhance quality of life, prevent complications (particularly those associated with treatment) and improve mortality.

- **Management.** Management requires a multi-disciplinary team and is best provided in centres that specialize in CF.
- **Clinic visits.** Spirometry, blood tests (including vitamins and *Aspergillus* precipitins), CXR and a physiotherapy and dietician review should be carried out.
- **Respiratory management.** The aim of respiratory therapy is to decrease the number and pathogenicity of the infecting organism and suppress the lung's hyper-responsive immune system. This can be achieved with antibiotics, anti-inflammatory agents, bronchodilators and airway clearance techniques. There is no good clinical evidence for the use of **oxygen**. In hypoxic patients, oxygen may delay or prevent the complications of chronic hypoxia, as it does in COPD. Oxygen may also be used during exercise.

Antibiotics

Routine sputum cultures and sensitivities guide antibiotic therapy. There is no overall consensus on the use of prophylactic antibiotics and duration of treatment.

- **Acute respiratory exacerbations.** IV antibiotics may be required if there is bacterial resistance to all orally administered antibiotics and if oral antibiotics fail to resolve symptoms. FEV_1 and CRP can be used to monitor response to therapy.
  - **Staph. aureus.** Antibiotics (p. 77) such as continuous twice-daily oral **flucloxacillin** are usually prescribed if there is evidence of chronic colonization. Continuous prophylactic antibiotics are used in patients with frequent recurrent exacerbations. Despite prophylaxis, isolates of *Staph. aureus* require high-dose **flucloxacillin** and an additional antibiotic such as **sodium fusidate**, **azithromycin/erythromycin**, **clindamycin** or **rifampicin**. Patients with severe exacerbations should receive a second-generation **cephalosporin**, an **aminoglycoside** or **vancomycin** for at least 10–14 days.
  - **H. influenzae.** All isolates should be regarded as pathogenic. A 2-week course of a **macrolide** or **ampicillin** should usually treat *H. influenzae*, although resistance is common. Persistent infection can be treated with **cefuroxime**, **cefotaxime** or **ceftazidime**, which should be continued until there is a sustained improvement in symptoms. Patients with repeated isolates despite the above measures should receive continuous oral antibiotics chosen according to sensitivities.
  - **Pseudomonas aeruginosa.** Once isolates are identified, aggressive treatment must be initiated to delay chronic colonization. Strategies for the **first isolation** of *P. aeruginosa* include:
    a) **oral ciprofloxacin** 750 mg twice daily plus **nebulized colomycin** 1–2 MU twice daily or **tobramycin/gentamicin** for 3 weeks; a 2-week course of IV antipseudomonal antibiotics is given, delaying the introduction of continuous antibiotic inhalation until subsequent positive cultures *or*
    b) combined use of **nebulized colomycin** plus **gentamicin** or **tobramycin**, followed by intensive oral or IV antibiotic therapy. The exact duration of therapy is controversial. Many prescribe a 3-month course.

Management of **chronic infection** varies and includes a regular IV antibiotic, irrespective of clinical state. Antimicrobial sensitivities should be checked regularly for appropriate therapy.
  a) A **β-lactam** in combination with an **aminoglycoside** is recommended as first-line in patients colonized with *P. aeruginosa*. Treatments should be given for 10–14 days but may need to be continued for longer if the patient has persistent symptoms.
  b) **Combination therapy** reduces antibiotic resistance and can produce synergistic effects.
  c) **Oral ciprofloxacin** can be used to treat mild exacerbation but is not sufficient as monotherapy if there is concomitant *Staph. aureus* infection.
  d) **Nebulized antipseudomonal antibiotic treatment**, such as **tobramycin** 300 mg nebulized 12-hourly for 28 days, alternating with 28 days off, decreases *P. aeruginosa* colonization.

Many patients receive IV antibiotics at home, although a test dose is usually given in hospital first. **Colomycin** 1–2 MU twice daily can cause bronchoconstriction, so a test dose should always be given.

● Long-term management. **Azithromycin** 500 mg orally results in improved lung function and reduced exacerbations in patients colonized with *P. aeruginosa*. It has immunomodulatory and anti-inflammatory actions.

Bronchodilators

Airflow obstruction occurs in CF secondary to mucus plugs, bronchial wall thickening due to inflammation and airway destruction. In addition, bronchial hyper-reactivity is common. An improvement in FEV_1 can be seen in response to β_2 agonists such as **salbutamol** 2–4 puffs 2–4 times daily. Beta$_2$ agonists are also helpful prior to physiotherapy to facilitate clearance of airway secretions. Long-acting β_2 agonists should be reserved for patients who show clear benefit. Antimuscarinics, such as **inhaled ipratropium bromide** 2–4 puffs 2–4 times daily, can also be used.

Anti-inflammatory agents

● Corticosteroids. Corticosteroids, e.g. **prednisolone** 20 mg daily, can be helpful in patients with recurrent wheeze. Alternate-day prednisolone at a dose of 1 mg/kg or 2 mg/kg improves lung function over 24 months. **Side-effects** (p. 585) are many, so oral corticosteroids are not recommended for routine use. They are useful in patients with allergic bronchopulmonary aspergillosis (a common complication of CF) or resistant bronchospasm and in patients who are profoundly ill and not responding to maximal therapy. Osteopenia (p. 324) prophylaxis is given.

Airway clearance

● Recombinant DNase. DNase can be used to decrease sputum viscosity by cleaving long strands of DNA into smaller ones. The usual dose is **dornase alfa** 2500 U (2.5 mg) once daily via a jet nebulizer. The most common **side-effect** is voice alteration; others include pharyngitis, laryngitis, conjunctivitis and chest pain.

● Hypertonic saline. Short-term studies have shown benefit from inhaled hypertonic saline in concentrations of up to 7%. Beta$_2$ agonists should be inhaled prior to administration to limit bronchospasm.

● N-acetylcysteine. Although this can reduce sputum viscosity, there are no RCTs that show benefit from its use.

● NIV. This may be used to improve symptoms in chronic respiratory failure or as a bridge to lung transplantation. There is no evidence of a survival benefit.

● Lung transplantation. In CF FEV_1 can be used as a predictor of mortality. Once FEV_1 is < 30% predicted, mean survival is about 2 years and patients should be referred to a specialized unit for assessment for lung transplantation.

Respiratory complications

● Haemoptysis, which is usually mild, is common during exacerbations but massive haemoptysis also occurs (see Box 13.1).

● Allergic bronchopulmonary aspergillosis does not seem to affect the clinical course of most patients without an allergic component. A four-fold rise in total serum IgE, associated with IgG precipitins to *Aspergillus* and large fleeting changes on the CXR, favour allergic bronchopulmonary aspergillosis. **Treatment** is with **corticosteroids**. The role of **itraconazole** remains controversial; however, some transplant centres recommend its use for the suppression of *Aspergillus* prior to transplantation.

- Pneumothorax should be treated in the conventional way (p. 529). Pleural stripping procedures to prevent recurrence may be a contraindication to subsequent lung transplantation.

Extrapulmonary disease

Gastrointestinal disease

- **Pancreatic enzyme supplements.** Pancreatic enzyme supplements (enteric-coated microspheres and mini-tablets) contain lipase, protease and amylase, and are taken with meals and snacks. Most adults take 4–8 tablets with main meals and 2–4 tablets with snacks; however, they learn to adjust the dosage to achieve normal stools. **Pancreatin** is available in a number of different strengths depending on the amount of lipase in the preparation (e.g. 10000, 25000 and 40000 units). Large-bowel strictures have been associated with these high-strength preparations. Increasing the jejunal pH with a protein pump inhibitor or an H_2 antagonist can improve absorption.
- **Nutrition.** Patients should eat a normal healthy diet with a high calorie intake. If they are unable to maintain an adequate weight, overnight enteral feeding via a gastrostomy or naso-gastric tube can be used. Good nutritional status (multi-vitamin preparation daily) is associated with an improved prognosis and dietitians should be involved. **Vitamin supplementation** is given with **fat-soluble vitamins A, D, E and K** 10 mg daily. Iron-deficient patients should receive iron.
- **Distal intestinal obstruction (DIOS).** DIOS can be treated with a naso-gastric tube for decompression, IV fluids, correction of electrolytes, and a combination of enemas and laxatives. Mineral oil and fleet enemas may be used initially, as may oral laxatives such as **senna** and **lactulose**. In severe cases, **gastrograffin** or **N-acetylcysteine** is given orally or naso-gastrically and as an enema. Surgery is sometimes required. As DIOS is a recurring condition, the patient is given regular pancreatic supplements and regular laxatives once symptoms are relieved.

Liver disease

- **Ursodeoxycholic acid** leads to clinical and biochemical improvement but does not modify the course of chronic liver disease.
- **Gallstones** may require a laparoscopic cholecystectomy. However, anaesthesia is not without risk due to lung disease.

Endocrine disease

- **Diabetes.** Over 65% of patients have glucose intolerance by the age of 25. A blood glucose test should be performed 3-monthly. CF patients with diabetes are encouraged to eat a high-calorie diet to maintain growth and weight; insulin should be adjusted accordingly.
- **Fertility**
  - *Women.* Fertility is usually normal and the oral contraceptive pill works in normal doses. For pregnancy, ideally the FEV_1 should be > 50% predicted and patients with an FEV_1 < 30% should be advised against pregnancy. Partners should undergo DNA analysis prior to conception. Teratogenic drugs should be avoided. Quinolones, aminoglycosides and DNase should also be avoided.

- *Men.* Male patients (98%) are infertile. They should receive seminal analysis and their partner should have DNA analysis. In vitro fertilization using aspiration of sperm and intracytoplasmic gamete injection can be successful.

Non-pharmacological therapies

- Physiotherapy and airway clearance techniques. Physiotherapy should be performed at least twice a day and increased during exacerbations. A number of techniques and devices are employed including postural drainage with percussion, active cycle of breathing techniques and 'huffing'. Mechanical devices are also used, such as flutter valves, external oscillation thoracic jackets, and low-and high-pressure positive expiratory pressure devices. Exercise should be used in combination with physiotherapy, as it can help mobilize secretions and is part of patients' pulmonary rehabilitation.
- Other therapies
  - *Sodium chloride tablets.* These may be required in hot weather due to excess sodium chloride loss in sweat.
  - *Gene therapy.* This is currently unavailable, mainly due to problems with vectors and delivery, but may be a treatment of the future.
  - *Vaccinations.* Patients should receive **pneumococcal polysaccharide vaccine** 0.5 mL IM and a yearly influenza vaccination.

Prognosis

The current average age of death of patients with CF is about 30 years old. However, the life expectancy of a newborn baby with CF today is about 45–50 years old without gene therapy.

ASTHMA

Asthma is a chronic inflammatory disorder of the airways. It has three characteristics: airway hyper-responsiveness to a wide range of stimuli, reversible airflow limitation and inflammation of the bronchi. It is more common in developed countries and the prevalence is increasing, particularly in the second decade of life when the disease affects 10–15% of the population.

Pathophysiology

The development of asthma is likely to be due to a combination of genetic predisposition and environmental factors. **Extrinsic asthma** usually occurs in atopic individuals and is associated with a positive skin prick reaction to common inhalant allergens. **Late-onset asthma** in adults can be due to sensitization to chemicals or biological products at work, aspirin intolerance or stimulation following β-adrenoceptor blockers prescribed for hypertension or angina. **Intrinsic asthma** is often described as 'late-onset', as it usually starts in middle age. However, many patients developing late-onset asthma have a positive skin prick test and on close questioning actually had childhood symptoms compatible with asthma.

Clinical features

Cough, wheeze, shortness of breath and chest tightness occur. These symptoms are intermittent, variable, worse at night and provoked by triggers such as exercise. Cough variant asthma is cough without a wheeze. There is often a family history of asthma or other atopic disease, such as eczema or hay fever, and patients often know triggers that worsen symptoms.

Physical signs

There may be no signs of airflow obstruction present at the time of examination. If wheeze is not present, the patient is asked to do a forced expiratory manœuvre, which may provoke an audible wheeze. During an exacerbation there may be tachypnoea, use of accessory muscles, wheeze and pulsus paradoxus, but in a severe exacerbation the chest may be silent (i.e. no airflow). Eczema, hives or allergic rhinitis may be present, indicating other allergic disease. Nasal polyps may be found with or without an associated history of aspirin sensitivity.

Churg–Strauss syndrome is a triad of asthma (with rhinitis), eosinophilia and systemic vasculitis.

Investigations

- Respiratory function tests can be normal (if there is no airflow limitation) or show an obstructive airflow picture. There is a reduced FEV_1 and a proportionally smaller reduction in FVC, resulting in an FEV_1:FVC ratio of < 75%. The PEFR is also reduced, but variability of PEFR and/or FEV_1 over time is diagnostic of asthma.
    - PEFR meters are inexpensive and easy to use, and patients can therefore be taught to use them at home. Measurements of PEFR on waking (prior to taking a bronchodilator) and before bed (after a bronchodilator) are useful in showing diurnal variation (see Fig. 13.2). An increase of 20% in PEFR after inhalation of a short-acting β-agonist, e.g. 400 mcg of **salbutamol** via a metered dose inhaler or after a trial of oral steroids (**prednisolone** 30 mg/day for 14 days), occurs in asthma. Patients with severe chronic asthma may have little reversibility.
    - Patients should be encouraged to keep PEFR diaries. Those with possible occupational asthma should record PEFR for at least 2 weeks at work and 2 weeks off work.
    - **Exercise tests** show a reduction in PEF or FEV_1 after 6 mins exercise.
- Histamine or methacholine bronchial provocation tests can be used to indicate the presence of bronchial hyper-responsiveness.
- Blood and sputum tests may reveal increased eosinophils (> 0.4×10^9/L) and total IgE in the peripheral blood, indicating an allergic tendency. Eosinophils may also be elevated in the sputum. Radioallergosorbent tests (RAST) measure minute quantities of IgE antibody in the blood, which are specifically directed at particular antigens. However, they are expensive and less sensitive than skin prick tests.
- CXR shows no characteristic features. It is done at diagnosis and always in a severe exacerbation to exclude a pneumothorax.
- Skin prick tests should be performed in all cases to try to identify an allergic cause. Allergen provocation tests are useful if occupational asthma is suspected.
- Exhaled nitric oxide measurement indicates the degree of inflammation and is used as a test for the efficacy of corticosteroids.

Management

The aims of treatment are symptom control, reduction of exacerbations and restoration of normal or best possible lung function with minimal side-effects from medication, minimal absences from work or school, and no limitation on physical activity. In children treatment is to enable a normal growth pattern to occur.

Non-pharmacological therapies

Patient education

Patients and their families should be given information about the condition. Clinicians should regularly check their patients' inhaler technique and should teach patients to use a PEFR metre. Patients should learn to recognize signs of poor control, such as increasing need for short-acting β-agonists, increasing breathlessness on exertion and waking at night with symptoms.

Primary prophylaxis

There are currently no recommendations on pre-natal or post-natal **allergen avoidance**. Breast feeding should be encouraged, as there is an association with reduced infant wheeze. Microbial exposure — the 'hygiene hypothesis' — suggests that early exposure to microbial products may prevent allergic disease such as asthma by switching off allergic responses. There is currently no good evidence for this. Smoking during pregnancy and after the child is born is associated with increased infant wheeze.

Secondary prophylaxis

- Allergen avoidance. Measures should be taken to avoid causative allergens, such as pets, mould and certain foods, as this may be helpful in reducing the severity of disease. Measures to avoid house dust mites have been shown to be ineffectual. In observational studies asthma symptoms have improved after removal of a pet from the house. Aspirin, other NSAIDs and β-blockers should not be used.
- Smoking. Active and passive smoking should be avoided.
- Weight reduction. This is recommended in overweight asthma patients to improve symptoms.

Drug treatment (Table 13.3)

- The mainstay of treatment for asthma involves the use of inhaled therapies that are delivered as aerosols or powders directly into the lung; thus first-pass metabolism is avoided and unwanted systemic effects are minimized.
- Asthma treatment involves a stepwise approach, enabling patients and doctors to increase or decrease medication according to symptoms (Table 13.4). This approach is based on the appreciation that asthma is an inflammatory disease and that anti-inflammatory drugs should be started, even in mild cases. Short-acting bronchodilator therapy should be used to relieve breakthrough symptoms only. Increasing use of short-acting therapy implies deteriorating uncontrolled disease and the need to step up therapy. Treatment is stepped down if control is good.

Step 1: Mild intermittent asthma

These patients have infrequent symptoms and should use a short-acting β₂ agonist, such as a salbutamol inhaler 100–200 mcg (1–2 puffs), as required. Beta₂ agonists should only be used for breakthrough symptoms and are a useful guide to changes in severity of asthma. If a patient is using two or more canisters of a β₂ agonist a month (> 10–12 puffs a day), this suggests poorly controlled disease. Beta₂ agonists are very effective for symptom relief but have no effect on underlying disease.

Table 13.3 Drugs used in asthma*

Drug	Regimen
Inhaled drugs	
Inhaled short-acting β₂ agonists	
Salbutamol (called albuterol in USA) Aerosol and powder preparations available	100 mcg per puff (metered dose) Take 2 puffs as required
Terbutaline Powder and nebulized solutions available	500 mcg per puff Up to 4 times daily as required
Inhaled long-acting β₂ agonist	
Formoterol Powder and aerosol formulations available	12 mcg twice daily Up to 24 mcg twice daily
Salmeterol	50 mcg (2 puffs or 1 blister) twice daily Up to 100 mcg (4 puffs or 2 blisters) twice daily
Inhaled corticosteroids	
Beclometasone dipropionate Dry (in blisters) and aerosol preparations	50, 100 or 200 mcg per metered dose 100–400 mcg twice daily, rising to 0.4–1 mg twice daily
Budesonide Powder or aerosol preparations	100, 200, 400 mcg per metered dose 100–800 mcg twice daily
Fluticasone propionate	50 mcg metered dose (powder) and 125 mcg (aerosol) 100–500 mcg twice daily
Mometasone furoate	200–400 mcg (powder) as a single dose in evening or in 2 divided doses
Compound inhaled long-acting β₂ agonist and inhaled corticosteroids	
Budesonide and formoterol	100/6 combination 1–2 puffs, up to 4 puffs daily (combinations in higher concentrations available 200/6 and 400/12)
Fluticasone and salmeterol	100, 250 or 500 mcg 50 mcg 1–2 puffs twice daily
Other inhaled preventer therapy	
Antimuscarinic bronchodilators Ipratropium bromide Tiotropium	(Aerosol 20–40 mcg 3–4 times daily) (Nebulized solutions 250–500 mcg 3–4 times daily) 18 mcg (powder) once daily 2.5 mcg (solution) 2 puffs once daily
Sodium cromoglicate	10 mg (2 puffs) 4–8 times daily
Nedocromil sodium	2 puffs (4 mg) 2–4 times daily

Table 13.3 Continued

Drug	Regimen
Oral agents	
Leukotriene modifiers	
Montelukast	10 mg once daily (evening)
Zafirlukast	20 mg twice daily
Theophylline	
Theophylline modified release	200–400 mg every 12 hours (tablets) 250–500 every 12 hours (capsules)
Aminophylline	225 mg (tablets) twice daily, rising to 450 mg twice daily if necessary
Corticosteroids	
Prednisolone	5 mg tablets 30–60 mg daily for acute asthma attack
β_2 agonists	
Salbutamol	2–4 mg 3–4 times daily
Terbutaline	2.5 mg 3 times daily
Steroid-sparing agents, e.g. methotrexate, ciclosporin	Specialist centres only

*See Table 13.4.

Ipratropium bromide, an antimuscarinic bronchodilator, is used for short-term relief in chronic asthma 20–40 mcg 3–4 times daily by inhaler.

Step 2: Regular preventer therapy

Patients should be moved to step 2 if they are using their short-acting β_2 agonist more than 3 times a week, if they have nocturnal symptoms more than once a week, or if they have had an exacerbation in the last 2 years requiring systemic corticosteroids or nebulized bronchodilators.

- Inhaled corticosteroids are the most effective preventers. The usual starting dose for **beclometasone dipropionate** is 100–400 mcg twice daily. The dose should be titrated to the lowest possible that controls symptoms. When changing between **beclometasone dipropionate** and **budesonide**, a 1:1 ratio should be assumed. **Fluticasone** 100–500 mcg twice daily, **mometasone** 200–400 mcg as a single dose and **ciclesonide** 80–320 mcg daily as a single dose are also available. Inhaled steroids are the first-line preventer therapy.
- Sodium cromoglicate and nedocromil sodium prevent activation of many inflammatory cells, especially mast cells, eosinophils and epithelial cells. It is difficult to predict who will benefit from them, but they are less effective 'preventers' than inhaled corticosteroids. **Sodium cromoglicate** is given by aerosol inhalation 10 mg (2 puffs) 4 times a day, increased to 6–8 times a day in severe cases. The dose of **nedocromil sodium** is 4 mg (2 puffs) daily.
- Leukotriene receptor antagonists inhibit the cysteinyl L1 receptor, one of the principal asthma mediators. They may be beneficial in

Table 13.4 The stepwise management of asthma

Step	PEFR	Treatment
1 Occasional symptoms, less frequent than daily	100% predicted	**As-required short-acting β₂ agonists** If used more than once daily, move to step 2
2 Daily symptoms	≤ 80% predicted	**Regular inhaled preventer therapy** Anti-inflammatory drugs: inhaled low-dose corticosteroids up to 800 mcg daily. LTRAs, theophylline and sodium cromoglicate are less effective If not controlled, move to step 3
3 Severe symptoms	50–80% predicted	**Inhaled corticosteroids and long-acting inhaled β₂ agonist** Continue inhaled corticosteroid Add regular inhaled LABA If still not controlled, add either LTRA, modified-release oral theophylline or β₂ agonist If not controlled, move to step 4
4 Severe symptoms uncontrolled with high-dose inhaled corticosteroids	50–80% predicted	**High-dose inhaled corticosteroid and regular bronchodilators** Increase high-dose inhaled corticosteroids up to 2000 mcg daily Plus regular LABAs Plus either LTRA or modified-release theophylline or β₂ agonist
5 Severe symptoms deteriorating	≤ 50% predicted	**Regular oral corticosteroids** Add prednisolone 40 mg daily to step 4
6 Severe symptoms deteriorating in spite of prednisolone	≤ 30% predicted	Hospital admission

LABA, long-acting β₂ agonist; LTRA, leukotriene receptor agonist; PEFR, peak expiratory flow rate.

aspirin-induced asthma, exercise-induced asthma or associated rhinitis, particularly if used in addition to an inhaled corticosteroid. **Montelukast** 10 mg daily in the evening and **zafirlukast** 20 mg twice daily are the most common leukotriene receptor antagonists used.

● **Theophylline** is a bronchodilator and sustained-release preparations are used in combination with inhaled corticosteroids in some cases of asthma. Modified release theophyllines include **Slo-Phyllin** 250–500 mg, **Nuelin SA** 250–500 mg and **Uniphyllin Continus** 200–400 mg, all 12-hourly. Brand names must be stated on prescription.

Theophyllines have a narrow therapeutic window and interact with a number of other drugs. Plasma levels should be between 10 and 20 mg/L for optimal response.

Step 3: Add-on therapy

If 400–800 mcg a day of inhaled steroid fails to control symptoms with good compliance, a trial of add-on therapy is used, instead of increasing inhaled corticosteroid dose. The add-on therapy of choice is a long-acting β_2-agonist (LABA); when used in addition to inhaled corticosteroids, these agents have been shown to improve lung function and symptoms in symptomatic patients taking low- and moderate-dose inhaled corticosteroids. Choices include **salmeterol** 50 mcg (2 puffs) twice daily, increased up to 100 mcg (4 puffs) twice daily in severe disease, or **formoterol** 12 mcg 1–2 times daily, increased to 24 mcg daily in more severe disease. If there is an improvement but there are still symptoms, the LABA should be continued and the inhaled corticosteroid dose increased to 800 mcg a day. LABAs and inhaled corticosteroids can be given as **combination therapy**, which is more convenient for the patient. A combination of **fluticasone** and **salmeterol** and a combination of **budesonide** and **formoterol** are available. If there is no improvement in symptoms after addition of a LABA, it should be discontinued and the inhaled corticosteroid dose increased to 800 mcg daily. If control is still inadequate, one of the following is added: **leukotriene receptor antagonists**, **modified-release oral theophylline** or **modified-release oral β_2 agonist**.

Step 4: Persistent poor control

If there is persistent poor control despite the combination of a short-acting β_2 agonist as required, moderate-dose inhaled corticosteroid 800 mcg daily and add-on therapy (usually a LABA), one of the following can be used:

- Increase inhaled corticosteroids to 2000 mcg a day (monitor for side-effects).
- Do a 6-week sequential trial of one of the following: leukotriene receptor antagonist, modified-release oral theophylline or modified-release oral β_2 agonist.
- If the trial is ineffective, stop the medication; if inhaled corticosteroid is used, reduce to the original dose.

Step 5: Continuous or frequent use oral corticosteroids

Prednisolone is the oral corticosteroid of choice and should be used at the lowest dose that controls symptoms. Patients taking long-term steroids or 3–4 courses a year are at increased risk of side-effects (p. 324). Patients receiving steroids for more than 3 months should be prescribed a long-acting **bisphosphonate** to prevent osteoporosis. BP and blood glucose should be checked regularly. Methods of trying to decrease oral steroids include maximizing other therapy and using maximal doses of inhaled corticosteroids. Immunosuppressants (steroid-sparing agents), such as **methotrexate**, **ciclosporin** or **oral gold**, can be tried for 3 months.

Stepping down treatment

Patients who are well controlled for 2–3 months should start decreasing their therapy. This should be done slowly and, where possible, the patient should be maintained on the lowest dose of inhaled steroid that controls symptoms. Reduction should be considered every 3 months and the steroid dose should be reduced by 25–50% each time.

Recombinant humanized monoclonal antibodies

Recombinant humanized monoclonal antibodies (**omalizumab**) that form complexes with free IgE, blocking its interaction with mast cells and basophils, have been developed. However, although clinical trials have shown benefit in patients with severe asthma despite corticosteroids, omalizumab is not regularly prescribed. Omalizumab is given subcutaneously 2–4 times weekly.

Management of acute exacerbations of asthma

The best strategy for management of acute exacerbations of asthma is early recognition and prevention. Patients should have an action plan and know how to identify the onset of an exacerbation. The signs of an onset include worsening PEFR, increasing symptoms or greater use of inhaled short-acting β_2 agonists. Patients should, at this stage, avoid precipitating factors, use inhaled β_2 agonists for symptom relief and start on a course of oral corticosteroids. If there is no improvement or they are getting worse, they should immediately seek medical help.

History, examination and evaluation

Patients often present with increasing shortness of breath, wheeze, chest tightness or cough. Those at increased risk of severe acute exacerbations of asthma can be identified in the history. Previous near-fatal asthma attacks requiring ICU admission, previous hospital admissions within the last year, previous attacks requiring corticosteroids, a need for three or more classes of drug for asthma, increased use of β_2 agonists (more than 2 canisters a month), known brittle asthma and repeated A&E attendance within the last year indicate patients who are at risk. Patients who are non-compliant with treatment, fail to attend hospital appointments, usually self-discharge from hospital or have any psychological or behavioural illness are also at risk of developing severe exacerbations of asthma.

Severity of disease

- Moderate asthma exacerbation involves:
  - PEFR 50–75% predicted
  - increasing symptoms
  - no signs of acute severe or life-threatening asthma.
- Acute severe asthma typically involves one of:
  - PEF 33–50% predicted or best
  - inability to complete a sentence in one breath
  - respiratory rate > 25 breaths/min
  - tachycardia > 110 bpm.
- Life-threatening asthma has features including:
  - PEF < 33% predicted or best
  - a silent chest
  - cyanosis
  - feeble respiratory effort
  - exhaustion, confusion or coma
  - bradycardia or hypotension
  - normal Pa_{CO_2} (4.6–6 kPa)
  - Sp_{O_2} < 92% or Pa_{O_2} < 8 kPa.

Investigations

- CXR should be performed to exclude a pneumothorax or consolidation.
- PEFR is used to stratify patients according to disease severity (see above), and to inform decisions as to intensity of treatment and whether

patients should be treated in hospital or at home. Measurements should be repeated regularly to gauge response to therapy. Normal values vary according to size and age but a peak flow < 200 usually indicates severe airflow obstruction. Often patients with exacerbations are too breathless to perform a PEFR.

- **ABGs** should be measured in patients requiring hospital admission who have oxygen saturations < 92% or features of acute severe or life-threatening asthma. A normal $Paco_2$ is a sign of life-threatening asthma and impending respiratory failure, possibly requiring endotracheal intubation and mechanical ventilation.
- **Pulse oximetry** should be used to monitor oxygen saturations throughout admission.

Treatment

- Assess the patient. Tachycardia, a high respiratory rate and an inability to speak in sentences indicate a severe attack.
- Apply **high-flow oxygen** (usually 40–60%), to maintain saturation > 92%.
- If PEFR is < 150 L/min (in adults), administer **nebulized salbutamol** 5 mg or **terbutaline** 10 mg — driven via oxygen. (Use a low-reading meter, as ordinary meters measure from 60 L/min upwards.)
- Give 200 mg **IV hydrocortisone** or **prednisolone** 40–50 mg orally.

In severe asthma not responding to the initial nebulizer:

- Repeat the **salbutamol** or **terbutaline nebulizer** at 15–30 min intervals or give continuous nebulization of **salbutamol** at 5–10 mg/hour (a special nebulizer is required).
- Add nebulized **ipratropium bromide** 0.5 mg 4–6-hourly to the nebulized **salbutamol/terbutaline**.
- Measure ABGs; if $Paco_2$ is > 7 kPa, consider ventilation. If $Paco_2$ is normal, monitor closely, as mechanical ventilation may be required.
- Take a CXR to exclude pneumothorax.
- If there is no improvement, **magnesium sulphate** IV 1.2–2 g over 20 mins, **salbutamol** IV 3–20 mcg/min, **terbutaline** IV 1.5–5 mcg/min or **aminophylline** loading dose (if not on maintenance oral therapy) 5 mg/kg over 20 mins, followed by a maintenance dose of 0.5 mg/kg/ hour can be used.
- **Corticosteroids.** Steroid therapy is given to reverse the underlying airway inflammation. It is associated with an improved outcome in exacerbations of asthma and should be given as early as possible (Fig. 13.2). **IV steroids (hydrocortisone** 400 mg daily in 4 divided doses) are usually given. Oral steroids (prednisolone 40–50 mg daily) are as effective, provided the patient is able to swallow. Oral steroids should be continued until resolution of acute symptoms and a return to usual daily activities, and until a PEFR within 80% of the patient's best or predicted has been obtained. They do not need to be tapered if the course is shorter than 3 weeks, provided patients are on an appropriate dose of inhaled corticosteroids.
- **Antibiotics.** There is no evidence that antibiotics are beneficial, as exacerbations are usually caused by viruses. Antibiotics should be reserved for cases where bacteria are cultured from the sputum or blood, or there is consolidation on CXR.
- **IV fluids and correction of electrolytes.** Many patients are dehydrated and require fluid replacement. They may develop hypokalaemia due to β_2 agonists and this should be corrected.

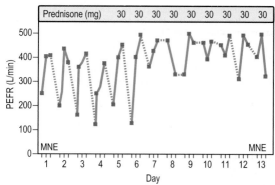

Fig. 13.2 Diurnal variability in PEFR in asthma, showing the effect of steroids. M, morning; N, noon; E, evening.

- **Helium oxygen mixtures.** These can be useful in exacerbations of asthma although evidence is lacking.
- **Intensive care.** Patients should be referred to ICU for possible endotracheal intubation and mechanical ventilation if they are not responding to treatment, i.e. there is persistent hypoxia, hypercapnia, confusion, drowsiness, deteriorating PEFR, increasing acidosis or respiratory arrest. NIV is not usually used in patients with severe exacerbations of asthma and should only be in an HDU/ICU setting.

Discharge

In moderate asthma, patients may quickly improve with nebulized therapy and may not require hospital admission. Their regular treatment should be increased and they should commence a 2-week course of oral prednisolone. If they are safe to discharge, follow-up must be arranged.

Hospitalized patients should be established on a drug regimen that they can safely take at home, and have a PEFR > 75% best or predicted and a diurnal variation of < 25% prior to discharge. Follow-up by a respiratory physician should be arranged.

Management of catastrophic sudden severe (brittle) asthma

This is a variant of asthma in which patients with well-controlled asthma suddenly develop severe asthma attacks and are at risk of sudden death. These patients require a detailed management plan for an exacerbation. On developing a wheeze they should go immediately to the nearest hospital and may require admission straight to ICU. Oxygen, resuscitation equipment, prednisolone 60 mg and nebulized β_2 agonists should be kept at home and at work. Patients should wear a MedicAlert bracelet and carry two self-injectable 0.3 mg **adrenaline (epinephrine)** syringes with them at all times.

PNEUMONIA

Pneumonia is an inflammation of the substance of the lungs. It can be classified by site (e.g. lobar, diffuse, bronchopneumonia) or by aetiological agent (e.g. bacterial, viral, fungal, aspiration, or due to radiotherapy or allergic mechanisms). Pneumonias can be community-acquired (CAP; commonest *Strep. pneumoniae*), hospital-acquired (often Gram-negative bacteria) or ventilator-associated (p. 548).

Causes

Strep pneumonia often follows a viral infection with influenza (p. 50) or parainfluenza viruses. Precipitating factors include cigarette smoking, alcohol excess, bronchiectasis, bronchial obstruction (e.g. carcinoma) or inhalation from oesophageal obstruction. IV drug users can contract a *Staph. aureus* infection and patients who are immunosuppressed (e.g. those having AIDS or receiving treatment with cytotoxic agents) develop pneumonia; the organisms include *Pneumocystis jiroveci*, *Mycobacterium avium intracellulare* and cytomegalovirus.

Community-acquired pneumonia (CAP)

The majority of patients with CAP are treated outside hospital with amoxicillin (see Fig. 13.4) but they should be reviewed at 48 hours. If the mild case has not improved or CAP is very severe, the patient should be admitted to hospital. There is a significant mortality, particularly in those over 65 years old. Overall mortality for those admitted to hospital is about 5%.

Strep. pneumoniae accounts for the majority of cases and for two-thirds of the mortality.

Clinical features

This varies according to the infecting agent (Table 13.5) or the immune state of the patient.

Following a radiological (Fig. 13.3) and microbiological (if possible) diagnosis of the pneumonia, an early assessment of the severity of the pneumonia must be made in order to admit the patient to a medical ward or to ICU. The CURB-65 (Box 13.3) is a useful guide for doing this.

Referral to ICU will be necessary if there is a failure to respond with a CURB-65 score of over 3 or if there is progressive hypercapnia, persistent hypoxia, severe acidosis, shock and depression of consciousness.

Investigations

All hospitalized patients should have the following:

- CXR. Repeat the CXR 6 weeks after discharge unless complications occur.
  - Strep. pneumoniae. Consolidation can lag behind clinical signs.
  - Mycoplasma. Usually one lobe is involved but infection can be bilateral.
  - Legionella. There is lobar and then multi-lobar shadowing, with the occasional small pleural effusion. Cavitation is rare.
- Blood tests. FBC, U&E, LFTs and CRP.
  - Strep. pneumoniae. White cell count is $> 15 \times 10^9/L$ (90% polymorphonuclear leucocytosis); ESR > 100 mm/hour; CRP > 100 mg/L.
  - Mycoplasma. White cell count is usually normal.
  - Legionella. There is lymphopenia without marked leucocytosis, hyponatraemia, hypoalbuminaemia and high serum levels of liver aminotransferases.
- Other tests
  - Sputum culture.
  - Blood culture.
  - Pulse oximetry and ABG analysis.

Table 13.5 Clinical features of community-acquired pneumonia

Pneumonia	Clinical features
Streptococcus pneumoniae	Patient is ill with a high temperature (39.5°C). Dry cough becomes productive, with rusty-coloured sputum after 1–2 days. Labial herpes simplex. Breathlessness. Pleuritic pain. Crackle and wheezes with signs of consolidation and pleural rub. CXR is shown in Fig. 13.3
Mycoplasma pneumoniae	Common in young. Cycles of 3–4 years. Headaches and malaise often precede chest symptoms by 1–5 days. Rare extrapulmonary complications include myocarditis, pericarditis, erythema multiforme, haemolytic anaemia, meningoencephalitis. Recovery usually in 10–14 days. Can be protracted, with cough and X-ray changes lasting for weeks; relapses occur. Lung abscesses and pleural effusions rare
Legionella pneumophila	Sporadic or in outbreaks in e.g. hotels or foreign travel, or in immunocompromised. Middle to old age. Males > females 2 : 1. Incubation period 2–10 days. Malaise, myalgia, headache, fever (up to 40°C), rigors. Nausea, vomiting, diarrhoea, abdominal pain. Can be acutely ill with mental confusion and other neurological signs. Haematuria, occasional renal failure and deranged liver function tests. Breathlessness with initially dry cough, which can become productive and purulent. CXR slow to resolve
Viral pneumonias	Uncommon in adults — influenza A virus or adenovirus infection is commonest cause. May predispose patients to bacterial pneumonia Cytomegalovirus pneumonia is seen in immunocompromised patients (p. 3) Influenza A (H5N1) (p. 50) Management is as for ARDS (p. 549)
Other pneumonias	
Haemophilus influenzae	Frequent cause of exacerbation of chronic bronchitis and can cause pneumonia in COPD patients. Pneumonia is diffuse or confined to one lobe. No special features to separate it from other bacterial pneumonias
Staphylococcus aureus	Rarely causes pneumonia, except after preceding influenzal viral illness. Patients are very ill. Patchy consolidation in one or more lobes, which break down to form abscesses. Pneumothorax, effusion and empyemas are frequent. Septicaemia develops with metastatic abscesses in other organs

Kumar & Clark's Medical Management and Therapeutics

Table 13.5 Continued

Pneumonia	Clinical features
Staphylococcal septicaemia	Areas of pneumonia (septic infarcts) frequently seen in IV drug users, and in patients with central catheters being used for parenteral nutrition. Infected puncture site is source of staphylococcus. Pulmonary symptoms often few but breathlessness and cough occur and CXR reveals areas of consolidation. Abscess formation is frequent

ARDS, acute respiratory distress syndrome; COPD, chronic obstructive pulmonary disease; SARS, severe acute respiratory syndrome.

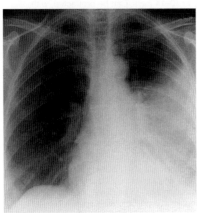

Fig. 13.3 Chest X-ray showing lobar pneumonia.

Specific tests for individual organisms are as follows:

- Pneumococcal antigen
  - Counter-immunoelectrophoresis (CIE) of sputum, urine and serum is 3–4 times more sensitive than sputum or blood cultures.
  - **Urinary antigen test** detects C-polysaccharide. This is rapid and unaffected by antibiotics; sensitivity is 65–80% and specificity about 80%.
- *Legionella* antigen
  - **Urinary antigen test** detects only serogroup 1, which accounts for most of these infections. Sensitivity (~80%) and specificity are high (almost 99%).
  - **Direct immunofluorescent staining** of organism in the pleural fluid, sputum or bronchial washings is carried out.
  - Serum antibodies are less reliable.
  - *Legionella* is not visible on Gram staining.
  - **Culture** on special media is possible but takes up to 3 weeks.

> **Box 13.3** CURB-65 criteria for the diagnosis of severe community-acquired pneumonia
>
> - **C**onfusion – defined as a mental test score of 8 or less or new disorientation in time, place or person
> - **U**rea > 7 mmol/L
> - **R**espiratory rate ≥ 30/min
> - **B**lood pressure: systolic < 90 mmHg or diastolic ≤ 60 mmHg
> - Age > **65** years of age
> - Score 0–1 — Treat as outpatient
> - Score 2 — Admit to hospital
> - Score 3+ — Often require ICU care
> - Mortality rates increase with increasing score
>
> **Other markers of severe pneumonia**
> - CXR — more than one lobe involved
> - $Pao_2 < 8$ kPa
> - Low albumin < 35 g/L
> - White cell count $< 4 \times 10^9$/L or $> 20 \times 10^9$/L
> - Blood culture — positive
>
> (Lim WS, et al 2003, with permission)

- **Retrospective** confirmation can be obtained by demonstrating a four-fold increase in antibody titre in the blood.
  - Nucleic acid sequence-based amplification (NASBA) tests on sputum samples are becoming available.
- Mycoplasma
  - Measure serum antibodies (IgM and IgG) in acute and convalescent samples. **Cold agglutinins** are present in 50% of cases. Other methods of identification include complement-fixing antibodies and PCR.
  - A kit for PCR is becoming available.
  - NASBA tests are becoming available.
- *Chlamydia* antibodies are sought by immunofluorescent complement fixation.

Management

Management of CAP is shown in Fig. 13.4.

The patient in hospital should be re-evaluated regularly by the nursing staff, depending on the severity of the illness (see MEWS, p. 2).

- Antibiotic therapy. Antibiotics should be started as soon as possible, preferably in the A&E department. The choice of the antibiotic is inevitably empirical and directed towards *Strep. pneumoniae*, as this is the commonest organism. Acquired antibiotic resistance is a concern but is still rare in the UK.
  - *Mild uncomplicated CAP* (CURB-65 0–1) is treated in the community with amoxicillin 500 mg 3 times daily (in the UK), or with **clarithromycin** 500 mg twice daily or doxycycline 200 mg followed by 100 mg daily (if penicillin-sensitive) for 5–7 days. The newer quinolones (e.g. **levofloxacin** 500 mg 1–2 times daily or **moxifloxacin** 400 mg once daily for 10 days) are used by some but increasing resistance is

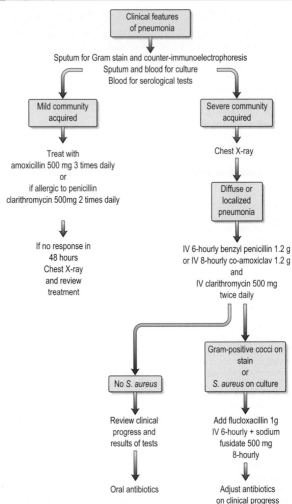

Fig. 13.4 Algorithm for management of community-acquired pneumonia.

a concern and these agents are best reserved for patients with co-morbidities.

- *More severe infections* require **amoxicillin** 500 mg–1 g 3 times daily plus **clarithromycin** 500 mg twice daily. If oral therapy is contraindicated, IV **amoxicillin** 500 mg 3 times daily or benzyl penicillin 1.2 g 4 times daily plus IV **clarithromycin** 500 mg twice daily is used. In patients with high severity pneumonia (CURB 65 3–5), **co-amoxiclav** 1.2g 6–8-hourly is combined with IV **clarithromycin** 500 mg twice daily.

- *If* Staph. aureus *infection is suspected* or is proven on culture, IV **flucloxacillin** 1–2 g every 6 hours by slow IV injection or infusion ± **sodium fusidate** 500 mg 3 times daily if over 50 kg by IV infusion should be added. Quinolones are recommended for those intolerant of penicillins or macrolides. Community-acquired meticillin-resistant *Staph. aureus* (CA-MRSA) can be treated with vancomycin or linezolid.
- *Parenteral antibiotics* should be switched to oral once the temperature has settled for a period of 24 hours and provided there is no contraindication to oral therapy.
- Mycoplasma *pneumonia* is treated with a macrolide, e.g. **clarithromycin** 500 mg twice daily (or **azithromycin**) for 7–10 days, or a tetracycline, e.g. **doxycycline** 100 mg twice daily.
- H. influenzae *pneumonia* is treated with oral **amoxicillin** 500 mg 3 times daily.
- Legionella pneumophila *pneumonia* is usually treated with one of the macrolides, **azithromycin** being the drug of choice. Quinolones are also effective and **rifampicin** can be added in very ill patients. Mortality can be up to 30% in elderly patients but most patients recover fully.

- **Oxygen.** All patients with hypoxaemia, acidosis and hypotension should receive oxygen. The aim is to keep the saturation (Sao_2) > 92% and a Pao_2 > 8 kPa (60 mmHg). If there is no history of COPD with hypercapnia, 35% humidified O_2 can be given. NIV (p. 485) may be useful. Criteria for referral to ICU are given above and referral should not be delayed.
- **Fluid balance/nutritional support.** Oral intake should encouraged but, if this is not possible, then IV fluids need to be given. Nutrition may be a problem for a longer illness and will need to be addressed (p. 542).

Hospital-acquired pneumonia

- It is commonly treated with **co-amoxiclav** 1.2 g 3 times daily but meropenem 1 g 3 times daily is also used.
- Co-morbidities require more aggressive antibiotic therapy. Management is the same as for severe CAP, once appropriate samples for culture and sensitivities have been taken.
- Gram-negative bacteria are common and aminoglycosides (e.g. **gentamicin** 5 mg/kg) are often added.
- Patients with **chronic chest infection** and others in whom *Pseudomonas* infection is suspected should receive an anti-pseudomonal penicillin (e.g. piperacillin plus tazobactam) or **ciprofloxacin** 200–400 mg IV over 30–60 mins or **ceftazidime** 2 g bolus IV 8-hourly.
- **Immunosuppressed patients** may require very high-dose broad-spectrum antibiotics, as well as antifungal and antiviral agents.
- **Aspiration pneumonia** is relatively common in hospital and usually involves infection with multiple bacteria, including anaerobes. The oral route is usually inappropriate in these patients. A combination of **metronidazole** (IV or rectal) and **co-amoxiclav** is recommended.

TUBERCULOSIS

Tuberculosis (TB) is a systemic granulomatous disease caused by *Mycobacterium tuberculosis*. It is more common in developing countries, in particular sub-Saharan Africa and South-East Asia. However, in the developed countries, following many years of steady decline, the incidence of TB is rising due to AIDS, the growing use of immunosuppressive drugs and increased immigration of people from areas of high endemicity. TB is transmitted between people by aerosol and therefore the most common site of infection is the lung.

- **Primary TB** is the first infection with TB and occurs in those without immunity. It is usually subpleural and a small lung lesion known as the Ghon focus may be seen in the mid- or upper zones within 4 weeks of infection. Hilar lymphadenopathy may be present as the tubercle bacilli drain into the lymphatics. Primary TB is often asymptomatic; there may be a mild cough, wheeze or erythema nodosum, and a transient pleural effusion. The bacilli will continue to proliferate and spread until an effective cell-mediated immune response is mounted (3–8 weeks), the spread of infection is arrested and the tuberculin skin test is positive. Tubercle bacilli remain dormant within calcified lesions but are capable of reactivation.

- **Post-primary TB** refers to all forms of TB that occur after the first few weeks of primary infection when immunity to *Mycobacterium* has developed. It occurs as a result of reactivation of a previously dormant focus in patients who have infection with HIV, diabetes mellitus, kidney disease, malnutrition, silicosis, malignancy and other forms of immunosuppression. **Common symptoms** include cough (often productive), fever, night sweats and weight loss.

- **Disseminated TB** occurs if there is unchecked proliferation and spread of bacteria due to a failure of the host to mount an effective cell-mediated immune response. Miliary TB is a form of disseminated TB in which the lesions on CXR resemble millet seeds.

TB is an **AIDS-defining illness**. It may arise in a patient with HIV from rapid progression of primary infection, reactivation of disease or re-infection (p. 115).

Diagnosis

- **Sputum staining.** Acid-fast bacilli in the sputum can be seen by staining with Ziehl–Neelsen (ZN) stain; alternatively, an auramine-phenol fluorescent test is performed. For patients who are unable to expectorate, a bronchoscopy can be performed and a bronchoalveolar lavage (BAL) or bronchial washing taken from the affected lobe.

- **Transbronchial biopsies.** These can be obtained for histological and microbiological assessment. Specimens for microbiology should be placed in 0.9% saline and not formalin. The presence of granulomas is virtually diagnostic of TB.

- **Culture.** Sputum is cultured on Ogawa or Lowenstein–Jensen medium for 4–8 weeks. Liquid cultures are often used, as they have shorter culture times. Antibiotic sensitivity should be performed on all cultures.

- **Pleural fluid and biopsy.** Pleural fluid culture is positive for *M. tuberculosis* in about 40% of patients, whereas pleural biopsy culture is positive in about 60% of patients with pleural TB. Pleural fluid adenosine

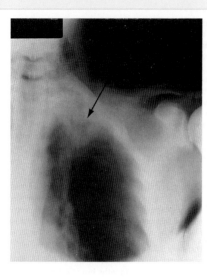

Fig. 13.5 Chest X-ray showing TB of the left upper lobe with cavitation (arrowed).

deaminase is elevated in tuberculous pleural effusions and may aid diagnosis.

- **Imaging.** The typical CXR findings are upper lobe infiltrates with or without cavitations (Fig. 13.5). The infiltrates are often fibronodular and irregular. CT scans are sensitive at identifying earlier disease and may show clusters of nodules or a 'tree in bud' appearance.

Treatment (p. 86)

Treatment must include more than one drug to which the organism is susceptible; drugs must be taken at the appropriate doses and must be taken regularly; and therapy must be continued for a sufficient period of time.

Treatment can be taken at home. However, patients who are ill, smear-positive, highly infectious (especially with multi-drug resistant TB), non-compliant or those in whom the diagnosis is uncertain may require a short period of hospitalization.

- **The initial phase** should consist of four drugs — **rifampicin, isoniazid** and **pyrazinamide** plus **ethambutol** or rarely **streptomycin** for 2 months. Ethambutol can be omitted in patients who are thought to be at low risk for isoniazid resistance. This regimen is for patients with previously untreated TB, who are HIV-negative, are not immunosuppressed and have not been in contact with anyone with drug-resistant TB. Neither should they have come from an area with a high prevalence of drug-resistant TB. The drugs are best given as a combination preparation to aid compliance.

- **The continuation phase** starts after drug sensitivities are known (6–8 weeks) and should consist of two drugs to which the organism is susceptible, given for a further 4 months. **Rifampicin** and **isoniazid** are usually standard treatment for adults with pulmonary TB (for doses see p. 87). **Pyridoxine** 10 mg daily is not routinely required but should be given as prophylaxis against isoniazid neuropathy in patients at increased risk, such as diabetics, alcoholics and those with dietary deficiencies.

- Directly observed therapy (DOT) is used for patients who are unlikely to be compliant with treatment, such as the homeless, those dependent on alcohol and IV drug users. Special clinics are used and patients are observed taking their tablets. Some clinics use incentives such as free meals and cash payments to improve attendance. DOT can be given daily but intermittent regimens such as 3 times weekly are often more convenient. However, the effectiveness of DOT therapy is variable and compliance is still an issue. For doses, see p. 87.

Pregnant patients
These women should be given standard treatment. Pyrazinamide and streptomycin should be avoided. Patients can breast feed normally whilst taking anti-tuberculous chemotherapy. Those on anti-tuberculous therapy containing rifampicin should be informed of the reduced effectiveness of the oral contraceptive pill.

Treatment of extrapulmonary TB (see specific chapters)
In patients with infected peripheral nodes, bones and joints or pericarditis, the treatment is as for pulmonary TB for 6 months but is extended if the infection is more advanced or extensive. In tuberculous meningitis, isoniazid and rifampicin are given for 9 months, supplemented with pyrazinamide, streptomycin or ethambutol for the first 2 months. Adjuvant corticosteroids for 3 weeks are recommended.

Drug-resistant organisms
Primary drug resistance occurs in people exposed to others with drug-resistant organisms. **Secondary drug resistance** is the development of resistance after initial drug sensitivity and usually occurs as a result of poor compliance.

WHO define two categories of drug resistance:
- multi-drug resistance (MDR) — **isoniazid**, **rifampicin**
- extensive drug resistance (XDR) — **isoniazid**, **rifampicin**, **quinolones** and at least one of the following second-line drugs: **capreomycin** and **amikacin**.

MDR and XDR are major therapeutic problems worldwide, having a high mortality and occurring mainly in HIV-infected patients. Transmission of MDR-TB to healthcare workers and to other patients poses a major public health problem. The drug treatment of suspected drug resistance in both HIV-positive and HIV-negative patients is as follows:
- With MDR use at least three drugs to which the organism is sensitive.
- With resistance to one of the four main drugs, use the other three.

Therapy should be continued for up to 2 years, or for at least 12 months after negative cultures in HIV-positive patients. Second-line drugs available for treatment of resistant *M. tuberculosis* infection are **capreomycin**, **cycloserine**, **clarithromycin**, **azithromycin**, **ciprofloxacin**, **ofloxacin**, **kanamycin**, **amikacin**, **moxifloxacin** and **rifabutin**.

Monitoring response to therapy
Patients with smear-positive TB should have regular (every 1–2 weeks) sputum examination for acid-fast bacilli with smear and culture. Once

sputum becomes negative for acid-fast bacilli, patients should have a monthly sputum examination until culture is also negative. This is the most reliable indicator of a response to therapy. If, after 3 months of treatment, symptoms have not resolved or sputum smear or culture is still positive, either there is non-compliance with medication or drug resistance has immerged. Specialist TB nurses and health visitors should monitor patients' compliance with treatment. If drug resistance occurs, the addition of a single drug is not recommended. If new drugs are added, at least two or preferably three should be commenced which the patient has not already received. Subsequent treatment should be fully supervised.

Follow-up

Patients should receive baseline blood tests, including renal and liver function, prior to commencing therapy. They should be informed of the possible side-effects of treatment and the indications for stopping medication and seeking advice. They should be seen in clinic regularly for the duration of chemotherapy to ensure symptoms are improving and that there are no adverse drug reactions. A CXR should be taken at the end of treatment.

Chemoprophylaxis

In tuberculous disease the skin test is usually positive and there is either radiological evidence and/or symptoms of TB. Latent tuberculous infection is when a patient is asymptomatic, with a normal CXR but a positive tuberculin skin test. The Mantoux test and whole-blood interferon (IFN)-γ assay are used to check for TB infection (current or past). The Mantoux test is an intradermal injection of tuberculin purified protein derivative (PPD). A second visit is required for the test to be read (induration > 10 mm is positive) at 72 hours. Whole-blood IFN-γ assay requires only a blood test and remains negative after bacille Calmette–Guérin (BCG).

Chemoprophylaxis consists of **isoniazid 300 mg** daily for 6 months or **isoniazid 300 mg + rifampicin 600 mg** daily for 3 months. Chemoprophylaxis should only be prescribed after active disease has been fully ruled out. In the USA there are annual screening tests for asymptomatic patients who are thought to be at high risk and who would benefit from treatment of latent TB. These include patients with HIV, residents of long-term care facilities, those with medical conditions that increase the risk of active TB and people with ongoing contact with patients who may have active TB, such as healthcare workers.

Chemoprophylaxis is used in the following groups of patients:

- those with CXR appearances compatible with previous TB who are due to start immunosuppressive agents, such as anti-tumour necrosis factor (TNF)α, or treatment that has an immunosuppressive effect, such as renal dialysis or corticosteroids
- tuberculin-positive children identified in the BCG schools programme who have a history of contact with infectious TB or have been resident in a country with a high prevalence of TB within the last 2 years
- adults between the ages of 16 and 34 found at new immigrant screening without BCG history
- adults with latent TB who have risk factors for progression to active TB disease including those with documented recent tuberculin conversion, those with a history of untreated TB, and those with chronic disease and immunosuppressive disease
- close contacts of patients with active disease and a positive tuberculin test

- patients with HIV who have been in close contact with a person who has active TB; this should be irrespective of the tuberculin test, as in HIV there may be a loss of response to tuberculin.

Contact tracing

Contact tracing helps to prevent the spread of disease and to identify new cases at an early stage. All close family members, other individuals who share a kitchen or bathroom, or close contacts at school or work are screened. Those with symptoms are thoroughly investigated for TB and asymptomatic individuals are sent for CXR and a tuberculin skin test.

DIFFUSE PARENCHYMAL LUNG DISORDERS

Diffuse parenchymal lung disorders (DPLD; also known as interstitial lung disease) are a heterogeneous group of disorders consisting of over 200 entities and accounting for about 15% of respiratory clinical practice. They are characterized by chronic inflammation and progressive fibrosis of the pulmonary interstitium.

Clinical features

Patients may be asymptomatic or present in one of the following ways:

- progressive onset of increasing shortness of breath or a persistent non-productive cough
- pulmonary symptoms associated with another disorder, such as an autoimmune rheumatic disease
- an abnormal CXR or abnormal lung function or spirometry, usually showing a restrictive defect
- rarely, haemoptysis, pleurisy or a pneumothorax.
- Signs. Clubbing suggests idiopathic pulmonary fibrosis, DPLD secondary to rheumatoid arthritis or asbestosis. Auscultation reveals fine end-inspiratory or more sporadic crackles and wheezes. There may be signs of pulmonary hypertension in patients with severe disease, or extrapulmonary signs, e.g. ocular features in sarcoidosis or vasculitis; skin disease may suggest a rheumatological disorder; erythema nodosum sarcoidosis or a mononeuritis multiplex may indicate a vasculitis.

Investigations

- Routine blood tests are rarely diagnostic but may aid the process.
  - *FBC*, including differential, may show anaemia, e.g. chronic disease (e.g. rheumatoid arthritis), an iron deficiency secondary to alveolar haemorrhage, or peripheral blood eosinophilia ($> 1.5 \times 10^9/L$) secondary to pulmonary eosinophilia or drug reactions.
  - *IgE level* is useful to discriminate between chronic forms of pulmonary eosinophilia in which IgE levels will be low and allergic forms.
  - *Hypercalcaemia* might be present in patients with sarcoidosis.
  - *ACE concentrations* are helpful in monitoring sarcoid treatment, although raised levels are not diagnostic of sarcoidosis.
  - *Serological tests.* **Antinuclear antibodies** may be present in autoimmune rheumatic diseases. Antineutrophil cytoplasmic antibodies (ANCA) and anti-glomerular basement antibodies point towards a systemic vasculitis. **Serum precipitins** suggest a hypersensitivity pneumonitis secondary to farming or pigeon breeding.
  - *Raised ESR and hypergammaglobulinaemia* may be present but are not diagnostic.

- Pulmonary function tests may be normal initially, but as disease progresses they show a restrictive pattern: reduction in total lung capacity (TLC), residual volume (RV), functional residual capacity (FRC) and flow rate (reduced FEV_1 and FVC with a normal or increased ratio).
- ABGs may be normal or show hypoxia with a respiratory acidosis. Carbon dioxide retention is unusual until end-stage disease. If ABGs are normal, exercise assessment must be performed, as arterial oxygenation frequently falls on exercise.
- Imaging with CXR and high-resolution computed tomography (HRCT) should be carried out. All radiology should be compared to previous films if available.
- Echocardiography assesses for pulmonary hypertension and the presence of cardiac failure that may be contributing to the diffuse shadowing on CXR.
- ECG to look for conduction defects, e.g. sarcoidosis.

Invasive diagnostic procedures
- Bronchoscopy and bronchoalveolar lavage (BAL) do not usually have a role in diagnosis or disease monitoring but are helpful if a surgical biopsy is not possible.
- Transbronchial biopsy taken during bronchoscopy. Biopsies are most useful in granulomatous diseases, such as sarcoidosis, and malignant disease, such as lymphangitis carcinomatosis.
- Lung biopsy is frequently required when the diagnosis remains uncertain.
- Surgical biopsy can be obtained from more than one site, guided by the HRCT results. Two approaches are commonly used: video-assisted thoracoscopic surgery (VATS) or a limited thoracotomy. VATS is preferred, as it is less invasive and is associated with lower morbidity and mortality.

Monitoring
Regular assessment of symptoms, spirometry, exercise tolerance, oxygenation and radiological changes is needed in order to follow progression of disease and response to therapy.

General treatment
This varies according to the underlying aetiology. Infection, malignancy and pulmonary oedema should be excluded. Histological confirmation is required in most cases prior to commencement of specific treatment. In general, drug regimens usually include corticosteroids, **azathioprine, cyclophosphamide** or **mycophenolate**.

Sarcoidosis
- This multi-system granulomatous disorder of unknown aetiology usually presents with bilateral hilar lymphadenopathy, pulmonary infiltrations, and skin and eye lesions.
- It commonly affects young adults, particularly women, with the peak incidence in the third and fourth decades.
- More than 90% of patients have involvement of the lungs and thoracic lymph nodes.
- The most common presentation is with respiratory symptoms, such as cough, dyspnoea and chest pain, or abnormalities found on the CXR (50%).

- Peripheral lymphadenopathy occurs in 5%, fatigue or weight loss in 5%, and fever in 4%.
- Extrapulmonary manifestations include:
  - skin disorders: erythema nodosum, lupus pernio — 10%
  - ocular lesions: anterior uveitis, posterior uveitis, conjunctivitis, retinal lesions, uveoparotid fever (bilateral uveitis, parotid enlargement with occasional development of facial nerve palsy) and keratoconjunctivitis sicca
  - metabolic manifestations: hypercalcaemia (10% of cases) and hypercalciuria, which can result in the development of renal calculi and nephrocalcinosis
  - CNS disorders: rare — 2%; can cause chronic meningoencephalitis, spinal cord lesions, cranial nerve palsies, polyneuropathy and myopathy
  - bone and joint involvement: arthralgia and bone cysts
  - hepatosplenomegaly
  - cardiac involvement: rare (3%), including arrhythmias, conduction defects and cardiomyopathy with congestive cardiac failure.

Diagnosis

- **CXR** characteristically shows bilateral hilar lymphadenopathy (BHL). The differential diagnosis for BHL includes lymphoma, TB, enlarged pulmonary arteries, metastatic carcinoma and histoplasmosis. There are four stages of pulmonary involvement based on the radiological stage of the disease. The stage of disease provides prognostic information.
  - *Stage I:* BHL alone
  - *Stage II:* BHL with pulmonary infiltrates
  - *Stage III:* pulmonary infiltrates without BHL
  - *Stage IV:* fibrosis.
- **HRCT chest** shows enlarged hilar and mediastinal lymph nodes, and diffuse lung involvement with nodules along the bronchi and blood vessels and in sub-pleural regions. There is beading and irregular thickening of broncho-vascular bundles and bronchial wall thickening. Fibrosis and traction bronchiectasis occur late in the disease.
- **Other investigations** are as for DPLD. The tuberculin test is negative in 80% of cases but is of no diagnostic value. Serum ACE is raised in 75% of cases.

Treatment

- **Patients with no symptoms**, normal lung function and only hilar lymphadenopathy on CXR (stage I) require no treatment. Spontaneous resolution commonly occurs within a year or two of diagnosis.
- **Corticosteroids** are the mainstay of treatment for patients with infiltrates on CXR and abnormal lung function (stages II and III) and those with chronic progressive disease (stage IV). Systemic steroids should also be prescribed for ophthalmic symptoms not responding to topical steroids, cardiac or neurological symptoms, and hypercalcaemia.
  - **Prednisolone** is usually started at 30 mg a day for 6 weeks and, in those who respond, treatment is gradually tapered down to 5 or 10 mg a day or alternate-day treatment. Treatment should be continued for a minimum of 1 year, keeping patients on the lowest possible dose that controls symptoms.

- Severe or persistent erythema nodosum and uveoparotid fever due to sarcoid will respond to a 2-week course of prednisolone 5–15 mg daily.
- Topical steroids can be beneficial for skin lesions, uveitis/iritis and nasal polyps. There is no clear evidence for the benefit of inhaled steroids.

- **Ophthalmic reviews** are carried out regularly for patients with eye signs, as uveitis can occasionally lead to blindness.
- **Other forms of treatment** clearly benefit some patients and drugs can be useful as steroid-sparing agents, although the evidence remains unclear. **Methotrexate** can be prescribed in chronic or refractory sarcoid at a dose of 10–25 mg once a week. **Side-effects** include gastrointestinal symptoms, hepatotoxicity, pulmonary oedema, interstitial pneumonitis and pulmonary fibrosis. **Hydroxychloroquine** can be used in acute and chronic disease at a dose of 200–400 mg/day. **Side-effects** include gastrointestinal disturbances, visual changes and retinal damage, headache and skin reactions. **Azathioprine** is used in chronic and refractory disease at a dose of 50–200 mg/day; for **side-effects**, see Table 6.3. **Cyclophosphamide** is given in chronic and refractory cases at a dose of 50–150 mg/day orally; **side-effects** include gastrointestinal disturbances, haemorrhagic cystitis and haematological toxicity.

Mortality is usually < 5% in the UK but can be up to 10% in black Americans.

Respiratory involvement in autoimmune rheumatic disorders

See p. 315.

Idiopathic interstitial pneumonias (IIPs)

These account for about 40% of DPLD and are characterized by diffuse inflammation and fibrosis in the lung parenchyma. There are a number of subtypes, of which the commonest is idiopathic pulmonary fibrosis (IPF).

Idiopathic pulmonary fibrosis

Patients have progressive breathlessness, non-productive cough and cyanosis, which eventually leads to respiratory failure, pulmonary hypertension and cor pulmonale.

Investigations (p. 516)
- *CXR* initially shows a ground glass appearance, followed by irregular reticulo-nodular shadowing maximal in the lower zones and finally a honeycomb lung (thick walled cysts 0.5–2 cm in diameter).
- *HRCT* shows bilateral predominantly lower lobe changes with basal and subpleural reticular abnormalities associated with honeycombing and traction bronchiectasis. There is minimal ground glass attenuation.
- *Brain natriuretic peptide* levels are raised in patients with pulmonary hypertension.
- *Respiratory function tests* show a restrictive pattern (p. 517).
- *Invasive diagnostic procedures* – see p. 517.
- **Treatment.** Treatment is with **prednisolone**, **azathioprine** and **N-acetylcysteine** unless there are contraindications. Domiciliary oxygen is given for disabling disease. If there is no response, other therapies such as **cyclophosphamide** may be tried.
- **Prognosis.** The median survival is about 5 years.

Hypersensitivity pneumonitis

Hypersensitivity pneumonitis (previously called extrinsic allergic alveolitis) is due to inhalation of organic dusts, e.g. microbial spores found in contaminated vegetable matter like straw or hay (farmer's lung), or in the feathers or excreta of birds, e.g. pigeons (bird fancier's lung). Fever, malaise, cough and shortness of breath occur after exposure.

- Diagnosis. Lung function tests show a restrictive pattern and precipitating antibodies to the antigen are found in the serum.
- Treatment. Treatment is by removal of the antigen, if possible, dust masks or, in acute cases, **prednisolone**.

Drugs and radiation-induced respiratory reactions

Drugs can produce a wide variety of respiratory problems. Mechanisms include direct toxicity (e.g. **bleomycin**), immune complex formation with arteritis, hypersensitivity and autoimmunity. TB reactivation is seen with immunosuppressive drugs, e.g. monoclonal antibodies. Table 13.6 gives some drugs and their respiratory reactions. For further interactions see www.pneumotox.com.

Irradiation damage following radiotherapy can cause a radiation pneumonitis. Patients present with breathlessness and a dry cough. They have a restrictive lung defect and corticosteroids can be used in the acute stage.

PULMONARY HYPERTENSION

Definition

Pulmonary hypertension is defined as a mean pulmonary arterial pressure of > 25 mmHg at rest. It may present spontaneously with no apparent underlying disease (idiopathic pulmonary hypertension) or it can occur in association with other diseases, e.g. COPD, pulmonary thromboembolism or left-sided heart disease (mitral stenosis).

Classification WHO

Group I is characterized by increased pulmonary artery pressure, i.e. pulmonary artery hypertension (PAH), followed by right ventricular failure. Groups II–V are classified as having pulmonary hypertension (PH).

- Group I: PAH. This consists of idiopathic, familial and pulmonary artery hypertension due to disease of the small muscular arterioles. The latter include autoimmune rheumatic diseases, congenital systemic to pulmonary shunts (e.g. congenital heart disease), portal hypertension, HIV infection and drug toxicity (e.g. dexfenfluramine). This group also includes diseases associated with significant venous or capillary involvement, e.g. pulmonary veno-occlusive disease.
- Group II: PH owing to left-sided heart disease. This describes increased pulmonary venous pressure due to left ventricular dysfunction or mitral valve disease.
- Group III: PH owing to lung diseases and/or hypoxia. This includes COPD, interstitial lung disease of sleep-disordered breathing, alveolar hypoventilation disorders, chronic exposure to high altitude and developmental abnormalities.
- Group IV: Chronic thromboembolic pulmonary hypertension (CTEPH). This includes thrombosis of the proximal or distal pulmonary vasculature and also non-thrombotic pulmonary embolism (tumour, parasites, foreign material).

Table 13.6 Some drug-induced respiratory reactions

Disease	Drugs
Bronchospasm	Penicillins, cephalosporins
	Sulphonamides
	Aspirin/NSAIDs
	Monoclonal antibodies, e.g. infliximab
	Iodine-containing contrast media
	β-Adrenoceptor-blocking drugs (e.g. propranolol)
	Non-depolarizing muscle relaxants
	IV thiamine
	Adenosine
Diffuse parenchymal lung disease and/or fibrosis	Amiodarone
	Anakinra (interleukin-1 receptor antagonist)
	Nitrofurantoin
	Paraquat
	Continuous oxygen
	Cytotoxic agents (many, particularly busulfan, CCNU, bleomycin, methotrexate)
Pulmonary eosinophilia	Antibiotics (penicillin, tetracycline)
	Sulphonamides, e.g. sulfasalazine
	NSAIDs
	Cytotoxic agents
Acute lung injury	Paraquat
Pulmonary hypertension	Fenfluramine, dexfenfluramine, phentermine
SLE-like syndrome including pulmonary infiltrates, effusions and fibrosis	Hydralazine
	Procainamide
	Isoniazid
	Phenytoin
	ACE inhibitors
	Monoclonal antibodies
Reactivation of TB	Immunosuppressant drugs, e.g. steroids
	Biological agents, e.g. tumour necrosis factor blockers

CCNU, chloroethyl-cyclohexyl-nitrosourea (lomustine); NSAIDs, non-steroidal anti-inflammatory drugs; SLE, systemic lupus erythematosus.

- Group V: PH with unclear multi-factorial mechanisms. This includes sarcoidosis, Langerhans' cell histiocytosis, lymphangioleiomyomatosis and compression of pulmonary vessels (adenopathy, tumour or fibrosing mediastinitis).

Pathophysiology of cor pulmonale

There is increased pulmonary vascular resistance due to changes in the pulmonary vessels caused by remodelling, vasoconstriction, hypoxia and acidosis with thrombosis. This eventually leads to PH and an increase in right ventricular afterload, with right ventricular hypertrophy and heart failure.

Clinical features and diagnosis of PH

These are mainly breathlessness, fatigue, chest pain and syncope. A similar classification to the New York scheme for heart failure (p. 417) is used for assessment.

- CXR, ECG and transthoracic echocardiography are used to assess severity of PH; appropriate investigations to exclude causal problems is essential.
- HRCT is used to assess lung fields and size of the pulmonary artery.
- Cardiac MR with contrast provides high-quality images of the pulmonary circulation.

Treatment

This involves addressing any underlying disease, with **diuretics** for fluid overload and anticoagulation with **warfarin** for pulmonary thromboembolism. **O$_2$ therapy** is necessary for patients with hypoxia at rest or after exercise.

Vasodilatation therapy is being used in PAH; **bosentan**, **sildenafil** and **inhaled iloprost** have all shown some benefit. Atrial septostomy and lung transplantation is used for patients unresponsive to therapy.

N.B. There is no evidence for the use of angiotensin receptor blockers, ACE inhibitors or α-blockers.

Pulmonary embolism (PE) (pulmonary thromboembolism)

Thrombi from systemic veins, e.g. pelvic, abdominal or deep femoral veins, or rarely from the right heart can dislodge and embolize into the pulmonary arterial system. Thrombi can form due to sluggish blood flow, local injury, compression of the vein or a hypercoaguable state. Tumour or fat can also embolize.

Embolism results in the lung tissue being unperfused but ventilated, producing an intrapulmonary dead space and resulting in impaired gas exchange.

Clinical features

- **Small to medium PEs** cause a sudden onset of breathlessness, with pleuritic chest pain and haemoptysis.
- **Multiple recurrent PEs** can lead to breathlessness over weeks or months. They can cause fatigue, syncope on exertion and occasionally angina. The signs are those of PH.
- **Massive PE** is rare but a medical emergency. The patient may suddenly collapse with severe central chest pain, shock (pale and sweaty), tachypnoea and tachycardia. There may be cyanosis and syncope, and death can occur rapidly. On examination the patient is hypotensive, with signs of right ventricular overload (a right ventricular heave and a loud pulmonary second sound).

The revised Geneva score (Table 13.7) gives the clinical probability of a PE.

Table 13.7 Revised Geneva score for the clinical prediction of a pulmonary embolism

Criterion	Score
Risk factors	
Age > 65 years	+1
Previous deep venous thrombosis or pulmonary embolism	+3
Surgery or fracture within 1 month	+2
Active malignancy	+2
Symptoms	
Unilateral leg pain	+3
Haemoptysis	+2
Clinical signs	
Heart rate (bpm)	
75–94	+3
≥ 95	+5
Pain on leg deep vein palpation and unilateral oedema	+4
Clinical probability	
Low	0–3
Intermediate	4–10
High	≥ 11

(Righini M, et al 2008, with permission)

Investigations

- Small/medium or recurrent emboli
  - *CXR.* This is often normal. Linear atelectasis, blunting of a costophrenic angle (due to a small effusion) and a raised hemidiaphragm may be seen after some time. Rarely, a wedge-shaped pulmonary infarct is seen. Previous infarcts are seen as opaque linear scars, and enlarged pulmonary arterioles with oligaemic lung fields indicate advanced disease.
  - *ECG.* This is usually normal, except for sinus tachycardia. Sometimes atrial fibrillation or another tachyarrhythmia occurs.
  - *Blood tests.* There is a polymorphonuclear leucocytosis, a raised ESR and increased serum lactate dehydrogenase levels.
  - *Plasma D-dimer.* This is positive. If undetectable, it excludes a diagnosis of PE.
  - *CT.* Contrast-enhanced, multi-detector CT angiograms (CTAs) have a sensitivity of 83% and specificity of 96%, with a positive predictive value of 92% (higher with 64-multislice scanners). This is the investigation of choice.
  - *Radionuclide ventilation/perfusion scanning ($\dot{V}/\dot{Q}$ scan).* This is a good initial test after measurement of D-dimers. It demonstrates ventilation/perfusion defects, i.e. areas of ventilated lung with perfusion defects. Pulmonary ^{99m}technetium scintigraphy demonstrates

the under-perfused areas, while a scintigram, performed after inhalation of radioactive xenon, shows no ventilatory defect. A matched defect may, however, arise with a PE that causes an infarct, or with emphysematous bullae. This test is therefore conventionally reported as a probability (low, medium or high) of PE and should be interpreted in the context of the history, examination and other investigations.

- **US.** This is used for detection of clots in pelvic or ilio-femoral veins.
- **MRI.** This gives similar results and is used if CTA is contraindicated.

● Massive pulmonary emboli

- **CXR** may show pulmonary oligaemia, sometimes with dilatation of the pulmonary artery in the hila. Often there are no changes.
- **ECG** shows right atrial dilatation with tall peaked P waves in lead II. Right ventricular strain and dilatation give rise to right axis deviation, a degree of right bundle branch block, and T wave inversion in the right precordial leads. The 'classic' ECG pattern with an S wave in lead I, and a Q wave and inverted T waves in lead III (S1, Q3, T3), is rare.
- **ABGs** show arterial hypoxaemia with a low arterial CO_2 level, i.e. type I respiratory failure pattern.
- **Echocardiography** shows a vigorously contracting left ventricle, and occasionally a dilated right ventricle and a clot in the right ventricular outflow tract.
- **Pulmonary angiography** has now been replaced by CT and MR angiography.

Acute treatment (See Ch. 20 p. 716)

- Give high-flow oxygen (60–100%), unless there is significant chronic lung disease. Bed rest and analgesia are prescribed for patients with pulmonary infarcts.
- Severe cases require:
  - Resuscitation with IV fluids with or without inotropic agents to improve the pumping of the right heart. Very ill patients will require care on the ICU.
  - Fibrinolytic therapy is indicated with persistent hypotension. Alteplase 10 mg IV over 1–2 mins, followed by IV infusion of 90 mg over 2 hours; or streptokinase 250 000 units by IV infusion over 30 mins, followed by streptokinase 100 000 U IV hourly for up to 12–72 hours according to manufacturer's instructions. This can clear pulmonary emboli more rapidly and confer a survival benefit.
  - Rarely, surgical embolectomy, when there is no alternative for very severe haemodynamic problems.

Prevention of further emboli (p. 243)

- Start low molecular weight heparin (LMWH).
- Give oral anticoagulants immediately and taper off heparin as the oral anticoagulant becomes effective (INR 2-3). Oral anticoagulants are continued for 6 weeks to 6 months, depending on the likelihood of recurrence of venous thrombosis or embolism. Recurrent embolism requires lifelong treatment. As an alternative to warfarin, oral thrombotic drugs are available (p. 71). They do not need preliminary heparin treatment.
- Vena cava filters (temporary or permanent) can be inserted percutaneously. They are designed to prevent clots passing through them from

the legs to the lungs. They are used for recurrent emboli with the patient already on warfarin. Warfarin can subsequently be stopped.

PLEURAL EFFUSION

An effusion is an excessive accumulation of fluid within the pleural space.

Causes

Pleural effusions can be caused by pleural, pulmonary or extrapulmonary disease. They are usually divided into transudates and exudates.

- **Transudates** occur due to increased hydrostatic or decreased oncotic pressures. Common causes include heart failure, cirrhosis and hypoproteinaemia.
- **Exudates** occur due to an increase in capillary permeability when the pleural surface or lung is damaged. Common causes include pulmonary emboli, malignancy, a post-pneumonia effusion and TB.

Clinical features

- Small effusions are often asymptomatic.
- Patients with larger effusions usually present with shortness of breath, with or without pleuritic chest pain, or with symptoms associated with the underlying disease.
- **Clinical examination** shows reduced expansion, a stony dull percussion note, reduced or absent breath sounds, and reduced or absent vocal fremitus on the affected side. In massive pleural effusions the trachea can be deviated.

Investigations

CXR

Over 300 mL of pleural fluid can be detected on a CXR (Fig. 13.6). Small effusions can be seen as obliteration of the costophrenic angle, whilst large

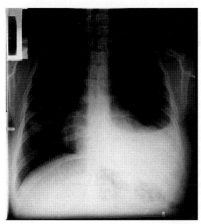

Fig. 13.6 Chest X-ray showing pleural effusion.

effusions produce a dense homogeneous shadow occupying part of the hemithorax.

US

This can detect smaller effusions.

Pleural aspiration

Simple aspiration can be performed safely at the bedside or in the clinic. Removal of large amounts of fluid should be done under ultrasound guidance which reduces the risk of pneumothorax and other complications. It is not necessary if the likely diagnosis is a transudate, e.g. left ventricular failure.

- Diagnostic aspiration is usually performed with a green needle and a 50 mL syringe under aseptic conditions. The best position for aspiration is posteriorly, about 10 cm lateral to the spine. Local anaesthetic lidocaine 1% should be infiltrated prior to aspiration.
- Fluid should be sent for microbiological, biochemical and cytological analysis.

Pleural fluid analysis

- Appearance and odour
  - Clear straw-coloured fluid that does not clot on standing indicates a transudate.
  - An exudate may look the same but is usually more turbid due to the presence of cells.
  - Blood-tinged fluid is non-diagnostic but a uniformly bloody effusion is likely to be secondary to a malignancy, PE with infarction or trauma. If the haematocrit in the pleural fluid is more than half that of the patient's peripheral blood haematocrit, the diagnosis is a haemothorax.
  - Purulent, viscous, unpleasant-smelling yellow fluid suggests pus and an empyema.
- Protein content. Under 30 g/L of protein is a transudate; > 30 g/L indicates an exudate. However, if the patient has an abnormal serum protein concentration or the pleural protein is between 25 and 35 g/L, Light's criteria should be used to differentiate between the two.
- Light's criteria and lactic dehydrogenase (LDH). The pleural fluid is an exudate if:
  - fluid to serum ratio of total protein is > 0.5
  - fluid to serum ratio of LDH is > 0.6 *and/or*
  - the pleural fluid LDH is more than two-thirds of the upper limit of normal serum LDH.
- Cell type. The white cell count can be helpful but is often not diagnostic.
  - *Neutrophilia* suggests infection, e.g. post pneumonia.
  - *Lymphocytosis* indicates TB or malignancy, e.g. lymphoma.
  - *Eosinophilia* is not diagnostic.
  - *Red cells* suggest trauma, malignancy or pulmonary emboli.
  - *Malignant cells* may be present.
- Glucose and pH. Glucose of < 3.3 mmol/L suggests malignancy, TB or rheumatoid arthritis. A low pH < 7.2 is usually due to infection (requiring drainage) or malignancy.
- Amylase pleural fluid/serum ratio. A ratio > 1 suggests acute pancreatitis, pancreatic pseudocyst, ruptured oesophagus or pleural malignancy (especially adenocarcinoma).

- **CT chest.** CT chest with contrast may be useful in cases of difficult drainage to delineate the size and location of loculations.
- **Percutaneous pleural biopsy.** This is performed for patients with an undiagnosed exudative pleural effusion when there is a clinical suspicion of malignancy or TB. It can be done blind with an Abram's needle or under CT guidance. Samples should always be sent for TB testing, in sterile saline and not formalin. All biopsy and aspiration sites should be marked with Indian ink; if the final diagnosis is mesothelioma, patients will require radiotherapy to the biopsy site within 1 month to prevent seeding in the biopsy track.
- **Bronchoscopy.** This should only be performed if there is haemoptysis or any evidence to suggest bronchial obstruction.
- **Video-assisted thoracic surgery (VATS).** VATS allows direct visualization of the pleura and should be performed if all other, less invasive tests fail to provide a diagnosis. It is very effective for the diagnosis of malignant effusions.

Management

- **Transudates** usually resolve with treatment of the underlying condition. Occasionally, pleurodesis and shunts are required to control symptoms.
- **Symptomatic pleural effusions** may require drainage of a large amount of pleural fluid. Re-expansion pulmonary oedema is a rare complication that can occur when more than 1 L is drained. For frequent recurrent re-accumulations of fluid an intercostal drain is used and, provided there is a confirmed diagnosis, pleurodesis may be necessary.
- **Indications for chest tube drainage** include frankly purulent or turbid fluid on pleural aspiration, positive pleural fluid Gram stain or culture, a pleural fluid pH < 7.2, loculated pleural collections and large non-purulent effusions that are causing symptoms. If there is a poor response to antibiotics alone, chest tube drainage may be required. If the chest tube becomes **blocked** it can be flushed with 20–50 mL of 0.9% saline to ensure patency. If drainage still remains poor, repeat imaging should be used to confirm the position and look for the presence of loculations.

Empyema

This is the presence of pus in the pleural cavity. It usually arises via bacterial spread from a severe pneumonia or rupture of a lung abscess into the pleural space. There is usually infection with an anaerobic organism (in 70%), and the patient is very ill and has a high temperature.

Investigations

Investigations are as above for the investigation of pleural fluid. A blood culture is performed to rule out septicaemia. FBC, U&E and liver biochemistry are performed routinely.

Management

- **Antibiotics (BTS guidelines).** Antibiotics should be given according to culture results and sensitivities for up to 6 weeks. They should cover both aerobic and anaerobic organisms, e.g. IV **cefuroxime** 1 g 6–8-hourly and IV **metronidazole** 500 mg 8-hourly for 5 days. This should be followed with **oral cefaclor** and **metronidazole**. If no culture results are available, a broad-spectrum antibiotic with metronidazole is given intravenously.

- Intercostal drainage. Intercostal drainage under US or CT guidance is required to drain the empyema.
- Surgery. Patients with persistent sepsis and a persistent pleural collection despite antibiotics and chest tube drainage for 7 days should be referred to a thoracic surgeon.

Management of malignant pleural effusion

- Intercostal drainage and pleurodesis prevents pleural fluid re-accumulation. A chest drain is inserted and the pleural effusion drained to dryness in a controlled manner so as to prevent re-expansion pulmonary oedema. A CXR should be performed to confirm drainage of pleural fluid, re-expansion of the lung and the position of the intercostal drain. A chemical is then instilled into the pleural space, leading to inflammation and formation of adhesions between the two layers of the pleura. **Lidocaine** 3 mg/kg is instilled into the pleural space, followed by the sclerosing agent. The chest drain should then be clamped for 1 hour and the patient rotated if talc slurry has been used. The chest drain can be unclamped and, provided the lung remains fully re-expanded and there is satisfactory drainage of pleural fluid, should be removed within 12–72 hours. Success rates are usually > 60%. Side-effects include pleuritic pain and fever. There are a number of sclerosing agents available, e.g. **tetracycline**, **bleomycin** and **doxycycline**. Talc is usually the preferred agent, as it is inexpensive, widely available and effective. However, < 1% of patients may develop respiratory failure post instillation. The recommended dose is 2–5 g.
- Thoracoscopy can be used to deliver talc poudrage, which has a mean pleurodesis success rate of > 90%.
- Pleural abrasion or partial pleurectomy can also be performed via thoracoscopy in patients who have a good prognosis.
- Other measures include chronic indwelling pleural catheters, pleuroperitoneal shunts, chemotherapy and radiotherapy.

PNEUMOTHORAX

Pneumothorax means air in the pleural space. A **primary** spontaneous pneumothorax occurs in patients with no underlying lung disease. They are usually found in young, tall, thin men and are caused by the rupture of a pleural bleb, which is usually apical. A **secondary** spontaneous pneumothorax occurs in individuals with underlying lung disease, such as COPD. Traumatic pneumothorax is the result of blunt or penetrating chest wounds.

History and examination

Patients present with sudden onset of unilateral chest or shoulder tip pain, with progressively increasing shortness of breath and occasionally a cough. The history may reveal an underlying disease process or history of trauma.

Patients with a small pneumothorax have no signs on clinical examination. In a larger pneumothorax there is reduced expansion, reduced or absent breath sounds, reduced vocal fremitus, and normal or hyperresonant percussion note on the affected side. If the pneumothorax is under tension the patient will be distressed, tachypnoeic, cyanosed and hypotensive, and the trachea is deviated away from the affected side.

> **Box 13.4** Simple aspiration of a pneumothorax
>
> 1. Explain the nature of the procedure and obtain consent
> 2. Infiltrate 2% lidocaine down to the pleura in the second intercostal space in the mid-clavicular line
> 3. Push a 3–4 cm 16 French gauge cannula through the pleura
> 4. Connect the cannula to a three-way tap and 50 mL syringe
> 5. Aspirate up to 2.5 L of air. Stop if resistance to suction is felt or the patient coughs excessively
> 6. Repeat CXR (in expiration) in the X-ray department

Investigations

- **Imaging.** A CXR usually makes the diagnosis by showing a pleural line. In a tension pneumothorax there may be deviation of the trachea and mediastinal shift away from the affected side. If a pneumothorax is clinically suspected but the PA film looks normal, a lateral radiograph may help detection. CT scans are useful in patients with severe bullous lung disease, as they help to differentiate an emphysematous bulla from a pneumothorax.
- **ABGs.** These may show hypoxia, particularly in patients with underlying chest disease. Hypercapnia may be present in COPD. Acute respiratory alkalosis may occur if there is pain, anxiety or severe hypoxia.

Treatment of primary pneumothorax (see Emergencies in Medicine p. 715)

- If the patient has no symptoms and the CXR shows a rim of air < 2 cm between the lung margin and the chest wall, no treatment is necessary. These patients can be discharged and reviewed in outpatients in 2–4 weeks. They should be advised not to travel by air or go diving.
- If a patient is breathless and/or has a rim of air of > 2 cm between the lung margin and the chest wall, high-flow oxygen should be given and aspiration of air should be attempted (Box 13.4).
- Repeated aspiration is performed if the first attempt was unsuccessful and < 2.5 L of air was aspirated.
- If the above measures fail and the lung does not re-expand and/or the patient remains breathless, an intercostal drain should be inserted and connected to an underwater seal or a Heimlich flutter valve (one-way valve). If, after 24 hours, the lung has fully expanded and there is no ongoing air leak, the drain can be removed.
- A bubbling chest drain should never be clamped. Some experienced chest physicians support the clamping of non-bubbling chest drains prior to removal to detect small air leaks. This should only be done under the supervision of a respiratory physician, on a specialist ward with experienced nurses. If the patient's symptoms get worse or subcutaneous emphysema develops, the drain should be unclamped immediately.
- Suction can be applied to the intercostal drain if, 48 hours after insertion, the lung has failed to re-expand fully or there is an ongoing air leak. This should be performed on a specialist ward using a high-volume, low-pressure (–10 to –20 cmH$_2$O) system.

- **Surgical referral** is indicated if the lung fails to re-expand or there is an ongoing air leak after 5–7 days. Surgical referrals should also be made for patients with a second ipsilateral pneumothorax, a first contralateral pneumothorax, bilateral spontaneous pneumothorax or spontaneous haemothorax, and for those in a profession at risk, such as pilots and divers. Surgical treatment includes inspection of the lung and pleura under VATS for blebs, bullous areas or breaches in the parietal pleura; these are dealt with by staple resection, electrocautery or ligation. At the same time, a procedure that creates pleurodesis can be performed. The options to prevent recurrence include pleurectomy, pleural abrasion with a scourer, or talc pleurodesis.

Treatment of secondary pneumothorax

- Observation alone is recommended only for asymptomatic patients with a small pneumothorax of < 1 cm or a small apical pneumothorax. These patients should be observed in hospital. All other cases require intervention.
- Simple aspiration is recommended only in patients under the age of 50 who have minimal shortness of breath and a small pneumothorax of < 2 cm. Treatment of the underlying lung disease may also be required.
- Intercostal drain insertion is recommended for most patients with secondary pneumothorax, except for those described above. As for primary pneumothorax, if, after 24 hours, the lung is fully re-expanded and there is no ongoing air leak, the drain can be removed. Suction is as for primary pneumothorax.
- A surgical referral should be made if the lung fails to re-expand or there is an air leak after 3 days. Surgical options are as for primary pneumothorax.

Tension pneumothorax

This is thought to develop when air is sucked into the pleural space during inspiration and cannot be expelled on expiration. This leads to increasing accumulation of air within the pleural space, positive intrapleural pressure throughout breathing, deflation of the lung, mediastinal shift, decreased venous return to the heart, and ultimately respiratory and cardiac embarrassment that can lead to a cardiac arrest. It is more common in patients on positive pressure ventilation and should be considered in those with respiratory/cardiovascular compromise post chest trauma or post any procedure in which the thorax is pierced with a needle. Treatment is with immediate decompression by placing a 14-gauge cannula into the second intercostal space in the mid-clavicular line. The diagnosis is confirmed if there is release of air with immediate improvement in symptoms. A chest drain should then be inserted on the affected side.

For all pneumothoraces, air travel should be avoided until full resolution.

Further reading

Calvaley PMA, Walter P: Chronic obstructive pulmonary disease, *Lancet* 362:1053–1081, 2008.

Jaff MR: Management of massive and sub-massive pulmonary embolism. A scientific statement from the American Heart Association, *Circulation* 123:1–43, 2011.

Lim WS, et al: Defining community acquired pneumonia severity on presentation to hospital, *Thorax* 58:377–382, 2003.

National Collaborating Centre for Chronic Conditions: Chronic obstructive pulmonary disease. National clinical guideline on management of chronic obstructive pulmonary disease in adults in primary and secondary care, *Thorax* 59(Supp 1):1–232, 2004.

Nava S, Hill N: Non-invasive ventilation in acute respiratory failure, *Lancet* 374:250–259, 2009.

Puhan MA, Garcia-Aymerich J, Frey M, et al: Expansion of the prognostic assessment of patients with chronic obstructive pulmonary disease: the updated BODE index and the ADO index, *Lancet* 374(9691):704–711, 2009.

Righini M, Le Gal G, Aujesky G, et al: Diagnosis of pulmonary embolism by multidetector CT alone or combined with venous ultrasonography of the leg: a randomized non-inferiority trial, *Lancet* 371:1343–1352, 2008.

Schünemann H: From BODE to ADO to outcomes in multimorbid COPD patients, *Lancet* 374(9691):667–668, 2009.

Simonneau G, et al: Clinical classification of pulmonary hypertension, *J Am Coll Cardiol* 43:5S–12S, 2004.

Tapson VF: Acute pulmonary embolism, *New Engl J Med* 358:1037–1052, 2008.

Van De Poll T, Opal SM: Pathogenesis, treatment and prevention of pneumococcal pneumonia, *Lancet* 374:1543–1556, 2009.

Wedzicna JA: Choice of bronchodilator therapy for patients with COPD, *NEJM* 64:1167–1168, 2011.

Further information

http://www.brit-thoracic.org.uk
British Thoracic Society

http://www.goldcopd.com
Global Initiative for Chronic Obstructive Pulmonary Disease working report

CHAPTER CONTENTS

INTRODUCTION

Critically ill patients are those with acute, severe and potentially life-threatening organ dysfunction and/or failure. The critical care environment provides continuous monitoring, organ-supportive therapies and a high staff to patient ratio. End-of-life care is often provided in this environment and requires additional skills.

SEVERITY OF ILLNESS SCORING SYSTEMS

A number of severity of illness scoring systems exist. Most can be used to generate estimates of mortality in the intensive care unit (ICU) but cannot predict outcomes in individual cases. All are complex algorithms based on physiological patient data. They have been used to monitor and compare the performance of individual ICUs but their accuracy remains controversial.

- Acute Physiology and Chronic Health Evaluation II (APACHE II) rates the most deranged values in the first 24 hours of ICU admission, of 12 physiological variables. The total score is added to two further scores for age and chronic organ insufficiency. **APACHE III** has added additional variables. It is best validated in the USA.
- Simplified Acute Physiology Score II (SAPS II) is significantly simpler than the APACHE III system but its applicability has been questioned.
- Sequential Organ Failure Score (SOFA) is not a prediction score but a simple daily score that can accurately track severity of illness. Although the higher the SOFA score, the worse the outcome, there is a much stronger association with poor outcome and a static or increasing score.

INITIAL ASSESSMENT: ABCDE

In any critically ill patient, assessment and resuscitation start with the **a**irway, followed by **b**reathing and **c**irculation, the so-called ABC approach. Over time, this has been extended to include **D** for **d**isability and **E** for **e**xposure and **e**xamination.

- The patency of the upper airway should be assessed by looking for any visible obstruction, listening for stridor or silence, and feeling for air movements. If the airway is partially or completely obstructed, institute a jaw thrust and/or chin lift manœuvre. Check whether the patient is at risk of cervical spine injury and, if so, institute immobilization precautions. If airway patency remains suboptimal, carefully insert an oral or naso-pharyngeal airway adjunct, paying attention to size and effectiveness.
- Administer oxygen at the highest available concentration. Assess the breathing by looking for symmetrical or asymmetrical movements of the chest rising and falling, listening for breath sounds and feeling for any chest movement.
- Simultaneously feel for a carotid pulse and, if present, obtain a BP measurement as soon as practical. If there is **no pulse**, call for assistance, initiate chest compressions and follow basic and advanced life support algorithms (p. 704, 705). If there is **a pulse, but no respiratory effort**, call for assistance and supply rescue ventilation, ideally with a bag mask valve system connected to high-flow oxygen. Again, follow life support algorithms. If there is **some respiratory effort**, determine the adequacy by clinical examination, by attaching a pulse oximeter and, if practical, by obtaining an arterial blood gas (ABG) specimen. Be aware of the limitations of pulse oximetry, especially in hypotensive patients. Arterial blood needs to be sampled into an anticoagulated syringe and any air in the sample should be expelled before the sample is safely capped. The sample should be analysed immediately or transported in ice to minimize cellular metabolism in the sample from consuming oxygen and producing carbon dioxide.

The immediate management of cardiovascular and neurological abnormalities is discussed in later sections.

GUIDELINES FOR INITIAL AND DAILY PATIENT ASSESSMENT

Initial assessment

- Age, number of days on the unit.
- A brief history and update. This should be comprehensive, chronological and concise, and should include:
  - a main diagnosis and the reason for ICU admission, with details of injuries/surgical procedures
  - current problems/progress over the last 24 hours (with the results of any imaging/investigations)
  - relevant co-morbidities and the pre-morbid level of function.
- Examination. Full detailed examination should be made of all systems, particularly cardiovascular and respiratory, and level of consciousness (p. 624).
- A complete list of medications. Stopping/restarting any of the patient's chronic medications may be necessary.

- Any abnormal blood test results.
- **The plan.** This should cover physiological/biochemical targets, investigation requests and any other instructions. Relevant details must be communicated to the nurse caring for the patient and recorded on the paper or electronic observation chart at the bed space, with legible handwriting.

Daily investigations

- Full blood count (FBC), clotting (including fibrinogen if coagulopathy is suspected), urea and serum electrolytes (U&E), liver biochemistry, troponin T (or I), calcium, phosphate, albumin, magnesium and glucose should all be documented on a flow chart.
- Patients receiving once daily aminoglycosides and/or continuous infusions of glycopeptides (vancomycin) require daily random blood levels.
- Patients receiving digoxin, aminophylline or phenytoin may require frequent blood level monitoring. As many critically ill patients have markedly reduced serum protein levels, especially albumin, total drug levels that would normally be considered sub-therapeutic or therapeutic may actually be toxic.
- If a patient is likely to require blood products or is going to theatre, ensure that a serum sample is, or has been, sent to the blood bank.
- Screening swabs for colonizing multi-resistant bacteria, in particular meticillin-resistant *Staphylococcus aureus* (MRSA), are usually sent on admission and on a fixed day of the week thereafter.
- Patients receiving mechanical ventilation may require a daily CXR (preferable erect) during the acute phase of their illness and after any relevant procedures, such as central venous line insertion or percutaneous tracheostomy, have been performed.
- Any patient with known or suspected cardiac problems should have a daily 12-lead ECG.

Radiological investigations

Discuss all requests with a radiologist and clarify that the optimal investigation has been requested to address the question raised.

Some radiological investigations may require the need for IV and/or oral contrast. Most IV contrast agents are nephrotoxic. The mainstay of prevention is good hydration. An additional bolus of an appropriate crystalloid is often required prior to giving the contrast agent. IV **N-acetylcysteine** (NAC) is used (p. 686) as a prophylactic agent against contrast-induced nephropathy. Prophylactic pre-procedural haemofiltration appears to be effective in patients with severely diminished renal function.

Communication

Make every effort to communicate, at least daily, with the patient's relatives and admitting teams; all discussions must be documented. Consent for procedures should be sought.

Discharge from the critical care environment

- Ensure that a concise but comprehensive discharge summary is completed prior to the patient's discharge. This should include diagnosis, clinical state, and drug and nutrition therapy.
- Speak to a senior member of the team who will be taking over the care of the patient, emphasizing any continuing problems and the current management plan.
- Avoid discharging patients outside 'normal hours', unless essential.

Kumar & Clark's Medical Management and Therapeutics

DYING PATIENTS AND END-OF-LIFE CARE

- In the terminal phase of a patient's illness, ensure optimal palliation of any/all sources of distress. Ensure that the family are fully aware of the situation.
- After discussion, withhold/withdraw any unnecessary interventions, including continuous monitoring.
- If appropriate, always discuss organ/tissue donation and adhere strictly to protocols (p. 562).
- If uncertain how to complete the death certificate, discuss this with a senior colleague. In the UK, many patients will require discussion with the coroner prior to completion of the death certificate.
- Whenever possible, inform the patient's GP/primary care physician.

TRANSPORTATION OF THE CRITICALLY ILL PATIENT

Transfer of any critical ill patient out of the critical care environment requires planning and specialist skills. Even short journeys may provoke significant deterioration.

- The team escorting the patient must ensure that all necessary equipment is taken on the transfer, including sufficient supplies to deal with all predictable adverse events. In particular, the quantity of oxygen and battery power required for ventilators, monitors and infusion pumps must be in place.
- Patients who are intubated should always be escorted by a doctor with established airway skills and a nurse.
- Try to minimize the amount of equipment taken with the patient. For example, disconnect from feeding pumps and non-essential infusions.
- Prior to leaving, work through the NEWS (**n**ecessary, **e**nough, **w**orking, **s**ecure) checklist.

GENERAL CONSIDERATIONS FOR PATIENT CARE IN THE CRITICAL CARE ENVIRONMENT

Many of the items detailed below are being brought together in so-called care bundles. This approach has been shown to increase compliance.

- Take a holistic approach.
- Always introduce yourself to patients and their visitors, and explain what you are about to do. The patient's comfort and dignity should be everybody's priority; be conscious of the loss of the patient's privacy and autonomy.
- Review the effectiveness of management plans at frequent intervals. If you initiate or change something, record it in the notes/chart and decide when you will need to review the patient's response.

Infection control

- Before entering a critical care environment, remove white coats and jackets. Roll up sleeves to above the elbow and remove all hand and wrist jewellery. Wash hands and/or use an alcohol gel-based disinfectant.
- Before approaching the patient, hands should be washed or disinfected, and a plastic disposable apron or non-sterile gown and non-sterile

gloves should be put on. When finished with a patient, remove gloves/gowns/aprons and wash or disinfect your hands again.

- To avoid cross-contamination between patients, all equipment should be dedicated for specific bed space use only.
- Barrier nursing is sometimes used for patients who are thought to have, or are colonized with, a communicable infection. Whenever practical, the patient should be isolated and the above guidelines strictly observed.

Patient care

- To prevent passive aspiration and enhance respiratory mechanics, all sedated patients should be positioned at least 30° head up. As soon as practical, sit patients out of bed for a portion of every day. Prescribe a simple eye ointment 6-hourly for all unconscious, sedated and/or mask/helmet-ventilated patients. Check the eyes daily for injury or inflammation in sedated or unconscious patients.
- Always examine the mouth and nose of patients with endotracheal and naso-gastric/naso-jejunal tubes. Look for signs of pressure necrosis, oral colonization and sinusitis. Start a **chlorhexidine mouthwash** with or without oral **nystatin** (topical antifungal) and discuss changing the offending tube. *Topical antiseptics are increasingly being adopted as primary prophylaxis and added to existing care bundles.*

Gastrointestinal care

- Oro-/naso-gastric tubes. All intubated patients, those receiving mask/helmet positive pressure ventilatory assistance and any other patient not able to eat should have either an oro-gastric or a naso-gastric tube.
- Stress ulcer prophylaxis. This is used for patient who are not receiving naso-gastric feeding, are shocked or on vasopressors, have a coagulopathy (including uraemia) or are anticoagulated, or are receiving gastric mucosal irritants, e.g. steroids, NSAIDS. Patients with burns/polytrauma or those who have had prolonged intubation and are sedated should also receive prophylaxis.
  - *Regimen.* Oral **ranitidine** 150 mg 12-hourly; IV **ranitidine** 50 mg 8-hourly is given (reduce to 12-hourly in renal failure) if the enteral route is unavailable.
  - *High-risk patients or those with proven untreated peptic ulcer disease.* Use an oral proton pump inhibitor (PPI), e.g. omeprazole 20 mg daily. For IV PPIs in patients with proven upper gastrointestinal bleeding, see p. 145.
- Bowel care. Constipation and diarrhoea are common complications of critical illness and most patients benefit from stool softeners, e.g. **sodium docusate** 200 mg twice daily, and mild aperients, e.g. **sennakot** 5–10 mL twice daily. Osmotic laxatives, e.g. **lactulose**, are avoided, as they can significantly contribute to bowel gas formation.

Nutritional support

Early enteral feeding

- Early initiation (within 12 hours) is the significant nutritional factor influencing clinical outcome, as 'late' feeding (i.e. feeding commenced within 36 hours of admission) is associated with increased gut permeability and an increase in late multi-organ failure.

- Timing, rather than amount/volume of feed administered, is the key factor.

Prokinetic therapy/enteral feeding failure

- If delayed gastric emptying is present (gastric aspirates > 200 mL after 4 hours), commence prokinetic therapy, e.g. metoclopramide 10 mg IV 8-hourly; erythromycin 250 mg IV 8-hourly is an alternative.
- Prokinetics should be stopped once patients have been absorbing for 24 hours.
- If enteral feeding cannot be established within 12 hours of admission, use a hypertonic glucose IV infusion, either 25 mL/hour of 20% or 10 mL/hour of 50% into a large vein.
- Post-pyloric feeding is used if gastric aspirates remain > 200 mL every 4 hours, or > 48 hours with regular prokinetic administration.

Total parenteral nutrition (TPN)

- To be of benefit, TPN has to given for a minimum of 10–14 days. It should only be used if enteral feeding cannot be successfully established.
- A dedicated central line or lumen should be set aside for TPN. Closely monitor electrolytes, liver biochemistry (for cholestatic jaundice) and line-related sepsis (p. 129).

Maintenance fluids — IV and enteral

Inputs

Patients with normal losses will require 2000–3000 mL per day. Whenever possible, this should be administered enterally. Additional losses are usually replaced intravenously to maintain adequate intravascular volume, patient hydration and normal electrolyte concentrations.

Losses

Losses may take place via normal routes (quantities may be low, normal or high): renal, gastrointestinal, respiratory and intact skin (sweat). Additional losses occur with bleeding, wounds/burns and third space accumulation due to leaky microvasculature and reduced oncotic pressure.

Assessing the adequacy of fluid replacement

- For intravascular volume, see the later section on cardiovascular support (p. 552).
- Plasma/serum biochemistry should be measured at least daily.
- Urine output should be at least 0.5–1 mL/kg/hour, except in oliguric or anuric renal failure.
- Accurate measurement of fluid input and output is very helpful but difficult to achieve.
- Achieving the target balance may require regular low doses or continuous infusion of loop diuretics or renal replacement therapy.
- Serum concentrations of sodium and chloride are monitored. Both tend to accumulate as a result of IV fluids and drugs, e.g. piperacillin. Iatrogenic hyperchloraemic acidosis is a common problem.
- Daily electrolyte requirements for a normal adult are: sodium 1–1.5 mmol/kg/day and potassium 1 mmol/kg/day.

Packed red cell transfusion

- The optimal haemoglobin (Hb) concentration is a balance of rheology and oxygen-carrying capacity. A target value is usually set at 8–10 g/dL, even in patients with critical myocardial or other organ ischaemia.
- A transfusion trigger of 7.5 g/dL is common. Most blood gas analysers are significantly less accurate at Hb measurement than formal haematology laboratories (errors as much as ± 2 g/dL).
- Try to minimize iatrogenic losses, in particular from blood sampling and during line insertion. Be conscious of the effects of iatrogenic haemodilution.
- Transfusion is not a benign intervention. Stored red blood cells become 2,3 diphosphoglycerate (2,3-DPG)-depleted, resulting in higher O_2 avidity, which causes a leftward shift in the oxygen dissociation curve, i.e. a reduction in oxygen release to the tissues. In addition, cells lose their highly deformable biconcave morphology and come to resemble spiky balls, which fail to enter capillaries and can become impacted, obstructing the micro-circulation. There is also the potential risk of disease transmission and allergic reactions.

Glycaemic control

- There is evidence now to suggest that tight glycaemic control (blood glucose levels between 4.0 and 6.0 mmol/L) in all critically ill patients is detrimental; instead, the blood sugar should be controlled < 10 mmol/L or 180 mg/dL. IV insulin infusion should be used with glucose as required.
- Keep a close watch on serum potassium concentration and supplement intake to maintain levels > 4.0 mmol/L.
- Avoid hypoglycaemia; if present, treat aggressively. Continuous feeding regimes, or dextrose infusions, should be used to reduce/avoid this problem.

Thrombo-prophylaxis

- All patients should receive an appropriate prophylactic dose of low molecular weight heparin (LMWH), unless they have a coagulopathy/thrombocytopenia or are receiving therapeutic anticoagulation or **heparin/epoprostenol** as anticoagulation for renal replacement therapy.
- Patients with severe acute, chronic or acute on chronic renal impairment should have unfractionated heparin 5000 U SC 12-hourly, as LMWHs accumulate in renal failure.
- Once daily LMWH should be prescribed at 18:00 h, so that any necessary surgical procedures (e.g. removal of epidural catheters, tracheostomies, line insertions or removals) are not delayed the following day.
- Appropriately sized TED stockings should be fitted to all patients where possible. Compression boots are also useful.

ANALGESIA AND SEDATION

Analgesia, with or without sedation, is an essential component of the holistic care of critically ill patients. With the exception of immediate life-saving interventions, patient comfort should be the priority. Ideally, patients should be calm, co-operative, and able to communicate and to sleep when undisturbed.

Guidelines

- The commonest indication for the initiation of analgesia/sedation is endotracheal intubation and ventilation. Some patients may tolerate this without any drugs but most will require analgesia and suppression of airway reflexes.
- Most ICUs employ continuous infusions of opiates and sedatives. The choice of agents depends on a number of factors, including drug pharmacokinetics, cost and personal preference (Tables 14.1a and b).
- Start with a small bolus dose prior to commencing an infusion. If this is insufficient to achieve the desired level of analgesia/sedation, repeat the small bolus prior to each increase in infusion rate. This is to allow steady state drug levels to be achieved more quickly and reduces total cumulative dosage.
- Neuromuscular blockade (Table 14.2) should only be used in patients when sedation/analgesia does not achieve the defined goals: most commonly, failure to achieve adequate ventilation or as part of a cooling

Table 14.1a Continuous infusion sedative analgesic regimens

Drug	Regime	Notes
Morphine	Loading 5–15 mg Maintenance 1–12 mg/hour	Slow onset. Long-acting. Active metabolites. Accumulates in renal and hepatic impairment
Fentanyl	Loading 25–100 mcg Maintenance 25–250 mcg/hour	Rapid onset. Modest duration of action. No active metabolites. Renally excreted
Alfentanil	Loading 15–50 mcg/kg Maintenance 30–85 mcg/kg/hour (1–6 mg/hour)	Rapid onset. Relatively short-acting. Accumulates in hepatic failure
Remifentanil	Maintenance 6–12 mcg/kg/hour	Rapid onset and offset of action, with minimal if any accumulation of the weakly active metabolite. Significant incidence of problematic bradycardia. Expensive
Clonidine	Maintenance 1–4 mcg/kg/hour	An α_2 agonist. Has marked sedative and atypical analgesic effects
Ketamine	Analgesia Induction 0.2 mg/kg/hour Maintenance 0.5–2.0 mg/kg 1–2 mg/kg/hour	Atypical analgesic with hypnotic effects at higher doses. Sympathomimetic; associated with emergence phenomena when given at hypnotic doses when usually co-administered with a benzodiazepine. Contraindicated in raised intracranial pressure

Table 14.1b Continuous infusion sedative regimens

Drug	Regime	Notes
Propofol 1%	Loading 1.5–2.5 mg/kg Maintenance 0.5–4 mg/kg/hour (0–200 mg/hour)	IV anaesthetic agent. Causes vasodilatation and hence hypotension. Extrahepatic metabolism, thus does not accumulate in hepatic failure. Has no analgesic properties
Midazolam	Loading 30–300 mcg/kg Maintenance 30–200 mcg/kg/hour (0–14 mg/hour)	Short-acting benzodiazepine. Used with morphine. Active metabolites accumulate in all patients, esp in renal failure

protocol. Intermittent bolus dosing is usually preferable to IV infusions. If given by infusion, daily cessation is mandatory. Prolonged use of neuromuscular blocking agents is associated with a higher incidence of critical illness neuromyopathy.

- Sedative drugs do not achieve physiological sleep (as assessed by EEG); sleep deprivation is probably one of the principal causes of ICU delirium.
- Prolonged use of sedation/analgesia drugs is associated with a degree of neurochemical dependence/withdrawal syndromes. Weaning from prolonged use may require staged reduction over a period of days.
- Over-sedation is associated with a higher incidence of ventilator-associated pneumonia, prolonged weaning from mechanical ventilation, colonization with multiply resistant organisms, an increased requirement for neurological investigations, prolonged ICU stay and death.

RESPIRATORY FAILURE

There are two principal functions of the respiratory system: uptake of oxygenation and elimination of carbon dioxide; respiratory failure can result in hypoxaemia, hypercapnia or both.

- Arterial oxygen tension is principally determined by the fraction of inspired oxygen (Fio_2), ventilation/perfusion matching and the oxygen-carrying capacity of the blood (essentially Hb concentration).
- Arterial carbon dioxide tension is primarily determined by minute volume, i.e. the tidal volume × the respiratory rate.

Respiratory support

Continuous positive airway pressure (CPAP)

This is used for patients with an acute exacerbation of chronic obstructive pulmonary disease (COPD) or those in respiratory failure with a Pao_2 of < 8 kPa (60 mmHg). The patient must be conscious and co-operative. CPAP may delay (or avoid) the necessity for invasive ventilation. CPAP has also been demonstrated to be efficacious in the management of atelectasis, pneumonia and pulmonary oedema.

- A tight-fitting helmet, nasal or full-face mask is used. The patient interface device is the primary determinant of patient tolerability.

Kumar & Clark's Medical Management and Therapeutics

- CPAP is a high-flow circuit providing a variable fraction of inspired oxygen (Fio_2) delivered at a set pressure.
- The pressure remains constant during the patient's respiratory cycle, providing positive end expiratory pressure (PEEP). The advantage of this system is that it recruits and retains the patency of smaller airways and alveoli by splinting them open. This process principally improves oxygenation.
- Failure to achieve a sustained clinical **improvement within 1 hour** should prompt the clinician to change therapy, usually by intubation and mechanical ventilation.
- Therapy is usually commenced at +5 cmH_2O and escalated to a maximum of +15 cmH_2O.
- Insert a naso-gastric tube if necessary to mitigate against aerophagia and gastric distension, which can result in nausea, vomiting, aspiration and ventilatory failure secondary to diaphragmatic splinting.
- Problems and complications include impediment to patient communication, ocular injury, nasal injury, facial injury (from straps), and secretion drying and retention. The latter may result in proximal airway obstruction.
- Contraindications to CPAP include a Glasgow coma score < 14, an uncooperative patient, recent upper airway or upper gastrointestinal surgery, and severe respiratory acidosis (commonly pH < 7.2).

Non-invasive ventilation

Non-invasive ventilation is used in patients with acute exacerbations of COPD and as a weaning strategy from invasive ventilation. The broad indications are mild to moderate hypercapnia with or without hypoxaemia.

- This technique adds some form of ventilatory assistance to CPAP. Most commonly, this takes the form of patient-triggered inspiratory pressure support (PS). Alternatively, a time-cycled bilevel of CPAP is delivered (BiPAP).
- All of the same precautions and contraindications for CPAP apply.
- There are a wide range of delivery devices available, ranging from small domiciliary units that merely provide a set expiratory and inspiratory pressure (EPAP and IPAP respectively), to full ICU ventilators, which have the ability to deliver a set Fio_2, higher levels of IPAP, continuous monitoring and alarms. At the simplest end of this range, supplemental oxygen can be provided by mask entrainment.
- Therapy is usually commenced with an IPAP of 8–10 cmH_2O and an EPAP of 4–5cmH_2O. These settings are then incremented, based upon efficacy and tolerability.

N.B. *Non-invasive ventilation and CPAP provide supportive care; you must determine the cause of the respiratory failure and initiate definitive therapy.*

Endotracheal intubation (Box 14.1)

Unless you are experienced in advanced airway skills, call for assistance whilst maintaining airway patency, delivering high-flow oxygen at maximal concentration and providing rescue ventilation as described above. Ensure all necessary equipment is available and functioning.

- Indications. Indications for endotracheal intubation include:
  - protection of the airway
  - preventing or relieving airway obstruction
  - respiratory failure requiring mechanical ventilation.

- Sedation and suppression of the airway reflexes. The choice of drug/s with which to sedate the patient for intubation must be tailored to the individual patient's needs. Many critically ill patients require minimal, and sometimes no, sedation. Whichever drug/s are used, be very familiar with their pharmacodynamics, pharmacokinetics and side-effects. Be prepared to deal with immediate haemodynamic instability, in particular hypotension, by having fluid resuscitation and vasopressor therapy immediately available. Drugs include **propofol**, **thiopentone**, **ketamine**, **fentanyl** and **alfentanil** (see Table 14.1 a and b).
- Muscle relaxants. Onset and duration of action and side-effects are shown in Table 14.2.

Table 14.2 Neuromuscular blocking drugs

Drug	Onset	Duration	Side-effects
Suxamethonium	30 s	5 mins	Depolarization. Histamine release. Elevation of plasma K^+ by ~1 mmol/L, hence contraindicated in hyperkalaemia
Rocuronium	30–60 s	20–60 mins	Risk of anaphylaxis
Cis-atracurium	90–120 s	20–60 mins	Broken down by serum esterases, hence predictable pharmacokinetics in renal and hepatic failure. Causes histamine release, hence contraindicated in acute severe asthma
Atracurium	90–120 s	60 mins	Racemic mixture. Broken down by serum esterases, hence predictable pharmacokinetics in renal and hepatic failure. Causes histamine release, hence contraindicated in acute severe asthma. Inactive metabolite, laudanosine, lowers seizure threshold
Vecuronium	60–120 s	20–60 mins	Accumulates
Pancuronium	90–120 s	60–180 mins	Noradrenaline (norepinephrine) re-uptake inhibition. Eliminated unchanged in urine, hence contraindicated in renal failure

Kumar & Clark's Medical Management and Therapeutics

> **Box 14.1** Endotracheal intubation and tracheostomy
>
> **Technique**
> - Pre-oxygenate the patient with 100% oxygen and a tight-fitting face mask. This should take at least 3 mins and is intended to achieve complete nitrogen washout. Ensure that the patient is optimally positioned, and if practical, is placed in the 'sniffing the morning air' position
> - Ask an assistant to apply cricoid pressure to reduce the risk of aspiration. Be prepared to deal with secretions, passive regurgitation and vomiting
> - To visualize the larynx, insert an appropriately sized laryngoscope into the right side of the mouth and sweep the tongue to the left. While advancing the scope blade, be careful not to damage the teeth or lips. By advancing the scope blade along the tongue, the epiglottis should come into view. Gently apply pressure along the axis of the handle until the optimal view of the vocal cords is achieved
> - Insert the cuffed endotracheal tube through the cords, noting the distance the cuff is below them. Inflate the cuff and manually ventilate to check endotracheal location and optimal position above the main carina (bilateral chest movement, equal air entry, absence of gastric ventilation and a classic capnograph trace)
> - A bougie or airway exchange catheter can be used if the view of the vocal cords is limited. If this is successfully placed, a lubricated endotracheal tube may be placed over the bougie
> - The cuff balloon inflation pressure should be checked. High inflation pressures may lead to tracheal injury
> - A naso-gastric tube should be passed and a CXR ordered to check endotracheal and naso-gastric tube position
>
> **Tracheostomy**
> - In patients who require prolonged support (> 5–7 days), tracheostomy is often performed. This can invariably be done by utilizing a percutaneous technique on the ICU. The optimal timing and individual patient's risks and benefits are assessed daily

Mechanical ventilation

The mainstay of respiratory support is intermittent positive pressure ventilation (IPPV).

Modern ICU ventilators are complex devices, which provide continuous monitoring. Alarms must be checked regularly for appropriate settings.

The value of regular review, including respiratory examination, cannot be overstated. Minimizing ventilator-induced lung injury (VILI), rather than trying to normalize gas exchange, should be the main priority.

Regional lung ventilation and perfusion are not homogenous and this heterogeneity increases in disease. Positive pressure ventilation can cause lung injury via over-distension (volutrauma), excessive pressure (barotrauma), and cyclical recruitment and derecruitment.

- **Patient position.** Sit the patient up as far as possible to maximize functional residual capacity; turn the bad side down to ventilate it or the good side down to maximize oxygenation in severe hypoxaemia. In resistant hypoxaemia, the patient can be ventilated in the prone position.
- **Types of ventilation.** IPPV can be set up as either volume-controlled (pressure-monitored) or pressure-controlled (volume-monitored) (Table 14.3). This somewhat arbitrary distinction has become blurred with the advent of complex software in modern ventilators and the development of such concepts as volume-targeted pressure control, pressure-limited volume control, volume support, proportional assist and assisted spontaneous ventilation. In essence it does not matter which mode of ventilation you select as long as you understand what you need to set and what you need to monitor.
- **Goals of supportive care.** The goal is a spontaneously breathing, conscious patient who is able to cough and protect his/her airway with a $Pa_{O_2} > 8$ кPa (> 60 mmHg) and a $P_{CO_2} < 6$ кPa (< 45 mmHg).
- **To treat hypoxaemia**
  - Increase the Fi_{O_2}.
  - Increase the CPAP/PEEP.
  - Increasing the I:E ratio.
  - Perform a recruitment manœuvre.
  - Change the patient's position.
- **To fix hypercapnia**
  - *Do not* proceed if the pH is normal or within acceptable limits (permissive hypercapnia).
  - Increase tidal volume and/or respiratory rate — watch the effect on peak pressures and on inspiratory and expiratory flows. Remember that the volume of dead space ventilation is fixed; hence increasing the rate at the expense of tidal volume will result in a reduction in alveolar minute ventilation and a rise in Pa_{CO_2}.
- **Unconventional ventilation:**
  - *Time-cycled, bilevel pressure ventilation* provides two levels of CPAP sequentially. It can be useful in patients who exhibit ventilator dyssynchrony or as a weaning mode.
  - *Airway pressure release ventilation (APRV)* provides CPAP, often at a high level, with periodic, very short reductions in distending pressure to facilitate the washout of dead-space gas. It can be useful as a form of recruitment manœuvre, as a method of minimising VILI or as a weaning mode. It is most effective when there is some spontaneous breathing effort and especially if the tidal volumes are small.
  - *High-frequency oscillatory ventilation (HFOV)* requires a specialist ventilator. CPAP is provided with the addition of a piston-driven diaphragm in the circuit, which oscillates at frequencies of 3–6 Hz. This results in the generation of multiple forms of gas diffusion and effective ventilation. HFOV is currently used as a second-line therapy in severe lung injury, although its optimal use remains controversial.

Complications associated with mechanical ventilation

- **Airway complications.** There may be complications with tracheal intubation or with additional local complications of a tracheostomy (see above).

Table 14.3 Mechanical ventilation guidance

Settings	Guidance notes
Part A	
Fio_2	Start high and reduce gradually Minimize to achieve Pao_2 8–10 kPa/Spo_2 88–92%
Modes *(what effort is the patient making?)*	**Mandatory ventilation (MV)** – referred to as assist/control. The ventilator delivers a set number of breaths per minute. The inspiratory flow rate and pattern, the length of inspiration, the presence and duration of any inspiratory pause, and the length of expiration are all set **Synchronized intermittent mandatory ventilation (SIMV)** delivers a set number of breaths per minute, which the ventilator will try to synchronize with the patient's inspiratory efforts, if any. In addition, if the patient initiates a breath in between the SIMV breaths, pressure support can be given. In SIMV, the minimum rate is set. Use this mode if patients are making some but not enough respiratory effort **'Pressure support + CPAP'/'Spont'/'Assisted spontaneous breathing'** are all the same mode. A pressure support alone is set for each patient-initiated breath. No rate is set
Cycling *(decide what to set and what to measure)*	Pressure-cycled or pressure control: peak pressure is set, volume achieved is measured. Keep end-inspiratory pressures ≤ 30 cm H_2O Volume-cycled or volume control: volume is set, peak/plateau pressure is measured/limited. Inspiratory flow pattern set to continuous, decelerating (mimicking pressure control) or sinusoidal. In continuous flow, a variable-length end-inspiratory pause must be set
Tidal volume target	6–8 mL/kg ideal body weight in injured lungs Otherwise ≤ 10 mL/kg ideal body weight
Set rate	Set rate to achieve target minute volume and $Paco_2$ (4.5–6.5 kPa or higher as long as pH > 7.2)
I:E ratio	1:2 normally Consider 1:1–2:1 to recruit/optimize oxygenation (termed inverse ratio ventilation) Consider 1:3–1:4 in the presence of expiratory airflow imitation/high intrinsic PEEP/air trapping
Pressure support	Initially set pressure support to the same level as peak inspiratory pressure and titrate to desired tidal volume

Table 14.3 *Continued*	
Settings	**Guidance notes**
Part B	
PEEP	**Externally applied PEEP** is used to recruit and retain alveolar units. Thus PEEP is used to improve oxygenation See section below for rough guide but remember high PEEP can compromise cardiovascular function The determination of the optimal level of PEEP in a patient at a particular time point remains controversial. In patients with potentially recruitable lung units consider performing a recruitment manœuvre, usually a single or series of sustained inspiratory pauses, e.g. 35 cmH_2O for 30–60 s, followed by a decremental PEEP trial starting at either 10 or 12 cmH_2O. The optimal PEEP is set at the level above which derecruitment is deemed to have occurred, often judged by a deterioration in dynamic compliance and/or peripheral oxygen saturations Remember that total PEEP delivered is the sum of any intrinsic PEEP and any externally applied PEEP. Patients with airflow limitation due either to disease (e.g. asthma, COPD) or to ventilator settings (e.g. too short an expired time to reach zero flow) will develop intrinsic PEEP. The optimal setting of extrinsic PEEP in the presence of significant intrinsic PEEP is often a matter of trial and error

Fio_2	0.3	0.4	0.4	0.5	0.5	0.6	0.7	0.7	0.7	0.8	0.9
PEEP	5	5	8	8	10	10	10	12	14	14	14

- Disconnection, failure of gas or power supply, mechanical faults. These are unusual but dangerous. A method of manual ventilation, such as a self-inflating bag, and oxygen must always be available by the bedside.
- Cardiovascular complications. The application of positive pressure to the lungs and thoracic wall impedes venous return and distends alveoli, thereby 'stretching' the pulmonary capillaries and causing a rise in pulmonary vascular resistance. Both these mechanisms can produce a fall in cardiac output.

- Respiratory complications:

  - **Ventilator-induced lung injury (VILI) and barotrauma.** Mechanical ventilation can be complicated by a deterioration in gas exchange because of $\dot{V}/\dot{Q}$ mismatch and collapse of peripheral alveoli. Traditionally, the latter was prevented by using high tidal volumes (10–12 mL/kg), but high inflation pressures, with over-distension of compliant alveoli, perhaps exacerbated by the repeated opening and closure of distal airways, can disrupt the alveolar–capillary membrane. There is an increase in microvascular permeability and release of inflammatory mediators, leading to **VILI**. Extreme over-distension of the lungs during mechanical ventilation with high tidal volumes and PEEP can rupture alveoli and cause air to dissect centrally along the perivascular sheaths. This '**barotrauma**' may be complicated by pneumomediastinum, subcutaneous emphysema, pneumoperitoneum, pneumothorax and intra-abdominal air. The risk of pneumothorax is increased in those with destructive lung disease (e.g. necrotizing pneumonia, emphysema), asthma or fractured ribs.

  - **Tension pneumothorax.** A tension pneumothorax can be rapidly fatal in ventilated patients. Suggestive signs include the development or worsening of hypoxia, hypercarbia, respiratory distress and an unexplained increase in airway pressure, as well as hypotension and tachycardia, sometimes accompanied by a rising CVP. Examination may reveal unequal chest expansion, mediastinal shift away from the side of the pneumothorax (deviated trachea, displaced apex beat) and a hyper-resonant hemithorax. Although, traditionally, breath sounds are diminished over the pneumothorax, this sign can be extremely misleading in ventilated patients. If there is time, the diagnosis can be confirmed by CXR prior to definitive treatment with chest tube draining.

  - **Ventilator-associated pneumonia.** Hospital-acquired pneumonia occurs in as many as one-third of patients receiving mechanical ventilation and may be associated with a significant increase in mortality. It can be difficult to diagnose. Multiple organisms have been isolated, such as aerobic Gram-negative bacilli, e.g. *Pseudomonas aeruginosa*, *Klebsiella pneumoniae*, *Escherichia coli*, *Acinetobacter* spp and *Staphylococcus*. Leakage of infected oro-pharyngeal secretions past the tracheal cuff is thought to be largely responsible. Bacterial colonization of the oropharynx may be promoted by regurgitation of colonized gastric fluid and the risk of pneumonia can be reduced by nursing patients in the semi-recumbent, rather than the supine, position and by oro-pharyngeal decontamination. Treatment is complicated by multiple drug resistance to many antibiotics and mortality is high.

- **Gastrointestinal complications.** Initially, many ventilated patients will develop abdominal distension associated with an ileus. The cause is unknown, although the use of opiates may in part be responsible.

- **Salt and water retention.** Mechanical ventilation, particularly with PEEP, causes increased ADH secretion and possibly a reduction in circulating levels of atrial natriuretic peptide. Combined with a fall in cardiac output and a reduction in renal blood flow, these can cause salt and water retention.

Weaning from IPPV

The weaning process starts the moment IPPV is initiated.

- Allow the patient to make spontaneous breathing efforts (albeit assisted) at the earliest possible stage of respiratory support.
- As oxygenation improves, wean FiO_2 and PEEP sequentially.
- As hypercapnia improves, wean from mandatory ventilation (MV)/ synchronized intermittent mandatory ventilation (SIMV) to PS. Then gradually reduce PS.
- Once established on PS, consider a daily trial of support withdrawal. This needs to be coordinated with daily sedation holds. Three methods are widely used:
  - CPAP +5 cmH$_2$O
  - PS +5–7 5 cmH$_2$O with 0 PEEP
  - just a T-piece.

  The usual duration is a maximum of 15 mins; if successful, it should prompt extubation.
- In tracheostomized patients, 'training periods' of reduced or absent support can be employed as part of a daily weaning routine. The routine should be reviewed at least daily and titrated according to progress. Complete rest overnight and establishing a day/night cycle are essential.

ACUTE LUNG INJURY (ALI) AND ACUTE RESPIRATORY DISTRESS SYNDROME (ARDS)

ALI and ARDS are syndromes and represent a spectrum of disease. The syndrome is defined as a specific form of lung injury with diverse causes, characterized pathologically by diffuse alveolar damage and pathophysiologically by a breakdown in both the barrier and gas exchange functions of the lung, resulting in proteinaceous alveolar oedema and hypoxaemia.

Diagnostic criteria

- Hypoxaemia (usually refractory to supplemental oxygen).
- Bilateral, diffuse, interstitial and alveolar infiltrates on CXR (and/or CT).
- Reduced respiratory compliance (optional).
- No evidence for cardiac factors as the principle cause of the pulmonary oedema (pulmonary artery occlusion pressure (PAOP) ≤ 18 mmHg).
- Pulmonary hypertension (common).
- ALI — PaO_2/FiO_2 < 40 kPa; ARDS — PaO_2/FiO_2 < 26 kPa.

Outcome

Mortality is 35–60%, possibly falling due to improved general care. ARDS/ ALI is still the commonest cause of death in multiple organ failure. It is the failure to improve over the first 7 days and not the initial severity that indicates prognosis. In survivors the long-term lung function returns to pre-morbid levels. However, the long-term quality of life and morbidity are worse than severity-matched critically ill patients without ARDS.

Pathophysiology

Changes include alveolar flooding with proteinaceous fluid (exacerbated by reduced clearance); decreased surfactant production, resulting in atelectasis and decreased compliance; and hyaline membrane formation and interstitial oedema, leading to impaired gaseous diffusion. There is increased intrapulmonary shunt and loss of mechanical defence barrier; hence the high risk of sepsis.

Management

- Early and aggressive treatment of the underlying condition.
- Optimal cardiovascular support with fluid restriction, diuretics and, if necessary, haemofiltration in order to achieve a consistently negative fluid balance.
- Early enteral nutrition.
- Minimal sedation and neuromuscular blockade is usually recommended although a recent trial has shown benefit of neuromuscular blockade given for 48 hours early in the disease.
- Adherence to the ventilator care bundle.
- Ventilatory strategy: 'open the lung and keep it open' and minimize VILI.
  - Low tidal volumes 6–8 mL/kg ideal body weight
  - 'Adequate' (high) PEEP
  - Minimal peak/plateau pressures (≤ 30 cmH$_2$O)
  - Minimal Fio$_2$
  - Maintenance of spontaneous breathing.
- Unproven ventilatory rescue therapies: unconventional ventilation, in particular HFOV; extracorporeal lung assist.
- Adjunctive therapies with *no* evidence of benefit: inhaled nitric oxide, nebulized **prostacyclin**, **almitrine** and **recombinant surfactant.**
- Adjunctive therapies under active investigation: **sildenafil** and **salbutamol**.
- Controversies: whether an open lung biopsy should be performed and the role of high-dose corticosteroids.

CARDIOVASCULAR FAILURE

The principal roles of the cardiovascular system are to deliver oxygen and glucose to the tissues and to remove carbon dioxide and other waste products. Failure to do this is termed 'shock'.

- Clinical manifestations of cardiovascular insufficiency/shock include:
  - low-volume peripheral pulses
  - cold peripheries, especially with proximal extension/peripheral capillary refill > 2 s (except in distributive shock states, where peripheries may be warm with capillary refill time < 2 s)
  - tachycardia and hypotension (not invariable and the least reliable signs)
  - altered mental function, confusion or diminished level of consciousness (cerebral hypoperfusion)
  - urine output < 0.5 mL/kg/hour (renal hypoperfusion).
- Cardiovascular support is achieved by assessing and optimizing four key components of the cardiovascular system in strict order (Table 14.4). More than one component failure may exist. Inotropic and/or vasopressor support should only be instituted after volume resuscitation. Exceptions to this suggestion include severe or drug-induced hypotension.
- At an organ level, shock may result in micro-circulatory failure. This complex phenomenon arises from, among other processes, endothelial cell damage, formation of capillary occlusive micro-thrombi and neutrophil margination. This results in arterio-venous shunting and tissue

Table 14.4 The four key assessable and treatable components of shock

Assessable and treatable components of shock	Aetiology of shock	Therapy	Physiological targets
Heart rate (HR) and rhythm	Bradyarrhythmia	Positive chronotropic drugs/pacing	Optimal HR is ~90/min in sinus rhythm
	Tachyarrhythmia	Anti-arrhythmic drugs/ cardioversion	
Preload (intravascular volume status)	Hypovolaemic shock	20 mL/kg fluid bolus (crystalloid or colloid)	CVP ≥ 8 cmH$_2$O Negative response to dynamic fluid challenge. Hb 8–10 g/dL, haematocrit > 0.3
	Haemorrhagic shock	*Stop* the bleeding 20 mL/kg fluid bolus (crystalloid or colloid) Red blood cells, platelets and clotting factors	
Cardiac contractility	Cardiogenic shock	Inotropic drugs Intra-aortic balloon pump Re-vascularization Structural repair	Cardiac index (output per m^2 body surface area) 3.0–5.0 L/min/m^2
Afterload or vascular resistance (both pulmonary (PVR) and systemic (SVR))	Obstructive shock (pulmonary embolism, tamponade)	Relieve obstruction	Systolic BP ≥ 90 mmHg Mean arterial pressure (MAP) ≥ 60 mmHg
	Distributive shock (septic, spinal, anaphylactic)	Vasopressor drugs	

ischaemia. This phenomenon is hard to monitor in almost all organs and no specific therapy exists to treat it.

- Measures of global oxygen delivery (Do_2) and consumption (Vo_2) are useful in assessing the adequacy of resuscitation and include the direct measurements of Do_2 and Vo_2, central or mixed venous oxygen saturations ($Scvo_2$ and Svo_2 respectively) and blood pH, lactate levels and calculated base excess.

Terminology and normal values

Note that these are normal value ranges for healthy human adults at rest. There are no normal ranges for shocked patients. Therapeutic targets are best considered by assessing the dynamic response to an intervention and using all available measures of both organ-specific and global hypoperfusion.

- Stroke volume = 70–100 mL.
- Cardiac output = Stroke volume × heart rate (normal range at rest 4–6 L/min).
- Oxygen delivery (DO_2) is the total amount of oxygen delivered to the tissues per minute.
  - DO_2 = Cardiac output × arterial oxygen content.
  - DO_2 = CO × ((SaO_2 × [Hb] × 1.34) + (PaO_2 × 0.003)).
  - DO_2 = 950–1300 mL/min.
- Oxygen consumption (VO_2) is the amount of oxygen consumed by the tissues per minute.
  - VO_2 = Cardiac output × (arterial oxygen content) – (mixed venous oxygen content – SvO_2).
  - VO_2 = 180–320 mL/min.
- Mixed venous saturation (SvO_2) is a guide to the difference between oxygen being delivered to the tissues and its extraction or use. This is measured by taking a sample of blood from the distal port of a pulmonary artery catheter (PAC) and measuring the saturation using a blood gas analyser. If a PAC is not available, samples from a central venous catheter in the superior vena cava will provide an approximate guide. This variable is called central venous oxygen saturation ($ScvO_2$). The normal value is 70–75%. This measurement has been successfully used to guide resuscitation, resulting in improved morbidity and mortality.

Methods of continuous haemodynamic monitoring

The insertion of peripheral arterial and central venous lines is the first step in the monitoring of critically ill patients.

Invasive arterial and venous pressure monitoring

- Arterial cannulation. Insert arterial cannulation. This allows real-time BP measurement and beat-to-beat display of the arterial waveform, and facilitates regular arterial blood sampling.
  - A modified Seldinger technique or direct cannulation can be used.
  - Favoured sites are the radial and femoral arteries.
  - The complication of distal ischaemia is rare. Infection is always a risk with invasive lines. Suspicion of colonization should prompt early line cultures and removal/change of lines if possible.
- CVP line. Insert a CVP line (Fig. 14.1), guided by US. The CVP line provides information on right heart filling pressures; allows estimation of mixed venous saturations; and acts as a vascular access.
  - Central venous pressures should correlate well with left ventricular filling pressures; however, this is not always so in the critically ill. Ischaemic cardiomyopathy, valvular pathology, pulmonary hypertension and pulmonary embolism are potential causes of disparity.
  - The **Seldinger technique** is routine for multi-lumen catheters. Strict aseptic technique should be employed. Skin preparation with 2% chlorhexidine in 70% alcohol is recommended. Exit sites should be dressed so as to prevent contamination. Prior to any use, any access

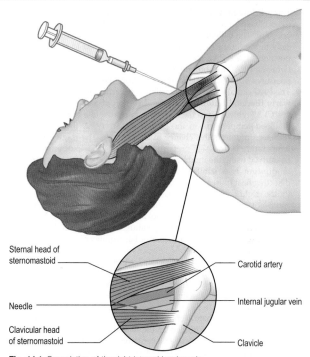

Fig. 14.1 Cannulation of the right internal jugular vein.

port should be cleaned with chlorhexidine. Lines should be removed at the earliest opportunity.

• Favoured sites are the internal jugular and subclavian. The latter has a lower risk of line-related bacteraemia but is associated with a high risk of complications at insertion and chronic stenosis and thrombosis. The femoral site should be avoided in the first instance.

Pulmonary artery catheterization and thermodilution

This is still the gold standard technique for measurement of haemodynamic status (see below).

● An introducer sheath is first placed into a central vein using the Seldinger technique. The flotation pulmonary artery catheter (PAC) is then inserted via the sheath into the cannulated vein. The PAC has a balloon on its tip. This is inflated in the cannulated vessel and the PAC is advanced slowly, its direction and location guided by the direction of blood flow. The pressure, measured at the tip of the PAC, is continuously transduced and should successively show the pressures within the right atrium, the right ventricle and the pulmonary artery. The PAC is further advanced until the balloon occludes a branch of the pulmonary artery, which is noted by a sudden change in pressure waveform.

The pressure now transduced, known as the pulmonary artery wedge (or occlusion) pressure (PAWP or PAOP), should represent left atrial pressure. The balloon should be deflated and only re-inflated periodically to measure PAOP. A CXR should be obtained to ensure optimal position of the PAC tip. Optimal position is within West's zone III (where the PAC tip communicates continuously with the distal vascular pressures during diastole) and < 5 cm from the hilum.

- The PAC can also provide an estimate of **cardiac output** using **cold or warm thermodilution techniques**. Injection of a 10 mL bolus of **cold** (~4°C) 5% glucose into the right atrium results in a transient decrease in blood temperature in the pulmonary artery. A thermistor at the catheter tip detects this change in temperature. The mean decrease in temperature is inversely proportional to the cardiac output, which can be derived using the modified Stewart–Hamilton equation. **Warm thermodilution** is a similar technique, with a downstream thermistor detecting heat pulses sent in binary code from a thermal filament placed in the right ventricle. The latter method is automated and semi-continuous. Thermodilution has its limitations. There are inaccuracies in both high and low cardiac output ranges, often as a result of operator error or errors from injectate temperature calibration. This is especially true when a patient is hypothermic or has significant tricuspid regurgitation or dysrhythmias.

- Svo_2 can be measured intermittently by blood sampling from the pulmonary artery or continuously using a specialist catheter.

- Complications of PACs, over and above central venous cannulation, include pulmonary infarction, pulmonary artery rupture and sustained arrhythmias.

- Due to the invasive nature of the PAC, a lack of evidence to demonstrate the benefit of therapy guided by the data that it can provide, and the development of less invasive alternative techniques of monitoring cardiac output, use of the PAC has declined dramatically over recent years. There is, however, overwhelming evidence that use of the PAC is safe.

Oesophageal Doppler

- This technique relies on the phenomenon that sound undergoes a frequency shift with respect to a fixed receiver when the source is moving at a different speed to the receiver. The degree of frequency shift is directly proportional to the speed of the sound source (the Doppler effect).

- A probe inserted 30–40 cm down the oesophagus and a US beam is focused on the blood flow in the descending aorta. In this area the aorta lies parallel to the oesophagus and has a predictable cross-sectional area. The frequency of reflected sound waves undergoes Doppler shift dependent on the speed of blood flow. By quantifying this shift and incorporating the estimated cross-sectional area and ejection time (stroke distance), the stroke volume can be calculated. The aortic stroke volume is a percentage of the actual cardiac output, which can be derived from patient nomograms based on height and weight.

- The advantages of this system include relative ease of use, minimal invasiveness and the fact that this is the only method of haemodynamic monitoring to provide real-time data based on the actual (and not derived) cardiac output.

- Conditions prohibiting use include severe aortic pathology, an intra-aortic balloon pump (IABP) and oesophageal disease.

Pulse contour analysis

The pressure wave displayed by an invasive arterial line is amenable to pulse contour analysis. The pressure waveform is converted to a volume–time waveform. The area under the curve gives a derived estimate of beat-to-beat stroke volume. Combination with the heart rate is used to calculate cardiac output. For accuracy, several of the systems calibrate the estimates of cardiac output using trans-pulmonary dilution methods.

Cardiovascular supportive therapies

Rate and rhythm control

- The target pulse rate is 90/min.
- If the patient is haemodynamically unstable, treat as per the Advanced Life Support algorithm. DC cardioversion is relatively straightforward in intubated patients and can be performed early.
- If the patient is haemodynamically stable, correct electrolytes and perform a dynamic fluid challenge prior to drug treatment and/or DC cardioversion.
- The commonest arrhythmia in critically ill patients is atrial fibrillation (AF). In the majority of cases there is an identifiable iatrogenic precipitant (e.g. furosemide, insulin, salbutamol, inotropes). Aim to keep serum Mg^{2+} > 0.9 mmol/L and K^+ > 4.4 mmol/L to prevent arrhythmias.
- If the onset of AF is known to have been within 12–24 hrs, DC cardioversion is used. If the AF has been paroxysmal, has been present for > 24 hours or fails DC cardioversion, **digoxin** (may control rate), **esmolol, metoprolol, sotalol** or **amiodarone** is used. **Verapamil** and **flecainide** should be avoided, as they are both profoundly negatively inotropic.

IV fluid resuscitation, the dynamic fluid challenge or pre-load optimization

- These techniques are used to describe the assessment of fluid responsiveness rather than assessment of the adequacy of intravascular volume. They are performed by administering a rapid 100–500 mL bolus of IV fluid and measuring the instantaneous response in heart rate and stroke volume (and hence cardiac output), CVP and MAP. Of all of these variables, stroke volume is most useful measure.
- There is no proven benefit in using any particular crystalloid or colloid.
- With regard to CVP, three patterns of response (see Fig. 11.1) are looked for, in patients with a starting CVP in the normal range of 4–8 cmH_2O (caution in interpretation is required in patients receiving positive pressure ventilation).
- A rapid fluid bolus should not be given via an automated volumetric pump, which is too slow to assess volume responsiveness properly. (N.B. Do it yourself)
- In patients receiving positive pressure ventilation, who demonstrate no inspiratory effort and are in sinus rhythm, a maximum variation in systolic or pulse pressure of > 15% over each respiratory cycle is a validated method of predicting volume responsiveness.
- There is evidence to support the idea that early and aggressive fluid resuscitation is beneficial. In the short term, fluid administration is simple, quick and often effective; iatrogenic fluid overload is rare. In

Kumar & Clark's Medical Management and Therapeutics

responsive patients, fluid therapy increases global oxygen delivery for the smallest increase in myocardial work.

Inotropes, vasopressors and other vasoactive drugs

- If rate and rhythm are acceptable and/or resistant to fluid and electrolyte resuscitation, estimation and continuous monitoring of cardiac output are highly desirable to guide pharmacological therapy.
- If there is a low or inadequate cardiac output and/or perfusion pressure (MAP), then vasoactive drugs should be commenced (Tables 14.5 and 14.6).
- **Dobutamine** is probably the inotrope of first choice. It is a strongly positive chronotrope and an arterial vasodilator. Alternatives include the inodilators, **milrinone** and **levosimendan** (available in some countries). Inodilators exert positive inotropic effects and induce systemic vasodilatation. Due to the vasodilatation that these drugs

Table 14.5 Cardiovascular effects of vasoactive drugs and devices

Drug	Receptor avidity				Physiological effects				
	DA	α	β₁	β₂	HR	MAP	CI	SVR	MOD
Dopamine									
< 5 mcg/kg/min	+++	+	+	+	=/+	=/+	=/+	=	+
5–10 mcg/kg/min	+++	++	++	+	+	+	+	+	+
> 10 mcg/kg/min	+++	+++	++		++	++	+	++	++
Dobutamine		+	+++	++	+	–/=	++	–/=	+++
Dopexamine	++		+	+++	++	–/=	+	–/=	++
Adrenaline (epinephrine)									
< 0.2 mcg/kg/min		+	+	+	+	=/+	+	=/+	++
> 0.2 mcg/kg/min		+++	++	+	++	++	++	++	+++
Noradrenaline (norepinephrine)									
< 0.2 mcg/kg/min		++	+	+	=/+	+	–/+	++	++
> 0.2 mcg/kg/min		+++	+	+	=/+	++	–/+	+++	++
Milrinone					++	– –	++	– –	++
Levosimendan					+	– –	++	– –	?=
Vasopressin/ analogues					=	+++	– –	+++	++
Methylene blue					=	++	– –	++	++
IABP (device)					=	–/+	+	– –	– –

α β₁ β₂, adrenergic receptor types; CI, cardiac index; DA, dopamine receptors; HR, heart rate; IABP, intra-aortic balloon pump; MAP, mean arterial pressure; MOD, myocardial oxygen demand; SVR, systemic vascular resistance.

+ increased, = unchanged, – decreased.

Table 14.6 Dosage regimens of commonly used vasoactive drugs

Drug	Dosage range	Notes
Dopamine	1–20 mcg/kg/min	Dominant effect dependent on dose. Some evidence of worse outcome compared to other drugs, therefore out of favour
Dobutamine	5–20 mcg/kg/min	Inodilator (positive inotropic and causes systemic vasodilatation)
Dopexamine	0.25–2.0 mcg/kg/min	Positive chronotrope/inodilator/anti-inflammatory?
Adrenaline (epinephrine)	0.01–1 mcg/kg/min	Inoconstrictor (positive inotropic causing systemic vasoconstriction)
Noradrenaline (norepinephrine)	0.01–1 mcg/kg/min	Vasoconstrictor (some inotropic activity), first-line vasopressor
Milrinone (phosphodiesterase inhibitor)	150–750 ng/kg/min	Inodilator. Significantly longer onset and elimination half-life than dobutamine. Accumulates in renal failure. Do not give loading dose
Levosimendan (Ca sensitizer and K channel opener)	0.05–0.2 mcg/kg/min	Inodilator. Active metabolite with long elimination half-life, hence 24-hour infusion will have measurable effects for up to 7 days. Do not give loading dose
Vasopressin	0.01–0.05 U/min	Vasoconstrictor. Second-line vasopressor in noradrenaline-resistant shock (*see also* functional hypoadrenalism)
Terlipressin (vasopressin analogue)	0.25–2 mg bolus	Vasoconstrictor. Duration of action 4–6 hours. Alternative to vasopressin
Methylene blue (nitric oxide antagonist)	2 mg/kg loading 0.25–2 mg/kg/hour	Vasoconstrictor. 2nd/3rd line vasopressor in norepinephrine resistant shock (*see also* functional hypoadrenalism)

cause, combination with a vasopressor is often required. All are pro-arrhythmogenic.

- **Dopamine** and **adrenaline (epinephrine)**, both inoconstrictors, are not so frequently used.
- In ischaemic cardiogenic shock, inotropic drugs should be used to provide a temporal bridge to definitive revascularization and/or mechanical support, most commonly an IABP.
- **Noradrenaline (norepinephrine)** is the first-choice vasoconstrictor with a weakly positive chronotropic and inotropic activity. Vasopressin analogues and methylene blue are also used. Excessive doses of vasopressors can lead to increased over-centralization of the circulation, left ventricular failure, and splanchnic and distal extremity ischaemia/infarction.
- In immediate resuscitation, **ephedrine**, **phenylephrine**, **metaraminol** and 1 : 100 000 **adrenaline (epinephrine)** can be given in small bolus doses to maintain BP.
- In the immediate management of decompensated left ventricular failure, **IV nitrates** are a useful first-line agent in offloading the left side of the heart. This is predominantly via venodilatation. Second-line agents in hypertensive cardiovascular crises include hydralazine and labetalol.

'Low-dose' corticosteroids and functional hypoadrenalism in shock

There is some evidence to suggest that a proportion of patients with distributive shock have functional hypoadrenalism. This is manifested as vasopressor resistance, with patients requiring rapidly escalating or high-dose infusions. Whether such patients have functional hypoadrenalism and/or peripheral resistance is unclear. 'Physiological replacement' dose hydrocortisone 200–240 mg/24 hrs, with or without fludrocortisone, has been demonstrated to be beneficial in some patients, both in terms of attenuating vasopressor requirements and outcomes.

In order to determine whether or not a patient is likely to benefit from such therapy, a short adrenocorticotrophic hormone (ACTH) stimulation test can be performed. A low baseline cortisol level, coupled with an attenuated or negligible response to ACTH, predicts patients who benefit from 'low-dose' corticosteroids. Outside of this profile, interpretation of the test remains an area of controversy.

Post-operative care of patients with a high risk of morbidity and mortality

The more extensive the surgery and the more physiologically deranged the patient, be it acute, acute on chronic or merely chronic, the higher the risk. Many such patients are often referred to critical care environments for their immediate post-operative care.

Survivors have a different physiological profile to non-survivors. The median value of DO_2I (I = index) in survivors was 600 mL/min/m². Maximizing a high-risk patient's DO_2I in the immediate post-operative period (8 hours) using the therapies described above, in particular intravascular fluid responsiveness, with the addition of low-dose inodilators where necessary, in an attempt to reach 600 mL/min/m² has been demonstrated to be a successful strategy in reducing morbidity and mortality.

SYSTEMIC INFLAMMATORY RESPONSE SYNDROME (SIRS), SEPSIS, SEVERE SEPSIS AND SEPTIC SHOCK

Definitions

SIRS is triggered by localized or generalized infection, trauma, thermal injury or sterile inflammatory processes, e.g. acute pancreatitis. It is considered to be present when patients have more than one of the following clinical findings:

- body temperature > 38°C or < 36°C
- heart rate > 90/bpm
- hyperventilation evidenced by respiratory rate > 20/min or Pa_{CO_2} < 4.2 kPa
- white blood cell count > 12×10^9/L or < 4×10^9/L.

Sepsis is defined as SIRS with a documented or suspected infection. **Severe sepsis** is sepsis with evidence of organ dysfunction (as defined by SOFA or equivalent, p. 31). **Septic shock** is defined as severe sepsis with hypotension despite adequate fluid resuscitation. Severe sepsis and septic shock are the commonest conditions requiring critical care. Their incidence is high and increasing. They are associated with a very high morbidity and an overall mortality of 30–60%.

The Surviving Sepsis campaign's recommendations (2004) may be found at www.survivingsepsis.org.

Initial resuscitation: goals during the first 6 hours

- Measure serum lactate.
- Obtain blood cultures prior to antibiotic administration.
- Administer broad-spectrum antibiotic(s), within 1 hour of admission, e.g. IV **cefotaxime**.
- In the event of hypotension and/or a serum lactate > 4 mmol/L:
  - Deliver an initial minimum of 20 mL/kg of crystalloid or an equivalent.
  - Commence vasopressors for hypotension not responding to initial fluid resuscitation to maintain MAP > 65 mmHg.
- In the event of persistent hypotension despite fluid resuscitation (septic shock) and/or lactate > 4 mmol/L:
  - Continue fluid resuscitation until CVP ≥ 8 mmHg.
  - Continue resuscitation until Scv_{O_2} ≥ 70% and Sv_{O_2} ≥ 65%.

Management goals within the first 24 hours (see Emergencies in Medicine, p. 718)

- Administer **low-dose steroids** for septic shock in accordance with a standardized ICU policy.
- Administer **drotrecogin alfa** (recombinant human activated protein C) in accordance with a standardized ICU policy (see below).
- Maintain blood glucose at < 10 mmol/L (< 180 mg/dL).
- In mechanically ventilated patients, maintain the inspiratory plateau pressure at < 30 cmH_2O.
- Activated protein C or drotrecogin alfa. In severe sepsis/septic shock there is activation of the coagulation cascade, including the fibrinolytic pathway. This leads to a depletion of activated protein C; lower levels are associated with a worse outcome.
  - Recombinant human activated protein C **(rhAPC)**, **drotrecogin alfa**, is used in patients with severe sepsis and septic shock. Controversy

continues over its use, as some trials and observational studies have raised doubts regarding both the safety and the efficacy of rhAPC.

- Current indications for its use are patients at high risk of death (APACHE II ≥ 25) from sepsis-induced multiple organ failure (two or more organs). It must be administered within 24 hours of the onset of organ dysfunction.

- It is contraindicated in patients with active internal bleeding, intracranial pathology, concurrent heparin use or significant thrombocytopenia (platelet count ≤ 30 × 10^9/L).

BRAIN INJURY

Regardless of the nature of the brain injury, certain universal principles of care apply; minimize secondary brain injury and optimize any chance of penumbral recovery.

- Take an ABC approach to resuscitation.
- Aim for normoxia, normocarbia, normotension, normothermia, normoglycaemia and normonatraemia. In particular, hypercarbia, hyperthermia and both hypo- and hyperglycaemia are associated with secondary brain injury. There is no therapeutic benefit in hypocarbia. Mild hypothermia may be of benefit.
- Position the patient 30° head up. This is the best compromise between the increased gravitational gradient placed on the arterial pressure and enhanced gravitational gradient for venous drainage. Try to avoid any intervention that may reduce or obstruct cerebral venous return, e.g. internal jugular lines, or high intrathoracic pressures (high mean airway pressures) created by mechanical ventilation.
- As regards blood pressure, the concept of cerebral perfusion pressure (CPP) (mean systemic pressure − intracranial pressure (ICP)) is helpful. A minimum target CPP of 70 mmHg is optimal. A lower CPP is associated with a higher incidence and extent of secondary brain injury. If possible, measure and continuously monitor ICP.
- Medical management of raised ICP includes:
  - aggressive normalization of PaCO_2 and core temperature
  - patient positioning (see above)
  - high-dose propofol or thiopentone infusion (barbiturate coma) to reduce cerebral metabolic demand
  - aggressive management of seizures
  - hypertonic saline and/or mannitol.
- Surgical management of raised ICP includes:
  - CSF drainage (placement of an extraventricular drain)
  - decompressive craniectomy.

Brainstem death

This is an emotive area that is often difficult to communicate and for family and staff at the bedside to understand.

The term may have different definitions in different countries. In the UK this term refers to 'the irreversible loss of the capacity for consciousness combined with the irreversible loss of the capacity to breathe'. This may be anatomically defined as brainstem death. In some states in the USA brain death also encompasses cardiopulmonary death as part of the definition.

The process of diagnosing brain death is divided into three parts: pre-conditions, exclusions and tests.

Pre-conditions

- The patient must be in an apnoeic coma and on a ventilator, unable to make spontaneous breathing effort.
- The presence is required of irremediable structural brain damage contributing to brainstem death, e.g. traumatic head injuries or haemorrhage.

Exclusions

- Hypothermia: core temperature must be > 35°C.
- Metabolic or endocrine derangement must be excluded (e.g. hypoglycaemia).
- Poisoning and use of neuromuscular drugs and sedatives must be excluded and taken into account.

Brainstem death tests

These should be performed and repeated by two separate senior doctors (ideally one should be a consultant or equivalent). This may be done on separate occasions or together. The two doctors should not be part of a transplantation team and should be competent in the area. The time of death is when the first set of tests confirms the presence of brainstem death.

- **Oculo-cephalic reflex.** This should be absent. It is tested by rolling the head from side to side. In a functioning brainstem the eyes will move relative to the orbit (doll's eyes present). In brainstem death the eyes move with the head in the direction of travel of the movement (doll's eyes absent).
- **Pupillary reflex.** Pupils are fixed and unresponsive to light stimulus. Direct and consensual light reflexes are absent. Pupils may or may not be dilated.
- **Corneal reflex.** Cotton wool may be used to elicit a response to corneal stimulation by light touch. This response will be absent in brainstem death.
- **Vestibulo-ocular reflexes.** Caloric testing is used to assess function of the labyrinth; it is essential that the tympanic membrane is visualized prior to the test. Fifty mL of ice-cold water is injected into the left ear over 1 min. Intact brainstem response will elicit nystagmus with fast movements to the right (away from the injected ear). The opposite response will take place in the intact brainstem of an individual if water is injected into the right ear. In patients with brainstem death no response to ice-cold water injection is seen.
- **Gag and cough reflex.** Pharyngeal, laryngeal (throat spatula) and tracheal (suction catheter down the endotracheal tube to the carina) stimulation would normally elicit a cough/gag response. This is absent in brainstem death.
- **Motor reflex.** Centrally or peripherally applied painful stimulus would normally elicit a motor response in the cranial nerve territory. In brainstem death this is absent.
- **Apnoea testing.** Intact brainstems will initiate spontaneous respiratory effort in the presence of hypercarbia. The patient is placed on 100% oxygen on the ventilator and pre-oxygenated for 10 mins. The minute volume should be reduced to achieve a $Pa_{CO_2} > 5$ kPa before the test. The patient is then disconnected from the ventilator and oxygen is attached to the endotracheal tube at 6 L/min (to maintain oxygenation

in the presence of hypercarbia). The $Paco_2$ must rise to > 6.65 kPa. The chest is visualized and inspected for movements. In brainstem death no movements are present and the patient is then re-connected to the ventilator.

Organ and tissue donation

Individual countries have their own processes. In the UK, organ and tissue donation are governed by the Human Tissue Act 2004 (see http://body.orpheusweb.co.uk/HTA2004/20040030.htm). Always consider donation in dying patients, especially in those with brainstem death and, in particular, if the brain injury is the sole organ failure. In the UK, to discuss any aspect of donation, contact your local transplant coordinator.

ACUTE KIDNEY INJURY

Acute kidney injury (p. 348) is a common complication of critical illness. Kidney injury is associated with increased morbidity and mortality regardless of the primary pathology, with a direct correlation between the severity of renal injury and poor outcome.

● Clinically, oliguria is the first presenting sign. This may lead promptly to anuric renal failure.
● Prevention, by maintaining intravascular volume and adequate renal perfusion pressure, together with the avoidance of nephrotoxic drugs, e.g. NSAIDs, in the at-risk population is well established.
● X-ray intravascular contrast is another potent precipitant of acute kidney injury (p. 351).

Medical management of acute oliguric/anuric renal failure

● **'Low-dose' dopamine** is not helpful in the prevention or treatment of acute kidney injury.
● **Furosemide** may aid in the management of fluid overload in non-oliguric patients but has no effect on disease progression or outcome of acute oliguric/anuric kidney injury.
● Optimize renal perfusion (intravascular volume, cardiac output, perfusion pressure).
● Initiate renal replacement therapy early, specifically to manage acidosis (pH < 7.2, in particular, acidosis associated with cardiovascular compromise), hyperkalaemia ($K^+ > 6.5$), uraemia (urea > 35 mmol/L) or fluid overload. Other indications include encephalopathy, hyperpyrexia, and possibly vasopressor-resistant septic shock.

Renal replacement therapy (p. 357)

● Continuous renal replacement therapy (CRRT) is performed either as haemofiltration (convection — CVVHF) or as haemodiafiltration (convection and diffusion — CVVHDF), i.e. haemofiltration with a counter-current for solutes to diffuse down.
● Higher rates of filtration produce better outcomes in patients with severe sepsis. Aim for 35 mL/kg/hour minimum, or more if the patient will tolerate it. A good starting point is 2000–2500 mL/hour of CVVHF.
● Replacement fluids are usually **bicarbonate-based buffer solutions** with a fixed concentration of potassium. Alternatives includes acetate-buffered solutions. If using high-volume replacement, increasing ventilatory demands on the patient, hypomagnesaemia and hypophosphataemia can develop.

- Make a fluid balance plan indicating how much, if any, fluid to take off.
- Intermittent haemodialysis (iHD) is helpful in haemodynamically stable patients. In the acute phase of critical illness, daily iHD has been shown to be of greater benefit than alternate-day treatment. Patients must have their hepatitis B and C status established prior to commencing therapy, as there is a risk of cross-infection.
- Approximately 80–90% of patients with acute kidney injury who require renal support will recover some if not all renal function at 3 months

Further reading

Adhikari NKJ, Fowler RA, Bhagwanjee S, Rubenfeld GD: Critical care and the global burden of critical illness in adults, *Lancet* 376:1339–1346, 2010.

Curtis J Randall, Vincent J-L: Ethics and end-of-life care for adults in the intensive care unit, *Lancet* 376:1347–1353, 2010.

Vincent J-L, Singer M: Critical care: advances and future perspectives, *Lancet* 376:1354–1361, 2010.

PITUITARY DISORDERS

The hypothalamus regulates many vital functions, including appetite, thirst, thermal regulation and sleep. It controls pituitary function by stimulatory and inhibitory factors and by hormones released via the pituitary stalk.

- Anterior pituitary produces hormones necessary for growth, stress response, reproduction and metabolism.
- Posterior pituitary stores antidiuretic hormone (ADH) and oxytocin.

Many hormones are released in either a pulsatile or a circadian pattern and are regulated by feedback systems. Endocrine tests on serum/plasma take advantage of natural peaks and troughs in secretion, while stimulatory or suppression tests are used to investigate hormone deficiency or excess further.

Pituitary tumours

Pituitary tumours are a relatively common incidental finding in the general population; only a minority cause clinical problems, either due to uncontrolled secretion of pituitary hormones, or due to local compression effects. Tumours may be small (micro-adenomas, < 10 mm diameter) or large (macro-adenomas, > 10 mm) and the vast majority are benign.

- Local compression effects of a pituitary tumour include:
  - failure of pituitary function due to compression of normal gland
  - bitemporal hemianopia due to pressure on the optic chiasm
  - diplopia and III, IV and VI cranial nerve palsies secondary to tumour compression at the cavernous sinus
  - high prolactin levels due to compression of the pituitary stalk with loss of dopaminergic inhibitory control
  - headache
  - if very large, altered hypothalamic control of appetite, thirst and somnolence.
- Uncontrolled hormone release occurs with tumours arising from:
  - corticotroph cells: Cushing's syndrome (adrenocorticotrophic hormone (ACTH) excess)
  - somatotroph cells: acromegaly or gigantism (growth hormone excess)
  - lactotroph cells: (prolactin excess)
  - thyrotroph cells: rarely hyperthyroidism (thyroid-stimulating hormone (TSH)-releasing tumours)

- gonadotroph cells: ovarian hyperstimulation and testicular enlargement (rare luteinizing hormone (LH) or follicular stimulating hormone (FSH) excess).

Treatment

The aim of therapy is to:

- reduce tumour bulk and relieve pressure on local structures where appropriate
- restore excess hormone secretion to normal levels
- eliminate associated co-morbidities and increased mortality resulting from hormone excess
- preserve or restore pituitary function.

Treatment (Table 15.1) options include surgery, radiotherapy and medical therapy, depending on the aetiology of the pituitary mass. Post-operative

Table 15.1 Comparison of primary treatment for pituitary tumours

Treatment method	Advantages	Disadvantages
Surgical		
Trans-sphenoidal adenomectomy or hypophysectomy	Relatively minor procedure Potentially curative for micro- and smaller macro-adenomas	Some extrasellar extensions may not be accessible Risk of CSF leakage and meningitis
Trans-frontal	Good access to suprasellar region	Major procedure; danger of frontal lobe damage High chance of subsequent hypopituitarism
Radiotherapy		
External (40–50 Gy)	Non-invasive Reduces recurrence rate after surgery	Slow action, often over many years Not always effective Possible late risk of tumour induction
Stereotactic	Precise administration of dose to lesion	Long-term follow-up data limited
Yttrium implantation	High local dose	Only used in few centres
Medical		
Dopamine agonist (e.g. bromocriptine)	Non-invasive; reversible	Usually not curative; significant side-effects in minority
Somatostatin analogue (octreotide)	Non-invasive; reversible	Usually not curative; expensive
Growth hormone receptor antagonist (pegvisomant)	Highly selective	Usually not curative; very expensive

radiotherapy is used if significant tumour bulk remains after surgery or the underlying disease is still active. Radiotherapy results in a gradual decline of residual pituitary function over many years and must be monitored.

Hypopituitarism

Compression of the pituitary gland by a mass lesion results in progressive loss of function. Growth hormone and gonadotrophins are usually the first hormones to be affected, followed by TSH and finally ACTH (panhypopituitarism). Prolactin levels may rise due to compression of the pituitary stalk and loss of dopaminergic inhibitory control.

Clinical features

Secondary hypothyroidism (p. 571) and adrenal failure (p. 582) both lead to tiredness and general malaise:

- **Hypothyroidism** causes slowness of thought and action, dry skin and cold intolerance.
- **Hypoadrenalism** causes mild hypotension, hyponatraemia and ultimately cardiovascular collapse during severe intercurrent stressful illness.
- **Gonadotrophin deficiency** causes loss of libido, loss of secondary sexual hair, amenorrhoea and impotence.
- **Hyperprolactinaemia** causes galactorrhoea and hypogonadism.

Examination

- **Fundoscopy** (with dilatation) and visual acuity testing are carried out to exclude optic atrophy, retinal vein engorgement and papilloedema associated with expansion of a tumour mass.
- **Visual field assessment**, by formal perimetry or by confrontation using a red pin, is used to assess for optic chiasmal compression causing bitemporal hemianopia.

Investigation of pituitary function

- Basal serum investigations
  - *ACTH and 09:00 h cortisol.* Individuals with normal diurnal rhythm (that is not disrupted by shift work or travel across time zones) show an early morning peak of cortisol > 500 nmol/L, which excludes ACTH deficiency. Cortisol values < 100 nmol/L at 09:00 h are strongly suggestive of hypothalamic–pituitary–adrenal (HPA) insufficiency. Levels lying between these values should be further investigated by dynamic testing of the HPA axis (see below).
  - *TSH, free T_4, total T_3.* Low thyroid hormone values with a low TSH suggest secondary hypothyroidism.
  - *LH, FSH, oestrogen/testosterone, sex hormone-binding globulin (SHBG).* Secondary hypogonadism is suggested by low LH and FSH, despite low levels of free circulating sex hormones (oestrogen and testosterone).
  - *Prolactin.* Prolactin may be high, indicating stalk compression, or low due to compression of the normal pituitary. Very high levels (typically > 5000 mU/L) indicate a prolactinoma, which is likely to respond well to medical therapy (see p. 578).
  - *Insulin-like growth factor (IGF)-1.* IGF-1 is produced by many tissues, including the liver, muscle and kidney, in response to growth hormone and is frequently used as a surrogate indicator of growth hormone levels. However, IGF-1 levels are also influenced by factors

such as nutritional status, insulin resistance and age, complicating its interpretation.

- *Paired serum and urine osmolality.* Failure of posterior pituitary function and diabetes insipidus manifest as polyuria and raised serum osmolality.

- Dynamic tests
  - *Insulin tolerance test.* 0.15 U/kg of short-acting insulin, administered intravenously to achieve a fall in plasma glucose to < 2.2 mmol/L (confirmed by a laboratory measurement), initiates a classical stress response with release of cortisol and growth hormone. Glucose, cortisol and growth hormone levels are measured at baseline, 30, 45, 60, 90 and 120 mins. ACTH levels are also measured at baseline. A **cortisol rise** to > 550 nmol/L confirms an intact HPA axis; a **growth hormone rise** to > 20 mU/L (10 ng/L) confirms an intact growth hormone axis. The test should not be used if the 09:00 h cortisol has been shown to be < 100 nmol/L (this confirms that the patient has ACTH deficiency) or if the patient is hypothyroid. A similar response is seen after **1 mg glucagon SC**. **Contraindications**: patients with epilepsy, unexplained losses of consciousness and ischaemic heart disease ideally should not have this test.
  - *Short tetracosactide test.* This does not directly assess pituitary reserve and is more useful for evaluating adrenal function. Where

Table 15.2 Replacement therapy for hypopituitarism	
Axis	**Usual replacement therapies**
Adrenal	Hydrocortisone 15–40 mg daily (starting dose 10 mg on rising/5 mg lunchtime/5 mg evening) (Normally no need for mineralocorticoid replacement)
Thyroid	Levothyroxine 100–150 mcg daily
Gonadal Male Female Fertility	Testosterone IM, orally, transdermally or implant Cyclical oestrogen/progestogen orally or as patch HCG plus FSH (purified or recombinant) or pulsatile GnRH to produce testicular development, spermatogenesis or ovulation
Growth	Recombinant human growth hormone used routinely to achieve normal growth in children Also advocated for replacement therapy in adults where growth hormone has effects on muscle mass and well-being
Thirst	Desmopressin 10–20 mcg 1–3 times daily by nasal spray or orally 100–200 mcg 3 times daily Carbamazepine, thiazides and chlorpropamide are very occasionally used in mild diabetes insipidus
Breast (prolactin inhibition)	Dopamine agonist (e.g. cabergoline 500 mcg weekly)

FSH, follicle-stimulating hormone; GnRH, gonadotrophin-releasing hormone; HCG, human chorionic gonadotrophin.

dynamic pituitary stimulation tests are impossible, it may be used as a surrogate. Injection of 250 mcg **synthetic ACTH** is given intravenously, with measurement of ACTH at baseline, and **cortisol** at 0, 30 and 60 mins. An increase from baseline to cortisol levels > 550 nmol/L suggests normal adrenal function. A sluggish rise at 30 mins is indicative of reduced pituitary function.

● Imaging. Gadolinium-enhanced MRI scanning of the pituitary is the investigation of choice, giving the most information regarding size and extension of the tumour.

Management
Options for hormone replacement regimes are given in Table 15.2.

THYROID DISORDERS

The thyroid hormones, T_4 and T_3, are produced within the thyroid gland. Synthesis and release are stimulated by TSH, which is released from the pituitary gland in response to the hypothalamic factor, TRH (thyrotrophin-releasing hormone) (Fig. 15.1). Predominantly, T_4 is produced, but this is converted in the peripheral tissues (liver, kidney, muscle) to the more

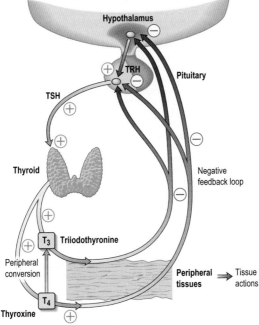

Fig. 15.1 The hypothalamic–pituitary–thyroid axis. TRH, thyrotrophin-releasing hormone; TSH, thyroid-stimulating hormone.

active T_3. More than 99% of T_4 and T_3 circulate bound to plasma proteins, mainly thyroid-binding globulin (TBG).

Diagnosis of thyroid disease includes the clinical features, together with measurement of plasma TSH and thyroid hormones T_4 and T_3.

Thyroid function tests

- Measurement of plasma TSH is the single most useful assessment of thyroid function, even for the detection of mild disease. Levels will increase in response to falling levels of circulating active thyroid hormones and fall with high levels of thyroid hormone. Exceptions include pituitary disease and 'sick euthyroid syndrome', in which TSH may be low without hyperthyroidism.
- Measurement of plasma free T_4 and free T_3, along with TSH, has simplified the interpretation of thyroid function tests.
- Accurate diagnosis requires two tests, e.g.:
  - TSH plus free T_4 or free T_3 for suspected hyperthyroidism
  - TSH plus free T_4 for hypothyroidism

Problems in interpreting thyroid function tests

- **Serious acute or chronic illness.** Failure of conversion of T_4 to T_3 (in favour of reverse T_3) causes a reduction in hypothalamic–pituitary production of TSH, resulting in low/normal measurements of all factors.
- **Pregnancy or oral contraceptive use.** Increased levels of TBG lead to higher levels of **total** T_4 and T_3. Levels of **free** hormone are unaffected. The TSH can be low.
- **Heterophile antibodies.** These interfere with assay measurements of hormone levels and lead to bizarre thyroid function tests that have no obvious clinical explanation. The laboratory should be able to confirm this with additional testing.
- **Amiodarone.** This prevents generation of T_3 from T_4, resulting in an increase in T_4 levels. Tissue perception of this is of 'reduced' active T_3 levels, and TSH levels may therefore increase. Amiodarone also provides a significant iodine load, up to 100 times the daily recommended amount. This can have two effects on thyroid function. The iodine load can:
  - precipitate thyrotoxicosis by unmasking subclinical hyperthyroidism in an iodine-deplete individual (amiodarone-induced thyrotoxicosis type 1) *or*
  - precipitate hypothyroidism due to blockade of intrathyroidal hormone production from excess iodine.

  Alternatively, amiodarone results in a destructive thyroiditis with the release of thyroid hormone (amiodarone-induced thyrotoxicosis type 2).

Treatment

While amiodarone-induced hypothyroidism is relatively straightforward to treat, with **thyroxine**, hyperthyroidism is more difficult. The destructive thyroiditis is best managed with **prednisolone** 40 mg/day, while type 1 hyperthyroidism is best managed with **antithyroid drugs**. In practice it can be difficult to tell the two apart and both treatments may be offered in tandem.

Hypothyroidism

- **Primary hypothyroidism** is confirmed by high levels of TSH. '**Compensated**' hypothyroidism comprises a slightly raised TSH (typically < 10 mU/L) with normal levels of T_4 and T_3. Further failure of the thyroid gland results in increasing TSH and falling levels of T_4 and T_3 below the normal range.

- **Secondary hypothyroidism** is due to pituitary–hypothalamic failure; there is no increase in TSH despite falling levels of thyroid hormone.

Clinical features

Hypothyroidism can produce the classic picture of a slow, dry-haired, thick-skinned, deep-voiced patient with weight gain, cold intolerance, bradycardia and constipation; however, symptoms are usually minimal and non-specific, and biochemical testing is essential in any suspected case.

Investigations

- There is raised TSH with low/normal T_4 and T_3.
- Thyroid antibodies may be positive.
- Additional features may include anaemia, typically normochromic normocytic, but possibly either microcytic due to menorrhagia or macrocytic due to autoimmune pernicious anaemia.
- There are raised serum aspartate aminotransferase (AST) levels from muscle and liver, raised creatine kinase (CK) levels, hypercholesterolaemia, hyponatraemia due to increased ADH and impaired free water clearance.

Treatment

- Thyroxine (T_4) replacement is lifelong, with the aim of reducing the TSH level to the lower half of the normal range. A typical replacement dose is **levothyroxine** between 100 and 150 mcg per day. Starting doses range between 25 mcg and 100 mcg, depending on existing co-morbidity.
- Patients with **heart disease** benefit from slow increments of thyroxine, and adjustments to anti-anginal therapy may be required. In severe cardiac disease treatment may be initiated with a small dose of T_3 (**liothyronine**) 2.5 mcg every 8 hours, doubling the dose every 48 hours until a maximal dose of 10 mcg 3 times daily is achieved. T_4 is then commenced at this point and the T_3 discontinued 5 days later.
- Fluctuating levels of TSH on replacement therapy typically reflect poor compliance but may result from malabsorption. Dose alterations should be reassessed after at least 6 weeks and then yearly.

Myxoedema coma

Myxoedema coma (rare) is profound hypothyroidism with a fall in core temperature, ECG changes (low voltage, prolonged QT interval, flat T waves and heart block), hypoglycaemia and altered mental status.

- **General management** includes maintenance of airway and body warmth (but not active rewarming, which risks peripheral vasodilatation and cardiovascular collapse), restriction of free water and glucose supplementation.
- **IV hydrocortisone** replacement 100 mg every 8 hours should be initiated, after blood tests have been taken for ACTH and cortisol.
- Thyroid hormone should be given without waiting for biochemical confirmation of hypothyroidism. There is no consensus on method of thyroid hormone replacement. Some advocate the use of 300–500 mcg **levothyroxine** IV followed by 50–100 mcg daily (either orally or IV). Others advocate a lower-dose regimen of 25 mcg **levothyroxine** daily, increasing on a weekly basis.
- **Liothyronine** (T_3) IV may be used if there are concerns regarding impaired conversion of T_4 to T_3, but this risks cardiac decompensation. Doses of T_3 range between 5 and 20 mcg daily.

Kumar & Clark's Medical Management and Therapeutics

Hypothyroidism and pregnancy

Maternal hypothyroidism impairs fertility and may lead to intellectual deficit in the developing child. An average increase of 50% in **levothyroxine** dose requirement is typical in pregnancy.

Hyperthyroidism

Hyperthyroidism is common and is characterized by high levels of T_3 and T_4 with suppression of plasma TSH. Nearly all cases are due to intrinsic thyroid disease.

Clinical features

Weight loss, increased appetite, irritability, tremor and heat intolerance are classic symptoms of hyperthyroidism. A tachycardia with or without atrial fibrillation is a frequent presentation, particularly in the elderly. A goitre with a bruit occurs. Apathetic thyrotoxicosis occurs in elderly patients, in whom the clinical picture is more like hypothyroidism with few clinical signs of thyrotoxicosis.

- **Graves' disease.** This autoimmune disease is the commonest form of thyrotoxicosis. In addition to symptoms and signs of hyperthyroidism, there may be ocular changes (exophthalmos and ophthalmoplegia), pretibial myxoedema and thyroid acropathy. Other autoimmune diseases, such as pernicious anaemia and myasthenia gravis, are also associated. The degree of thyrotoxicosis may fluctuate and the typical picture is of relapses and remissions. Ultimately many patients become hypothyroid.
- **Toxic solitary nodule/toxic multinodular goitre.** Although typical thyrotoxicosis can occur, autonomy within a nodule may not cause complete suppression of TSH.
- **De Quervain's thyroiditis.** A transient episode of hyperthyroidism can occur with acute inflammation of the thyroid, secondary to viral infections such as mumps, Coxsackie, influenza, adenoviruses and echoviruses. Toxicosis may last for some weeks and may be followed by a period of hypothyroidism. In its acute phase it is accompanied by fever, malaise and local thyroid tenderness, and the ESR is often raised. Symptomatic treatment is with **NSAIDs** or **aspirin**, with the option of short-term **prednisolone** starting at 40 mg per day, reducing over 6 weeks.

Treatment (Table 15.3)

Propranolol is used to gain rapid control of thyrotoxic symptoms. High doses (up to 160 mg 3 times daily) may be required due to increased metabolism of the drug.

There are three main options and preference varies widely.

- **Antithyroid medications. Carbimazole** initially 20 mg 3 times daily is the drug most commonly used in the UK. Its active metabolite, methimazole, is used preferentially in the USA. These drugs inhibit the formation of thyroid hormone and the clinical benefits can take up to 2 weeks to become apparent. **Propylthiouracil** 300–600 mg daily is occasionally used as an alternative, particularly during pregnancy and breast feeding. It has additional theoretical benefits in that it prevents peripheral conversion of T_4 to T_3. The major **side-effect** of these medications is agranulocytosis, and prior to commencing treatment patients should be told to seek medical help should severe mouth ulcers, sore throat or febrile illness occur. A white blood cell count is then urgently required.

Table 15.3 Drugs used in the treatment of hyperthyroidism

Drug	Usual starting dose	Side-effects	Remarks
Antithyroid drugs			
Carbimazole	20–40 mg daily 8-hourly, or in single dose	Rash, nausea, vomiting, arthralgia, agranulocytosis (0.1%), jaundice	Active metabolite is thiamazole (methimazole) Mild immunosuppressive activity
Propylthiouracil	100–200 mg 8-hourly	Rash, nausea, vomiting, agranulocytosis	Additionally blocks conversion of T_4 to T_3
Beta-blocker for symptomatic control*			
Propranolol	40–80 mg every 6–8 hours	Avoid in asthma	Use agents without intrinsic sympathomimetic activity, as receptors highly sensitive

*May need higher doses than normal.

Antithyroid medication also reduces the immune processes and thus a trial of therapy for up to 18–24 months may result in remission of autoimmune thyrotoxicosis. Initially doses of antithyroid medications are high. There is then the option of dose reduction as the thyroid tests normalize, or the option of adding thyroxine to high-dose anti-thyroid medication ('block and replace regimen'). A fall of T_4 and T_3 in response to treatment guides initial dose reductions (gradually reduce dose to 5 mg over 6 to 24 months if hyperthyroidism is controlled), as the TSH may remain suppressed for some time. Antithyroid medications will never lead to remission in toxic nodular disease, and while long-term antithyroid medications are an option, more definitive treatment is required.

- Radioactive iodine. This is increasingly accepted as a safe treatment option in the management of adults with thyrotoxicosis. It provides definitive treatment for toxic nodular disease and can be used in Graves' disease, although there are concerns that antibody levels rise following treatment and these can exacerbate dysthyroid eye disease. Patients should be made euthyroid prior to therapy but anti-thyroid medications should be discontinued at least 4 days before. A pregnancy test is performed in young females. Following treatment with ^{131}iodine 200–550 MBq, patients must be monitored for a short-term 'flare' of thyrotoxicosis (transient hypothyroidism may also occur) and for longer-term development of hypothyroidism. The presence of a large goitre with potential for airway compromise is a contraindication. Radioactive iodine is contraindicated in pregnancy and lactation.
- Surgery. Subtotal thyroidectomy is performed when anti-thyroid medications are not tolerated, when radioactive iodine is contraindicated, or for cosmetic reasons. All patients must be rendered euthyroid, stopping the antithyroid drugs 1–2 weeks before surgery and giving 60 mg of **potassium iodide** 3 times daily to reduce the vascularity of the gland.

Kumar & Clark's Medical Management and Therapeutics

• *Transient hypocalcaemia* is relatively common following surgery due to trauma to the parathyroid glands and disruption to the blood supply. This resolves with oral or IV **calcium** supplementation. Long-term replacement with **alfacalcidol** 0.25–1 mcg/day is occasionally required. Damage to the recurrent nerve and permanent loss of parathyroid gland function can occur. Function from the residual gland may be sufficient to avoid thyroid hormone replacement.

Thyroid storm

Fever (> 38.5°C), liver dysfunction, confusion and delirium are seen in this rare disorder. Systolic hypertension and high-output cardiac failure are also present.

Treatment
● Corticosteroids. **Hydrocortisone** IV 100 mg is given since this will further inhibit peripheral conversion of T_4 to T_3. Any precipitant cause, e.g. infection, should be treated.
● High-dose anti-thyroid drugs. (e.g. **propylthiouracil** 250 mg 8-hourly) is given.
● Chlorpromazine. **Chlorpromazine** 50–10 mg IM is given for agitation and may help with hyperpyrexia as a result of its central action.

Goitre

Assessment is made of its pathological nature and the patient's thyroid status. **Acute pain** within a goitre suggests an acute viral thyroiditis (de Quervain's), which may be associated with transient hyperthyroidism. Pain may also herald bleeding into a cyst and is rarely associated with thyroid cancer.

Investigations
● Thyroid function tests and thyroid antibodies allow assessment of function and diagnosis of autoimmune thyroiditis.
● Ultrasound can help monitor gland size and nature, and identify whether any nodules are cystic or solid. US does not identify malignant lesions but calcification raises the suspicion of cancer. Multiple small nodules may be demonstrated within a goitre associated with Graves' disease.
● Thyroid isotope scans can identify hot or cold nodules; a hot nodule reduces concerns of malignancy.
● Fine needle aspiration (FNA) of solitary nodules or of dominant nodules within a multinodular gland helps diagnose malignancy and has replaced isotope scans and reduced the necessity for surgery. There is, however, a 5% false negative rate and follow-up is essential.

Treatment
Surgery is only required in some cases:
● Possibility of malignancy. There may be a history of rapid growth, cervical lymphadenopathy or neck irradiation. The finding of a hard, craggy nodule should prompt referral for FNA but any dominant nodule within a gland may harbour a malignancy. Surgical resection is required if doubt persists.
● Local pressure symptoms. Retrosternal extension should be assessed by CT of the neck.
● Cosmetic reasons. If the patient is euthyroid and the goitre is small, simple reassurance may be all that is required. However, if surgery is needed, the patient is rendered euthyroid prior to it.

REPRODUCTION AND SEXUAL DISORDERS

Normal puberty in the male begins between 10 and 14 years with acceleration of growth velocity and development of secondary sexual characteristics. In girls sexual development starts a year earlier and normal menses begin between the ages of 11 and 15.

Investigation of gonadal function

- Serum LH, FSH, SHBG, oestrogen or testosterone. A low free testosterone or oestradiol indicates gonadal failure. If associated with high LH and FSH, this failure is primary. Low LH and FSH values indicate hypothalamic–pituitary failure.
- Serum prolactin. Hyperprolactinaemia is associated with reduced sexual function.
- Luteal phase progesterone. High levels of serum progesterone in the second phase (typically measured on day 21) of the menstrual cycle confirms ovulation.
- Semen analysis.

Male disorders

Hypogonadism

- Treatment. There are increasing options for testosterone replacement, including topical preparations, injections and tablets; IM depot preparations, e.g. **testosterone mixed esters** 250 mg every 3 weeks or **testosterone propionate** 50–100 mg 2–3 times per week are the preferred long-term therapy. Adequacy of replacement is assessed by return of normal libido and secondary sexual characteristics, such as a requirement to shave. Serum levels of testosterone, LH and FSH should also be monitored. Maintenance of bone density is a further goal of therapy. Haemoglobin and prostate surface antigen should also be measured on treatment. Fertility may be achieved with gonadotrophin injections, e.g. **gonadorelin analogues**, provided testicular maturity has been reached.

Erectile dysfunction

Psychogenic, vascular, neurogenic and endocrine factors, diabetic mellitus, drugs and alcohol may lead to erectile dysfunction.

- Treatment. Management requires avoidance of alcohol, withdrawal of drugs that may be compounding the problem, exclusion of endocrine causes and cardiovascular/neurological assessment. Drugs such as the phosphodiesterase inhibitors (e.g. **sildenafil 50 mg**) are the treatment of choice but must not be given with nitrates, as the combination causes severe hypotension. Intracavernosal injections, penile implants and vacuum expanders are less frequently used.

Female disorders

Hypogonadism

- Primary amenorrhoea is the failure of menarche by the age of 16.
- Secondary amenorrhoea is a cessation of menses for over 6 months.
- Oligomenorrhoea is defined as fewer than 9 menstrual cycles per year.

Symptoms of oestrogen deficiency include hot flushes, vaginal dryness and dyspareunia, mood changes and sleep disturbance.

Amenorrhoea

Pregnancy should be excluded in all cases as a cause of amenorrhoea.

Polycystic ovarian syndrome (PCOS)

PCOS consists of oligomenorrhoea, hirsutism, acne and weight gain. Hyperandrogenism, insulin resistance and features of the metabolic syndrome (p. 429) are frequently seen. The syndrome probably arises from a combination of environmental and genetic interactions. Increased numbers of ovarian follicles may be found on US, but this is also seen in women without the syndrome.

- Investigations
  - *Serum androgens — testosterone, dehydroepiandrosterone (DHEAS), androstenedione, SHBG.* Testosterone levels may be within normal limits, but in the context of a low SHBG (reflecting an insulin-resistant state) the free testosterone ratio may be high. Androgens are secreted by the ovary, and the adrenal glands. If the androgen levels are very high, an adrenal or an ovarian tumour is the likely source. Suppression of testosterone with a low-dose **dexamethasone** suppression test should be undertaken in these cases. A reduction of testosterone by more than 40% helps exclude an androgen-secreting tumour. Suppression of cortisol during the same test excludes Cushing's disease, another cause of menstrual disturbance, weight gain and hirsutism. If suspicion of adrenal or ovarian tumour is high, imaging of the adrenal glands and ovaries is indicated.
  - *Serum gonadotrophins.* Raised LH:FSH ratio to > 2 is seen, but not always on a random sample.
  - *17α hydroxyprogesterone.* An elevated 17α hydroxyprogesterone (17 OHP) measured in the follicular phase of the menstrual cycle indicates late-onset congenital adrenal hyperplasia (CAH), particularly in the context of low cortisol levels and raised ACTH. A very high rise of 17 OHP in response to a short tetracosactide stimulation test confirms the diagnosis of CAH.
  - *Consensus/Rotterdam criteria 2003* for diagnosis of PCOS stipulate at least two of:
    a) clinical or biochemical evidence of hyperandrogenism
    b) evidence of oligo- or anovulation
    c) presence of polycystic ovaries on US.
- Treatment. Weight loss, exercise and non-medical management of hirsutism, e.g. shaving, waxing, laser and electrolysis, are used. A topical cream, **eflornithine** (an antiprotozoal), has become available and reduces hair growth.
  - *Prevention of endometrial hyperplasia and the risk of malignancy.* In order to avoid this, regular withdrawal bleeds with the **oral contraceptive pill** (OCP) or progesterone (e.g. **medroxyprogesterone** 5 mg for 10 days) are used.
  - *Reduction in insulin resistance.* Weight loss and exercise help the metabolic features of the disorder and may improve ovulatory function and androgen excess. **Metformin** 500 mg 3 times daily is being increasingly used.
  - *Anti-androgen therapy.* Suppression of ovarian function with the OCP reduces serum androgen levels, while the oestrogen component increases SHBG levels, thereby lowering free testosterone. A commonly used OCP is **co-cyprindiol**, which has additional benefits

since it contains the long-acting progesterone **cyproterone acetate** 50–100 mg daily, which also possesses anti-androgen activity. Additional cyproterone acetate may be given for the first 10 days of each OCP cycle to maximize its effect. Other anti-androgens include **5α-reductase inhibitors**, e.g. **finasteride** 5 mg/day or **dutasteride** 500 mcg daily. **Spironolactone** 200 mg daily also has anti-androgenic properties and can help hirsutism. **Flutamide** 250 mg 3 times daily is less commonly used because of hepatic side-effects. Risks of teratogenicity mean that anti-androgen treatments should only be offered with adequate contraception.

* *Restoration of ovulation.* Weight management alone may help restore ovulation and **metformin** has been beneficial in some women. Reverse circadian **prednisolone** (2–2.5 mg prednisolone taken on rising in the morning and 4–5 mg prednisolone on retiring) can help with anovulation by suppressing androgen release. **Clomiphene** 50–100 mg daily on days 2–6 of the cycle and low-dose **gonadotrophins** are used with US surveillance.

Menopause

Menopause is diagnosed with loss of menses for 12 months, occurring at an average age of 50 years.

Premature menopause occurs with loss of menses before the age of 40. Chromosomal abnormalities and autoimmune ovarian failure account for the majority of cases, while chemotherapy and radiotherapy can also result in early gonadal failure.

* Investigation of premature menopause. Serum LH, FSH and oestradiol are performed. A low oestrogen level with high gonadotrophins confirms ovarian failure. Autoimmune screen, thyroid function tests, prolactin and karyotype are required in selected cases.
* Treatment
  * *Premature menopause.* Exogenous oestrogens with progestogen are required to alleviate symptoms and maintain bone strength. Replacement should continue until the woman reaches the average age at which natural menopause occurs (around 50 years).
  * *Hormone replacement therapy (HRT).* Following **natural menopause** at or around the age of 50 years, HRT is controversial. Hot flushes and vaginal dryness are helped by HRT. There are increases in bone strength. However, HRT increases the risk of breast cancer, venous thrombosis, and cardiovascular and cerebrovascular disease. Endometrial cancer can be avoided by giving progesterone with oestrogen treatment in women with an intact uterus. If amenorrhoea has been present for some time, the starting dose of oestrogen should be low and titrated upwards. In patients with an intact uterus, progesterone should be offered for 10–14 days each month to prevent endometrial hyperplasia. Replacement options include implants and transdermal, intravaginal and oral preparations. Oral oestrogens undergo extensive first-pass metabolism and should be avoided in liver disease. For alternatives to HRT for prevention of osteoporosis, see p. 324.
* Examples of HRT
  * *Continuous oral preparations.* Conjugated **oestradiol** 0.625 mg + **medroxyprogesterone acetate** 2.5 mg. Bleeding may be unpredictable but should reduce within the first year of use.

Kumar & Clark's Medical Management and Therapeutics

- *Cyclical preparations.* Conjugated **oestradiol** 0.625 mg + **medroxy-progesterone acetate** 5–10 mg on days 1–10 each month. A daily dose of between 0.3 and 2.5 mg **conjugated oestradiol** is required for symptom control. **Medroxyprogesterone** is the favoured progester-one, being the least androgenic.

Hyperprolactinaemia

Prolactin stimulates breast milk production and inhibits the gonado-trophin axis, resulting in oligomenorrhoea and reduced libido.

- Marginally raised serum levels of prolactin (400–600 mU/L) may be seen with stress (including phlebotomy) and drugs.
- Higher levels of prolactin may be associated with pituitary stalk compression and disinhibition of dopaminergic tone on lactotroph cells.
- Very high levels (> 5000 mU/L) suggest a prolactin-secreting adenoma. Assay interference by 'macroprolactin', a prolactin–IgG complex that lacks biological activity, should be excluded.
- **Investigations.** Pituitary function tests are required:
  - blood (09:00 h cortisol, thyroid function tests, LH/FSH, oestradiol/testosterone, prolactin)
  - pregnancy test
  - macroprolactin: should be excluded
  - visual fields and MRI of pituitary.
- **Treatment.** The presence of a pituitary tumour with raised prolactin levels (> 5000 mU/L) is indicative of a prolactin-secreting tumour rather than disinhibition. Continuous medical therapy with a dopamine agonist is the treatment of choice rather than surgery. It not only reduces prolactin levels but may also achieve tumour shrinkage.
  - **Bromocriptine** 2.5–15 mg in divided doses is well established but associated with gastrointestinal side-effects. **Cabergoline** 500 mcg taken once or twice each week or **quinagolide** 75–150 mcg daily is an alternative.
  - **Response** to treatment is monitored by serum prolactin measure-ments and MRI of the pituitary.
  - **Side-effects** of these dopamine agonists may include pulmonary, retroperitoneal and pericardial fibrotic reactions and patients should be constantly monitored.

ACROMEGALY

Growth hormone acts in the liver to synthesize and secrete insulin-like growth factor (IGF)-1, which promotes growth and soft tissue growth. Growth hormone excess will result in gigantism prior to epiphyseal fusion, and acromegaly following puberty.

Acromegaly is due to excess growth hormone release, usually from a benign pituitary adenoma.

Somatotroph tumours are frequently large (> 1 cm diameter) and are associated with local compression effects, including chiasmal compres-sion causing visual field defects and ophthalmoplegia. Compromise of normal pituitary function can result initially, with loss of libido or oligomenorrhoea.

Excess growth hormone results in a change of bodily appearance with coarsening of the features and an increase in shoe, glove and in particular ring size. Increased sweating is a common symptom, as is generalized lethargy and weakness — which may result from loss of ACTH but may also reflect loss of intrinsic muscle power despite increasing muscle bulk.

Acromegaly is associated with increased mortality from cardiovascular, respiratory and metabolic complications, e.g. diabetes. Obstructive sleep apnoea is commonly recognized. The incidence of colorectal carcinoma is also higher.

Investigation of growth hormone levels

- **IGF-1 levels.** These are almost always raised. IGF-binding protein 3 (IGF-BP3) is less useful, as there is overlap with normal levels.
- **Growth hormone day curve.** Growth hormone release is pulsatile in nature, making single measurements difficult to interpret. The absence of undetectable levels of growth hormone at intervals of the day is abnormal and suggestive of growth hormone excess.
- **Glucose tolerance test (GTT).** Failure of suppression of growth hormone levels to < 1 mU/L supports a diagnosis of acromegaly.
- **Further pituitary function tests.** The presence of a pituitary tumour should prompt exclusion of functional deficits affecting the other pituitary hormones (see 'panhypopituitarism', p. 567). Prolactin should be measured, and if high, may reflect dual secretion from the tumour or disinhibition from pituitary stalk compression.
- **Neuro-ophthalmological assessment.** Visual field defects are common.
- **Imaging.** Pituitary MRI is the investigation of choice. Pituitary CT is also used.

Treatment

Trans-sphenoidal surgery remains the treatment of choice, with medical therapy used to optimize the patient for anaesthesia and to achieve a reduction in tumour bulk to facilitate removal. Normal growth hormone dynamics are rarely achieved with surgery and therefore disease control rather than cure is sought. Following surgery, medical therapy may once more be required to achieve satisfactory growth hormone control — patients with uncontrolled levels are offered radiotherapy, which should improve growth hormone levels over subsequent months and years. A nadir of growth hormone levels following a GTT of < 5 mU/L, and normalization of serum IGF-1 level are predictive of good outcome in the long term.

- Medical therapies
  - *Somatostatin analogues.* Injectable **octreotide** 100–200 mcg SC 3 times daily and **lanreotide** 60 mg every 28 days are somatostatin analogues, which are the treatment of choice in resistant cases and employed as a short-term treatment, while other modalities, e.g. surgery/radiotherapy, become effective.
  - *Dopamine agonists.* These agents are available for oral administration but have limited efficacy and dose requirements are large. **Bromocriptine** (doses up to 20–30 mg may be required) is frequently associated with side-effects, e.g. hypotension, headaches and dyskinesia, limiting its use. Longer-acting alternatives such as **cabergoline** may have a better side-effect profile, but again large doses are required (1 mg/day). Both drugs are associated with an increased incidence of gallstone disease.
  - *Growth hormone antagonists.* **Pegvisomant**, a genetically modified analogue of growth hormone, prevents binding of growth hormone

Kumar & Clark's Medical Management and Therapeutics

to its receptor. IGF-1 levels are normalized in 90% of cases. It is used after failure of other therapies.

CUSHING'S SYNDROME

Cortisol, secreted from the adrenal cortex under the influence of pituitary ACTH, is the principle endogenous glucocorticoid. It enhances gluconeogenesis, fat deposition, protein catabolism, sodium retention and potassium loss, and attenuates the immune response.

Cushing's syndrome is due to glucocorticoid excess, which is seen most frequently following the therapeutic administration of exogenous synthetic steroids.

Clinical features consist of weight gain, change of appearance, depression, lack of libido, excess hair growth, acne and psychosis. **Signs** include plethora, thin skin, bruising, hypertension, pathological fractures (particularly involving the vertebrae and ribs), striae (purple or red) and a proximal myopathy. Moon face is characteristic.

Diagnosis

Exogenous steroid use should be excluded. Medications such as oestrogen will increase cortisol-binding globulin and result in misleadingly high total cortisol measurements. Such medications should be stopped 6 weeks prior to investigations.

- **Timed cortisol measurements.** In health, cortisol levels fluctuate throughout the day; thus random measurements of cortisol are meaningless. Measurements are taken to coincide with the normal peak morning secretion, to exclude deficiency syndromes, while measurements taken during the natural trough at midnight exclude excess. Loss of the normal circadian rhythm of cortisol secretion with measurable levels, asleep at midnight, is indicative of Cushing's syndrome. False positives occur in depression and intercurrent illness. Simultaneous measurement of ACTH aids interpretation; confirmation of reduced ACTH levels in the context of high cortisol values suggests adrenal disease, while raised ACTH levels result from pituitary disease or ectopic sources, and further investigation seeks to differentiate between all these.
- **24-hour urinary free cortisol measurements.** This is a useful screening tool for outpatient investigation. Repeatedly normal values make the diagnosis of Cushing's syndrome unlikely.
- **Low-dose dexamethasone suppression test.** Individuals with Cushing's syndrome are resistant to suppression of the HPA axis seen with administration of exogenous steroid. Dexamethasone 0.5 mg, taken strictly every 6 hours (starting at 09:00 h following a baseline measurement of serum cortisol and ACTH) for 48 hours, should result in suppression of serum cortisol to < 50 nmol/L (sensitivity > 97%). Hepatic enzyme inducers, such as phenytoin, will reduce plasma dexamethasone levels, invalidating the test.
- **High-dose dexamethasone test.** Pituitary disease retains an element of feedback control that ectopic sources of ACTH will not have. Thus, excess cortisol from pituitary disease will tend to suppress with 2 mg dexamethasone given every 6 hours for 48 hours. Ectopic ACTH secretion or adrenal tumour will not be suppressed with dexamethasone.

- **CXR or CT.** This is done to exclude bronchial carcinoma or carcinoid as the source of ectopic ACTH.
- **Adrenal CT or MRI.** This is used to exclude adrenal adenoma or carcinoma. A unilateral cortisol-secreting adenoma may result in atrophy of the contralateral gland. Any adenoma > 5 cm in diameter must be viewed as potentially malignant and resected for histological examination. Bilateral nodular hyperplasia may reflect ACTH excess from either a pituitary or ectopic source, or may be ACTH-independent.
- **Pituitary MRI.** This is done to exclude corticotroph adenoma. Images must be interpreted in the context of biochemistry since roughly 10% of people harbour an incidental pituitary adenoma; adenomas associated with Cushing's disease may only be a few millimetres in diameter, so are easily missed.

Treatment

- **Control of cortisol levels.** Uncontrolled cortisol levels lead in the long term to glucose intolerance, hypertension and cardiovascular disease. In the shorter term, high levels of cortisol compromise tissue healing and immune response, so levels are controlled medically prior to more definitive (surgical) therapy. The most commonly used agents inhibit steroid biosynthesis in the adrenal cortex. Serum levels of cortisol must be monitored at several time points through the day at the start of treatment to establish adequate control (cortisol 150–300 nmol/L) and to avoid over-treatment. Examples of **adrenolytic agents** include:
  - **metyrapone** 750 mg–4 g daily in divided doses
  - **ketoconazole** 200 mg 3 times daily
  - **mitotane** 1 g 3 times daily is used for inoperable adrenocortical carcinoma.

Cushing's disease (pituitary-dependent hyperadrenalism)

- **Trans-sphenoidal surgery** is the treatment of choice, with selective removal of the adenoma where a pituitary lesion has been identified on MRI. Lateralization with inferior petrosal sampling can guide the surgeon to a hemi-hypophysectomy while preserving pituitary function. Post-operative dependence on steroid replacement is indicative of good outcome, although such patients must remain under surveillance for both re-emergence of the suppressed HPA axis and for recurrence.
- **External beam radiotherapy** is unsatisfactory as primary therapy but is used following surgery where cortisol levels have not been controlled.
- **Bilateral adrenalectomy** may be used as a last resort to control pituitary-dependent Cushing's disease.

Adrenal adenomas and carcinoma

Surgical resection of adenomas, and tumour debulking in the case of carcinoma, are primary management. Suppression of the contralateral adrenal gland may take years to recover.

Ectopic ACTH-secreting tumours

Surgery, chemotherapy or localized radiotherapy is indicated, depending on the nature of the tumour suppression.

Nelson's syndrome

Enlargement of a pituitary corticotroph tumour can occur following bilateral adrenalectomy, resulting in pressure on residual normal pituitary, with loss of function and with high levels of α-melanocyte stimulating hormone (derived from the ACTH precursor peptide, pro-opimelanocortin, POMC), which causes darkening of the skin.

The incidence of Nelson's syndrome has reduced as radiotherapy is now offered to patients with pituitary-dependent Cushing's in whom surgery has failed to control cortisol burden.

Management is difficult and frequently unsuccessful. Options include surgery and radiotherapy.

ADRENAL INSUFFICIENCY

Adrenal insufficiency may result from primary adrenal disease, pituitary disease with failure of ACTH production or, very rarely, hypothalamic disease (failure of corticotrophin-releasing hormone (CRH)). In practice, adrenal insufficiency is most commonly seen in the context of stopping exogenous glucocorticoid therapy for inflammatory diseases such as rheumatoid arthritis or asthma.

Clinical features are often vague and non-specific, but include weight loss, anorexia, weakness, fever, depression, diarrhoea, abdominal pain and constipation. Signs include pigmentation (especially of new scars and palmar creases) and postural hypotension. Loss of body hair and vitiligo also occur.

Addison's disease (primary adrenal failure)

Autoimmune destruction of the entire adrenal cortex leads to failure of glucocorticoid, mineralocorticoid and adrenal sex steroid production. Patients with autoimmune destruction of the adrenal gland are prone to other autoimmune endocrine disorders, including type 1 diabetes, thyroiditis and premature ovarian failure.

Secondary adrenal failure

Insufficient ACTH production from pituitary disease, or HPA axis suppression following long-term exogenous steroid therapy, leads to failure of adrenal glucocorticoid production. Adrenal mineralocorticoid function is mainly preserved, being stimulated predominantly by angiotensin II rather than ACTH.

Assessment of the HPA axis

- 09:00 h ACTH and cortisol measurement: the patient should be relaxed.
- Insulin tolerance test/glucagon stimulation test: see p. 568.
- Short tetracosactide test: see p. 568. Variations exist, which extend the test to last up to 2 days. These tests help differentiate between primary, secondary and tertiary (hypothalamic) failure. Primary adrenal failure will fail to respond to ACTH, while secondary and tertiary adrenal failure will exhibit a delayed response to exogenous ACTH.

Management of adrenal failure (Table 15.4)

In primary adrenal failure, both glucocorticoid and mineralocorticoid replacement is required.

Table 15.4 Replacement therapy for primary hypoadrenalism

Drug	Dose
Glucocorticoid	
Hydrocortisone	20–30 mg daily e.g. 10 mg on waking, 5 mg at 12:00 h, 5 mg at 18:00 h
or	
Prednisolone	7.5 mg daily 5 mg on waking, 2.5 mg at 18:00 h
rarely	
Dexamethasone	0.75 mg daily 0.5 mg on waking, 0.25 mg at 18:00 h
Mineralocorticoid	
Fludrocortisone	50–300 mcg daily

- **Hydrocortisone** is the glucocorticoid of choice at a dose of 20 mg per day in 3 divided doses (e.g. 10 mg on waking, 5 mg at midday and 5 mg at 18:00 h). Hydrocortisone has some inherent mineralocorticoid activity, but additional **fludrocortisone** about 0.1 mg daily may be required to maintain intravascular volume and to prevent sodium loss and hyperkalaemia. In pituitary ACTH deficiency, replacement with mineralocorticoid agents is unnecessary. Adequacy of hydrocortisone dose is assessed by measurements of hydrocortisone through the day, while fludrocortisone is assessed by absence of postural hypotension and suppression of plasma renin levels to the upper half of the normal range.
- Alternatives to hydrocortisone include **prednisolone** 5–7.5 mg/day and **dexamethasone** 0.25–0.75 mg/day. These preparations are less physiological, being longer-acting, and therefore may be associated with signs of glucocorticoid excess.

Emergency management of adrenal failure (Box 15.1) (also see Emergencies in Medicine p. 720)

- Fluid resuscitation with 0.9% saline is required, as sodium and water deficit is significant.
- Glucocorticoid replacement with **hydrocortisone** 100 mg IV is followed immediately with **hydrocortisone** 100 mg IM every 6 hours. At these doses, an additional mineralocorticoid agent is not required.
- IM hydrocortisone is also used perioperatively until the patient is eating and drinking normally. Over periods of illness or physical stress (e.g. minor operative procedures), the oral hydrocortisone dose is increased to double the normal dose.
- All patients dependent on adrenal replacement therapy should wear a 'MedicAlert' bracelet and carry with them a steroid alert card. They should also have immediate access to a single dose of 100 mg IM **hydrocortisone** and be trained in its use.

Kumar & Clark's Medical Management and Therapeutics

> **Box 15.1** Management of acute hypoadrenalism
>
> - Clinical context: hypotension, hyponatraemia, hyperkalaemia, hypoglycaemia, dehydration, pigmentation often with precipitating infection, infarction, trauma or operation. The major deficiencies are of salt, steroid and glucose
> - Assuming normal cardiovascular function, the following are required:
>   - 1 L of 0.9% saline should be given over 30–60 mins with 100 mg of IV bolus hydrocortisone
>   - Subsequent requirements are several litres of saline within 24 hours (assessing with central venous pressure line if necessary) plus hydrocortisone 100 mg IM 6-hourly, until the patient is clinically stable
>   - Glucose should be infused if there is hypoglycaemia
>   - Oral replacement medication is then started, unless the patient is unable to take oral medication: initially hydrocortisone 20 mg 8-hourly, reducing to 20–30 mg in divided doses over a few days (Table 15.4)
>   - Fludrocortisone is unnecessary acutely as the high cortisol doses provide sufficient mineralocorticoid activity — it should be introduced later

The incidental adrenal adenoma

The incidental finding on CT or MRI of an adrenal adenoma occurs with increasing frequency. Assessment of function should include a low-dose dexamethasone test, measurement of urinary catecholamines and, if the patient is hypertensive, measurement of serum potassium and plasma aldosterone/renin activity ratio. Patients with an adenoma > 5 cm should undergo surgery, since these tumours have a higher risk of malignancy. Adenomas of < 3 cm diameter and no evidence of function can be monitored.

LONG-TERM STEROID THERAPY

Long-term therapy with supra-physiological doses of **exogenous steroids** results in adrenal failure and compromise of the adrenal response to stress if the glucocorticoid therapy is abruptly withdrawn.

- **Suppression.** This may be seen with topical and inhaled steroid preparations, as well as oral therapy.
- **Synthetic glucocorticoids.** These vary in their relative glucocorticoid or mineralocorticoid potency — **hydrocortisone** possesses glucocorticoid and mineralocorticoid activity, **prednisolone** has predominantly glucocorticoid properties, and **dexamethasone** exclusively glucocorticoid effects.
- **Side-effects.** While steroid replacement therapy at physiological doses is not associated with side-effects (Box 15.2), high-dose treatment is frequently associated with unwanted effects. In the short term, high-dose steroid therapy may be associated with mood swings and sleep disturbance. Longer-term therapy may lead to adrenal suppression, osteoporosis and cushingoid appearance. Glucose intolerance can also

---

Box 15.2 Adverse effects of corticosteroid treatment

Physiological
- Adrenal and/or pituitary suppression

Pathological

Cardiovascular
- Increased BP

Gastrointestinal
- Pancreatitis

Renal
- Polyuria
- Nocturia

CNS
- Depression
- Euphoria
- Psychosis
- Insomnia

Endocrine
- Weight gain
- Glycosuria/hyperglycaemia/diabetes
- Impaired growth
- Amenorrhoea

Bone and muscle
- Osteoporosis
- Proximal myopathy and wasting
- Aseptic necrosis of the hip
- Pathological fractures

Skin
- Thinning
- Easy bruising

Eyes
- Cataracts (including inhaled drug)

Increased susceptibility to infection
- Septicaemia
- Fungal infections
- Reactivation of TB
- Skin (e.g. fungi)

---

be seen with high-dose steroid therapy, as can hypertension and hypokalaemia.
- Stopping long-term steroid therapy. A gradual dose reduction not only diminishes the risk of deterioration of the underlying disease, but also prevents adrenal crisis.
    - Once physiological replacement dose has been reached (e.g. 7.5 mg **prednisolone**, 20 mg **hydrocortisone** and 0.75 mg **dexamethasone**), further reductions hold the risk of adrenal insufficiency so reduction in dose must be slow and carefully monitored.

- Options for assessing the adrenal axis include measurement of pre-dose 09:00 h cortisol levels, short tetracosactide testing and response to insulin-induced hypoglycaemia.

DIABETES INSIPIDUS

Fluid homeostasis, i.e. thirst and water regulation, is largely controlled by antidiuretic hormone (ADH, also called vasopressin); this is synthesized in the hypothalamus and released from the posterior pituitary in response to rising serum osmolality or perceived hypovolaemia. Other factors influencing ADH release include nausea, hypothyroidism and hypercortisolaemia.

Polyuria and loss of free water (as much as 10–15 L/24 hours) can result from loss of ADH action, either through failure of secretion secondary to hypothalamic damage, or renal insensitivity to ADH. Any cause of polyuria, including psychogenic polydipsia, will give mild renal resistance to ADH. Relative protection from overwhelming dehydration in diabetes insipidus is maintained by an intact thirst axis, which will ensure an adequate fluid intake. Cranial diabetes insipidus may be masked by cortisol deficiency resulting from pituitary damage, since glucocorticoids are necessary for renal handling of free water.

Clinical features

Deficiency of vasopressin or insensitivity to its action leads to polyuria, nocturia and compensatory polydipsia. This in turn causes dehydration, which may be severe if the thirst mechanism or consciousness is impaired so that the patient is deprived of fluid.

Investigations

- High or high–normal plasma osmolality with low urine osmolality (in primary polydipsia plasma osmolality tends to be low).
- Resultant high or high–normal plasma sodium.
- High 24-hour urine volumes (< 2 L excludes the need for further investigation).
- Failure of urinary concentration with fluid deprivation.
- Restoration of urinary concentration with vasopressin or an analogue.
- **Water deprivation test** (ensure the patient is fully hydrated, with normal thyroid and adrenal function, or on adequate replacement therapy).

In normal subjects, plasma osmolality remains normal while urine osmolality rises > 600 mosmol/kg. Plasma osmolality rises while the urine remains dilute in both cranial and nephrogenic diabetes insipidus, only concentrating after desmopressin is given in the former.

Treatment

- Cranial diabetes insipidus is treated with **desmopressin** (synthetic ADH), available as tablets (100–200 mcg 3 times daily), SC injection or nasal spray. Adequacy of treatment is monitored by urine volumes, thirst, serum sodium and osmolality measurements. Rehydration should be with 5% glucose rather than saline, to avoid worsening hypernatraemia.
- Nephrogenic diabetes insipidus will respond to correction of electrolyte imbalances; high doses of **desmopressin**, **thiazide diuretics**, or **prostaglandin synthase inhibitors** such as **indometacin** may occasionally be required.

SYNDROME OF INAPPROPRIATE ADH SECRETION (SIADH)

Inappropriate secretion of ADH results in retention of water and subsequent hyponatraemia. Mild symptoms of confusion, irritability and nausea occur as sodium levels fall below 125 mmol/L (125 meq/L); fitting and coma occur as the sodium falls below 115 mmol/L. A diagnosis of SIADH can only be made in a patient who is clinically normovolaemic with normal thyroid and adrenal function.

Investigations

There is low serum sodium (< 135 mmol/L) and osmolality (< 270 mOsm/kg), urine that is not maximally dilute (osmolality > 100 mOsm/kg) and renal sodium loss (> 20 mmol/L). Ensure normal adrenal and thyroid function.

Treatment

- Fluid restriction to as little as 500 mL/day may be required.
- Rarely, demeclocycline 600–1200 mg daily (antagonizes action of ADH on the renal tubules) may be indicated.
- In exceptional circumstances, e.g. when the patient is disorientated and the onset acute, saline infusion is used to correct sodium levels slowly (correct at a rate of approximately 1 mmol/L per hour (a total of 8 mmol/L during the first day, p. 372) to avoid central pontine myelinolysis, which can be seen on MRI. This can be achieved giving 0.9% saline slowly (1 L over 12 hours), promoting free water excretion with the use of **furosemide**. **Hypertonic saline 3%** is only necessary when the hyponatraemia is acute and very severe.
- Conivaptan, a vasopressin V_{1A} and V_2 receptor antagonist, may also be used to increase the serum sodium level.

HYPERCALCAEMIA

The major causes of hypercalcaemia are primary hyperparathyroidism and malignancies (> 90% of cases).

Clinical features

- Mild hypercalcaemia (e.g. adjusted calcium < 3 mmol/L) is frequently asymptomatic, but more severe hypercalcaemia can produce a number of symptoms: tiredness, malaise, dehydration, depression, renal colic from stones, polyuria/nocturia, haematuria and hypertension. The polyuria results from the effect of hypercalcaemia on renal tubules, reducing their concentrating ability — a form of mild nephrogenic diabetes insipidus. There may be bone pain.
- Hyperparathyroidism mainly affects cortical bone; bone cysts and locally destructive 'brown tumours' occur, but only in advanced disease. Abdominal pain occurs and there may also be symptoms from the underlying cause.
- Malignant disease is usually advanced by the time hypercalcaemia occurs, typically with bony metastases. True ectopic parathyroid hormone (PTH) secretion is rare and most cases of hypercalcaemia are due to raised levels of PTH-related protein. The common primary tumours are bronchus, breast, myeloma, oesophagus, thyroid, prostate, lymphoma and renal cell carcinoma.

Investigations and differential diagnosis

- Biochemistry. Primary hyperparathyroidism causes hypercalcaemia and hypophosphataemia with detectable or elevated intact PTH levels during hypercalcaemia. When this combination is present in an asymptomatic patient, further investigation is usually unnecessary. **When PTH is undetectable or equivocal**, a number of other tests may lead to the diagnosis:
  - *Protein electrophoresis/immunofixation:* to exclude myeloma
  - *Serum TSH:* to exclude hyperthyroidism
  - *09:00 h cortisol and/or ACTH test:* to exclude Addison's disease
  - *Serum ACE:* helpful in the diagnosis of sarcoidosis
  - *Hydrocortisone suppression test:* **hydrocortisone** 40 mg 3 times daily for 10 days leads to suppression of plasma calcium in sarcoidosis, vitamin D-mediated hypercalcaemia and some malignancies.
- Imaging
  - *US:* though insensitive for small tumours, is simple and safe.
  - *High-resolution CT scan or MRI:* more sensitive.
  - *Radioisotope scanning using* $^{99m Tc}$-sestamibi: ~90% sensitive in detecting parathyroid adenomas.

Treatment of hypercalcaemia (see Emergencies in Medicine p. 719)

Details of emergency treatment for severe hypercalcaemia are given in Box 15.3. Thereafter, treatment is management of the underlying disease.

> **Box 15.3** Treatment of acute severe hypercalcaemia
>
> Acute hypercalcaemia often presents with dehydration, nausea and vomiting, nocturia and polyuria, drowsiness and altered consciousness. The serum Ca^{2+} is > 3 mmol/L and sometimes as high as 5 mmol/L. While investigation of the cause is under way, immediate treatment is mandatory if the patient is seriously ill or if the Ca^{2+} is > 3.5 mmol/L.
>
> - Rehydrate at least 3–4 L of 0.9% saline on day 1, and 3–4 L for several days thereafter. CVP may need to be monitored to control the hydration rate
> - IV bisphosphonates are the treatment of choice for hypercalcaemia of malignancy or of undiagnosed cause. Pamidronate is preferred (60–90 mg as an IV infusion in 0.9% saline or glucose over 2–4 hours or, if less urgent, over 2–4 days). Levels fall after 24–72 hours, lasting for ~2 weeks. Zoledronate is an alternative
> - Prednisolone 30–60 mg daily is effective in some instances (e.g. in myeloma, sarcoidosis and vitamin D excess) but in most cases is ineffective
> - Calcitonin 200 U IV 6-hourly has a short-lived action and is little used
> - Oral phosphate (sodium cellulose phosphate 5 g 3 times daily) produces diarrhoea

Treatment of primary hyperparathyroidism

- **Medical management.** There are no effective medical therapies for primary hyperparathyroidism, but a high fluid intake should be maintained, a high calcium or vitamin D intake avoided, and exercise encouraged. New therapeutic agents that target the calcium-sensing receptors (e.g. **cinacalcet** 30 mg daily (max. 180 mg daily)) are of proven value in parathyroid carcinoma and in dialysis patients (p. 355).
- **Surgery.** Surgery is indicated for:
  - patients with renal stones or impaired renal function
  - bone involvement or marked reduction in cortical bone density
  - unequivocal marked hypercalcaemia (in the UK, typically > 3.0 mmol/L; USA guidelines state > 1 mg/dL above reference range)
  - the uncommon younger patient, below the age of 50 years
  - a previous episode of severe acute hypercalcaemia.

  The situation where plasma calcium is mildly raised (2.65–3.00 mmol/L) is more controversial. Most authorities feel that young patients should be operated on, as should those who have reduced cortical bone density or significant hypercalciuria, as this is associated with stone formation.
- **Surgical technique and complications.** Parathyroid surgery should be performed only by experienced surgeons, as the minute glands may be very difficult to define, and it is difficult to distinguish between an adenoma and normal parathyroid. In expert centres over 90% of operations are successful, involving removal of the adenoma or removal of all four hyperplastic parathyroids. Minimal access surgery is increasingly used, and some centres measure PTH levels intra-operatively to ensure that the adenoma has been removed.
- **Post-operative care.** The major danger after operation is hypocalcaemia, which is more common in patients with significant bone disease — the 'hungry bone' syndrome. Some authorities pre-treat such patients with **alfacalcidol** 2 mcg daily from 2 days pre-operatively for 10–14 days. Chvostek's and Trousseau's signs are monitored, as well as biochemistry. Plasma calcium measurements are performed at least daily until stable — with or without replacement — as a mild transient hypoparathyroidism often continues for 1–2 weeks. Depending on its severity, oral or IV calcium needs to be given only temporarily, as only a few patients (< 1%) will develop longstanding surgical hypoparathyroidism.

Endocrine causes of hypertension

Endocrine causes account for < 5% of all cases of hypertension. Patients that warrant investigation for secondary causes of hypertension include those under the age of 35 years and those with accelerated hypertension, evidence of kidney disease including proteinuria, hypokalaemia preceding diuretic therapy, resistance to conventional antihypertensive therapy and association with symptoms such as sweating, weakness and premonitions of doom.

Primary hyperaldosteronism

Angiotensin is generated in response to increased renin levels, which occur due to reduced renal perfusion. It causes vasoconstriction and aldosterone release. Aldosterone leads to renal sodium and water retention with potassium loss.

Kumar & Clark's Medical Management and Therapeutics

Adrenal adenomas (**Conn's syndrome**) and bilateral adrenal hyperplasia account for the majority of cases of primary hyperaldosteronism.

Investigations

Prior to investigation, drugs such as β-blockers, **spironolactone**, **diuretics** and ACE inhibitors should be stopped. Hypokalaemia should be corrected with oral supplements, since low potassium levels will suppress aldosterone release. Oral salt loading (120 mmol sodium per day) helps to unmask hypokalaemia by facilitating sodium and potassium exchange in the kidney. **Sodium loading** will, itself, tend to suppress aldosterone in the healthy individual — failure of which helps make the diagnosis.

- Hypernatraemia, hypokalaemia and metabolic alkalosis. These reflect renal reabsorption of sodium with loss of potassium and hydrogen.
- Plasma aldosterone : plasma renin activity ratio. An undetectable renin level should raise suspicion of primary hyperaldosteronism but is neither sensitive nor specific. Thus a ratio of plasma aldosterone to renin activity confers better specificity and sensitivity.
- Postural studies. Adenomas are not usually responsive to changes in posture, while adrenal hyperplasia retains some renin responsiveness and levels will increase on standing.
- Adrenal venous sampling. Measurement of aldosterone levels within the adrenal veins helps to distinguish patients with unilateral or bilateral disease to guide definitive therapy.

Treatment

- **Aldosterone antagonists** such as **spironolactone** 200 mg daily are the treatment of choice for hyperaldosteronism not amenable to surgical cure. Spironolactone can be associated with significant side-effects in men, e.g. gynaecomastia, due to antagonism of testosterone synthesis and action. An alternative is **eplerenone** 25–50 mg daily, which does not affect testosterone synthesis. Further agents can be added as required to achieve BP control, including thiazide diuretics, ACE inhibitors, calcium channel blockers and angiotensin II antagonists.
- **Surgery** is the treatment of choice for a unilateral adenoma. BP response to spironolactone offers an insight into the potential benefits with surgery — there may be persistent hypertension due to established changes in the renovasculature.

Phaeochromocytoma

Phaeochromocytomas are tumours arising from the adrenal medulla, although 10% occur in extramedullary chromaffin tissue and are referred to as paragangliomas. Around 90% of cases are sporadic and these are typically solitary lesions. The majority are benign, although significant morbidity and mortality can be associated with them. Most phaeochromocytomas release noradrenaline (norepinephrine), some release noradrenaline and adrenaline (epinephrine), and occasionally they release adrenaline alone or dopamine. They are associated with sustained or paroxysmal hypertension; symptoms include headaches, palpitations and sweating.

Investigations

- Plasma measurements
  - *Plasma metanephrines.* These products of noradrenaline and adrenaline metabolism are the most reliable method to diagnose phaeochromocytoma.

- *Plasma catecholamines.* Sensitivity is increased if plasma sampling coincides with a symptomatic episode.
- Urine collections. Twenty-four-hour urine collections for metanephrines are the most sensitive and specific. Measurement of dopamine has limited value, since much is generated from the kidneys; if, however, it is high, this may increase suspicion of malignancy.
- Imaging. The majority of tumours lie within the abdomen; a small minority occur in the thorax, pelvis, head and neck. CT and MRI are both suitable imaging modalities. [123]I meta-iodobenzyl guanidine (MIBG) is taken up by phaeochromocytomas and facilitates whole-body screening, but is not sensitive. Other options include PET scanning and venous sampling for localization.

Management

Surgical resection of a localised tumour is the treatment of choice, with careful medical preparation before. Both α- and β-receptor blockade is required, with α-blockade using IV **phenoxybenzamine** achieved first to avoid hypertensive crisis due to unopposed α-stimulation. Alpha-blockade and relief of chronic vasoconstriction is often associated with a fall in BP that responds to IV fluids, and a dilutional anaemia. Beta-blockade can then be added, using drugs such as **propranolol**, **atenolol** or **metoprolol**.

If long-term oral blockade is required, alternative oral α-blocking drugs such as **doxazosin**, **prazosin** and **terazosin** are used.

Further reading

Bahn RS: Graves ophthalmology, *NEJM* 362:726–738, 2010.

DeGroot LJ, Jameson JL, editors: *Endocrinology*, ed 5, Philadelphia, 2006, Elsevier Saunders.

Klibanski A: Prolactinoma, *NEJM* 362:1219–1226, 2010.

Ross DS: Radio-iodine treatment of hypothyroidism, *NEJM* 364:542–555, 2011.

Further information

www.endobible.com

www.endotext.org

Diabetes mellitus and hyperlipidaemia 16

DIABETES MELLITUS

Diabetes mellitus (DM) is characterized by a failure of glucose homeostasis leading to hyperglycaemia. This may result from a lack of insulin secretion, from a failure of insulin effect, or from both. It is associated with disturbances not only in carbohydrate metabolism but also in that of fat and protein.

Insulin is an anabolic hormone that is secreted from pancreatic β-cells into the portal vein after a rise in blood glucose. Other hormones involved in glucose homeostasis include glucagon and gut peptides such as glucagon-like peptide (GLP)-1 and gastric inhibitory peptide (GIP), which are also released in response to food.

- Carbohydrate metabolism. Basal levels of insulin, present when fasting and between meals, inhibit hepatic enzymes that control the critical limiting steps in both gluconeogenesis (glucose synthesis from amino acids and lactate) and glycogenolysis. Thus hepatic glucose production, a major contributor to fasting glycaemic levels, is reduced by insulin. Post-prandial peaks of insulin stimulate glucose uptake into skeletal muscle (where it is used for energy) and adipose tissue (where it is used for the synthesis of triglycerides.)
- Fat metabolism. Insulin promotes triglyceride synthesis and inhibits its breakdown into free fatty acids and ketone bodies.
- Protein metabolism. Insulin inhibits protein breakdown into amino acids, which are precursors for hepatic gluconeogenesis.

WHO CLASSIFICATION OF DIABETES

Type 1 diabetes mellitus

Type 1 DM (~10% of total) results from pancreatic β-cell destruction, which is usually autoimmune. This leads to failure of insulin secretion. It typically presents with a brief history of malaise and weight loss in a child or young adult. Its cardinal features are hyperglycaemia, dehydration, ketogenesis and uncontrolled breakdown of fat and muscle. Insulin replacement is crucial for the survival of these individuals.

Type 2 diabetes mellitus

Type 2 DM (> 90% of total) results from a progressive fall in insulin secretion with, in addition, resistance to the action of insulin. It is frequently associated with obesity and the 'metabolic syndrome' (p. 429). Early in the disease, there may be high levels of circulating insulin, in contrast to type 1 diabetes. Hyperglycaemia results from a progressive failure of the pancreatic β-cells to maintain high levels of insulin secretion to overcome peripheral resistance. The diagnosis is therefore often delayed since endogenous insulin levels are initially sufficient to prevent ketogenesis and a catabolic state. Intercurrent illness, with increased insulin resistance secondary to release of stress response hormones, is associated with worsening glycaemic control and consequent dehydration. The presentation is often with a concurrent illness in an adult with a history of polyuria, polydipsia and malaise over some weeks.

Higher-risk population groups that may benefit from **screening** for type 2 diabetes include:

- those with a first-degree relative with diabetes, the obese, patients on glucocorticoid therapy
- those with markers of cardiovascular disease, such as hypertension, ischaemic heart disease and hypercholesterolaemia.

Although insulin therapy is sometimes required in the short term following diagnosis, the mainstay of treatment for patients with type 2 diabetes is advice on diet, exercise, weight loss and healthy lifestyle. Oral antidiabetic therapy is frequently successful, particularly for the first few years, but many patients ultimately require insulin to achieve satisfactory glycaemic control.

Other types of diabetes

- **Pancreatic disease.** Chronic pancreatitis with progressive destruction of the β-cells results in diabetes that requires insulin in about one-third of patients. Simultaneous loss of α-cells with failure of glucagon secretion can result in profound hypoglycaemia, particularly in poorly nourished individuals; this is typically seen in patients with chronic alcohol abuse. Acute pancreatitis may be associated with transient hyperglycaemia.
- **Genetic diseases.** Genetic diseases such as cystic fibrosis and haemochromatosis have pancreatic damage which may lead to insulin-deficient diabetes, similar in clinical nature to type 1 diabetes.
- **Genetic defects of β-cell function.** A number of different genetic abnormalities produce type 2 diabetes at a young age (formerly called maturity onset diabetes of the young (MODY)). Presentation is before the age of 25, without features of type 1 diabetes. There is a strong family history of early-onset diabetes. The diabetes is often managed with oral antidiabetic agents alone, although insulin may be needed in some cases.
- **Gestational diabetes.** Glucose intolerance may develop during pregnancy due, in part, to increases in maternal insulin resistance resulting from circulating placental hormones. Tight control of maternal blood glucose levels in these patients reduces stillbirth rates, macrosomia, hydramnios and pre-eclampsia. Abnormal glucose tolerance returns to normal following delivery. It can be difficult to exclude pre-existing type 2 diabetes presenting for the first time in pregnancy. Gestational

diabetes itself is a predictor of diabetes in later life and regular follow-up is required.

Diagnosis

The diagnosis of diabetes should never be made on a single high blood sugar reading, unless the clinical history is strongly suggestive of the diagnosis. During periods of intercurrent illness (such as myocardial infarction) the stress response hormones may result in a transient rise in blood sugar; follow-up blood sugar levels will help to exclude type 2 diabetes. A glucose tolerance test is only required for borderline cases and to detect impaired glucose tolerance (IGT).

Diagnostic criteria
- DM
  - Fasting plasma glucose > 7 mmol/L (126 mg/dL) after overnight fast. Repeat × 1.
  - Symptoms of diabetes and random plasma glucose of > 11.1 mmol/L (200 mg/dL).
  - An HbA1C of > 6.5% (48 mmol/mol) has recently been suggested as being diagnostic of diabetes but has not yet been ratified by WHO.
- Impaired glucose tolerance (IGT)
  - Fasting plasma glucose < 7 mmol/L (126 mg/dL) and at 2 hours following a 75 g glucose oral load levels of between 7.8 and 11 mmol/L (140–200 mg/dL).
  - Plasma glucose >11.1 mmol/L (> 200 mg/dL) at 2 hours is diabetic.
- Impaired fasting glucose (IFG). American Diabetes Association criterion is a plasma glucose level of 5.6–6.9 mmol/L (110–126 mg/dL).

Both IFG and IGT are not clinical entities but are risk factors for developing diabetes and are markers of increased cardiovascular risk. These groups require annual screening for type 2 diabetes and lifestyle changes to be introduced in order to reduce the risk of progression to diabetes. Early treatment with metformin has also been shown to reduce the incidence of diabetes in patients with IGT or IFG. It also reduces the risk of developing cardiovascular disease in these groups.

MANAGEMENT OF DIABETES

Patients must take the lead in the management of their diabetes. Their general care must be multi-disciplinary and involve all healthcare workers. Educational programmes are available and should be emphasized continuously.

The aims of management are to:
- alleviate symptoms
- achieve glycaemic and metabolic control
- prevent complications of diabetes — both acute and long-term.

There is good evidence to suggest that good glycaemic control is associated with the lowest risk for long-term complications in type 1 as well as type 2 diabetes.

Insulin therapy

Insulin is the only therapy suitable for the treatment of type 1 diabetes and in cases where endogenous insulin production has been significantly reduced, such as haemochromatosis. Interruptions in insulin therapy

Table 16.1 Insulin preparations: time of action following SC injection

Insulin	Onset of action	Peak	Duration
Rapid			
Insulin Lispro*			
Insulin Aspart*	5–15 min	45–75 min	2–4 h
Insulin Glulisine*			
Short			
Soluble (neutral) insulin	15–30 min	1–3 hr	4–8 h
Intermediate			
Isophane (NPH)† insulin	1–2 h	2–8 h	18–20 h
Long-acting			
Insulin zinc suspension	2–4 h	6–16 h	20–24 h
Protamine zinc insulin	3–8 h	12–24 h	≅24 h
Insulin Detemir*	≅2 h	No peak	6–24 h
Insulin Glargine*	2–4 h	No peak	≅20 h
Biphasic			
Biphasic insulin aspart*	–	–	–
Biphasic insulin lispro*	–	–	–
Biphasic isophane insulin	–	–	–

*Analogue insulins.
†NPH = neutral protamine Hagedorn.

render these individuals at risk of ketosis. Insulin is also used to cover periods of intercurrent illness in type 2 diabetes when insulin resistance is increased, or there are concerns that hepatic or renal clearance of an oral drug may be impaired. Progressive β-cell failure is seen in type 2 diabetes and thus oral antidiabetic agents may with time fail to control glycaemia adequately. While there is often resistance to injectable therapy, either through patient preference or a fear of weight gain, initiation of insulin in this group of patients should not be delayed.

Insulin formulations (Table 16.1)

In developed countries most patients use human insulin rather than animal-derived insulin preparations. Insulin in the UK is provided at a concentration of 100 U/mL, although some countries use 40 U/mL. Diabetics who travel should be aware of this. Very rarely, insulin five times this strength, at 500 U/mL, is used in cases of severe insulin resistance.

- Short-acting 'soluble'/rapid human insulins are administered intravenously, subcutaneously or intramuscularly. These insulin preparations are typically clear fluids with an onset of action within 15–30 mins when injected subcutaneously. They are therefore used to control mealtime glycaemic swings. They are the only insulins used for IV infusions and SC insulin pumps. The rapid-acting analogue insulins, which have an altered amino acid structure, are more rapidly absorbed than soluble (regular) insulin.

- Longer-acting insulins have a speed of absorption that is prolonged by complexing insulin to compounds such as **protamine** and **zinc**. The resulting cloudy crystalline solution is absorbed over a period of hours. These are administered by SC injection only and are used to provide steady levels of background insulin through the day and overnight. Pre-mixed (biphasic) formulations, containing fixed amounts of short- and longer-acting insulins, are available.
- Analogue insulin preparations offer improved profiles, with the rapid-acting insulin being absorbed more quickly, and the longer-acting insulin showing a smoother profile of action. These are intended for SC use. All are clear solutions, which can cause confusion with biosynthetic human short-acting insulin preparations.

Principles of insulin treatment

Absorption of insulin will be influenced by the site of injection (fastest from the abdomen, then from the arm and slowest from the thigh). The speed of insulin effect will also be increased in the context of increased local blood flow, such as during exercise. Insulin regimens vary, having an emphasis on either simplicity or flexibility. The most successful regimen would mimic normal physiological release of insulin, with a low level of basal insulin present at all times and superimposed prandial peaks of insulin.

- Basal bolus regimen. This incorporates a background of longer-acting insulin and prandial short-/rapid-acting insulin. It typically requires four injections per day. This regimen is flexible in that the individual can alter injection times and doses to take into consideration activity levels, portion size, food type and time of eating.
- Pre-mixed insulin. Two injections per day of pre-mixed short-/rapid-acting and longer-acting insulin reduce flexibility and quality of blood sugar control compared to basal bolus, but are more convenient and therefore compliance may be improved. The fraction of short-acting insulin is usually indicated in the name of the mixture preparation (e.g. biphasic insulin aspart 30 contains 30% rapid-acting insulin aspart and 70% aspart protamine).
- Once-daily insulin. A single injection of long-acting insulin helps in the management of those unable to inject themselves, or as a short-term measure to encourage conversion to insulin from oral therapy. It is also added to oral therapy as an additional agent to help control fasting hyperglycaemia.
- Continuous SC insulin infusion. To achieve this, a small portable insulin device is worn at all times, providing a continuous infusion of insulin at a basal rate designed to control background glycaemic levels. Additional mealtime boluses can be provided through the device by pressing a button, avoiding the need for additional injections. This technique should only be used by patients prepared to monitor their blood glucose levels regularly, as these patients have no protective reservoir of depot insulin.
- Continuous IV insulin infusions (in hospital management of hyperglycaemia). IV insulin infusions are used following admission with hyperglycaemic crises (see below) or when a patient with diabetes is unable to eat or drink. Choice lies between a variable rate of insulin ('sliding scale') and a steady rate of insulin infusion (glucose/potassium/insulin 'GKI' infusion). When the patient is otherwise stable,

e.g. pre-operatively, good glycaemic control may be achieved by fixed rate infusion of soluble insulin and potassium. The variable rate, or sliding scale, of insulin infusion tends to be unsatisfactory on general wards, although it offers flexibility with close monitoring, such as in intensive care. The problem is that the rate of insulin is adjusted frequently in response to glycaemic excursions, rather than to avoid them, and can result in wild fluctuations in blood sugar without achieving good baseline control.

Side-effects of insulin

Side-effects include hypoglycaemia, weight gain, lipodystrophy at injection sites and insulin antibodies (if animal insulins are used). Transient peripheral oedema due to salt and water retention occurs. Local allergy is rare.

Equipment required by patients

Patients should be informed about how to dispose of needles, syringes and lancets safely. Containers for safe disposal of contaminated waste must be given, e.g. sharps bins. The following are also needed:

- Fingerprick devices for checking blood sugar — single use, sterile lancets, manual or automatic.
- Needles, sterile for single use for syringes, or pre-filled and reusable pen injectors.
- Syringes — calibrated glass syringes, pre-set U100 insulin syringes, disposable syringes.
- Injection devices — a variety are available, allowing adjustments of doses of insulin in multiples of 0.5 or 1 U of insulin. These include jet injectors and pen-like devices.

Oral antidiabetic drugs (Table 16.2)

Insulin secretagogues

- Sulphonylureas stimulate insulin release from the pancreatic β-cells, with a peak of insulin levels within 1–2 hours and a duration of action that varies between drugs. They reduce both fasting and post-prandial glucose by 2–4 mmol/L (36–72 mg/dL). They rely on a functional β-cell population, so efficacy may wane with time. Most are taken twice daily. The longer-acting agents are useful as once-daily preparations to aid compliance but hypoglycaemia, especially in the elderly or those with chronic kidney disease (CKD), is frequent. Therapy is associated with weight gain, largely due to the anabolic effects of higher insulin levels increasing appetite and the reduction in urinary glucose loss. Therefore these drugs are used as first-line agents in non-obese patients or those intolerant of metformin.
  - *Cautions/contraindications:* avoid the longer-acting preparations in CKD, pregnancy and breast feeding.
- Meglitinides act via a similar cellular mechanism as the sulphonylureas to induce pancreatic insulin release but action is augmented by glycaemia. This, together with a rapid onset of action (30–60 mins), makes them a good medication to take at mealtimes to counteract post-prandial blood glucose excursions. They are primarily metabolized in the liver. so have a better safety profile for use in CKD.
  - *Cautions/contraindications:* severe hepatic impairment, pregnancy and breast feeding.

Insulin sensitizing agents

- Metformin, a biguanide, is not associated with weight gain and is the drug of choice in the overweight diabetic person. It improves insulin sensitivity and significantly reduces hepatic gluconeogenesis. It is not an insulin secretagogue and will not, therefore, cause hypoglycaemia when used in isolation. It has a similar impact on glycaemia and HbA_{1C} to the sulphonylurea agents. Treatment is associated with gastrointestinal **side-effects**, e.g. diarrhoea, which can be minimized by a slow dose titration on initiation (e.g. starting dose of 500 mg daily with main meal, increasing by 500 mg increments each month). Anorexic side-effects may be viewed as beneficial in those trying to reduce food intake.
  - *Caution/contraindications:* there is a small risk of lactic acidosis due, at least in part, to inhibition of hepatic gluconeogenesis, which consumes lactate. Situations where lactate production is increased (cardiac and respiratory failure), where lactate clearance is reduced (hepatic failure) or where metformin excretion is reduced (renal failure) predispose to lactic acidosis. Metformin should be stopped where creatinine clearance is < 60 mL/min. Metformin should be stopped for 48 hours after administration of iodinated contrast media to avoid consequent renal dysfunction.
- Thiazolidinediones (glitazones) influence glycaemic control at the level of gene transcription via nuclear receptors, so their maximal effect is not seen for up to 8 weeks after initiation of therapy. They enhance glucose utilization by skeletal muscle and adipocytes, and act via the peroxisome proliferator-activated receptor (PPAR) family, which is also implicated in the control of many genes, including those involved in lipid metabolism.
  - *Cautions/contraindications:* avoid in pregnancy and breast feeding. This group of drugs should not be used in hepatic impairment, and liver biochemistry should be assessed prior to therapy and every 2 months for the first 12 months. Fluid retention and exacerbation of cardiac failure are also seen. Rosiglitazone is no longer recommended for general use.

Intestinal enzyme inhibitors

- Alpha-glucosidase inhibitor, e.g. acarbose 50 mg daily, increasing to a maximum of 200 mg daily, reduces post-prandial hyperglycaemia by inhibiting intestinal breakdown of complex starches and thus delaying carbohydrate absorption. It should be chewed with the first mouthful of food or swallowed whole with a little liquid before the meal. It is not as efficacious as other oral antidiabetic agents. **Side-effects** include abdominal bloating and diarrhoea.
  - *Cautions/contraindications:* hepatic and renal failure, pregnancy and lactation.

Other therapies

- Incretins
  - *Glucagon-like peptide (GLP)-1.* This is produced from the L-cells of the small intestine and is secreted after a meal. Oral glucose stimulates insulin secretion more than an IV glucose load (the incretin effect), partly due to GLP-1 release. **Exenatide** and **liraglutide** are GLP-1 analogues and bind to the GLP receptor. These drugs increase insulin secretion, inhibit glucagon secretion and slow gastric emptying. They are given by SC injection to patients with type 2 diabetes

Table 16.2 Antidiabetic drugs

(a)

	Dose	Dosage/Day	Duration of action	Metabolism and excretion	Main adverse side-effect
Sulphonylureas					
Chlorpropamide	250–500 mg	Once daily	24–72 h	K > L	Severe hypoglycaemia, seldom used
Glibenclamide	5–15 mg	Once daily			Hypoglycaemia; weight gain
or Glyburide in USA	5–20 mg	1–2 times daily	16–24	L > K	Hypoglycaemia; weight gain
Gliclazide	40–320 mg	Once daily (but divided higher doses)			Hypoglycaemia; weight gain
Glimepiride	1–4 mg	Once daily	24 h	L > K	Hypoglycaemia; weight gain
Glipizide	2.5–20 mg	1–2 times daily	12–24 h	L > K	Hypoglycaemia; weight gain
Gliquidone	15–180 mg	2–3 times daily			Hypoglycaemia; weight gain
Tolbutamide	0.5–2 g	2–3 times daily	12 h	L > K	Hypoglycaemia; weight gain
Meglitinides					
Repaglinide	500 mcg–16 mg	2–4 times daily	< 4 h	L > K	Hypoglycaemia; weight gain
Nateglinide	60–180 mg	3 times daily	< 4 h	K > L	Hyperinsulinaemia
Biguanides					
Metformin	0.5–2 g	2–3 times daily	6–12 h	K	Anorexia, diarrhoea, rarely lactic acidosis

Thiazolidinediones				
Rosiglitazone	4–8 mg	1–2 times daily	12–24 h	Possible increased cardiac deaths, not currently recommended
Pioglitazone	15–45 mg	Once daily	24 h	Hepatotoxicity, increased fracture risk
Alpha glucosidase inhibitors				
Acarbose	50–300 mg	3 times daily	N/A	Diarrhoea, abdominal discomfort, flatulence
Voglibose	0.3 mg with meals	3 times daily	N/A	–
Lipase inhibitors				
Orlistat	120–360 mg with meals		N/A	Liquid oily stools
(b) New drugs available				
Incretins				
Glucagon-like-peptide 1				
Exenatide	5 mcg SC	Twice daily		Persistent nausea, GI side-effects, pancreatitis
Liraglutide	1.2 mg SC	Once daily		
DDP-4 inhibitors				
Sitagliptin	100 mg oral	Once daily		GI disturbances, nausea, peripheral oedema.
Vildagliptin	50 mg oral	Twice daily		Rare — liver toxicity
Saxagliptin	5 mg oral	Once daily		
Amylin analogue				
Pramlintide	15–60 mcg SC	3–4 times daily		Nausea, severe hypoglycaemia

K, kidney; L, liver.

on metformin, sulphonylurea or both, if glycaemic control is poor. They produce weight loss, which is beneficial. **Side-effects** include persistent nausea and pancreatitis. Long-term studies are awaited.

- *Dipeptidyl peptidase (DPP)-4 inhibitors.* DPP-4 deactivates both glucose-dependent insulinotropic peptide (GIP) and GLP-1. **Saxagliptin**, **sitagliptin** and **vildagliptin** inhibit this enzyme to increase insulin secretion and lower glucagon. They can be given orally with metformin in type 2 diabetes. There is no associated hypoglycaemia.

- Amylin analogue. Amylin is stored in the pancreatic β-cells and is secreted along with insulin. It is deficient in type 1 diabetes and also, to a lesser extent, in type 2 patients requiring insulin. It decreases gastric emptying, suppresses glucagon secretion and decreases appetite. **Pramlintide** is an amylin analogue and is given at mealtimes as an SC injection. It is used in poorly controlled type 1 diabetic patients taking insulin and in type 2 patients when they are overweight and not well controlled on insulin. **Side-effects** include severe hypoglycaemia and nausea.

- Orlistat. Orlistat is a lipase inhibitor that reduces the absorption of fat from the diet. It promotes weight loss in patients on a low-fat diet, thus indirectly benefiting the diabetes. The low-fat diet is necessary to avoid unpleasant steatorrhoea.

- Bariatric surgery, e.g. gastric banding, gastric bypass surgery, roux-en-Y, is used in patients with type 2 diabetes and gross obesity unresponsive to 6 months of intensive attempts at dieting and graded exercise. One-third of patients become non-diabetic after surgery, those with recent onset of diabetes benefiting the most.

Practical management of type 1 DM

Diet

Patients should be on a healthy diet with flexibility to allow for the lifestyle of this younger group of patients. Regular home blood glucose monitoring is required. Carbohydrate intake can be made more flexible to vary with glycaemic control, weight and serum lipids. Pregnant and lactating women, as well as children, require further dietary advice. Most patients find diets difficult and require support from dietitians. Type 1 diabetics who regularly monitor their glucose levels can vary the amount of carbohydrate consumed or their mealtimes, with an adjustment of their insulin therapy — DAFNE (**d**ose **a**djustment **f**or **n**ormal **e**ating regimens). DAFNE involves high-quality training courses for diabetic patients, which allow them to self-manage their diabetes with insulin dosage being varied according to lifestyle, which gives better blood glucose control and less risk of hypoglycaemia.

Monitoring

- Self-monitoring of blood glucose levels should be done regularly by all type 1 diabetics.
- Fasting blood glucose measurements indicate a background glycaemic control and should lie between 4 and 7 mmol/L (72–126 mg/dL). Measuring blood glucose 2 hours post-prandially gives an indication of glycaemic swings following food and levels should be < 10 mmol/L (180 mg/dL).
- HbA_{1c} is a glycosylated haemoglobin reflecting glycaemia over the preceding 3 months. It should be measured every 2–6 months,

depending on stability of the disease and changes in treatment. Good glycaemic control benefits both microvascular and macrovascular complications of diabetes. The aim is to achieve an HbA_{1c} between 6.5 and 7.5% (48–59 mmol/mol), which requires good compliance with therapy with an increased risk of iatrogenic hypoglycaemia.

● Ketonuria is measured by using a ketostix when the patient is ill or has a febrile illness. It reflects ketonaemia. This is useful with persistent hyperglycaemia, particularly if the patient has symptoms of nausea, vomiting and abdominal pain — signs of impending diabetic ketoacidosis.

Pharmacotherapy

● Insulin therapy (p. 595). All type 1 patients require insulin therapy. All need careful training for a life with insulin. This is best achieved outside hospital, provided that adequate facilities exist for outpatient diabetes education.

  • A **multiple injection regimen**, with short-acting insulin and a longer-acting insulin at night, is appropriate for most younger patients (Fig. 16.1b). The advantages of multiple injection regimens are that the insulin and the food go in at roughly the same time, so that mealtimes and sizes can vary without greatly disturbing metabolic control. The flexibility of multiple injection regimens is of great value to patients with busy jobs, shift workers and those who travel regularly.

  • Some recovery of endogenous insulin secretion may occur over the first few months (the 'honeymoon period') in type 1 patients and the insulin dose may need to be reduced or even stopped for a period. Requirements rise thereafter.

  • Some type 1 diabetes patients will opt for twice-daily mixed insulin injections (Fig. 16.1a) and put up with the lifestyle restrictions that this imposes (with twice-daily regimens, the size and timing of meals are fixed more rigidly). Target blood glucose values should normally be 4–7 mmol/L before meals, 4–10 mmol/L after meals.

● When to use insulin analogues. Hypoglycaemia between meals and particularly at night is the limiting factor for many patients on multiple injection regimens. The more expensive rapid-acting insulin analogues (Fig. 16.1c) are a useful substitute for soluble insulin in some patients. They reduce the frequency of nocturnal hypoglycaemia due to reduced carry-over effect from the daytime. They are often used on grounds of convenience, since patients can inject shortly before meals, but this is illogical since standard insulins injected at the same time give equivalent overall control. High or erratic morning blood glucose readings can prove a problem for about a quarter of all patients on conventional multiple injection regimens because the bedtime intermediate-acting insulin falls and the absorption is variable. The long-acting insulin analogues, insulin glargine and insulin detemir, help to overcome these problems and reduce the risk of nocturnal hypoglycaemia.

Risk factor reduction (Table 16.3)

● BP control (see also p. 335): BP of below 130/80 mmHg should be achieved using lifestyle changes, e.g. dietary control for reduction in weight, stopping smoking, reduction in intake of alcohol and salt, and taking exercise. If necessary, an ACE inhibitor, e.g. lisinopril 20 mg daily

Kumar & Clark's Medical Management and Therapeutics

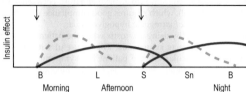

(a) Twice-daily mixed soluble and intermediate insulins

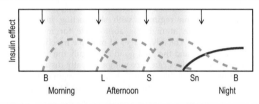

(b) Three-times-daily soluble with intermediate- or long-acting insulin given before bedtime

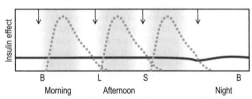

(c) Three-times-daily rapid-acting analogue with long-acting analogue insulin given before bedtime

Fig. 16.1 Insulin regimens. Profiles of soluble insulins are shown as dashed lines; intermediate- or long-acting insulin as solid lines (purple); and rapid-acting insulin as dotted lines (blue). The arrows indicate when the injections are given. B, breakfast; L, lunch; S, supper; Sn, snack (bedtime).

Table 16.3 Treatment targets in diabetic patients		
Parameter	**Ideal**	**Reasonable**
HbA$_{1c}$	< 7%	< 8%
BP (mmHg)	< 130/80	< 140/80
Total cholesterol (mmol/L)	< 4.0	< 5.0
LDL	< 2.0	< 3.0
HDL*	> 1.1	> 0.8
Triglycerides	< 1.7	< 2.0

*In women > 1.3 mmol/L.
HDL, high-density lipoprotein; LDL, low-density lipoprotein.

Kumar & Clark's Medical Management and Therapeutics

maintenance, or an angiotensin receptor II antagonist, e.g. candesartan 8–32 mg daily, is prescribed.

- **Lipid monitoring.** A total cholesterol of < 4.0 mmol/L (< 150 mg/dL), low-density lipoprotein cholesterol (LDL-C) of < 2.00 mmol/L (< 76 mg/dL), a fasting triglyceride of < 1.7 mmol/L (< 150 mg/dL) and a high-density lipoprotein (HDL) cholesterol of > 1 mmol/L (> 38 mg/dL) should be aimed for as ideal goals. To achieve these levels most diabetics require statin therapy (p. 617–8).

- **Aspirin.** Low-dose aspirin 75–150 mg/daily should be given as a secondary prevention strategy in those with a history of cardiovascular events, e.g. myocardial infarction, stroke, peripheral vascular disease or angina. Its benefits in primary prevention are less clear but it should be used in patients with a high cardiovascular risk. Patients allergic to aspirin or with a bleeding tendency should use clopidogrel. Aspirin is not recommended for patients under the age of 21 years because of an increased risk of Reye's syndrome.

- **Exercise.** Exercise improves insulin sensitivity and 30 mins of moderate physical activity, 5 days a week, is recommended. In the young type 1 diabetic, both diet and insulin doses will require adjustment. Prior to undertaking a new exercise programme, individuals should receive a cardiovascular assessment, including physical examination, BP and ECG. Peripheral nervous system and vascular supply to the feet should be looked at and advice given on adequate footwear. Diabetic complications, such as autonomic neuropathy, should be excluded, as they make exercise more hazardous.

- **Smoking.** Patients must stop smoking and referral for help to special clinics is often necessary.

Practical management of type 2 DM

Diet

Advice on a healthy diet should be given. For patients with a normal BMI, the total energy intake should remain constant, with a higher carbohydrate and lower fat (particularly saturated fat) intake. In general, the composition of the diet should be:

- **Protein:** 1 mg/kg ideal bodyweight.
- **Total fat:** < 35% of energy intake (with saturated fat < 10%, n-6 polyunsaturated fat < 10%, n-3 no absolute quantity but more oily fish intake, cis-monosaturated fat 10–15%).
- **Total carbohydrate:** 40–60% of total energy intake. The glycaemic index (GI) describes the rise in blood glucose after carbohydrate ingestion. For example, the blood glucose peak level after eating pasta is much flatter (low GI) than that seen after eating the same amount of white potato (high GI). Low GI foods are encouraged.
- **Vitamins and antioxidants:** best taken as fruit and vegetables (five portions per day).

Alcohol is not forbidden but its energy content should be taken into account. Salt should be restricted to < 6 g per day or lower in hypertension. Cholesterol intake should be < 300 mg per day.

Obese patients require low-energy, weight-reducing diets with a daily calorie reduction of about 2100 kj (500 kcal) (in conjunction with moderate exercise), leading to a gradual weight loss of 0.5–1 kg per week. It should be remembered that sulphonylureas, thiazolidinediones and insulin cause weight gain by increasing appetite.

Lifestyle
- Weight reduction. Even a 4 kg weight reduction can reverse hyperglycaemia.
- Exercise.
- Stopping smoking.

Although these measures are effective initially, they are difficult to adhere to in the long term. Most patients therefore require drug therapy.

Monitoring
- **Fasting blood glucose measurements** are as for type 1 diabetes (p. 602), with glycaemic control to lie between 4 and 7 mmol/L (72–126 mg/dL).
- **HbA$_{1c}$** can be used for longer-term glycaemic monitoring every few months, depending on the stability of the disease. HbA$_{1c}$ < 6.5% 48 mmol/mol is suggested but this means tight control and an increased chance of hypoglycaemia; it is inappropriate in those with cardiovascular disease.
- **Urine glucose** is not usually used for monitoring unless patients are unable to measure blood glucose. It correlates poorly with blood glucose and also depends on the renal glucose threshold (150–300 mg/dL).

Choosing an oral antidiabetic agent
Metformin is the first-line agent, particularly if BMI > 25 kg/m². If metformin is not tolerated or the person is not overweight, a sulphonylurea is used as first-line agent. Failure of a single agent should prompt addition of further agents rather than substitution. Metformin and a secretagogue (a sulphonylurea agent in the first instance) are recommended as initial combination therapy. Shorter-acting sulphonylurea agents are recommended in the elderly or if flexibility of lifestyle is an issue. DPP4 inhibitors or a thiazolidinedione may be used in addition if the above combination is not tolerated or does not control HbA$_{1c}$. Failure of oral hypoglycaemic agents indicates insulin therapy. Metformin should be continued in conjunction with insulin. Continuing sulphonylurea agents with background insulin injections or inhaled insulin may also be useful in those intolerant of metformin.

Risk factor reduction (Table 16.3)
BP control, lipid monitoring, aspirin, exercise and lifestyle changes should be encouraged, as with type 1 diabetes. Aspirin 75–162 mg/day is used for primary prevention and in patients with type 2 diabetes who are at increased risk of cardiovascular disease.

Indications for hospital admission
Newly diagnosed type 2 diabetics seldom need admission unless they have concurrent serious illnesses. However, most newly diagnosed type 1 diabetics sometimes require admission for institution of insulin therapy, education about their condition, self-administration of insulin and monitoring blood glucose. Other situations requiring admission include:
- Diabetic ketoacidosis (DKA, p. 608). This occurs mainly in type 1 DM, with a mortality in developed countries of 5–10%. Cardinal features are hyperglycaemia (> 11 mmol/L; 250 mg/dL), or known diabetes mellitus and metabolic acidosis (pH < 7.3; bicarbonate < 15 mmol/L or < 5 mEq/L). Any diabetic with heavy ketonuria should be monitored closely.

- Hyperosmolar hyperglycaemic state (HHS) (p. 610). There is severe hyperglycaemia (> 22 mmol/L; > 400 mg/dL) and an elevated serum osmolality (> 320 mosm/kg). There is no significant hyperketonaemia or acidosis (pH > 7.3). It is characteristic of type 2 uncontrolled diabetes.
- Hypoglycaemia (p. 612). If this is severe, it may cause confusion, fits or coma. It may be prolonged following sulphonylurea therapy.

Diabetics required to fast for surgery and other procedures

The diabetic control of patients admitted to hospital often deteriorates due to many factors, e.g. illness, effects of medication (e.g. corticosteroids, thiazide diuretics, β-blockers) and a change in their diet. Smooth control of diabetes minimizes the risk of infection and balances the catabolic response to anaesthesia and surgery.

The procedure for **insulin-treated patients** is simple:

- Patients whose diabetic control is inadequate and for whom surgery is not an emergency should have their diabetic control reassessed and therapy adjusted with HbA_{1c} < 8.5%, if possible pre-operatively.
- Pre-operative glucose levels should be in the range of 7–11 mmol/L.
- The patient's usual insulin is given the night before the operation and, whenever possible, diabetic patients should be first on the morning procedure/operating list.
- An infusion of glucose, insulin and potassium is given during the procedure/surgery. The insulin can be mixed into the glucose solution or administered separately by syringe pump. A standard combination is 16 U of soluble insulin with 10 mmol of KCl in 1 L of 5–10% glucose, infused at 125 mL/hour. The insulin dose is adjusted:
  - Blood glucose < 4 mmol/L — 8 U/L.
  - Blood glucose 4–15 mmol/L — 16 U/L.
  - Blood glucose 15–20 mmol/L — 32 U/L.
- Post-operatively, the infusion is maintained until the patient is able to eat. Other fluids needed in the peri-operative period must be given through a separate IV line and must not interrupt the glucose/insulin/potassium infusion. Glucose levels are checked every 2–4 hours and potassium levels are monitored. The amount of insulin and potassium in each infusion bag is adjusted either upwards or downwards according to the results of regular monitoring of the blood glucose and serum potassium concentrations.
- The same approach is used in the emergency situation, with the exception that a separate variable-rate insulin infusion may be needed to bring blood glucose under control before surgery.

Non-insulin-treated patients should stop medication 2 days before the procedure. Patients with mild hyperglycaemia (fasting blood glucose < 8 mmol/L) can be treated as non-diabetic. Those with higher levels are treated with soluble insulin prior to the procedure/surgery, and with glucose, insulin and potassium during and after the procedure. Be careful of hypoglycaemia due to the additive effect of medications taken previously. Post-operatively, patients should return to their normal management regimen when they begin eating and drinking.

Diabetes and pregnancy

Glycaemic control should be optimized prior to conception to reduce the risk of congenital malformations. Women on oral hypoglycaemic agents should be switched to insulin, although metformin may be continued. Poorly controlled diabetes in pregnancy is associated with stillbirth, preeclampsia, fetal macrosomia and hydramnios. Women should be monitored intensively by both the diabetic and the obstetric teams.

DIABETIC KETOACIDOSIS

Diabetic ketoacidosis (DKA) is the hyperglycaemic crisis usually associated with type 1 diabetes, but increasingly being seen in type 2 obese diabetes. It stems from a failure of pancreatic insulin production, resulting in hyperglycaemia, dehydration, ketosis and acidosis. It can present as a new diagnosis of DM.

Risk factors

These include the interruption of insulin therapy, the stress of illnesses, myocardial infarction, pregnancy, sepsis and trauma. Insulin should never be stopped, even when the intake of food is reduced during an illness in type 1 diabetics, as insulin requirements may even increase due to rising peripheral insulin resistance resulting from counter-regulatory stress hormones such as glucagon.

Diagnosis and management

Diagnosis and management are shown in Box 16.1. The patient should be closely monitored until stable.

● Water depletion. Insulin deficiency leads to hyperglycaemia with resultant osmotic diuresis and dehydration. Uncontrolled lipolysis and production of ketone bodies result in a metabolic acidosis that may be associated with nausea and vomiting, exacerbating the level of dehydration. The typical fluid deficit seen in DKA is between 5 and 7 L for an average adult patient. Assessment may be complicated by pre-existing autonomic neuropathy leading to BP instability.

Box 16.1 Guidelines for the diagnosis and management of diabetic ketoacidosis

Diagnosis
- Hyperglycaemia: measure blood glucose
- Ketonaemia: test plasma with ketostix. Fingerprick sample for β-hydroxybutyrate measurement
- Ketonuria: measure urinary ketone levels where plasma ketone measurements are not available
- Acidosis: measure pH on arterial blood or bicarbonate on venous blood (< 12 mmol/L — severe acidosis)

Investigations
- Blood glucose
- U&E
- FBC
- Blood gases
- Blood and urine culture
- CXR
- ECG
- Cardiac enzymes

Box 16.1 Continued

Phase 1 management

- Admit to HDU
- Insulin: soluble insulin IV 0.1 U/kg/hour by infusion, or 20 U IM stat, followed by 6 U IM hourly
- Fluid replacement: 0.9% sodium chloride with 20 mmol KCl per litre. An average regimen would be 1 L in 1 hour, then 1 L in 2 hours, then 1 L in 4 hours, then 1 L in 8 hours
- Adjust KCl concentration depending on results of 2-hourly blood K^+ measurement

If:

- BP < 80 mmHg, give 500 mL 0.9% sodium chloride over 15 mins

Phase 2 management

- When blood glucose falls to 14 mmol/L, change infusion fluid to 1 L 10% glucose 8-hourly *plus* 0.9% sodium chloride with 20 mmol KCl 6-hourly. Continue fixed-rate insulin infusion, increasing the rate of glucose infusion to maintain blood glucose levels

Phase 3 management

- Once patient is stable and able to eat and drink normally, and blood ketone levels < 0.3 mmol/L or venous pH > 7.3, transfer to 4 times daily SC insulin regimen (based on previous 24 hours' insulin consumption, and trend in consumption)

Special measures

- Broad-spectrum antibiotic if infection likely
- Bladder catheter if no urine passed in 2 hours
- Naso-gastric tube if drowsy
- Consider CVP monitoring if shocked or if previous cardiac or renal impairment
- Give SC prophylactic low molecular weight heparin

Subsequent management

- Monitor glucose hourly for 8 hours
- Monitor electrolytes 2-hourly for 8 hours
- Adjust K replacement according to results

Note: The regimen of fluid replacement set out above is a guide for patients with severe ketoacidosis. Excessive fluid can precipitate pulmonary and cerebral oedema; inadequate replacement may cause acute kidney injury. Fluid and electrolyte replacement must therefore be tailored to the individual and monitored carefully throughout treatment.

- Electrolytes (Box 16.2). Total body potassium will be depleted by about 350 mmol (mEq) but the measured serum potassium may be within the normal range, or even high as a result of acidosis. Potassium should therefore be replaced even when the serum level is within the normal range, but not if the serum potassium is > 6.5 mmol/L, particularly if there is acute kidney injury. There is hyponatraemia with total body sodium being depleted by 500 mmol (mEq).

Box 16.2 Electrolyte changes in diabetic ketoacidosis and the hyperosmolar hyperglycaemic state

Examples of blood values

	Severe ketoacidosis	Hyperosmolar hyperglycaemic state
Na$^+$ (mmol/L)	140	155
K$^+$ (mmol/L)	5	5
Cl$^-$ (mmol/L)	100	110
HCO$_3^-$ (mmol/L)	5	25
Urea (mmol/L)	8	15
Glucose (mmol/L)	30	50
Arterial pH	7.0	7.35

The normal range of osmolality is 285–300 mOsm/kg. It can be measured directly, or can be calculated approximately from the formula:

Osmolality $= 2(Na^+ + K^+) + $ glucose $+$ urea.

For instance, in the example of severe ketoacidosis given above:

Osmolality $= 2(140 + 5) + 30 + 8 = 328$ mOsm/kg

and in the example of the hyperosmolar hyperglycaemic state:

Osmolality $= 2(155 + 5) + 50 + 15 = 385$ mOsm/kg.

The normal anion gap is less than 17. It is calculated as $(Na^+ + K^+) - (Cl^- + HCO_3^-)$. In the example of ketoacidosis the anion gap is 40, and in the example of the hyperosmolar hyperglycaemic state the anion gap is 25. Mild hyperchloraemic acidosis may develop in the course of therapy. This will be shown by a rising plasma chloride and persistence of a low bicarbonate even though the anion gap has returned to normal.

- Insulin therapy. An IV insulin infusion is commenced at a fixed rate of 0.1 U/kg/hour via an infusion pump. If the blood ketone measurements or venous bicarbonate levels are not normalizing, the fixed rate may be increased. Blood ketone levels should fall by at least 0.5 mmol/hour; venous bicarbonate levels should increase by 3 mmol/L/hour. Do not stop insulin IV until SC insulin is started. If the patient is using a long-acting analogue insulin as part of the normal regime, this should be continued alongside the insulin infusion. If facilities for IV infusion are not available, give 20 U insulin IM, followed by 6 U IM every hour. When blood glucose concentration falls to 10 mmol/L (180 mg/dL) give IM injections every 2 hours. **N.B.** Absorption may be variable, particularly with hypotension; watch for late hypoglycaemia.
- Frequency of monitoring. This depends on the severity. In severe DKA, glucose should be monitored hourly and electrolytes 2-hourly for 8 hours.

HYPEROSMOLAR HYPERGLYCAEMIC STATE

Hyperosmolar hyperglycaemic state (HHS) is the hyperglycaemic crisis associated with type 2 diabetes. It is due to a reduction in effective circulating insulin levels, exacerbated by elevated levels of counter-regulatory hormones such as cortisol, growth hormone and catecholamines. Thus hepatic glucose production is increased but there is sufficient insulin to prevent significant ketosis. Mortality rates for HHS are as high as 15%, increasing with age and co-morbidity.

Clinical features

One-fifth of cases present with a new diagnosis of type 2 diabetes. Urinary and respiratory tract infections, a high glucose intake and drugs are common precipitants. A background history of polyuria and polydipsia over several weeks or months and recurrent superficial infections is a feature. Although the patient is typically obese, a history of recent weight loss is common. On examination, dehydration with hypotension, tachycardia and an altered mental state is seen.

Investigations (see Box 16.2)

- Blood glucose is often > 50 mmol/L (900 mg/dL); bedside capillary blood glucose testing kits are extremely inaccurate at this level of glycaemia.
- A 25% deficit in total body water is usual, which for a 70 kg man equates to about 10 L of fluid. The severity of dehydration correlates with the patient's mental state.
- Measurement or calculation of serum osmolality is useful. Reduced consciousness would be unexpected with a serum osmolality < 340 mosmol/kg, and if present in such a situation, an alternative cause should be sought.
- Since the brain is relatively permeable to both glucose and urea, serum sodium alone may give a more accurate indication of the degree of cerebral dehydration. However, measured sodium is a poor indicator of sodium status since intravascular hyperglycaemia results in movement of free water from the intracellular space to the extracellular space with a consequent dilution effect. The measured sodium level may be corrected for the degree of hyperglycaemia by increasing the measured sodium level by 1.6 mmol/L for every 5.6 mmol/L increment of serum glucose above the normal level.
- Mild ketosis and acidosis reflect a degree of insulin insufficiency but HHS is not typically associated with significant acid–base disturbance, which if present may indicate additional factors (e.g. a raised anion gap acidosis may suggest lactic acidosis in someone on metformin).

Management

- Rehydration is the mainstay of treatment; it must be undertaken slowly in patients with coexistent cardiac failure. Isotonic 0.9% saline is the fluid of choice.
- Gradual reduction in serum glucose is largely achievable with rehydration; about 3 mmol/L per hour is the aim. Slow insulin replacement (< 3 U/hour) avoids precipitous falls in serum glucose. Glucose levels initially should be repeated half-hourly. The osmotic pressure exerted by glucose within the intravascular space helps maintain circulating volume in severely dehydrated patients and rapid reductions in glucose without adequate fluid replacement can result in circulatory collapse.

Kumar & Clark's Medical Management and Therapeutics

- Hypokalaemia may be dilutional but it also results from potassium being driven into cells following insulin therapy and rehydration. Electrolytes should be measured every 1–2 hours initially and potassium added to the saline infusion as necessary.
- Mental status must be monitored. Rapid osmotic changes in the brain can lead to cerebral oedema and an abrupt deterioration in conscious level. The brain attempts to control its intracellular water content in prolonged hyperglycaemia by accumulating intracellular electrolytes and other osmotically active substances. This process takes several hours and allows the brain to achieve osmotic equilibrium with the external environment, with minimal loss of water. These substances only slowly diffuse out of the brain, so in the event of rapid corrections in serum osmolality, water will accumulate within the brain cells, causing oedema.
- IV infusion of insulin is stopped following resolution of HHS, and SC insulin injections started. Ultimately, it may be possible to place the patient on oral antidiabetic agents. Insulin requirements will fall gradually following an episode of HHS and this must be closely monitored over several weeks to avoid iatrogenic hypoglycaemia.

HYPOGLYCAEMIA

Hypoglycaemic symptoms include hunger, sweating, tremor and tachycardia. Impaired cognition and agitation are frequently seen and hypoglycaemia may result in seizures. Marked neurological deficits such as hemiparesis can occur. These normally resolve, but profound hypoglycaemia resulting in coma and delay in resolution can lead to permanent deficit.

Immediate management includes oral glucose in the form of sugar-sweetened drinks or dextrose tablets, if the patient is conscious. This should be followed by ingestion of more complex carbohydrates. If the patient is unconscious, IM glucagon (1 mg) or IV glucose (15–20 g with either 10% or 20% glucose) is given. Repeated measurement of capillary blood glucose after 15 mins is imperative to ensure resolution of hypoglycaemia.

A single episode of hypoglycaemia can blunt the symptoms of subsequent events for some weeks, placing that individual at risk of further more serious episodes.

Iatrogenic hypoglycaemia results from injected insulin or from oral hypoglycaemic agents that raise circulating insulin levels, e.g. sulphonylureas. Common scenarios include dosage errors, inadequate food intake or delay in mealtimes. Hypoglycaemia in the early hours of the morning occurs as a result of unopposed high levels of insulin in a relatively fasted state. The only clues may be an inexplicably high blood sugar on waking (counter-regulatory hormones push the blood glucose up in response to hypoglycaemia) and poor glucose control as assessed by the HbA$_{1C}$ or fructosamine. The patient may complain of waking with a headache or of night sweats drenching the bed. The only way to exclude such hypoglycaemic events is for capillary blood glucose testing at 3 a.m.

Repeated episodes of hypoglycaemia in a previously well-controlled diabetic should raise the possibility of malabsorption, such as that seen in coeliac disease, a loss of counter-regulatory hormones as in Addison's disease, or chronic kidney disease with reduced clearance of hypoglycaemic agents, including insulin. Recurrent hypoglycaemia is sometimes treated with insulin pump therapy.

Exercise can have unpredictable effects on blood glucose. Exercise will hasten insulin absorption with the risk of hypoglycaemia. Short bursts of intense activity can result in short term increases in blood glucose due to release of stress hormones. More prolonged energy expenditure can result in hypoglycaemia, especially a few hours post exercise as the muscles replenish glycogen stores.

Poor nutrition can decrease hepatic glycogen stores and **alcohol** inhibits hepatic gluconeogenesis; hypoglycaemia can result.

COMPLICATIONS OF DIABETES

Macrovascular disease

Diabetes is an independent risk factor for atheroma and is additive to other cardiovascular risk factors, including hypercholesterolaemia, hypertension and smoking. These risk factors frequently occur together in type 2 diabetes as the 'metabolic syndrome' and should all be aggressively managed.

Management of hypertension

Hypertension predisposes to cardiovascular disease and also contributes to the deterioration in diabetic nephropathy and retinopathy. In type 1 diabetes hypertension may result from underlying nephropathy; in type 2 diabetes it occurs as part of the metabolic syndrome with associated dyslipidaemia and central obesity (p. 613).

Present guidelines suggest:

- a target BP of 130/80 mmHg, or 125/75 mmHg in patients with microalbuminuria, which is early evidence of nephropathy.

This is often achievable only with changes in lifestyle and with the use of multiple therapeutic agents. Reducing salt and alcohol intake and increasing activity may help in BP management in addition to aiding glycaemic control, weight management and dyslipidaemia. Initial drug therapy is with an ACE inhibitor, e.g. ramipril 5–10 mg daily, or angiotensin receptor blocking agents, e.g. valsartan 80–160 mg daily, since these drugs also slow progression of renovascular disease. These agents should be avoided in renal artery stenosis, which is relatively common in this group of patients. Other agents used include diuretics, calcium channel-blocking agents and β-blockers.

Management of dyslipidaemia

Dyslipidaemia compounds cardiovascular risk in diabetes and treatment aimed at lowering LDL cholesterol and triglycerides, as well as increasing HDL cholesterol, is beneficial. Cardiovascular risk assessment tables tend to underestimate cardiovascular risk, and assessment should incorporate smoking, family history, BP, glycaemic control and renal albumin excretion. Those with evidence of increased risk on these parameters should be offered pharmaceutical agents in addition to lifestyle modification.

All patients with known cardiovascular disease should be given therapy. For target levels see Table 16.3. This may require several agents in addition to statins, including fibrates, ezetimibe, nicotinic acid or omega-3 fatty acids.

Microvascular disease

Improved glycaemia control and risk factor reduction will reduce microvascular complications including nephropathy, retinopathy and neuropathy.

Nephropathy

Diabetic nephropathy is the commonest single cause of chronic kidney disease. Overt diabetic nephropathy occurs when there is a persistent urinary albumin excretion rate (AER) of > 300 mg/day (normal urinary protein exertion is < 150 mg, of which 10 mg is albumin). However, much lower levels of albumin loss have prognostic implications and persistent urinary albumin losses of 30–300 mg/24 hours predict progression to nephropathy in type 1 diabetes and an increased cardiovascular risk in type 2 diabetes. At this level, albumin loss is not detected by routine urine dipsticks and is termed 'microalbuminuria'. A rising serum creatinine and BP suggests the progression of renal disease.

Investigations

A random urine sample (mid-stream, early-morning) reliably estimates urine albumin:creatinine ratio (ACR) and a ratio of > 3.5 in women and > 2.5 in men is abnormal. If ACR is raised, the test should be repeated; if it is still abnormal, an AER should be performed by a 24-hour urine collection.

Management

- Good glycaemic control for type 1 and 2 DM is required. In type 2, change to insulin if poorly controlled; if renal function is impaired, stop metformin and the renally excreted sulphonylureas, e.g. glibenclamide.
- Hypertension is controlled to a level of 125/75 mmHg. An ACE inhibitor/blocker is the drug of choice as it delays the progression of nephropathy. More than one antihypertensive may be required, e.g. a low-dose thiazide diuretic or calcium channel blocker.
- A normal protein diet is followed.
- Other risk factors, e.g. lipids, smoking, should be treated.
- Monitor for anaemia; ensure iron, B_{12} and folate are normal. All patients should already be on antiplatelet therapy.
- Referral to a renal physician for joint management is recommended when the serum creatinine is > 150 μmol/L.

Retinopathy

The eye can be affected in a variety of ways in diabetes: cataract formation, reduced visual acuity due to osmotic changes secondary to hyperglycaemia, and ocular nerve palsies. Diabetic retinopathy is the leading cause of blindness in people under the age of 60 in industrialized countries. Initial changes result from thickening of the basement membrane and increased vascular permeability, with subsequent aneurysm formation and vascular occlusion. Ischaemia encourages growth of new fragile blood vessels, which lie superficially and are therefore prone to damage and bleeding. The retina is susceptible to hypoxic damage from reduced blood flow in microvascular disease due to its high metabolic rate.

- **Non-proliferative background retinopathy** consisting of microaneurysms, hard exudates, and 'dot and blot' haemorrhages is not a threat to vision but may progress to **pre-proliferative retinopathy** with cotton wool spots (representing local infarction of retinal nerve fibre layer), venous beading and loops, and intra-retinal microvascular abnormalities.

- Maculopathy, with oedema or proliferative retinopathy, is a common cause of blindness and requires elective/urgent laser photocoagulation therapy.
- Advanced retinopathy, with vitreous haemorrhage or tractional retinal detachment, requires urgent referral to an ophthalmologist for treatment, e.g. vitrectomy.
- Annual screening with digital photography is necessary for all patients who are over 12 years of age or post-pubertal. Good digital imaging is the best screening modality.

Neuropathy

Diabetes-related neuropathies may be focal or diffuse, and both metabolic and microvascular factors may contribute.

- Diffuse symmetrical polyneuropathy, with sensory symptoms predominantly in a 'glove and stocking' distribution, is seen, although the feet and legs are typically more affected than the upper limbs. This is a diagnosis made after exclusion of other common causes of peripheral neuropathy that may be amenable to treatment, such as hypothyroidism, or vitamin B_{12} or thiamin deficiency. Patients may remain asymptomatic and thus annual foot assessment is imperative to detect an early sensory deficit that may predispose to trauma not perceived by the individual. Many patients, however, experience sharp, burning, or paraesthesic pains, which are typically worse at night.
- Acute painful neuropathy with sudden onset of severe sensory symptoms and allodynia requires treatment with e.g. **pregabalin** 50 mg 3 times daily, **duloxetine** 60 mg daily and **amitriptyline** 25 mg daily. **Mononeuritis and mononeuritis multiplex** can affect any nerve in the body and damage usually recovers spontaneously.
- Diabetic amyotrophy causes painful asymmetric wasting of the quadriceps muscles, typically in the older patient; improving blood glucose levels may help resolution.
- Autonomic neuropathy affects both the sympathetic and parasympathetic nervous system; this can be disabling to a minority of patients.

Other complications

Cardiovascular system

Postural hypotension, with a fall of systolic BP by 20mm Hg on standing for 2 mins, results from failure of sympathetically mediated increases in cardiac output and vasoconstrictor tone. Treatment is unsatisfactory.

Gastrointestinal tract

Dysphagia and gastric stasis result from vagal damage. These may be helped by **metoclopramide** or **erythromycin**. Intractable diarrhoea from abnormal colonic motility may be complicated by bacterial overgrowth, and rotational antibiotics are helpful, e.g. **tetracycline**, **ampicillin**.

Erectile dysfunction

This is common in diabetes and may be attributed to autonomic neuropathy, although contributory factors, including vascular insufficiency, drugs and other endocrine causes, as well as psychological factors and alcohol, play a role. Treatment is with a phosphodiesterase 5 inhibitor, e.g. **sildenafil** 50 mg. Do not use with nitrate therapy, as severe hypotension can be fatal.

The diabetic foot

Foot care is accomplished with education of the patient and support of a multi-disciplinary team. A combination of compromised vascular supply and neuropathy leads to increased risk of foot injury, infection and ultimately amputation.

Clinical manifestations

Foot ulceration occurs as a consequence of ischaemia and neuropathy, which frequently coexist. Loss of sensation to the foot risks unnoticed injury if regular visual examination is not made. Neuropathic foot ulcers occur at pressure points and are associated with a warm, numb foot. Ischaemic ulcers occur in the context of a cold pulseless foot and are typically painful. Polymicrobial infection occurs rapidly in poorly perfused tissue, and may spread to deeper tissue infection including bone.

Management

Management of any foot ulcer includes optimizing glucose control to aid healing and addressing vascular health with aspirin and cholesterol-lowering agents. Smoking should be stopped. Poor vascular supply may be improved with angioplasty.

- **Non-infected ulcers** should be dressed and weight-bearing should be avoided, e.g. by elevation or specially designed shoes.
- **Non-healing ulcers** with signs of active **infection** should be treated with broad-spectrum antibiotics. There is little evidence for any specific anti-microbial regimen. Penicillins, such as **flucloxacillin** and **amoxicillin** with **metronidazole** if anaerobic infection is suspected, are examples. IV administration of antibiotics should be offered in cases of cellulitis or systemic illness. Dead tissue should be removed by debridement — either surgical, chemical or other (larvae). If bone is seen at the base of an ulcer, an MRI is useful to look for osteomyelitis. A plain X-ray of the foot is less helpful.

HYPERLIPIDAEMIA

Hyperlipidaemia is diagnosed on a fasting blood test. Causes of secondary hyperlipidaemia must be excluded prior to deciding therapeutic options. These include hypothyroidism, alcohol, obesity, renal impairment, nephrotic syndrome, hepatic dysfunction, dysglobulinaemia, drugs, e.g. thiazide diuretics and corticosteroids, and poorly controlled diabetes mellitus.

- **Hypertriglyceridaemia.** The majority of these cases reflect a polygenic disorder with a moderate increase in triglyceride levels. Familial hypertriglyceridaemia is inherited in an autosomal dominant manner and there may be a history of pancreatitis or retinal vein thrombosis.
- Hypercholesterolaemia
  - *Familial hypercholesterolaemia* results in under-expression of the LDL cholesterol receptor in the liver, leading to high LDL levels. It is relatively common, occurring in 1 in 500 individuals. Homozygotes

have a total absence of LDL receptors and die in their teens from coronary artery disease if not aggressively treated. Heterozygotes may remain well, or develop coronary artery disease in their forties. Clinical features include tendon xanthomas and xanthelasmas.

- *Polygenic hypercholesterolaemia* results in modest elevations of cholesterol.
- Combined hyperlipidaemia. The most common cause of combined hyperlipidaemia is polygenic. Familial combined hyperlipidaemia affects 1 in 200 people and is characterized by raised cholesterol and triglyceride levels, with a family history of cardiovascular disease.

Treatment

Management includes addressing modifiable risk factors, including hypertension, smoking, obesity, lack of exercise and diabetes mellitus. Aspirin confers further benefits to cardiovascular risk management. High intake of saturated fatty acids and cholesterol impacts negatively on cardiovascular risk, while diets high in fruits, vegetables, whole grains and unsaturated fatty acids confer benefit.

- Goals of treatment
  - *Estimation of coronary heart disease risk* Prediction charts help identify individuals likely to benefit from lipid reduction therapy but will tend to underestimate risk in diabetes and those with a strong family history of premature cardiovascular disease or diabetes.
  - *Secondary prevention.* Therapy is recommended for individuals with known cardiovascular disease.
  - *Primary prevention.* Anyone with a 10-year risk of developing cardiovascular disease > 20%, as defined by a risk calculator (systolic BP total cholesterol:HDL ratio), or with strong predisposing factors such as diabetes should be offered therapy.
  - *Aim of treatment.* The aim is to reduce serum total cholesterol to below 5.0 mmol/L (190 mg/dL) (< 4.0 mmol/L, 150 mg/dL for patients with diabetes and hypertension) or by 20–25%, whichever will achieve the lower level. LDL should be reduced by 30% (or to below 3.0 mmol/L or 100 mg/dL) and triglyceride levels should fall below 2.3 mmol/L (200 mg/dL). HDL levels should be > 1.0 mmol/L (> 38 mg/dL).
- Therapy (Table 16.4)
  - *HMG CoA reductase inhibitors (statins).* Statins inhibit the rate-limiting step in cholesterol biosynthesis, reducing LDL levels by between 10 and 15%. Most statins undergo rapid first-pass metabolism in the liver. Efficacy is improved if they are taken with the evening meal or at bedtime. **Atorvastatin** is unusual in that it has a longer period of action and thus may be given in the morning if needed. It is possible that statins may hold benefits over and above reducing LDL cholesterol, including modulation of inflammatory, immune and coagulation responses. **Response to treatment** can be assessed 4 weeks after therapeutic changes. The dose response to dose increments is not linear and it is often better to combine agents to maximize effect.
  - *Ezetimibe* inhibits intestinal cholesterol absorption and interferes with the enterohepatic circulation of cholesterol synthesized in the liver. It is useful as an adjunct to statin therapy in reducing LDL cholesterol levels. The effect on clinical outcomes is unclear.

Kumar & Clark's Medical Management and Therapeutics

Kumar & Clark's Medical Management and Therapeutics

Table 16.4 Drugs used in the management of hyperlipidaemia

Drug	Dosage	Contraindications and adverse reactions	Expected therapeutic effect	Long-term safety
Statins, e.g.				
Simvastatin	20–80 mg daily	**Contraindications:** Active liver disease, pregnancy, lactation **Adverse effects:** Derangement of liver biochemistry, diarrhoea, myositis Stop if transferase levels ×3 normal Stop with clarithromycin or itraconazole Raised ciclosporin level in blood	30–60% reduction in LDL cholesterol Modest triglyceride lowering Tiny effect on HDL cholesterol Atorvastatin and particularly rosuvastatin have the most potent cholesterol-lowering effects (HMG CoA reductase)	Simvastatin, atorvastatin and pravastatin have good long-term safety in large-scale trials and in clinical practice. Avoid if possible in women of childbearing age
Pravastatin	40 mg daily			
Fluvastatin	20–80 mg daily			
Atorvastatin	10–40 mg daily			
Rosuvastatin	5–20 mg daily			
Cholesterol absorption inhibitors, e.g.				
Ezetimibe	10 mg daily	**Contraindications:** Lactation **Adverse effects:** Occasional diarrhoea, abdominal discomfort	Reduce LDL cholesterol by additional 10–15% if given with a statin Triglyceride concentrations reduced by 10% Increase HDL cholesterol by 5%	Mostly act in gut and little is absorbed Short-term safety good; long-term safety unknown

Bile acid sequestrants, e.g.			
Colestyramine	4 g daily max. 36 g	**Adverse effects:** Gastrointestinal side-effects predominate Palatability is a problem **Counselling:** Other drugs bind to resins and should be taken 1 h before or 4 h afterwards	8–15% reduction in LDL cholesterol Little or no effect on HDL cholesterol 5–15% rise in triglyceride concentration	Not systemically absorbed Safety profile is good Appear safe in women of childbearing age. Fat-soluble vitamin supplements may be required in children, pregnancy and breast feeding
Colestipol	5–30 g daily			
Colesevalam	3.75 g– 4.375 g daily			

Fibric acid derivatives, e.g.			
Gemfibrozil	0.9–1.2 g daily	**Contraindications:** Severe hepatic or renal impairment, gallbladder disease, pregnancy **Adverse effects:** Reversible myositis, nausea, predispose to gallstones, non-specific malaise, impotence	Reduction of LDL cholesterol by 10–15% and triglycerides by 25–35% HDL cholesterol concentrations increase by 10–50% (newer agents often have greater beneficial effect on HDL)	No knowledge of effect on developing fetus. Avoid in women of childbearing age Long-term safety appears good
Bezafibrate	200 mg 3 times daily			
Ciprofibrate	100 mg daily			
Fenofibrate	1 capsule daily			

Kumar & Clark's Medical Management and Therapeutics

Table 16.4 *Continued*

Drug	Dosage	Contraindications and adverse reactions	Expected therapeutic effect	Long-term safety
Nicotinic acid and derivatives, e.g.				
Modified-release nicotinic acid (also used with laropiprant which stops flushing)	375 mg to 2 g at night	**Contraindications:** Pregnancy, breast feeding **Adverse effects:** Value limited by frequent side-effects: headache, flushing, dizziness, nausea, malaise, itching, abnormal liver biochemistry. Glucose intolerance, hyperuricaemia, dyspepsia, hyperpigmentation may occur	Reduce LDL cholesterol by 5–10% Reduce triglycerides by 15–20% HDL cholesterol increased by 10–20%	Medium-term safety but marred by adverse effects listed Modified-release preparation reduces side-effect incidence
Acipimox	250 mg 2–3 times daily			
Fatty acid compounds				
Omega-3 acid ethyl esters	1 g 2–4 capsules daily	Occasional nausea and belching	Reduce triglycerides in severe hypertriglyceridaemia No favourable change in other lipids, and may aggravate hypercholesterolaemia in a few patients	Long-term safety is not yet known but seems unlikely to be poor
Omega-3 marine triglycerides	5 mL twice daily with food			

- *Bile acid sequestrants.* These agents pass unabsorbed through the gastrointestinal tract, binding bile acids and reducing enterohepatic recirculation, resulting in increased conversion of cholesterol into bile salts within the liver. This reduction in hepatocyte cholesterol leads to an increase in HMG CoA reductase activity, which is effectively blocked by combination therapy with a statin.
- *Fibric acid derivatives (fibrates).* The fibrates stimulate peroxisome proliferator activator receptor-α (PPAR-α). They enhance clearance of triglycerides and reduce very low-density lipoprotein (VLDL) synthesis. Fibrate therapy is associated with moderate reduction of cardiovascular risk and these drugs are therefore mainly used where high triglyceride levels confer a risk of pancreatitis, or in combination therapy with a statin (increased risk of rhabdomyolysis). Fibrates tend to be well tolerated.
- *Nicotinic acid.* This appears to reduce lipoprotein synthesis and inhibit peripheral production of free fatty acids. It benefits all aspects of the lipid profile but its use is limited by side-effects, which include flushing (reduced in some individuals by taking aspirin prior to administration), gastrointestinal effects, gout, hepatotoxicity and glucose intolerance. Nicotinic acid combined with laropiprant, which is a selective antagonist of prostaglandin D2 receptor Type 1, stops the flushing.
- *Omega fatty acids.* The omega fatty acids offer an alternative to fibrates and nicotinic acid for targeting hypertriglyceridaemia by reducing hepatic secretion of triglyceride-rich lipoproteins (VLDL). More clinical trials are needed to evaluate their place in the management of hyperlipidaemia further.

Further reading

American Diabetic Association: Diagnosis and classification of diabetes mellitus — position statement, *Diabetes Care* 33(Suppl 1):562–569, 2010.

Joint British Diabetes Societies Inpatient Care Group: *The management of diabetic ketoacidosis in adults*, 2010. Available from www.library.nhs.uk/diabetes/.

The International Expert Committee Report on the Role of the A1C Assay in Diagnosis of Diabetes, *Diabetes Care* 32:1327–1334, 2009.

Further information

www.diabetes.org.uk

www.endotext.org

Neurological disease 17

CHAPTER CONTENTS

APPROACH TO THE PATIENT

A detailed history and examination guide the choice of investigations that will enable you to answer the three questions that are key to formulating a diagnosis:

- 'Location, location, location': where is/are the lesion/s?
- Does the pattern of this presentation fit a recognizable disease pattern?
- What is the pathology?

Imaging plays a key role in diagnosis.

- CT is the investigation of choice in an acutely ill patient, particularly if intubated. It is quick and readily available. Acute haemorrhage is easily visualized. CT resolution is increased by using thinner slices but disadvantages include its failure to detect lesions whose attenuation is similar to that of the brain (e.g. subdurals and strokes during the isodense phase) or to that of the bone if the lesion is near the skull vault. Posterior fossa structures are poorly resolved. On modern scanners CT angiography is now the non-invasive neurovascular imaging modality of choice.
- MRI has great advantages over CT, with superior soft-tissue differentiation making it the best imaging modality to delineate brain parenchyma and spinal cord anatomy and pathology. Tumours, infarction, multiple sclerosis plaques and lesions of the cord and nerve roots are well demonstrated. Intracerebral and extracranial (carotid) blood vessels can be imaged without contrast. Diffusion-weighted imaging is sensitive for early infarction in stroke and allows differentiation between recent and old ischaemic lesions. Other advantages of MRI include multi-planar imaging in axial, sagittal and coronal planes, and absence of ionizing radiation. Disadvantages include longer imaging times than CT scanning, claustrophobia for some patients, inability to image patients with pacemakers and difficulty monitoring severely ill or ventilated patients while in the scanner.

ALTERATIONS IN CONSCIOUSNESS

- Consciousness is a state of wakefulness with awareness of self and surroundings.

Table 17.1 Glasgow Coma Score (GCS)		
Category	**Response**	**Score**
Eye opening (E)	Spontaneous	4
	To speech	3
	To pain	2
	Nil	1
Speech/verbal response (V)	Appropriate and orientated	5
	Confused	4
	Inappropriate words	3
	Incomprehensible sounds	2
	Nil	1
Motor response (M)	Obeys commands appropriately	6
	Localizes to pain	5
	Withdraws to pain	4
	Flexes to pain	3
	Extends to pain	2
	Nil	1

GCS = E + V + M. Minimum score 3, maximum score 15.

- Coma is a state of unrousable unresponsiveness (often defined as a Glasgow Coma Score (GCS) of 8 or less; Table 17.1). GCS is a useful and reliable standardized tool, especially for serial measurements, but be aware of limitations, e.g. tetraparetic patients or those with tracheostomy.
- State of arousal is influenced by the central reticular activating system (extends from brainstem to thalamus) and its interactions with cortex, hypothalamus, cerebellum and sensory stimuli. Consequently, coma results from two main processes:
  - diffuse metabolic/toxic/neurological dysfunction or other disorders affecting extensive areas of cortex (e.g. drugs, toxins or hypoxia)
  - brainstem (or thalamic) lesions that damage the reticular activating system, including pressure effects on the brainstem from cerebral mass lesions or oedema (coning).

Coma is a life-threatening emergency. Assessment must be swift and comprehensive, and occur in tandem with life support measures and initial investigations (Box 17.1, p. 624, and see Fig. 20.21 (p. 722)).

Initial assessment

- Assess vital signs and airway safety. Guedel airway insertion may be necessary. Is intubation/ventilation or circulatory support required?
- Capillary blood glucose and pulse oximetry
- History. Taking a history from relatives, witnesses and paramedics is crucial.
  - Onset?
  - How found?

> **Box 17.1** Management of the comatose patient
>
> This is a neurological emergency (*see also* Fig. 20.21). Enlist the help of an experienced nurse. The immediate priority is cardiorespiratory resuscitation.
> - Secure airway; give oxygen
> - Check pulse/BP and breathing. Resuscitate if necessary. Place on continuous cardiac and oximetry monitoring
> - Record Glasgow Coma Score
> - Perform primary survey: check head/spine for trauma; immobilize spine if necessary
> - Check breath: hepatic fetor, ketones, alcohol
> - Check rectal temperature with low-reading thermometer
> - Secure IV access and give **50 mL of 50% glucose**. In patients with suspected alcohol use, the glucose should be preceded by **250 mg thiamine IV** (to prevent Wernicke's encephalopathy)
> - Check pupils: if pinpoint, give **0.4–1.2 mg naloxone IV** to counteract possible opiate poisoning
> - Treat seizures (**lorazepam** and **phenytoin** — see Box 17.4) and suspected bacterial meningitis (p. 54)

- Any head/spinal injury?
- Past history of diabetes, epilepsy, opiate/alcohol use, suicide attempts?
- Any medication or prescriptions available?
- General examination. Look for clues to the cause of coma. Is there fever, purpuric rash, shock, anaemia, liver disease, melaena or renal disease, e.g. haemodialysis shunt or injection marks? Is there a MedicAlert bracelet? Is there evidence of trauma — blood or CSF in ears/nose or bruising (battle sign or 'racoon eyes' indicating skull fracture)? Neck stiffness can still be detected in unconscious patients and is indicative of meningeal infection or subarachnoid haemorrhage (SAH).
- Neurological examination. This is helpful to lateralize signs, to determine the level of pathology and to assess integrity of brainstem reflexes.
  - *Pupil size and reaction to light.* These are of great diagnostic significance in coma. **Unilateral fixed dilated pupil** indicates 3rd nerve compression or stretch, and suggests herniation of the uncus of the temporal lobe through the tentorial hiatus (coning) or posterior communicating artery aneurysm. **Bilateral fixed and dilated pupils** follow as coning progresses and indicate imminent death, but can also occur in deep coma of any cause, e.g. tricyclic overdose and hypothermia. **Bilateral pinpoint pupils** occur in opiate overdose and pontine lesions. **Small reactive pupils** are usually found in toxic and metabolic coma.
  - *Eye position and movements.* Conjugate deviation of eyes may indicate a frontal hemispheric lesion, e.g. stroke (eyes deviated towards lesion, away from hemiplegic side) or pontine lesion (eyes away from lesion). Disconjugate eye position may indicate a brainstem lesion. Roving eye movements ('windscreen wiper eyes') are seen in light metabolic coma or diffuse cortical injury.

- *Fundoscopy.* Look for papilloedema, hypertensive retinopathy and subhyaloid haemorrhage (in SAH).
- *Other brainstem reflexes.* Look for the corneal reflex, gag reflex (or cough reflex with suction catheter via endotracheal tube), (if spine is stable) doll's eye movements, and assess pattern and effort of respiration.
- *Limbs.* Check for asymmetric spontaneous movements, response to painful stimuli and extensor plantar responses. Focal motor signs usually suggest a structural cause, e.g. stroke or space-occupying lesion. Hypoglycaemia and hepatic coma occasionally cause focal signs.

Investigations where cause of coma is unknown after initial assessment

- CT brain is the priority once the patient is stabilized and glucose checked, especially if lateralizing neurological signs are present, e.g. hemiparesis. Note that raised intracranial pressure (ICP) cannot always be excluded with imaging; specialist review of imaging may be required to look for features of raised pressure such as early cerebral oedema or effacement of chiasmatic cisterns.
- Blood for:
  - FBC, U&E, creatinine, liver biochemistry, glucose, coagulation, thyroid function, cortisol
  - toxicology, including alcohol, paracetamol and salicylates
  - blood cultures.
- Urine toxicology, ABG, ECG and CXR
- Lumbar puncture (LP) and CSF examination should be performed only after risk assessment and if there is no CT evidence of a mass lesion or raised ICP.

   ⚠ **N.B.** Treat suspected bacterial meningitis with IV antibiotics and high-dose steroids immediately — BEFORE lumbar puncture.
  - Lumbar puncture is contraindicated in meningococcal septicaemia (p. 54). If viral encephalitis is a possibility (p. 55), start IV aciclovir 10 mg/kg 3 times daily (monitor renal function).
- EEG should be done if there is suspicion of non-convulsive status epilepticus.
- MRI brain should be performed if the cause of the coma is still uncertain, and obtain a neurological opinion.

Immediate management

- Immediate management is directed at treating the underlying cause.
- Nursing care of skin (pressure areas), eyes and mouth is essential.
- If the patient cannot swallow after 12 hours, insert a naso-gastric tube.
- Ensure adequate fluid and calorific intake.
- Only catheterize if absolutely necessary.

Acute confusional state (delirium)

Delirium is characterized by abnormalities of perception and cognition, often **without a decrease** in the level of consciousness. **Impairment in consciousness**, if present, can vary and fluctuates with confusion, usually being worse at night. It is very common, especially in elderly hospitalized patients. There are a wide variety of causes, often occurring in combination, in a patient vulnerable by virtue of age or impaired cognitive reserve. Common causes include systemic infection, hypoxia, electrolyte imbalance, liver or renal failure, and drug/alcohol intoxication or withdrawal (especially anticonvulsants, anxiolytics, opiates), as well as brain injury, encephalitis/meningitis or deficiency states such as Wernicke–Korsakoff encephalopathy.

Delirium should be distinguished from dementia, aphasia and psychosis. Dementia can also predispose to the development of periods of delirium with intercurrent illnesses. In dementia there is no clouding of consciousness, the patient is alert, and there is less likely to be agitation or rapid fluctuations.

Management

- Initial management and evaluation is similar to that of the comatose patient. Review the notes, take a history and examine the patient.
- General measures include nursing in moderately lit, quiet room, repeated reassurance, and correction of metabolic imbalance. Perform appropriate investigations to determine the cause and treat underlying disease. Sedation must be used judiciously, as occasionally paradoxical worsening of confusion can result, particularly with benzodiazepines. Give haloperidol 1 mg oral twice daily if patient presents risk to themselves or others.

Delirium tremens (DTs)

This is the most serious alcohol withdrawal state and occurs 1–3 days after alcohol cessation. Patients have disorientation, agitation, tremor and visual hallucinations. For treatment, see Box 17.2.

Box 17.2 Management of delirium tremens

General measures
- Admit the patient
- Correct electrolyte abnormalities and dehydration
- Treat any co-morbid disorder (e.g. infection)
- Give IV thiamine slowly (250 mg daily for 3–5 days in the absence of Wernicke–Korsakoff (W–K) syndrome)
- Give IV thiamine slowly (500 mg daily for 3–5 days with W–K encephalopathy)
- **N.B.** *Beware anaphylaxis with thiamine*
- Give prophylactic phenytoin if previous history of withdrawal fits.

Specific drug treatment
- One of the following orally:
  - Diazepam 10–20 mg
  - Chlordiazepoxide 30–60 mg
  - *Repeat 1 hour after last dose, depending on response.*

Fixed-schedule regimens
- Diazepam 10 mg every 6 hours for 4 doses, then 5 mg 6-hourly for 8 doses *or*
- Chlordiazepoxide 30 mg every 6 hours for 4 doses, then 15 mg 6-hourly for 8 doses

Provide additional benzodiazepine when symptoms and signs are not controlled.

STROKE

Stroke is characterized by the sudden onset of focal neurological symptoms caused by interruption of the vascular supply to a region of the brain (ischaemic stroke) or intracerebral haemorrhage (haemorrhagic stroke). It is a common cause of mortality and physical disability.

Paramedics and members of the public are encouraged to make the diagnosis of stroke on a history and simple examination (the 'FAST' test):
- **f**ace — sudden weakness of the face
- **a**rm — sudden weakness of one or both arms
- **s**peech — difficult speaking/slurred speech
- **t**ime — the sooner the treatment can be started, the better.

⚠ **N.B.** *Stroke is a medical emergency and prompt treatment can improve prognosis.*

Pathophysiology
- **Ischaemic stroke** (infarction of central nervous tissue) results from cerebral infarction secondary to either arterial thromboembolism or emboli arising from the heart (e.g. in atrial fibrillation, mural thrombus after acute myocardial infarction, or rarely from vegetations in infective endocarditis).
- **Cerebral haemorrhage** accounts for ~15% of strokes and is often caused by microaneurysm rupture in small penetrating arteries in hypertensive patients; occasionally by aneurysm or arteriovenous malformation rupture; or by amyloid angiopathy in older patients.
- Other causes of stroke in younger patients include arterial dissection, venous sinus thrombosis, thrombophilia, vasculitis and paradoxical embolization through a patent foramen ovale.

Clinical evaluation
Onset is acute (a gradual or stuttering onset may indicate a mass lesion) and characterized by negative rather than positive symptoms (e.g. numbness rather than tingling).

Ask about preceding trauma or neck/facial pain (may indicate dissection) and use of anticoagulants (cerebral haemorrhage). Identify vascular risk factors.
- **General physical examination**
  - Check for fever to exclude a possible infective aetiology; look for altered mental state (possible meningo-encephalitis).
  - Look for systemic signs of underlying disease, e.g. evidence of vasculitis, stigmata of infective endocarditis.
  - Cardiovascular examination should include pulse (atrial fibrillation?), BP, carotids for bruits and heart for murmurs.
  - Check fundi for hypertensive or diabetic retinopathy, Roth spots and papilloedema.
  - Horner's syndrome (partial ptosis with miosis) may indicate ipsilateral carotid artery dissection. The accompanying hemiparesis is contralateral to the dissection and due to embolic phenomena.
- **Neurological examination** localizes the lesion to anterior or posterior circulation territory.
  - *Anterior circulation.* **Middle cerebral artery (MCA)** or **anterior cerebral artery (ACA)** and **branches (carotid artery distribution)**. Hemispheric infarction typically causes a combination of contralateral limb/facial weakness and/or sensory loss, visual field defects,

dysphasia/aphasia or sensory inattention (especially in right hemi-sphere stroke). Initially the affected limbs are flaccid (hypotonia), but this progresses to spasticity with upper motor neurone (UMN) signs.

- *Posterior circulation.* **Vertebral, basilar and posterior cerebral arteries and branches.** Brainstem infarction may result in a combination of ataxia, long tract signs and cranial nerve palsies. The **lateral medullary syndrome** causes a characteristic clinical picture, which includes ipsilateral facial numbness, diplopia, nystagmus and ataxia. Posterior cerebral artery (PCA) infarction results in visual field defects. Posterior circulation stroke may lead to coma.
- *Lacunar infarcts.* Small infarcts in deep white matter, especially basal ganglia, may result in pure motor or pure sensory deficits or ataxic hemiparesis.

Stroke is primarily a clinical diagnosis, supported by imaging.

Immediate management (see Emergencies in Medicine p. 721)

- Resuscitate the patient, including administration of oxygen; establish IV access, oximetry and cardiac monitoring. Decide whether thrombolysis is appropriate.
- Take blood for FBC, ESR (raised in giant cell arteritis (GCA), infective endocarditis), U&E, creatinine and glucose; if appropriate, test for sickle cell disease.
- Perform ECG and CXR.
- Imaging in acute stroke
  - *Non-contrast CT* will demonstrate haemorrhage immediately but cerebral infarction is often not detected or only subtle changes are seen acutely (Fig. 17.1A).
  - *Diffusion-weighted MRI* (DWI) shows changes early in infarction (Fig. 17.1B) and may distinguish between acute and chronic areas of ischaemia. It is more sensitive than CT for small infarcts and for the detection of haemorrhage. If MRI is unavailable a CT should be performed so that there is no delay in giving thrombolysis.

Thrombolysis (Box 17.3)

⚠ *N.B. Every minute counts. The benefit of thrombolysis decreases with time, even within the 4.5-hour window.*

- Exclude patients with strokes due to haemorrhage, infection or other non-ischaemic pathologies (Box 17.3).
- Are there any contraindications to thrombolysis?
- Give alteplase after discussion with a senior doctor.

Thrombolysis improves long-term morbidity after an ischaemic stroke but is associated with an increased risk of acute haemorrhage. Maximal benefit of thrombolysis is achieved if it is given as soon as possible, although benefit may be derived if administered up to 4.5 hours after the start of symptoms. The short time window and need for prior MRI/CT to exclude haemorrhage or massive infarction require urgent action. Intra-arterial thrombolysis and mechanical disruption of clot are occasionally employed in specialist centres.

Further management

Subsequent management aims to reduce complications, lower the risk of further events and ensure adequate rehabilitation.

Kumar & Clark's Medical Management and Therapeutics

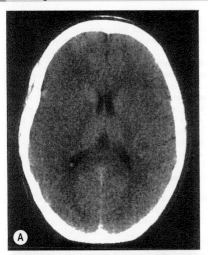

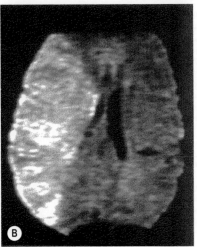

Fig. 17.1 Middle cerebral artery (MCA) infarction.
(A) CT performed initially shows only very subtle low-density changes in the right MCA territory.
(B) Diffusion-weighted MRI done at the same time shows the full extent of the area of ischaemia. (Courtesy of Dr Paul Jarman.)

Box 17.3 Thrombolysis in acute ischaemic stroke

Eligibility
- Age ≥ 18 years
- Clinical diagnosis of acute ischaemic stroke
- Assessed by experienced team
- Measurable neurological deficit
- Blood test results available
- CT or MRI consistent with acute ischaemic stroke
- Timing of onset well established
- Thrombolysis should commence as soon as possible and up to 4.5 hours after acute stroke

Exclusion criteria
Historical
- Stroke or head trauma within the previous 3 months
- Any prior history of intracranial haemorrhage
- Major surgery within 14 days
- Gastrointestinal or genitourinary bleeding within the previous 21 days
- Myocardial infarction in the previous 3 months
- Arterial puncture at a non-compressible site within 7 days
- Lumbar puncture within 7 days

Clinical
- Rapidly improving stroke syndrome
- Minor and isolated neurological signs
- Seizure at the onset of stroke if the residual impairments are due to post-ictal phenomena
- Symptoms suggestive of subarachnoid haemorrhage, even if the CT is normal
- Acute MI or post-MI pericarditis
- Persistent systolic BP ≥ 185 mmHg, diastolic BP ≥ 110 mmHg, or requiring aggressive therapy to control BP
- Pregnancy or lactation
- Active bleeding or acute trauma (fracture)

Laboratory
- Platelets ≤ 100×10^9/L
- Serum glucose ≤ 2.8 mmol/L or ≥ 22.2 mmol/L
- INR ≥ 1.7 if on warfarin
- Elevated partial thromboplastin time if on heparin

Dose of IV alteplase (tissue plasminogen activator)
- Total dose 0.9 mg/kg (maximum 90 mg)
- 10% of total dose by initial IV bolus over 1 min
- Remainder infused IV over 60 mins

(Amended from Adams HP, et al. 2007)

- Admit to a stroke unit. Specialist care, including nursing, physiotherapy, speech and language therapy and occupational therapy, on a dedicated stroke unit improves outcome. Maintain hydration, perform swallowing assessment for aspiration risk, and turn regularly to avoid pressure sores. Try to avoid catheterization if possible. Do not lower BP in the acute phase unless hypertensive encephalopathy or other acute complications of severe hypertension (e.g. hypertensive nephropathy, hypertensive cardiac failure/acute myocardial infarction, aortic dissection, eclampsia) are present. Hyperglycaemia is associated with poorer outcome, so maintain normoglycaemia with **insulin** if required. Treat infections.
- Secondary prevention
  - Do *not* give antiplatelet drugs within 24 hours of recombinant tissue-type plasminogen activator (rt-PA). Then start clopidogrel 75 mg per day. Treatment with modified release dipyridamole (200 mg × 2 daily) in combination with aspirin (300 mg/day loading dose, then 75–150 mg/day) is now recommended only if clopidogrel is contraindicated or not tolerated (see NICE guidelines 2010).
  - Modify risk factors, particularly hypertension, hypercholesterolaemia, diabetes and smoking. Sustained hypertension persisting beyond 2 weeks should be treated (target BP < 140/85 mmHg or 130/80 mmHg if diabetic). All patients should be on a statin (e.g. **simvastatin** 40 mg) unless cholesterol < 3.5, started 48 hours after stroke.
- Identification of embolic source
  - *Carotids.* All patients with anterior circulation stroke who are not severely disabled by the stroke should have carotid imaging with Doppler or MRI/CT angiography to identify symptomatic carotid stenosis. *Early* carotid endarterectomy greatly reduces the risk of further stroke if there is 70–99% stenosis on the affected side. Benefits for 50–69% stenosis and for asymptomatic > 70% stenosis are more modest.
  - *Cardiac source.* Perform echocardiography to identify a cardiac source of embolism if an embolic stroke is possible. Transoesophageal echocardiography (TOE) is appropriate in younger patients with cryptogenic stroke, e.g. to identify a patent foramen ovale (PFO) or if endocarditis is suspected. Twenty-four-hour ECG monitoring is used to identify paroxysmal atrial fibrillation. Anticoagulation should be initiated in atrial fibrillation or if cardiac thrombus is present — generally wait 2 weeks after the acute event before starting anticoagulation to reduce the risk of haemorrhagic transformation, unless dealing with a lacunar or small stroke.
  - *Thrombophilia screen.* This should be performed in cases of stroke in the young.
- Treat or prevent complications. DVT prophylaxis with SC low molecular weight heparin (LMWH), e.g. **enoxaparin 40 mg SC** daily (**N.B.** not in haemorrhagic stroke). Treat complications early, e.g. depression, seizures, pneumonia. If patient deteriorates neurologically, repeat brain imaging. Intracerebral haematoma, for example, might require urgent neurosurgical intervention.
- Rehabilitation. In severe stroke refer early for multi-disciplinary rehabilitation assessment. Discharge with a full plan for rehabilitation and having liaised with the patient's primary care physician.

Surgery in acute stroke

Decompressive craniectomy should be considered in cases of massive MCA infarction in patients under 60 years of age where there are clinical deficits compatible with MCA infarct. CT demonstrates infarction in at least 50% of the arterial territory without additional ipsilateral infarction in the anterior or posterior cerebral arterial territories. Surgery should be performed within 48 hours of symptom onset or in the event of a deteriorating clinical condition.

The National Institute of Health's Stroke Scale Score, which is comprised of 11 items with total scores of 0–42, is a useful validating system. A score of > 15 suggests a decrease in the level of consciousness.

Transient ischaemic attacks (TIAs)

This is a transient episode of neurological dysfunction caused by focal brain, spinal cord or retinal ischaemia without acute infarction. The previous definition with its arbitrary 24-hour time scale is no longer used, as the end point is now tissue injury. Examples include anterior circulation — sudden transient loss of vision in one eye (amaurosis fugax), aphasia, hemiparesis; or posterior circulation — diplopia, ataxia, hemisensory loss, dysarthria, transient global amnesia.

- Migraine aura can be difficult to distinguish from TIA when it occurs without headache.
- TIA is not a cause of loss of consciousness.
- **Examination for cause**: look for atrial fibrillation, hypertension, carotid artery bruit and valvular heart disease.
- TIAs may herald the onset of stroke (one-quarter of patients developing stroke have had a TIA, usually within the previous week).
- The **ABCD² score** can help to stratify stroke risk in the first 2 days.

  - **A**ge > 60 years   1 point
  - **B**P > 140 mmHg systolic and/or > 90 mmHg diastolic   1 point
  - **C**linical features
Unilateral weakness	2 points
Isolated speech disturbance	1 point
Other	0 points
  - **D**uration of symptoms (mins)
> 60	2 points
10–59	1 point
< 10	0 points
  - **D**iabetes
Present	1 point
Absent	0 points

  A score of < 4 is associated with a minimal risk, whereas > 6 is high-risk for a stroke within 7 days of a TIA.
- If patients are considered to have had a high-risk TIA, i.e. ABCD² score > 4, or have had two recent TIAs, especially within the same vascular territory, then they should be admitted for investigation and commencement of secondary prevention.
- *All* patients should be referred to a TIA clinic and ideally seen within 24 hours. Investigation and treatment should be regarded as **urgent** and should be **completed** within 2 weeks.

Investigations

- Look for the source of the embolus — carotids (Doppler) or cardiac echo, ECG + 24-hour tape.

Kumar & Clark's Medical Management and Therapeutics

- CT brain in the first instance. Further (MRI) imaging of the brain and vascular system may subsequently be required where pathology or vascular territory is uncertain.

Treatment

- Antiplatelet therapy as for stroke (p. 632).
- Modification of vascular risk factors — smoking, hypertension, statins as above.
- Early endarterectomy for symptomatic 70–99% carotid artery stenosis (within 1 week if possible).
- Anticoagulation for atrial fibrillation (p. 457) (aspirin 300 mg daily for 2 weeks, then anticoagulate with **heparin** and **warfarin** or **dabigatran**).

Intracerebral haemorrhage

- If stroke is secondary to an intracerebral bleed, management is primarily supportive. There is a limited role for surgical evacuation of haematoma.
- Stop antiplatelet therapy and reverse anticoagulation (if the patient has a mechanical cardiac valve, consult a cardiologist).
- Hypertension should be treated but not aggressively, as it may reduce cerebral perfusion. **Give antihypertensives** if BP is persistently > 200 mmHg systolic (p. 457). Cerebellar haematomas may progress to brainstem compression or obstructive hydrocephalus and require prompt neurosurgical evaluation.

Subarachnoid haemorrhage (SAH)

SAH usually results from arterial bleeding into the subarachnoid space following rupture of saccular berry aneurysms on the circle of Willis (70–80%). Arteriovenous malformations account for 5–10% of SAH.

Patients present with sudden onset of an explosive headache — thunderclap (< 30 secs from onset to maximal severity), often associated with vomiting. There may be loss of consciousness at the onset. Sentinel haemorrhage can cause warning headache a few days before the major bleed. **Examination** may reveal neck stiffness, reduced level of consciousness, focal neurological deficit, e.g. third nerve palsy (indicating ruptured posterior communicating artery aneurysm) or hemiparesis. Subhyaloid haemorrhage may be visualized on fundoscopy. Migraine and coital headache can also occasionally present with sudden onset of severe headache. In thunderclap headache always investigate for possible SAH.

Management

- Initially stabilize the patient, resuscitate, give O_2, site IV access, and place on cardiac and BP monitor (see management of coma, p. 627).
- Perform an urgent CT brain to look for subarachnoid or intraventricular haemorrhage (95% sensitivity on day 1, falling to 50% at 1 week and 30% at 2 weeks after the bleed).
- If the history is suggestive and CT is normal, perform lumbar puncture to look for blood-stained CSF and xanthochromia (bilirubin discoloration of CSF due to cell lysis). Xanthochromia may be detected from ~12 hours to 3 weeks after SAH. Visible inspection of a centrifuged sample is often sufficient to detect xanthochromia, but laboratory spectrophotometry is more sensitive.

- If SAH is confirmed, arrange for CT cerebral angiography to identify the source of bleeding.
- Definitive treatment is early endovascular coiling of the aneurysm or surgical clipping where endovascular treatment is not possible.
- **Nimodipine** (e.g. 60 mg orally 4-hourly for 2–3 weeks, or 1 mg/hour IV) can reduce arterial spasm and reduce further cerebral infarction.
- Avoid hypotension (it may worsen the ischaemic deficit). Treat hypertension if diastolic pressure is persistently > 130 mmHg. Aim for a very gradual decrease in BP with monitoring and frequent repeat neurological examination.
- Supportive measures include bed rest, analgesia and laxatives (avoid sudden rises in ICP or BP).
- Watch for complications, including hyponatraemia (SIADH), hydrocephalus (obstruction of cerebral aqueduct by blood) and vasospasm causing ischaemic deficits.

Subdural haemorrhage

Subdural haemorrhage is caused by venous bleeding from bridging veins between cortex and venous sinuses. The elderly, alcoholics and patients on anticoagulants or with epilepsy are particularly susceptible. Subdural haemorrhage often follows head trauma, which may be minor. The latent period between injury and symptoms can be several weeks.

Patients present with headache, drowsiness and confusion that may fluctuate, focal neurological deficits and/or personality change.

Conservative management may be appropriate in older patients without neurological deficit.

Extradural haemorrhage

Extradural haemorrhage results from arterial bleeding between bone and dura, usually at the site of skull fracture (often the middle meningeal artery). Following head injury there may be a lucid interval followed by a rapid reduction in the level of consciousness as the haematoma increases in size. Refer to a neurosurgeon.

EPILEPSY

Epilepsy is a predisposition to recurrent seizures. Seizures are classified as:

- Generalized seizures. These are due to diffuse electrical discharge within the brain. They are characterized by loss of awareness (e.g. absence seizures and generalized tonic clonic seizures) or myoclonic jerks.
- Partial seizures. Seizure activity is localized to one part of the brain (also known as localization-related epilepsy (LRE)):
  - *simple partial* (no loss of awareness, e.g. motor jerking of a body part, epigastric aura).
  - *complex partial* (alteration of awareness, frequently associated with stereotypical behaviour and automatisms). Partial seizures may become secondarily generalized.

Diagnosis

The diagnosis of epilepsy is predominantly clinical, but determining whether an episode of apparent loss of consciousness is due to epilepsy can be difficult. The main distinction is from syncope (p. 385). Witness descriptions or video recordings of the event are invaluable. Ask the patient and the witness what happened before, during and after the event. Ask about risk factors for epilepsy (e.g. family history, birth and developmental history, febrile convulsions in childhood, previous meningitis or encephalitis, significant head injury), arrhythmias and diabetes. Also enquire about drug use and alcohol excess.

- Syncope may be associated with precipitants, e.g. prolonged standing in a hot place, micturition, a bout of coughing, or distress such as pain or the sight of blood.
- Syncopal prodrome and rapid recovery are characteristic.
- Loss of consciousness while lying down is not likely to be syncope.
- Urinary incontinence may occur in both syncope and seizures, and is a poor discriminator.
- Even in simple syncope, isolated jerks of a limb or the whole body may be seen.

Examination is often normal.

Investigations and referral
- Lying and standing BP.
- FBC, electrolytes, glucose.
- ECG (look for conduction block, arrhythmia, long QT interval).
- For a probable epileptic event, brain imaging with MRI (especially if focal onset seizure) and EEG to classify epilepsy type. EEG is usually not helpful where diagnosis (syncope vs. seizure) is uncertain.

Use of anti-epileptic drugs (AEDs) (Table 17.2)
After a first seizure, patients should be seen in a specialist neurology clinic. AEDs are indicated when there is a firm diagnosis of epilepsy and a substantial risk of recurrent seizures (usually after second seizure or after first seizure with abnormal imaging or unequivocal abnormal EEG). The aim is monotherapy with seizure freedom and no side-effects. There is no role for trial of an AED where diagnosis of epilepsy is uncertain.

- Introduce AEDs at low dose and gradually titrate upwards until the seizures are controlled or side-effects become unacceptable.
- **Partial seizures or secondary generalized seizures** (LRE) are often treated with **carbamazepine retard, lamotrigine** or **levetiracetam**.
- **Generalized seizure types** may be treated with **sodium valproate, levetiracetam or lamotrigine** as first-line treatment. Phenytoin is now generally only used in emergency treatment of seizures to achieve a rapid therapeutic effect.
- Acute symptomatic seizures e.g. in the context of an intercurrent infection in patients with epilepsy can be treated with clobazam 10 mg twice daily for one week, 10 mg daily for one week and then stopped.
- If seizures are not controlled with the first AED, gradually introduce a second agent and slowly withdraw the first AED once the second is established. If the patient is still not seizure-free, then combination therapy may be required. **Levetiracetam** is increasingly used and is licensed as first-line therapy for all seizure types.
- Epilepsy is one of the few disorders where non-generic prescribing is justified to ensure consistent drug levels.
- Routine monitoring of AED levels is not needed and should be possibly reserved for assessing compliance and toxicity.

Table 17.2 Anti-epileptic drugs (AEDs) — indications and common side-effects

AED	Indication	Starting dose daily (all oral)	Dose increments	Usual daily therapeutic dose	Common side-effects*	Particular features
Carbamazepine (slow-release usually preferred)	LRE	200 mg (100 mg in elderly)	200 mg steps every 2 weeks	400–1200 mg	**Rash**, diplopia, unsteadiness, neutropenia, hyponatraemia	Enzyme inducer Interacts with OCP Can worsen myoclonus
Clonazepam	Myoclonus	1 mg	1 mg every 2 weeks	4–8 mg	Drowsiness	
Ethosuximide	Childhood absence seizures	0.5 mg ×2	250 mg every 2 weeks	1.0–1.5 g	Insomnia, ataxia, blood dyscrasias	Rarely used in adult practice
Gabapentin	LRE	300 mg	300 mg every 2–3 days	600–1200 mg 3 times daily	Ataxia, drowsiness	
Lamotrigine	LRE and generalized epilepsies JME	25 mg	25 mg steps every 2 weeks	Up to 500 mg (usual dose 100–200 mg)	**Rash** is common toxic epidermal necrosis (TEN) or Stevens–Johnson syndrome	Interactions with valproate — start at 25 mg alternate days and slowly increase if patient also on valproate Monitor levels closely during pregnancy
Levetiracetam	LRE and generalized epilepsies JME	250 mg	250 mg steps every 2 weeks	1000–2000 mg	Irritability, sometimes mood problems	Therapeutic window, initial benefit may be replaced by increased seizure frequency with higher doses No known drug–drug interactions

Kumar & Clark's Medical Management and Therapeutics

Table 17.2 *Continued*

AED	Indication	Starting dose daily (all oral)	Dose increments	Usual daily therapeutic dose	Common side-effects*	Particular features
Lacosamide	Adjunctive therapy in LRE with or without secondary generalization	50 mg once daily	50 mg every 2 weeks	400 mg	Nausea, dizziness, ataxia	New AED May prolong PR interval — avoid in second- or third-degree heart block
Oxcarbazepine	LRE	300 mg twice daily	300–600 mg every week	600–2400 mg	**Rash**. Similar to carbamazepine but can cause profound hyponatraemia	Enzyme inducer (less than carbamazepine) Interacts with OCP
Phenytoin	All forms of epilepsy Now generally only initiated in emergency setting	Start 150–300 mg See Box 17.4 for emergency use	N/A	300 mg/day (monitor levels)	**Rash**, gum hypertrophy, hirsutism, diplopia, unsteadiness, coarse facial features	If long-term AED needed, aim to switch to newer AED Enzyme inducer
Phenobarbital	All forms of epilepsy Now generally only initiated in emergency setting	60 mg	Gradual, e.g. 15 mg every 2 weeks	60–180 mg	**Rash**, drowsiness, ataxia, depression	Requires very gradual withdrawal and titration Rarely initiated, as may cause profound cognitive impairment

Pregabalin	Adjunctive therapy in LRE with or without secondary generalization	25 mg twice daily	50 mg every 1–2 weeks	300–600 mg	Drowsiness, dry mouth, peripheral oedema, weight gain	Also used for neuropathic pain and anxiety disorder
Sodium valproate	Generalized epilepsies JME	300 mg twice daily	200 mg steps every 3 days	1000–2500 mg	Weight gain, hair thinning, tremor, thrombocytopenia, encephalopathy, liver dysfunction, Parkinsonism	Teratogenicity — do not use in pregnancy
Tiagabine	LRE	5 mg twice daily	5–10 mg every week	30–40 mg	Headaches, psychosis, depression, leucopenia	No longer widely used
Topiramate	Generalised epilepsies and adjunct to LRE JME	25 mg	25 mg steps every 2 weeks	Up to 400 mg	Cognitive decline, weight loss, peripheral paraesthesiae, renal stones, rarely **rash**	Advise to hydrate well. If eye symptoms, consider acute closed-angle glaucoma
Zonisamide	Adjunctive therapy in LRE with or without secondary generalization	50 mg once daily	50 mg every 2 weeks	300–500 mg	**Rash**, nausea, drowsiness, ataxia, GI side-effects	Advise to hydrate well, as may associate with nephrolithiasis

*All AEDs can cause idiosyncratic side-effects. JME, juvenile myoclonic epilepsy; LRE, localization-related epilepsy (partial-onset seizures with or without secondary generalization); OCP, oral contraceptive pill; PCOS, polycystic ovarian syndrome; TEN, toxic epidermal necrolysis.

- In refractory epilepsy reconsider diagnosis, for example, non-epileptic attack disorder. Consider combination therapy with newer AEDs, vagal nerve stimulation and, in LRE, epilepsy surgery (e.g. temporal lobectomy for temporal lobe epilepsy secondary to hippocampal sclerosis).

Driving and epilepsy

Rules for this vary in different countries. In the European Union, patients with epilepsy are not legally permitted to drive motor vehicles unless they have been seizure-free for 12 months (with or without medication); this can be as little as 3 months in parts of the USA. Driving may be permitted by some licensing authorities if attacks occur solely in sleep. Similarly there may be more flexibility if an isolated seizure is considered 'provoked'. Rules are much more stringent for driving commercial vehicles and for some occupations, e.g. aircraft pilots, divers. In the UK it is an essential medical requirement to inform patients of the law. The patient should then inform the licensing authority.

Lifestyle issues

Patients should avoid known precipitants, e.g. sleep deprivation, recreational drugs or excess alcohol. Encourage full compliance with prescribed medication. Give safety advice, e.g. showers rather than baths, care when cooking, do not bathe infants alone, do not swim alone or in deep water, avoid strobe lighting in generalized epilepsies.

Women and epilepsy

Women of childbearing age should be informed of the risk of teratogenicity with AEDs (particularly high with sodium valproate and increased if multiple AEDs). Careful planning of pregnancy is essential. Enzyme-inducing AEDs increase oestrogen metabolism and reduce efficacy of the OCP (e.g. **carbamazepine**, **oxcarbazepine**, **phenytoin**, **phenobarbital**, **primidone**, **topiramate**; a higher dose of oestrogen is required). Give advice on contraception, including barrier methods (in combination with the OCP), intrauterine devices or depot injections. If the patient is planning pregnancy commence **folic acid** 5 mg daily to reduce the risk of neural tube defects and try to reduce medication to monotherapy at the lowest effective dose. If the patient is taking **valproate**, switch to another AED. Advise patients to seek medical attention as soon as they know they are pregnant.

Long-term use of AEDs, particularly in women, is associated with osteoporosis. Refer peri- and post-menopausal patients for bone mineral density scans at approximately 3-yearly intervals.

Withdrawal of AEDs

AED withdrawal should only be contemplated after at least 2 years of freedom from seizures. In **juvenile myoclonic epilepsy** (10% of patients in epilepsy clinics) patients usually require lifelong therapy.

Ensure that the patient is actively involved in decision-making. Probability of remaining seizure-free after AED withdrawal is increased if:

- the patient is seizure-free on monotherapy
- there is no structural lesion
- there has been a long seizure-free period.

If the patient is taking multiple AEDs, withdraw only one drug at a time.

EEG prior to or during drug reduction can be helpful in predicting seizure recurrence.

Advise patients not to drive during periods of drug reduction and for 6 months after reduction/withdrawal is completed. If they have a seizure during drug alteration the Driving Licence Authority regulations will apply.

Status epilepticus (SE)

Isolated seizures usually terminate spontaneously within 2 mins. SE is defined as seizures or multiple seizures occurring without full recovery of consciousness over a prolonged period (> 10 mins). It is a neurological emergency with high mortality. In young women presenting with SE, consider eclampsia.

Administer oxygen. The patient may need a naso-pharyngeal airway. Early administration of benzodiazepines (e.g. **lorazepam** IM or IV, **diazepam** 20 mg rectally, buccal **midazolam** 10 mg) can prevent frequent seizures from progressing to SE.

Acute management
This is shown in Box 17.4.

MOVEMENT DISORDERS

Movement disorders may be divided into:
- *hypokinetic* disorders, where there is too little movement, e.g. parkinsonism.
- *hyperkinetic* disorders, where there are additional involuntary movements (tremor, chorea, dystonia, tics and myoclonus).

Idiopathic Parkinson's disease (PD)

PD is a neurodegenerative disorder affecting nigrostriatal dopaminergic cells, as well as other brain cell populations.
- The diagnosis is clinical and based on the presence of distinctive motor features: tremor (resting, 'pill-rolling'), rigidity, hypokinesia (poverty of movement — the sine qua non of Parkinsonism) and postural changes (stooped posture, shuffling gait, reduced arm swing, impaired balance).
- Patients may have hypophonia, reduced facial expression and impaired dexterity, e.g. manifesting as micrographia. Non-motor features, such as anosmia, diffuse aches and pains and rapid eye movement (REM) sleep behaviour disorder, may precede development of motor symptoms by many years. Symptoms and signs are initially unilateral, becoming bilateral as the disease progresses. Check for use of neuroleptic, antiemetic or other drugs causing Parkinsonism, e.g. **valproate**. In patients under the age of 50, exclude Wilson's disease (p. 193).
- A dopamine transporter (DaT) scan may occasionally be useful to confirm nigrostriatal dopaminergic cell loss in patients with atypical tremor where diagnosis is uncertain.

Medical treatment (Table 17.3)
Dopamine replacement with a dopamine agonist or L-dopa (LD) (combined with a dopa decarboxylase inhibitor (DDI) — **benserazide, co-beneldopa**) is the mainstay of pharmacological therapy. There is no conclusive evidence that any of the currently available drugs is neuroprotective. Antiparkinsonian drugs should be initiated at low dose and titrated gradually to the minimum dose required for adequate symptom control.
- Initial medical treatment. Exercise and physiotherapy are useful. Initiate pharmacological treatment when there is impairment/disability resulting from symptoms. Early treatment with monoamine oxidase B

Kumar & Clark's Medical Management and Therapeutics

Box 17.4 Status epilepticus management

Remember:
- Accuracy of diagnosis — ensure not pseudo-status epilepticus
- Treat convulsions quickly
- Continued ICU monitoring and cardiorespiratory support

Several treatment schedules exist:
- At home, give immediate benzodiazepines, e.g. diazepam (10–20 mg) orally or buccal midazolam 10 mg, and repeat once if necessary. If oral route impossible, give rectal diazepam
- Arrange immediate admission to hospital
- Administer oxygen, monitor ECG, BP, routine bloods (include alcohol level, glucose, calcium, magnesium, drug screen, anticonvulsant levels)
- Correct hypoglycaemia if found
- Give thiamine IV (250 mg) if nutrition is poor or excess alcohol use suspected. (In the UK, give vitamin B and C, high-potency ampoules, one pair IV over 10 mins). Beware anaphylaxis with IV thiamine
- Anti-epileptic drugs (AEDs):
  1. Give lorazepam IV 4 mg at 2 mg/min
  2. Reinstate previous AEDs. Measure levels urgently. Has the patient had phenytoin recently?
  3. If status continues, IV phenytoin or fosphenytoin is used:
     a) Phenytoin: give 15 mg/kg IV diluted to 10 mg/mL in 0.9% saline into a large vein at ≤ 50 mg/min (Phenytoin 250 mg 5 mL ampoule)
     b) Fosphenytoin: this is a pro-drug of phenytoin and can be given faster than phenytoin. Doses are expressed in phenytoin equivalents (PE): fosphenytoin 1.5 mg = 1 mg phenytoin Give 15 mg/kg (PE) fosphenytoin (15 mg × 1.5 = 22.5 mg) diluted to 10 mg/mL in 0.9% saline at 50–100 mg (PE)/min (Fosphenytoin sodium 750 mg 10 mL ampoule)
  4. If status continues, give phenobarbital 10 mg/kg diluted 1 in 10 in water for injection at ≤ 100 mg/min. (Phenobarbital 200 mg/mL 1 mL vial in propylene glycol 90% with water for injection 10%.) IV clonazepam, valproate or levetiracetam are alternative AEDs that can be administered
  5. If status persists, use thiopental or propofol anaesthesia with assisted ventilation and transfer patient to ICU. Alternative sedatives include lorazepam or midazolam infusions
- EEG monitoring is valuable if there is doubt about the nature of status and to monitor for burst suppression pattern
- Search for an underlying cause and treat appropriately
- Complications of status epilepticus, including acidosis, aspiration pneumonia, rhabdomyolysis and acute kidney injury also need addressing
- Patients require continuous monitoring until status epilepticus is controlled
- Remember: 25% of apparent status turns out to be pseudo-status

Table 17.3 Drugs used in Parkinson's disease

Dopamine receptor agonists	Day dose		Major side-effects
	Initial	Maximum	
Ergot-derived			
Bromocriptine Cabergoline Pergolide	Non-ergot derivatives preferred		Ergot-derived; associated with pulmonary, retroperitoneal and pericardial fibrosis. Valvular fibrosis
Non-ergot-derived			
Pramipexole	88 mcg (base) 3 times daily (doubled every 5–7 days if tolerated) oral	3.3 mg 3 times daily	All cause sudden onset of sleep. Increase dose slowly. Hypotensive in first few days of treatment (pramipexole). Gastrointestinal — nausea, vomiting, abdominal pain, constipation, diarrhoea Hallucinations, dizziness. Behavioural changes — pathological gambling, increased libido. Do not withdraw abruptly
Ropinirole	250 mcg 3 times daily (double dose weekly to 3 mg) XL formulation now available	9–16 mg	
Rotigotine	*Monotherapy:* Oral 2 mg/24 hr patch applied to dry skin. Remove after 24 hr and replace on different site	4 mg/24 hr	
	Adjunctive therapy with levodopa 4 mg/24 hr patch	16 mg/24 hr	

Table 17.3 Continued

Dopamine receptor agonists	Day dose		Major side-effects
	Initial	Maximum	
Levodopa complex			
Co-beneldopa	50 mg 3–4 times daily (expressed as levodopa) Increase by 100 1–2 times weekly	100–800 mg	Nausea, vomiting (treat with domperidone). Dry mouth. Anorexia, postural hypotension. Drowsiness (sudden onset of sleep). Dementia, psychosis, depression. Response fluctuations and dyskinesis. 'On'/'off' periods. End-of-dose deterioration
Co-careldopa	100 mg 3 times daily Increase by 50–100 mg to at least 700 mg	800 mg	
Monoamine oxidase B inhibitors			
Rasagiline	1 mg		Dry mouth, dyspepsia, constipation, hallucinations, headache, weight loss. Urinary urgency (rasagiline)
Selegiline	10 mg		
Catechol-O-methyltransferase inhibitors			
Entacapone	200 mg	2 g	Nausea, vomiting, abdominal pain, constipation, diarrhoea, urine discoloration (reddish-brown), dizziness, confusion, dyskinesia. Hepatotoxicity — potentially life-threatening (tolcapone)
Tolcapone	100 mg 3 times daily	2 g	

(MAOB) inhibitors (**selegiline** or **rasagiline**) may delay the need for more definitive dopamine replacement therapy by several months.

- **Dopamine receptor agonists (DAs)** are used, particularly in younger patients (e.g. below age 70, but depends on individual patient needs). Although less efficacious in symptom control than LD and generally less well tolerated, initial DA monotherapy may be associated with fewer long-term motor complications. Start LD + DDI (**co-beneldopa** or **co-careldopa**) in older patients or those more severely affected at diagnosis.
- Non-ergot DAs (**pramipexole** and **ropinirole** oral 3 times daily, or once daily with slow-release formulations, **rotigotine** via transdermal patch) are used in preference to ergot-derived drugs.
- All patients with PD will eventually require treatment with LD, often in combination with a DA. A typical starting dose is 50 mg of LD (e.g. **co-careldopa** 62.5 mg) 3 times daily, increasing after 1 week to 100 mg 3 times daily.
- LD absorption after protein-rich meals is unpredictable and taking doses at least 40 mins prior to meals may be helpful.
- Use **domperidone** as an antiemetic (20 mg 3 times daily) when initiating DA therapy. Other antiemetics may exacerbate parkinsonism by blocking central dopamine receptors.

● **Subsequent medical treatment.** As the disease progresses, medical therapy for PD becomes more difficult. Higher doses of dopamine replacement therapy are required and response becomes more unpredictable with the development of motor fluctuations and dyskinesias. Approximately 10% of patients per year develop motor complications in the form of 'wearing off' (the duration of effect of individual doses of LD becomes progressively shorter), dyskinesias (involuntary choreiform movements) and, eventually, 'on/off' phenomenon (sudden, unpredictable transitions from mobile to immobile). Eventually, patients may alternate between the 'on' state with dopamine-induced dyskinesias and periods of complete immobility ('off').

● **Motor complications.** Management of the motor complications of treatment is difficult. Dose fractionation of LD, increasing dose frequency and introduction of a catechol-O-methyl transferase (COMT) inhibitor (**entacapone** or **tolcapone**) improve motor control for 'end-of-dose deterioration'. **Entacapone** is also available as a combined preparation with LD and carbidopa. Controlled-release preparations of LD are generally not used during the day owing to slow onset of action and unpredictable response. However, slow-release LD is still often used in the management of overnight symptoms.

Other drugs used to treat PD

● MAOB inhibitors such as **selegiline** and **rasagiline** have a mild symptomatic effect (see above).
● Amantadine 100–200 mg once or twice daily has a modest antiparkinsonian effect but may improve dyskinesias in advanced disease. Amantadine should not be taken after 2 p.m. as it may disturb sleep.
● Antimuscarinics (e.g. **trihexyphenidyl** up to 15 mg daily) may help tremor in particular but are now rarely used in PD except in younger patients. They often cause confusion in older patients.
● Apomorphine (SC pump 1–4 mg/hour during daytime; maximum dose 100 mg) is a potent, short-acting, DA administered subcutaneously by

Kumar & Clark's Medical Management and Therapeutics

an auto-injector pen as intermittent 'rescue' injection for 'off' periods or by continuous infusion pump. It is used in advanced PD.

● A formulation of LD administered by continuous infusion via a jejunostomy tube is used in patients with advanced disease but availability is limited by high cost.

Surgical treatment

Deep brain stimulation (DBS), particularly bilateral insertion of electrodes into the subthalamic nucleus or globus pallidus, is increasingly used to treat advanced PD where medical treatment causes severe motor fluctuations and dyskinesias. Efficacy is equivalent to LD treatment but drug-induced complications such as dyskinesias improve after drug reduction or withdrawal.

Non-motor complications

Eventually, postural instability, falls, swallowing problems and other LD-unresponsive problems may develop. **Fludrocortisone** may help with postural hypotension. Cognitive impairment and dementia become a significant problem in advanced disease and respond to cholinesterase inhibitors, e.g. **rivastigmine** (start 1.5 mg up to 3–6 mg twice daily). Treating depression (present in up to 50% of patients) with a selective serotonin reuptake inhibitor (SSRI) is one of the interventions that most improves quality of life in PD. Access to skilled physiotherapy, occupational therapy and nurse specialists is necessary throughout the course of the disease.

Hyperkinetic movement disorders

Benign essential tremor

This describes symmetrical postural tremor of hands e.g. holding a cup or cutlery; sometimes head or voice tremor occurs. There is usually a long history by the time of presentation and a family history is common. Tremor may improve with alcohol. **Treatment** is with a β-blocker, e.g. **propranolol** 80–240 mg of slow release or 40 mg 3 times daily, or **primidone** — start at 62.5 mg daily and gradually increase; maximum dose 750 mg daily, often poorly tolerated. Rarely, thalamic DBS is required if tremor is severe.

Chorea

Chorea is jerky, dance-like, involuntary movements that 'flit' from one body part to another. When chorea is mild, the patient may appear 'fidgety'. Causes include systemic disease (thyrotoxicosis, SLE, primary polycythaemia, rheumatic fever — Sydenham's chorea), drugs (e.g. LD and OCP), pregnancy and Huntington's disease. **Treatment** involves dopamine-blocking and depleting drugs, which may reduce chorea. **Tetrabenazine** depletes neurones of dopamine (starting dose 12.5 mg twice daily, increasing to 12.5–25 mg 3 times daily; maximum dose 200 mg/day) but may be limited by development of depression and parkinsonism. Neuroleptic drugs such as **sulpiride** 200–400 mg twice daily, which block dopamine receptors, are also used.

Dystonia

Dystonia is painless muscle spasms causing twisting movements and abnormal postures. Childhood-onset dystonia is often genetic or due to a structural brain abnormality (e.g. birth asphyxia) and is more likely to become generalized. Late-onset dystonia is commoner, usually sporadic and more likely to remain localized to one body part, particularly the cranio-cervical region, e.g. blepharospasm or torticollis. Task-specific forms may occur, e.g. writer's cramp or occupational dystonias, especially in musicians. **Treatment** of focal dystonia is by IM injection of **botulinum toxin**. Duration of effect is approximately 3 months.

- Dopa-responsive dystonia is a genetic disorder that responds dramatically to low doses of **LD**; a trial of treatment should be considered in cases of early-onset dystonia (< 30 years of age).
- Acute dystonic reactions (e.g. trismus, spasmodic torticollis, oculogyric crises) may occur after even a single administration of a dopamine receptor antagonist, e.g. phenothiazines, butyrophenones and metoclopramide. Treat with an IV antimuscarinic, e.g. **benzatropine** 1–2 mg IV or **procyclidine** 5–10 mg IV. Tardive dystonia may follow prolonged use of neuroleptic medications in psychiatric practice.

Myoclonus

Sudden involuntary jerks of a single muscle or a group of muscles may cause patients to drop what they are holding or fall to the floor (negative myoclonus). Myoclonus may be part of epilepsy (e.g. juvenile myoclonic epilepsy) or encephalopathies and a wide variety of neurological disorders. Drugs such as **clonazepam**, **levetiracetam** or **valproate** can be useful.

HEADACHE

The history is often sufficient to differentiate between common primary headache syndromes and more sinister, but rare, secondary headache.

Acute single episode of headache

If the headache is associated with drowsiness or neck stiffness, meningitis (p. 54), encephalitis (p. 55) and subarachnoid haemorrhage (p. 634) must be excluded. Sudden-onset thunderclap headache is suggestive of SAH. The incidence of serious secondary causes of headache is higher in A&E attenders than in general practice.

- Examination should include GCS, temperature, BP, neck stiffness, a check for any focal neurological signs, and fundoscopy (papilloedema is a late sign of raised ICP).
- Investigations include ESR, CT scan and lumbar puncture, if necessary (check opening pressure; send for microscopy, protein, glucose (with matched blood glucose for ?meningitis) and xanthochromia if SAH is a possibility)

Primary headache disorders

Migraine

There is a high population prevalence (~10–15%, F > M). Migraine usually starts in the teenage or early adult years and rarely starts after age 40. The headache is typically:

- moderate or severe
- throbbing
- hemicranial or holocranial
- made worse by head movements or exertion
- associated with features such as nausea, photophobia, phonophobia and osmophobia
- lasts usually from 4 hours to 3 days.

Migraine is due to changes in the brainstem blood flow which cause release of vasoactive peptides leading to neurogenic inflammation which produces the pain. Migraine without aura is more common than migraine with aura (25%) and those who experience auras usually do not have aura before each attack. Aura occurs before the onset of the headache and should last no longer than 1 hour. Visual aura is more common than sensory aura or dysphasia. Weakness (hemiplegic migraine) is rare. Typically, aura consists of positive and negative symptoms (shimmering, bright lights, fragmented images with scotomas or other visual field defects such as hemianopia) and usually evolves, changing over minutes. Migraine aura without subsequent headache (acephalic migraine) may occur in older patients and be confused with TIA.

- Acute treatment. **Paracetamol** 1 g, **aspirin** 900 mg (dispersible formulation) or an NSAID, e.g. **ibuprofen** 400–600 mg, **naproxen** 500 mg or **tolfenamic acid** 200 mg rapid release, is given, as early as possible during an attack. Gastric emptying is reduced during the attack so dispersible formulations are preferred. Antiemetics (e.g. **metoclopramide** 10 mg or **domperidone** 10 mg) are also usually required, both to promote absorption of analgesics and reduce nausea. Combined tablets are available. If these measures are ineffective, use a 5-hydroxytryptamine (5HT)$_{1B}$/$_{1D}$ serotonin receptor agonist (**triptan**). These drugs relieve both the pain and the nausea. Triptans should be avoided in patients with vascular disease or uncontrolled/severe hypertension. Triptans should not be given too early (e.g. during the aura phase), as they may be ineffective at that point. They should be given at the onset of the headache. There are several triptans available with a spectrum of efficacy, including:
  - *Sumatriptan* 25–100 mg at onset of headache, repeat if necessary after at least 2 hours, max. 300 mg in 24 hours; SC 6 mg sumatriptan produces highest efficacy and most rapid response.
  - *Zolmitriptan* 2.5 mg at onset, repeat if only partial response after 2 hours; 5 mg also available.
  - *Rizatriptan* 10 mg at onset, repeat after 2 hours if only partial response.
  - *Naratriptan* 2.5 mg at onset, repeat after 4 hours if only partial response; has placebo level side-effects but probably lower efficacy than other triptans. It is used when other triptans are not tolerated.
  - *Almotriptan* 12.5 mg at onset, repeat after 2 hours if necessary, max. 25 g in 24 hours.
  - *Eletriptan* 40 mg at onset, repeat after 2 hours if necessary, max. 80 g in 24 hours.
  - *Frovatriptan* 2.5 mg at onset, repeat after 2 hours if necessary, max. 5 g in 24 hours.
  - *Oro-dispersible formulations* exist for some triptans but absorption is slower. **Nasal spray** formulations also exist (but **sumatriptan** spray is not recommended in vomiting as absorption depends on ingestion; **zolmitriptan** spray is partially absorbed in the mouth).

If there is no response to an initial dose, do not persist with subsequent doses during the same attack; the drug may be effective in subsequent attacks, however. Ergotamine and derivatives are no longer recommended except in specialist headache clinics. Avoid the use of opiate-based drugs.

- Women and migraine
  - Combined oral contraceptives may provoke or exacerbate migraine, necessitating withdrawal or a switch to a progesterone-only pill. The OCP may be effective in menstrual migraine.

- Women with migraine and aura should not take an oestrogen-containing OCP and should be advised not to smoke owing to increased stroke risk.
- In pregnancy migraine may improve. Paracetamol is safe as acute treatment.

- **Treatment of frequent migraine and chronic migraine.** Trigger factors to be avoided include stress and 'let-down' after a stressful period, lack (or excess) of sleep, missing meals, alcohol and bright light. Individual foods are rarely a trigger. Analgesic overuse must be stopped (see below). Migraine suppression medication is underused and should be advised if frequency of migraine is more than twice per month or one disabling attack per month.
  - *Propranolol LA,* a β-blocker, 80 mg increasing according to response (**atenolol**, **metoprolol** and **bisoprolol** are also used).
  - *Sodium valproate* 200 mg twice daily, increasing after 1 week to 400 mg twice daily. Higher doses may be required. Women must be warned about potential teratogenicity.
  - *Topiramate* 25 mg at night, increasing by 25 mg every 2 weeks to 50 mg twice daily. Women must be warned about potential teratogenicity.
  - *Amitriptyline* 10 mg at night, increasing by 10 mg per week to 50–70 mg.
  - *Serotonin antagonists:* **pizotifen** is occasionally used but may cause weight gain.
  - *Methysergide* is rarely used because of side-effects (retroperitoneal, heart valve and pleural fibrosis). If methysergide is initiated, this should be under the supervision of a specialist headache clinic.

Medication overuse headache

Regular use of analgesics, especially codeine-containing combinations, on two or more days per week over several months will lead to chronic headache. This occurs particularly in those with a primary headache disorder such as migraine. It is a common problem in clinical practice and complete withdrawal from analgesics is needed for prophylactic drugs to be effective. Patients should be warned that their headache will worsen for 2–3 weeks after cessation of medication, before starting to improve.

Giant cell arteritis

See p. 319.

Cluster headache

- There is **severe, strictly unilateral** pain centred around one eye.
- It is more common in men.
- Associated autonomic features include lacrimation, red eye, rhinor-rhoea and ptosis.
- Patients are restless and agitated, tending to walk around with the pain (in contrast to migraine).
- Attacks last 15 mins to 3 hours and occur several times in 24 hours, typically at night ('alarm clock headache'). Attacks occur in clusters lasting weeks with long periods (up to years) of complete remission between.
- Analgesics are rarely helpful. Abortive treatment with SC **sumatriptan** or 100% oxygen at 7–12 L/min can be effective. A short course of high-dose steroids may also be tried at the start of a cluster. Prevention of the cluster is with **verapamil/lithium carbonate**. Patients should have an

Kumar & Clark's Medical Management and Therapeutics

ECG prior to starting verapamil and with each dose increase. Very high doses of verapamil may be required. Avoid alcohol during clusters.

- Paroxysmal hemicrania is a rare form of headache with shorter, more frequent, but also very severe bouts of headache and is a differential for cluster headache. It is more common in women. Unlike cluster headache, paroxysmal hemicrania is **indometacin**-responsive (25 mg 3 times daily, increased up to a maximum of 75 mg 3 times daily).

Idiopathic stabbing headache

There are paroxysms of sharp, well-localized, momentary pain. It may move from place to place or be localized to one spot. Idiopathic stabbing headache is common in migraineurs. Treatment is usually not required but responds to **indometacin**.

Idiopathic intracranial hypertension

This mainly affects young, overweight women who present with high-pressure headache (worse on lying flat) and visual obscurations or visual field deficits. Examination may reveal reduced acuity, visual field constriction and papilloedema on fundoscopy. Investigations include MRI/MR venography to exclude a mass lesion and venous sinus thrombosis. If lumbar puncture confirms high opening pressure (> 25 cmH$_2$O) with normal CSF constituents, then treat as idiopathic intracranial hypertension. Treatment is to advise weight loss and initiate acetazolamide 250 mg twice daily (may increase up to 500 mg twice daily). Bendroflumethazide 2.5 mg is an alternative. Repeated lumbar puncture is also used. If, despite these measures, visual acuity worsens, then refer for surgical intervention (e.g. ventriculo-peritoneal shunt, lumbo-peritoneal shunt, optic nerve fenestration).

Low-pressure headache

- This is similar to post-lumbar puncture headache but may occur spontaneously due to a CSF leak, e.g. after coughing, straining or exercise.
- The postural nature, with resolution immediately after lying flat, is the characteristic feature.
- Gadolinium-enhanced MRI may show meningeal enhancement; CSF radionuclide tracer studies may be needed to identify a leak.
- IV caffeine may be tried; an autologous epidural blood patch close to the site of the spinal leak can be helpful.
- Patients presenting with spontaneous low-pressure headache should be screened for autoimmune rheumatic disorders.

Facial pain

Trigeminal neuralgia

- Trigeminal neuralgia is usually primary but can be secondary to demyelination (MS) or other posterior fossa inflammatory/structural disorders.
- There are intense stabs of lancinating pain in the distribution of one or more branches of the trigeminal nerve. A facial trigger point is often present.
- **Carbamazepine** 100–400 mg/8 h or **oxcarbazepine** 300 mg twice daily (for more rapid titration) can be effective in reducing the frequency and severity of attacks. **Gabapentin**, **lamotrigine** and **phenytoin** are also used.

- MRI scanning with dedicated sequences to look for neurovascular compromise is useful.
- Surgery (trigeminal ganglion destructive procedures or posterior fossa microvascular decompression) is the treatment of choice if response to medication is inadequate or not maintained.

BENIGN PAROXYSMAL POSITIONAL VERTIGO

'Dizziness' means different things to different people. True vertigo indicates an illusion of movement, typically spinning. The commonest cause is benign paroxysmal positional vertigo, which may follow head injury or ear infection. The Hallpike test is diagnostic, with torsional nystagmus seen. The Epley particle repositioning manœuvre may be curative. Cawthorne–Cooksey exercises/vestibular rehabilitation are preferred to vestibular sedatives (http://www.dizziness-and-balance.com/disorders/bppv/bppv.html; www.dizziness-and-balance.com/treatment/rehab/cawthorne.html).

TRAUMATIC BRAIN INJURY

Head injury is common. Most cases are mild, but severe injuries carry a high morbidity and mortality.

Severe head injury

Immediate management

- Initially, ensure that the patient is resuscitated (see coma, p. 627). Site IV access. Immobilize the neck in a stiff collar. Avoid nasal intubation if there are facial fractures. Emergency tracheostomy may be needed. Avoid hypoventilation and hypotension, as these can worsen cerebral perfusion.
- Examination must include a search for penetrating injuries and wounds. CSF otorrhoea/rhinorrhoea suggests a base of skull fracture.
- Document GCS (Table 17.1) and any neurological deficits. Perform serial examinations to detect signs of deterioration early.
- Indications for immediate intubation include:
  - GCS < 8/15
  - loss of protective laryngeal reflexes
  - Pa_{O_2} < 9 kPa on air; Pa_{CO_2} > 6 kPa
  - spontaneous hyperventilation resulting in Pa_{CO_2} < 3.5 kPa.
- Immediate CT head, including bone windows, is needed to look for fractures or signs of intracranial haemorrhage if the patient exhibits any of the following:
  - GCS < 13 at any point since injury
  - GCS 13–14 at 2 hours post injury
  - suspected skull fracture — the risk of intracranial haemorrhage is increased with skull fracture
  - evidence of possible skull-base fracture, e.g. haemotympanium, CSF otorrhoea
  - more than one episode of vomiting
  - post-injury seizure
  - post-injury focal neurological deficit
  - post-injury retrograde amnesia of > 30 mins (requires imaging within 8 hours of event).

CT scanning is also required if the patient is > 65 years old or on antico-agulants, or if there was a dangerous mechanism of injury. Head injury is often associated with trauma to the cervical spine. Imaging of the cervical spine is essential to exclude fracture or dislocation.

Further management

Most patients with severe head injury and/or, for example, contusion, intracranial haematoma, cervical or skull fracture, penetrating injury (do not remove the foreign object), focal neurological deficit, persisting coma (GCS < 8), unexplained confusion > 4 hours, seizure without full recovery or CSF leak require prompt neurosurgical consultation and subsequent neurosurgical management.

- The aim is to maintain the patient with a well-perfused and well-oxygenated brain. Maintain cerebral perfusion pressure (mean arterial pressure minus intracranial pressure; estimate ICP at 30 mmHg if unknown) > 70 mmHg using ionotropes if necessary. Nurse the patient head up at a 10–15° angle. Keep Pao_2 > 15 kPa and $Paco_2$ < 4.5 kPa if possible.
- Duration of post-traumatic amnesia (PTA) is one of the most useful indicators of severity of brain injury and long-term prognosis. It presents as a confusional state and agitation following head injury and lasts until the patient is able to make and retain new memories. Nursing a confused patient in PTA is often difficult.

Late complications

Late complications following significant traumatic brain injury include incomplete recovery (hemiparesis, cognitive impairment), post-traumatic epilepsy, depression, benign paroxysmal positional vertigo, chronic sub-dural haematoma (p. 635), hydrocephalus and chronic traumatic encepha-lopathy. Patients with persisting deficits may require specialist rehabilitation on a dedicated rehabilitation unit.

Less severe head injury

Management

Some patients are discharged from A&E into the care of a responsible adult. These patients should have a GCS of 15 at time of discharge and give no cause for clinical concern. They should only be discharged when it is certain that there is someone to supervise them. The carer must be given written documentation on how to observe the patient and in which circumstances to return to the hospital.

Admission to hospital is indicated in patients with new, significant abnormalities on imaging, GCS < 15 after imaging, ongoing vomiting, severe headache or other concerns (e.g. drug or alcohol intoxication, men-ingism, CSF leak), or if the patient warrants CT imaging but this cannot be performed promptly.

Patients who are alert and awake with no neurological deficit are moni-tored in hospital for 24 hours. Observations should be recorded every 30 mins until GCS = 15 and then half-hourly for 2 hours, hourly for 4 hours and 2-hourly thereafter. Any neurological deterioration after head injury warrants further brain imaging to look for haemorrhage or expanding haematoma. MRI is more sensitive than CT and will better allow for detec-tion of shallow intrinsic and extra-axial blood collections, as well as diffuse axonal injury.

DISEASES OF THE SPINAL CORD

The spinal cord extends from C1 to the lower border of L1. Below L1 the spinal canal is occupied by the cauda equina and compressive lesions cause a radiculopathy (lower motor neurone syndrome). **Paraparesis** (weakness of both legs) is usually due to a spinal cord lesion (occasionally a parasagittal tumour). **Quadriparesis** (weakness of arms and legs) is often due to a cervical cord lesion.

Spinal cord syndromes

Presentation is with motor and sensory involvement below the level of the lesion. Compression causes weakness of both legs and the sphincters may be involved. Look for motor and sensory level; the lesion may be several segments above the sensory level. Pain and spinal tenderness (abscess or vertebral collapse) often occur at the level of the lesion and radicular pain may radiate bilaterally at the level of lesion. Acute lesions (trauma, infarction) cause initial spinal shock with flaccid paraparesis and areflexia. Spasticity and hyperreflexia take weeks to develop.

Acute cord syndrome presenting as an emergency

- Stabilize the neck and move the patient with extreme caution after trauma, until spinal instability is excluded.
- Urgent MRI of the **whole spinal cord** is necessary.
- Contact the neurosurgeons to forewarn them about a possible need for decompression.
- If cord compression is confirmed, start high-dose steroids pre-operatively, e.g. **dexamethasone** 10 mg IV, followed by 4 mg IV 4 times daily. If MRI is normal or suggests myelitis, proceed to lumbar puncture to look for inflammatory cells and elevated protein.

Patients need regular turning and skin care to prevent pressure sores. Urinary catheterization is usually required. Physiotherapy may help prevent contractures. In the chronic stage, spasticity may respond to **baclofen** 5 mg 3 times daily or **tizanidine** 2 mg daily (max. 36 mg).

Cauda equina syndrome

Cauda equina syndrome is a neurosurgical emergency. Central prolapse of a lumbar disc into the lumbar canal is the usual cause, but a chronic form may result from degenerative lumbar canal stenosis or benign tumours.

- Bilateral radicular pain radiating into both legs with severe low back pain is a 'red flag' symptom for cauda equina compression from disc prolapse, as is impairment of sphincter or sexual function in the context of back pain.
- **Examination** reveals bilateral foot weakness with weakness of hip extension and knee flexion, reflex loss in ankles and/or knees, saddle anaesthesia and a palpable bladder.
- Urgent (immediate) MRI of the lumbar spine and surgical decompression are required.

MULTIPLE SCLEROSIS

Multiple sclerosis (MS), an autoimmune disorder causing T- and B-cell dysfunction, is characterized by episodes of demyelination that are disseminated in time and space throughout the CNS. Patients usually present

Kumar & Clark's Medical Management and Therapeutics

with discrete episodes (relapsing–remitting type) and after many years may develop gradually progressive disability without relapses (secondary progressive). Clinical features of a relapse depend on the site affected but often consist of a combination of positive and negative sensory symptoms, weakness, ataxia, myelitis or episodes of optic neuritis, usually evolving over days and resolving fully or partially over weeks. Optic neuritis is inflammation of the nerve with disc swelling and causes visual loss. Retrobulbar neuritis refers to inflammation behind the disc causing visual loss but with no ophthalmoscopic signs.

Investigations

- MRI is very sensitive for the presence of demyelinating plaques in brain or spinal cord, most of which are clinically silent. Distinguishing white matter lesions on MRI from other pathologies e.g. ischaemic lesions, is occasionally difficult. In patients presenting with a clinically isolated syndrome suggestive of demyelination with no relevant previous neurological history, the presence of asymptomatic white matter lesions on brain MRI predicts the subsequent development of MS.
- Visual evoked potentials can be useful to detect subclinical optic nerve involvement.
- CSF analysis is seldom necessary. Mononuclear cells are raised. Oligoclonal IgG bands are present in 80% due to intrathecal synthesis.

Symptomatic treatment

Treat acute relapses with high-dose steroids (1 g **methylprednisolone IV** daily for 3 days with proton pump inhibitor (PPI) cover). Symptomatic treatment includes:

- **baclofen** 5 mg 3 times daily (max. 100 mg/day) or **tizanidine** 2 mg daily (max. 36 mg/day; monitor LFTs) for severe spasticity
- treatment of neuropathic pain, e.g. **gabapentin**
- antimuscarinics (e.g. **oxybutinin** or **tolterodine** 2 mg twice daily) for detrusor instability
- intermittent self-catheterization for incomplete bladder emptying.

Physiotherapy, occupational therapy and social worker input are necessary, as is education about the condition, often by nurse specialists.

Disease-modifying treatments

- Interferon-β or glatiramer acetate by injection (SC or IM) reduces relapse rate by one-third (severe relapses by half) but the effect on progression of disability is uncertain. Patients with relapsing–remitting MS who can still walk at least 100 metres unaided and who have had at least two clinically significant relapses in the previous 2 years should be referred to a specialist multiple sclerosis clinic for consideration of disease modifying drugs (DMD). Treatment with DMD after a clinically isolated syndrome delays time to second relapse but is not routine practice.
- Natalizumab is a monoclonal antibody that inhibits migration of leucocytes into the CNS via inhibitory α4 integrins on the surface of lymphocytes and monocytes. It is used in severe relapsing–remitting MS. There is an increased risk of progressive multifocal leucoencephalopathy with this treatment.
- Alemtuzumab, an anti-CD52 monoclonal antibody that destroys T- and B-cells, reduces disease activity.
- Mitoxantrone may be used in primary progressive MS in specialist centres. It is potentially cardiotoxic and myelosuppressive.

- New oral DMDs, e.g. **fingolimod**, a sphingosine-1-phosphate receptor modulator, and **cladribine**, an immunomodulator of lymphocytes, have shown benefit in ongoing trials.

DISORDERS OF THE NEUROMUSCULAR JUNCTION

Myasthenia gravis (MG)

MG is an acquired autoimmune disease involving antibody-mediated disruption of post-synaptic nicotinic acetylcholine receptors at the neuromuscular junction. Weakness principally affects extra-ocular, bulbar and limb muscles. The hallmark is **fatigability** (e.g. difficulty with prolonged upgaze, voice becomes weaker on counting to 50). It may be limited to ptosis and diplopia (ocular MG) or generalized, affecting limb and respiratory/bulbar muscles.

Diagnostic investigations

- Anti-acetylcholine receptor antibodies are found in up to 90% of cases with generalized MG (only 30% in pure ocular MG); anti-MuSK antibodies (antibodies against muscle-specific tyrosine kinase) are found in up to 50% of patients that are anti-acetylcholine receptor antibody negative.
- Neurophysiology studies show decrement in compound muscle action potential after repetitive motor nerve stimulation and jitter and block on single-fibre EMG.
- CT thorax is required to exclude thymoma.
- Tensilon test has a high incidence of false positives and is no longer used. Edrophonium is not available in many countries.

Treatment

- Plasmapheresis or IV immunoglobulin 0.4 g/kg for 5 days is used for immediate control of myasthenic crisis.
- Acetylcholinesterase inhibitors have a modest symptomatic effect. **Pyridostigmine** initiated at 30–60 mg × 4 daily can be gradually increased up to 1.2 g daily, although doses of > 450 mg/day may be associated with acetylcholine receptor down-regulation. Co-administration of **propantheline** 15 mg may be required to reduce muscarinic side-effects such as colic, diarrhoea and excess salivation.
- Immunosuppression is required in most cases of generalized MG. Owing to a dip in function shortly after commencement of steroids, initiation of steroids should generally be carried out with the patient admitted to hospital. Start steroids slowly, as rapid titration may also paradoxically exacerbate weakness. In generalized MG start **prednisolone** at 10 mg on alternate days, increasing 10 mg every alternate day to a ceiling dose of 1–2 mg/kg on alternate days. Once the patient enters remission (often after 2–6 months), wean prednisolone to the minimum therapeutic dose (usually 10–40 mg on alternate days). Steroids may be combined with acetylcholinesterase inhibitors. Initiate PPI and osteoporosis prophylaxis with steroid therapy (p. 324). **Azathioprine** (titrate up to 2–2.5 mg/kg/day) is a steroid-sparing immunosuppressive agent that takes up to 6 months for full effect. Measure thiopurine S-methyltransferase (TPMT) assay for susceptibility to toxicity before therapy. Monitor FBC and liver biochemistry (every week for 8 weeks, then every 3 months while on azathioprine). In refractory patients **ciclosporin**, **methotrexate** or **mycophenolate** are used.

● **Thymectomy** is required in patients < 60 years old and with moderate–severe disease once in remission. If thymoma is found on CT, always proceed to thymectomy; in these cases, however, thymectomy does not induce remission, as it does in patients with thymic hyperplasia.

Myasthenic crisis

Respiratory infection or other stressors, e.g. surgery, can precipitate crisis. Monitor respiratory function closely with lying and sitting FVC. Alert the ICU and ventilate if the FVC is < 15 mL/kg. If ventilation is required, withdraw anticholinesterases temporarily (this removes the uncertainty of a possible overdosage leading to cholinergic crisis and depolarizing block). If the patient is ventilated, it is possible to start steroids at high dose (start at 1.5 mg/kg/day; max. 100 mg daily). Plasmapheresis or IVIG is usually also required.

Botulism

Toxin produced by *Clostridium botulinum* leads to cranial nerve palsies, weakness and autonomic symptoms, e.g. dry mouth, due to parasympathetic block. Botulism may mimic MG. Food-borne botulism is now rare but wound botulism in IV drug users is on the increase due to 'skin popping' (injection of heroin contaminated with *C. botulinum* spores into anaerobic skin abscesses). Neutralize toxin by administration of the botulism antitoxin and debride abscesses.

DEMENTIA

Dementia is defined as progressive impairment of intellect, affecting more than one cognitive domain (usually including memory) and sufficient to impair day-to-day functioning. It is necessary to exclude clouding of consciousness, indicating delirium. The prevalence increases sharply with age, 25% of the over-80s being affected. Alzheimer's disease (AD) is by far the most common cause, followed by multi-infarct dementia.

Clinical assessment

This is directed at determining whether the patient has significant cognitive impairment, identifying treatable causes and attempting to make a clinico-pathological diagnosis to guide treatment and indicate prognosis.

A definitive diagnosis can only be made by pathological examination of brain tissue, which is not usually necessary.

Clinical diagnosis is based on history (particularly a corollary history from a family member, as patients may be unaware of their difficulties), examination (especially cognitive testing, including the mini-mental state examination (MMSE) or the more comprehensive Addenbrookes Cognitive Estimate) and investigations.

● **History.** Ask about temporal gradient in episodic memory ('forgets what happened yesterday but remembers what happened 40 years ago'), personality change (possible fronto-temporal dementia), language function, calculation, visuo-spatial function (e.g. 'do you get lost?'), praxis (e.g. dressing dyspraxia), visual hallucinations (dementia with Lewy bodies), effect on functioning, tempo of progression and family history.

● **Quantitative psychometric testing** by a psychologist is invaluable in identifying the cognitive domains affected and providing a baseline against which to measure future progression in mild cognitive impairment.

Treatable causes for dementia are rare. Investigate all patients (see below). Additional tests may be required in younger patients and those with rapid progression. Depression can present as 'pseudo-dementia' and is treatable.

Investigations
- All patients
  - *Bloods:* perform FBC, ESR, U&E, liver biochemistry, glucose, calcium, thyroid function tests, syphilis serology, B_{12} and folate.
  - *Brain imaging:* CT is sufficient to reveal hydrocephalus, diffuse cerebrovascular disease or a structural lesion, e.g. meningioma, but MRI may reveal a pattern of lobar or hippocampal (AD) atrophy.
- Selected patients
  - Autoimmune screen, including thyroid peroxidase antibodies.
  - Paraneoplastic antibodies (e.g. anti-Yo for cerebellar degeneration) ± PET scan.
  - Voltage-gated potassium channel antibodies, anti-NMDA (N-methyl D-aspartate) receptor antibodies.
  - HIV testing.
  - Genetic testing — e.g. Huntington's disease, Tau mutations in familial Alzheimer's disease, prion gene mutations.
  - EEG — exclude non-convulsive status; loss of alpha rhythm may occur in AD.
  - Lumbar puncture — to exclude infection, inflammation and to measure CNS-specific proteins.
  - Brain or tonsil biopsy in prion disease (sporadic and variant Creutzfeldt–Jakob disease respectively).

Management
Counselling, provision of social support to patient and carers, respite care and use of Enduring Power of Attorney may be required. Treat depression. Avoid the use of neuroleptics for agitation and behavioural disturbance if possible, and use atypical neuroleptics (e.g. risperidone or **quetiapine**) sparingly if needed. In multi-infarct dementia modify risk factors.

Cholinesterase inhibitors (e.g. **donepezil** 5–10 mg daily, **rivastigmine** 1.5–6 mg twice daily, **galantamine** 8–12 mg twice daily) provide modest benefits in improving cognition and behaviour in AD and fronto-temporal dementia and slow progression slightly. **Memantine**, an NMDA antagonist, is also used for treatment of moderate to severe AD (5–20 mg per day). Drugs should be introduced at low dose and titrated up gradually according to tolerance. The MMSE should be > 12 to initiate therapy, and should be monitored at least every 6 months and treatment stopped if there is no benefit or if there is marked progression.

MOTOR NEURONE DISEASE

Motor neurone disease (also called amyotrophic lateral sclerosis/Lou Gehrig disease in the USA) is caused by relentless destruction of the upper motor neurones and anterior horn cells in the brain and spinal cord. There is no involvement of the sensory system or motor nerves to the eyes and sphincters. The three main disease patterns are progressive muscular atrophy (mainly anterior horn cell), amyotrophic lateral sclerosis (mixed upper and lower motor neurone) and progressive bulbar/pseudobulbar palsy. There can be a mixture of upper and lower motor neurone signs.

Kumar & Clark's Medical Management and Therapeutics

Needle EMG characteristics shows extensive muscle denervation (including bulbar muscles, and abdominal or paraspinal muscles) with preserved motor conduction velocity.

Treatment should be in the context of a multi-disciplinary team, including nurse specialist and therapists.

- Symptomatic relief includes treatment of spasticity, saliva management, gastrostomy for dysphagia, and non-invasive ventilation for respiratory failure.
- **Riluzole** 50 mg twice daily is used to extend life or time to ventilation.
- FBC and liver biochemistry require checking prior to initiation of therapy and every 8 weeks thereafter.

PERIPHERAL NERVE DISEASE

This affects a single nerve (mononeuropathy) to several individual nerves (multiple mononeuropathy/mononeuritis multiplex), or causes a distal symmetrical polyneuropathy that may be due to either direct axonal damage or, less often, demyelinating disease (see Guillain–Barré, p. 659). Neuropathy usually involves both motor and sensory modalities, but occasionally only motor or only sensory nerves are affected. Since peripheral nerves have long axons, they are metabolically vulnerable and there are therefore many possible causes of neuropathy, especially axonal neuropathy. Many drugs cause a neuropathy (Table 17.4).

Axonal distal polyneuropathy

This typically produces length-dependent nerve involvement, the longest nerves (to the toes) being affected first with gradual proximal progression. A sock distribution of sensory loss, followed by eventual glove

Table 17.4 Drug-related neuropathies

Drug	Neuropathy	Mode/site of action
Amiodarone	S, M	D, A
Anti-retroviral drugs	S > M	A
Chloramphenicol	S, M	A
Chloroquine	S, M	A, D
Cisplatin	S	A
Dapsone	M	A
Disulfiram	S, M	A
Isoniazid	S, S/M	A
Metronidazole	S, S/M	A
Nitrofurantoin	S/M	A
Paclitaxel	S > M	A
Phenytoin	M	A
Suramin	M > S	D, A
Vincristine	S > M	A

A, axonal; D, demyelinating; M, motor; S, sensory.

and stocking sensory loss, results. Reflexes are usually absent and distal weakness and wasting may be seen. Proprioception, vibration sensation and cutaneous sensation (e.g. pinprick, light touch) are tested, starting distally in the limbs and moving proximally.

Investigations

Investigations are directed at delineating the underlying cause. Nerve conduction studies (NCS) are useful to confirm neuropathy and to distinguish between demyelinating and axonal neuropathy. Approximately 50% will remain idiopathic after investigation.

- Initial investigations
  - *All patients:* FBC, ESR, B_{12}, folate, U&E, LFTs, γ-glutamyl transpepidase, glucose, immunoglobulins, protein electrophoresis, urine for Bence Jones proteins, serum ACE, rheumatoid factor, ANA and CXR.
  - *Selected patients:* Hepatitis B and C, HIV, ANCA, ENAs (extractable nuclear antigens) antineuronal antibodies, cryoglobulins, antiganglioside antibodies, heavy metal screen, homocysteine, methylmalonate, vitamin E and genetic testing (chromosome 17p duplication/deletion for CMT1a/HNLPP (Charcot–Marie–Tooth/hereditary neuropathy with liability to pressure palsies). Connexin 32, transthyretin for familial amyloid polyneuropathy and mitofusin-2 are checked in selected cases. Lumbar puncture is often performed in cases of demyelinating neuropathy. Nerve biopsy (usually sural nerve) may be necessary, particularly if vasculitis, amyloid or chronic inflammatory demyelinating polyneuropathy is suspected.

Management

- Treat the underlying cause. Ensure good glycaemic control in diabetics and thiamine/multi-vitamin replacement in alcoholic-dependent patients.
- Offer appropriate therapeutic aids (e.g. ankle–foot orthoses for foot drop) and emphasize foot care.
- For neuropathic pain, give **amitriptyline** (e.g. start at 10 mg at night and increase weekly in steps of 10 mg to an initial ceiling dose of 60–70 mg). **Gabapentin** and **pregabalin** are also widely used.
- In immune-mediated neuropathy, e.g. chronic inflammatory demyelinating polyneuropathy (CIDP), IV immunoglobulin or immunosuppression is sometimes required.

Guillain–Barré syndrome (GBS)

Typically, a mild antecedent infection (e.g. *Campylobacter jejuni*-associated diarrhoea, Epstein–Barr virus, cytomegalovirus) is followed, after a latent period of several days, by an acute progressive, demyelinating, mainly motor polyradiculoneuropathy. It is usually demyelinating but axonal GBS is also seen. Unlike in other peripheral polyneuropathies, proximal weakness is prominent. Cranial nerves (especially VII) may be affected. Patients may complain of back pain and sensory symptoms. Areflexia is usually found on examination.

- Lumbar puncture typically demonstrates an acellular CSF with a high protein content. Early in the disease CSF may be normal.
- NCS are useful in confirming the diagnosis but may also be normal early in the disease. Generally there is a demyelinating pattern. Axonal GBS is associated with a poorer prognosis.

- Specific antibody tests include antiganglioside antibodies and anti-GQ1b (in Miller Fisher variant), as well as *Campylobacter* serology.
- Check FVC at least every 4–6 hours and have a low threshold for transfer to ICU with a view to ventilating (if FVC < 15 mL/kg).
- Monitor BP (prone to hypotension — give IV fluids) and ECG (arrhythmias — bradycardias or tachycardias due to autonomic involvement).

Treatment

Treatment is primarily supportive, with attention to nutrition, exposure keratitis, pressure areas, and physiotherapy of chest and limbs. DVT prophylaxis with LMWH is given. **IV immunoglobulin** 0.4 g/kg/day for 5 days is the standard treatment in patients who have significant impairment (e.g. unable to walk, respiratory compromise) or who deteriorate rapidly. Corticosteroids are *not* indicated.

Autonomic features, e.g. hypotension and tachyarrhythmias, require treatment (p. 403). Hyponatraemia occurs secondary to SIADH. Neuropathic pain may require neuromodulatory agents, e.g. gabapentin. Avoid amitriptyline in GBS, as it is potentially arrhythmogenic.

Prognosis

Most patients recover but some may be left with permanent disability; neuro-rehabilitation in a specialist unit is required to maximize recovery in severely affected patients.

Carpal tunnel syndrome (CTS)

CTS results from compression of the median nerve at the wrist, causing pain and tingling (especially at night), and later, weakness and wasting of the median-innervated hand muscles (particularly abductor pollicis brevis). Any cause of soft-tissue swelling can provoke CTS. Diagnosis is confirmed on NCS. **Treatment** is of the underlying cause (e.g. hypothyroidism, rheumatoid arthritis). Wrist splints or hydrocortisone injection may provide symptomatic relief. Unless self-limiting, e.g. in pregnancy, definitive treatment is surgical decompression.

Other common sites of compression neuropathy are the ulnar nerve at the elbow, common peroneal nerve at the fibula head, and radial nerve in the spiral groove.

Further reading

Adams HP Jr, del Zoppo G, Alberts MJ, et al: Guidelines for the early management of adults with ischemic stroke: a guideline from the American Heart Association/American Stroke Association Stroke Council, Clinical Cardiology Council, Cardiovascular Radiology and Intervention Council, and the Atherosclerotic Peripheral Vascular Disease and Quality of Care Outcomes in Research Interdisciplinary Working Groups: the American Academy of Neurology affirms the value of this guideline as an educational tool for neurologists, *Stroke* 38:1655–1711, 2007.

Hughes T: Stroke on the acute medical take, *Clin Med* 10:68–72, 2010.

CHAPTER CONTENTS

CARE OF THE UNCONSCIOUS PATIENT

- All self-ventilated patients should be nursed in the left lateral position with the lower leg straight and the upper leg flexed; in this position the risk of aspiration is reduced. A clear passage for air should be ensured.
- Nursing care of the mouth and pressure areas should be instituted. Immediate catheterization of the bladder in unconscious patients is usually unnecessary, as it can be emptied by gentle suprapubic pressure.
- Insertion of a venous cannula is usual, but administration of IV fluids is unnecessary unless the patient has been unconscious for more than 12 hours or is hypotensive.

Ventilatory support

- If respiratory depression is present, as determined by pulse oximetry or preferably by arterial blood gas (ABG) analysis, an oro-pharyngeal airway should be inserted and oxygen should be administered.
- Loss of the cough or gag reflex is the prime indication for intubation.
- The gag reflex can be assessed by positioning the patient on one side and making him or her gag using a suction tube.
- In many severely poisoned patients the reflexes are depressed sufficiently to allow intubation without the use of sedatives or relaxants. The complications of endotracheal tubes are discussed on p. 544.
- If ventilation remains inadequate after intubation, as shown by hypoxaemia and/or hypercapnia, intermittent positive-pressure ventilation (IPPV) should be instituted.

Cardiovascular support

- Although hypotension (systolic BP < 80 mmHg) is a recognized feature of acute poisoning, the classic features of shock — tachycardia and pale cold skin — are observed only rarely.
- In patients with marked hypotension, volume expansion with crystalloids should be used, guided by monitoring of central venous pressure (CVP).
- Urine output (aiming for 35–50 mL/hour) is also a useful guide to the adequacy of the circulation.
- If a patient fails to respond to the above measures, more intensive therapy is required (p. 555).

Other problems

- Hypothermia: rectal temperature below 35°C. The patient should be covered with a 'space blanket' and, if necessary, given IV and fluids at normal body temperature. The administration of heated (37°C), humidified oxygen delivered by face mask is also useful.

- **Skin blisters:** may be found in poisoned patients who are, or have been, unconscious. Such lesions are not diagnostic of specific poisons, but are sufficiently common in poisoned patients (and sufficiently uncommon in patients unconscious from other causes) to be of diagnostic value.

- **Rhabdomyolysis:** can occur from pressure necrosis in drug-induced coma, or it may complicate, for example, ecstasy (MDMA) use in the absence of coma. Patients with rhabdomyolysis are at risk of developing:
  - acute kidney injury from myoglobinaemia, particularly if they are hypovolaemic and acidotic
  - peripheral nerve damage from the development of a compartment syndrome.

- **Convulsions:** occur, for example, in poisoning due to tricyclic antidepressants, mefenamic acid or opioids. Usually the seizures are short-lived, but if they are prolonged, diazepam 10–20 mg IV or lorazepam 4 mg IV should be administered.

- **Stress ulceration and bleeding:** measures to prevent stress ulceration of the stomach should be started on admission in all patients who are unconscious and require intensive care. A proton pump inhibitor, e.g. omeprazole 40 mg, should be administered intravenously over 5 mins or as an infusion over 20–30 mins.

REDUCTION OF POISON ABSORPTION

- **Poison absorption** through the lungs is reduced by moving the person from the toxic atmosphere, without the rescuers themselves being put at risk.
- **Contaminated clothing** should be removed to reduce dermal absorption. In addition, contaminated skin should be washed thoroughly with soap and water.
- **The efficacy of current methods** for the removal of unabsorbed drugs from the gastrointestinal tract remains unproven. Efforts to remove small amounts of non-toxic drugs are not worthwhile or appropriate.

Gastric lavage

- The amount of marker removed by gastric lavage is highly variable and diminishes with time.
- Gastric lavage should not be used routinely. It is used if a patient has ingested a potentially life-threatening amount of a poison and the procedure is undertaken within 60 mins of ingestion. Even then, clinical benefit has not been confirmed in controlled studies.
- Gastric lavage is contraindicated if airway protective reflexes are lost, unless the patient is intubated.
- It is also contraindicated if a hydrocarbon with high aspiration potential or a corrosive substance (e.g. caustic soda) has been ingested.

Syrup of ipecacuanha

- **Do not use**. There is no evidence from clinical studies that syrup of ipecacuanha improves the outcome of poisoned patients and therefore its administration, even in children, should be abandoned.

Single-dose activated charcoal

- The effectiveness of activated charcoal decreases with time. (In volunteers the mean reduction in absorption was 40%, 16% and 21% at 1 hour, 2 hours and 3 hours.) Activated charcoal should therefore only be used in those who have ingested a potentially toxic amount of a poison (known to be adsorbed by charcoal) up to 1 hour previously. There are insufficient data to support or exclude its use after 1 hour.
- There is no evidence that the administration of activated charcoal improves clinical outcome.
- The administration of charcoal is contraindicated unless a patient has an intact or protected airway.

Cathartics

- There is no evidence to suggest that a cathartic, with or without activated charcoal, will reduce the bioavailability of drugs or improve the outcome of poisoned patients.

Whole bowel irrigation (WBI)

- This involves insertion of a naso-gastric tube to give polyethylene glycol solution 1500–2000 mL/hour until the rectal effluent is clear.
- There is no conclusive evidence that WBI improves the outcome of the poisoned patient.
- WBI can be used for potentially toxic ingestions of modified-release or enteric-coated drugs and can be of use for potentially toxic ingestions of iron, lead, zinc or packets of illicit drugs.

INCREASING POISON ELIMINATION

Once a poison has been absorbed, unless there is an antidote, it is reasonable to use treatments that might speed its elimination from the body.

Urine alkalinization

- This is used for salicylate poisoning when plasma concentrations are > 500 mg/L (3.62 mmol/L).
- Before commencing urine alkalinization, correct plasma volume depletion and hypokalaemia, as administration of sodium bicarbonate will exacerbate pre-existing hypokalaemia.
- Sodium bicarbonate, most conveniently administered as an 8.4% solution (1 mmol bicarbonate/mL), is infused intravenously to ensure that the pH of the urine, which is measured by narrow-range indicator paper or a pH meter, is > 7.5 and preferably close to 8.5. In most cases the administration of 225 mmol bicarbonate will be required to produce urine alkalinization initially.

N.B. Urine alkalinization requires medical and nursing expertise, as it is a metabolically invasive procedure requiring frequent biochemical monitoring. It should *not* be employed if expertise is not available.

Acid diuresis

- There is no evidence that this is of any clinical value in cases of poisoning.

Multiple-dose activated charcoal (MDAC)

- Multiple doses of activated charcoal aid the elimination of some drugs from the circulation by interrupting their entero-hepatic and enter-enteric circulations.

Kumar & Clark's Medical Management and Therapeutics

- MDAC should be used only if a patient has ingested a life-threatening amount of carbamazepine, dapsone, phenobarbital, quinine or theophylline.
- Current recommendations are that adults should receive 50–100 g initially, followed by 50 g 4-hourly or 25 g 2-hourly until charcoal appears in the faeces or recovery occurs.
- This therapy has not yet been shown in a controlled study in poisoned patients to reduce morbidity and mortality.

Haemodialysis, haemodiafiltration and haemofiltration (p. 358)

- Haemodialysis is used only infrequently to increase the elimination of poisons.
- Haemodialysis is of little value in patients who ingest poisons with large volumes of distribution, e.g. tricyclic antidepressants, because the plasma contains only a small proportion of the total amount of drug in the body.
- Haemodialysis is indicated in patients with severe features and high plasma concentrations of ethanol, ethylene glycol, isopropanol, lithium, methanol or salicylate.
- Although haemofiltration and haemodiafiltration are widely available and increase elimination of poisons such as ethylene glycol and methanol, haemofiltration is much less efficient than haemodialysis and therefore should not be used unless haemodialysis is unavailable. Haemodiafiltration is preferable to haemofiltration.

TOXICOLOGICAL INVESTIGATION

A timed blood sample should always be taken in suspected poisoning and sent to the reference laboratory with as much clinical detail as possible.

SPECIFIC POISONS

Specific management for each poison is set out below alphabetically. Antidotes are available for only a small number of poisons (Table 18.1) and dosage recommendations are given under each poison.

Acetaminophen

See paracetamol (p. 684).

Acetone

This is inhaled or ingested and absorbed through the lungs, gut or skin. It is exhaled unchanged or metabolized to glucose and subsequently liberated as carbon dioxide. A common source of acetone is nail varnish remover, which can be swallowed accidentally by children.

Clinical features

- Acetone has an irritating effect on the mucous membranes of the eyes, nose and throat, causing burning and erythema. It also causes reversible corneal injury.
- Nausea, vomiting, light-headedness, headache, excitement, restlessness, chest tightness and incoherent speech are characteristic of intoxication. Coma, convulsions and respiratory failure supervene in severe cases. Kidney and liver damage can also occur.
- Hyperglycaemia may develop and ABGs may show a high anion gap metabolic acidosis.

Table 18.1 Antidotes of value in poisoning

Poison	Antidote
Anticoagulants (oral)	Vitamin K$_1$
Arsenic	DMSA* Dimercaprol (BAL)
Benzodiazepines	Flumazenil
β-adrenoceptor-blocking drugs	Atropine Glucagon
Carbon monoxide	Oxygen
Copper	DMPS†
Cyanide	Oxygen Dicobalt edetate Hydroxocobalamin Sodium nitrite Sodium thiosulphate
Diethylene glycol	Fomepizole, ethanol
Digoxin	Digoxin-specific antibody fragments
Ethylene glycol	Fomepizole, ethanol
Iron salts	Desferrioxamine (deferoxamine)
Lead (inorganic)	Sodium calcium edetate DMSA*
Methaemoglobinaemia	Methylthioninium chloride (methylene blue)
Methanol	Fomepizole, ethanol
Mercury (inorganic)	DMPS†
Nerve agents	Atropine Pralidoxime, obidoxime
Opioids	Naloxone
Organophosphorus insecticides	Atropine Pralidoxime, obidoxime
Paracetamol	Acetylcysteine
Thallium	Berlin (Prussian) blue

*Dimercaptosuccinic acid (succimer).
†2,3-dimercaptopropanesulfonate (unithiol).

Treatment

- Administer oxygen if there is respiratory distress. Measure ABGs in symptomatic patients.
- Irrigation of the eyes with 0.9% saline should be carried out if ocular irritation is present.
- Give 50–100 g of activated charcoal in an adult who presents within 1 hour of a substantial ingestion, providing the airway is secure. In vitro studies suggest that acetone is adsorbed to activated charcoal.

- Monitor blood glucose 1–2-hourly in symptomatic patients and correct hyperglycaemia with insulin. Take blood for renal and liver function assessment and measurement of creatine kinase activity.
- Give IV crystalloids, e.g. 0.9% saline, if vomiting is severe. Treat agitation and convulsions with IV **diazepam** 10–20 mg.
- Since the parent compound has a small volume of distribution (0.82 L/kg) and is responsible for toxicity, haemodialysis or haemodiafiltration is used in the management of severely poisoned patients in whom the plasma acetone concentrations are high.

Amfetamines

The N-methylated derivative, metamfetamine, is now used widely; the crystalline form of this salt is known as 'crystal meth' or 'ice'. Ecstasy (MDMA) is discussed on page 675.

Clinical features

- Euphoria, extrovert behaviour, a lack of desire to eat or sleep, tremor, dilated pupils, tachycardia and hypertension are seen.
- More severe intoxication is associated with agitation, paranoid delusions, hallucinations and violent behaviour.
- Convulsions, rhabdomyolysis, hyperthermia and cardiac arrhythmias may develop in severe intoxication.
- Rarely, intracerebral and subarachnoid haemorrhage occur and may be fatal.
- Serotonin syndrome consists of clonus, agitation, tremor, hyperreflexia, diaphoresis, hypertonicity and hyperthermia.

Treatment

- IV fluids, e.g. 0.9% saline, should be given for dehydration.
- Monitor electrolytes, renal function, liver function and creatine kinase (because of rhabdomyolysis) activity.
- Do an ECG and monitor cardiac rhythm.
- Monitor core temperature.
- Agitation may be controlled by **diazepam** 10–20 mg IV or **haloperidol** 2.5–5.0 mg IV or IM in an adult.
- **Dantrolene** 1 mg/kg IV can be used for hyperthermia that persists despite cooling measures.
- The peripheral sympathomimetic actions of amfetamines (e.g. hypertension and arrhythmias) are antagonized by **β-adrenoceptor blocking drugs** (e.g. **propranolol** 40–80 mg orally or 1–5 mg IV slowly).
- Treat seizures with **diazepam** 10 mg IV in an adult.
- Treat rhabdomyolysis conventionally with aggressive IV fluids to maintain high urine flow. There are theoretical reasons why urine alkalinization (p. 663) may be helpful in preventing or reducing the severity of rhabdomyolysis-induced kidney injury.
- If the serotonin syndrome develops, agitation can be controlled with a benzodiazepine. Treat hyperthermia with tepid sponging and a fan; paralysis and IPPV is used if no response. Control seizures with diazepam 10–20 mg. Cyproheptadine and chlorpromazine are not helpful.

Anticonvulsants

See carbamazepine (p. 671), gabapentin (p. 677), lamotrigine (p. 679), phenytoin (p. 688) and sodium valproate (p. 691).

Antidepressants

See selective serotonin reuptake inhibitors (p. 690), mirtazapine (p. 681), monoamine oxidase inhibitors (p. 682), tricyclic antidepressants (p. 692) and venlafaxine (p. 693).

Barbiturates

Clinical features

- Impairment of consciousness, respiratory depression, hypotension and hypothermia are typical.
- Hypotonia and hyporeflexia are common.
- Skin blisters and rhabdomyolysis may develop.
- Most deaths result from respiratory complications.

Treatment

- The elimination of phenobarbital is increased by oral MDAC (p. 663).

Batteries

Mercuric oxide has now been removed from disc batteries in Europe and hence the concern for leakage has disappeared in European countries. Some batteries also contain lithium.

Clinical features

Most disc batteries will pass through the gut in 2 or 3 days without causing symptoms. Gastrointestinal obstruction, mainly in the oesophagus, can occur. Oesophageal perforation is rare.

Treatment

- Do an AXR and CXR to confirm battery ingestion.
- **Endoscopic removal** is used for batteries lodged in the oesophagus or batteries that remain in the stomach more than 48 hours after ingestion, as they are at greater risk of leaking.
- If a small battery lies within the stomach on the first X-ray and patients are asymptomatic, they can be observed at home and return if any gastrointestinal symptoms develop. The stools should be inspected to confirm successful passage.
- If larger or multiple batteries have been ingested and are seen on the initial X-ray, confirm successful passage through the pylorus by repeating the X-ray 48 hours after ingestion.
- Surgical removal should be undertaken if symptoms of intestinal obstruction or bleeding develop at any stage.

Beta$_2$-adrenoceptor agonists

Clinical features

- Patients who are poisoned with a β_2-agonist, e.g. salbutamol, have a feeling of excitement, often accompanied by tremor, sinus tachycardia, agitation, convulsions, and supraventricular and ventricular arrhythmias.
- Hyperglycaemia (rarely hypoglycaemia in severe poisoning) and ketoacidosis have been reported.
- Psychosis and hallucinations are observed uncommonly.

Treatment

- **Severe hypokalaemia** should be corrected as soon as possible, by administration of **potassium** 40–60 mmol/hour, diluted with 0.9%

saline. As patients given potassium may develop significant hyperkalaemia during recovery, potassium concentrations should be monitored closely.

- A non-selective β-blocker, e.g. **propranolol** 1–5 mg, can be administered by slow IV injection to reverse hypokalaemia and sinus tachycardia but may exacerbate pre-existing obstructive pulmonary disease. Propranolol is more effective than atenolol in reversing the metabolic effects of salbutamol.
- Supraventricular tachycardia has been treated successfully with **adenosine** 6 mg IV over 2 secs followed by 12 mg after 1–2 mins if no response. If myocardial ischaemia occurs as a result of a tachyarrhythmia, **propranolol** 1–5 mg IV should be administered.
- Convulsions are usually single and short-lived, but if they continue, **diazepam** 5–10 mg IV is given in an adult.

Beta-adrenoceptor-blocking drugs

Clinical features

- Sinus bradycardia and hypotension usually occur within 6 hours of ingestion.
- Widened QRS and ventricular dysrhythmias, first-degree heart block, intraventricular conduction defects, right and left bundle branch block, ST segment elevation, the Brugada syndrome, ventricular extrasystoles and absent P waves may also be seen on ECG.
- Coma and convulsions occur if the overdose is substantial.
- Bronchospasm and respiratory depression can occur. Cardiorespiratory arrest caused by asystole or ventricular fibrillation occurs.
- Mild hyperkalaemia can occur.
- Hypoglycaemia can complicate β-blocker toxicity in children but is observed rarely in adults.

Treatment

- Record a baseline ECG and monitor cardiac activity continuously.
- IV **glucagon** 10 mg (150 mc/kg) in an adult is the treatment of choice for significant **hypotension** that persists despite volume replacement. This dose can be repeated every 3–5 mins but if there is no response it is unlikely that further boluses will be helpful. IV glucagon at this dose causes vomiting and should be given slowly. It can be diluted in 5% glucose and infused over 15 mins if necessary.
- Standard inotropes e.g. dobutamine may be added. Insulin and glucose therapy (hyperinsulinaemic euglycaemic therapy) is used experimentally in severe poisoning.
- If **bradycardia** is refractory to **atropine** 0.6–1.2 mg IV, repeated as necessary, and IV **glucagon**, transcutaneous or transvenous pacing may be necessary.
- If there is a favourable response in BP and/or pulse rate to glucagon, commence a **glucagon infusion** 5–10 mg/hour depending on response. Monitor blood glucose during glucagon therapy.
- Convulsions are usually short-lived and treatment is seldom necessary, though **IV diazepam** 10–20 mg in an adult is very effective if seizures persist.
- Give a **β₂-agonist**, e.g. salbutamol 2.5–5.0 mg by nebulizer, if bronchospasm develops.

Benzodiazepines

Clinical features

- Benzodiazepines produce drowsiness, ataxia, dysarthria and nystagmus.
- Coma and respiratory depression develop in severe poisoning.

Treatment

- Maintain a clear airway and adequate ventilation.
- Measure ABGs if conscious level is reduced or the oxygen saturation on air is ≤ 95%.
- If respiratory depression is present, **flumazenil** 0.5–1 mg IV should be administered in an adult and this dose may be repeated, if necessary.
- If the patient does not respond to flumazenil 1 mg it is likely that another **respiratory depressant** has been co-ingested.
- Flumazenil should not be administered if the patient is benzodiazepine-dependent, has epilepsy or has ingested pro-convulsants concurrently. Hypoventilation in these circumstances should be treated by **mechanical ventilation** (p. 544).
- As flumazenil has a short half-life (about 1 hour), patients with severe poisoning may need repeated bolus doses or an IV infusion (0.5–4 mg/hour).

Calcium channel blockers

There are three classes of calcium channel blocker: phenylalkylamines, e.g. verapamil; benzothiazepines, e.g. diltiazem; and dihydropyridines, e.g. amlodipine, felodipine, nifedipine.

Dihydropyridines are predominantly peripheral vasodilators with little direct cardiac effect, while verapamil, and diltiazem to a lesser extent, have significant cardiac effects (both myocardial depression and impaired cardiac conduction), in addition to peripheral vasodilatation.

Calcium channel blockers are often prepared as sustained-release preparations, which both delays and prolongs toxicity in overdose.

Clinical features

- Hypotension occurs due to peripheral vasodilatation, myocardial depression and conduction block.
- The ECG may progress from sinus bradycardia through first, then higher, degrees of block, to asystole.
- When a sustained-release preparation has been ingested, the onset of severe features may be delayed for more than 12 hours.
- Cardiac and non-cardiac pulmonary oedema occurs in severely poisoned patients.
- Other features include nausea, vomiting, seizures and a lactic acidosis.

Treatment

- Observe with cardiac and BP monitoring for at least 12 hours following overdose of a non-sustained-release preparation and at least 24 hours following overdose of a sustained-release preparation.
- Treat hypotension initially with **IV crystalloid, 0.9% saline** at a rate and volume appropriate to the age and co-morbidity of the patient. Expanding the intravascular volume in this way may be the only measure required in patients with hypotension secondary to peripheral vasodilatation who do not have evidence of impaired cardiac conduction.

- Measure ABGs.
- Correct metabolic acidosis that persists despite fluid resuscitation and adequate ventilation with 50–100 mmol of 8.4% **sodium bicarbonate** IV.
- Treat bradycardia with **IV atropine** 0.6–1.2 mg in an adult. This dose can be repeated as required. The response to atropine may be improved following parenteral calcium administration (see below).
- If there is evidence of cardiac conduction block, give 10% **calcium chloride** 5–10 mL IV (at 1–2 mL/min), or **calcium gluconate** solution, 10–20 mL to an adult. The initial dose can be repeated every 3–5 mins but if there is no response in BP or pulse rate after three such doses it is unlikely that further boluses will be helpful.
- If there is an initial response to calcium, give a continuous infusion; this may be given as 10% **calcium chloride**, 1–10 mL/hour. Serum calcium should be measured but note that modest hypercalcaemia is the aim of treatment.
- If significant hypotension persists despite **volume replacement**, give **IV glucagon** (see p. 668 for details).
- If there is a favourable response in BP to glucagon, commence a **glucagon infusion** 5–10 mg/hour depending on response. Monitor blood glucose during glucagon therapy.
- If hypotension persists despite the above measures administer a sympathomimetic amine intravenously. If hypotension is thought to be mainly due to reduced systemic vascular resistance, high-dose **dopamine** 10–30 mcg/kg/min is a reasonable choice. Alternatively, administer **adrenaline (epinephrine)** 0.1–1 mcg/kg/min.
- **Insulin/glucose euglycaemia** improves myocardial contractility and systemic perfusion and is used as an adjunct to sympathomimetic amine therapy. Check serum potassium before commencing insulin/glucose and if it is < 3.0 mmol/L give 20 mmol K$^+$ over 30 mins. If there is severe hypotension, give a loading bolus of IV 50 mL 50% glucose plus insulin 1.0 U/kg. An infusion of 10% glucose should be given, along with an infusion of insulin 0.5–1.0 U/kg/hour. Check blood sugar every 20 mins to determine the patient's insulin and glucose requirements, then check hourly. Check serum potassium hourly and replace as necessary.
- **Cardiac pacing** is used if there is evidence of atrio-ventricular conduction delay but there may be failure to capture.
- If cardiotoxicity is unresponsive to above, 1.5 mL/kg of 20% intralipid IV bolus followed by 0.25–0.5 mL/kg/min for 30–60 mins can be used.

Cannabis (marijuana)

Clinical features

- Euphoria, distorted and heightened images, colours and sounds, altered tactile sensations, sinus tachycardia, hypotension and ataxia occur.
- Visual and auditory hallucinations, depersonalization and acute psychosis are particularly likely to occur after substantial ingestion in naïve cannabis users.
- Cannabis impairs memory, an effect that may persist for months, even after abstinence.
- Cannabis infusions injected intravenously may cause nausea, vomiting and chills within mins; after about 1 hour, profuse watery diarrhoea, tachycardia, hypotension and arthralgia may develop.

Treatment

- Most acutely intoxicated patients require no more than reassurance and supportive care.
- Sedation with **diazepam** 10 mg IV, repeated as necessary, should be administered to patients who are disruptive or distressed. **Haloperidol** 2.5–5 mg IM or IV, repeated as necessary, is occasionally required.

Carbamate insecticides

Carbamate insecticides inhibit acetylcholinesterase but the duration of this effect is comparatively short-lived since the carbamate–enzyme complex tends to dissociate spontaneously.

Clinical features

These are similar to those of organophosphorus insecticide poisoning (p. 684).

Treatment

- Treatment is supportive, though **atropine** 0.6–2 mg IV is occasionally required for bradycardia and may need to be repeated.
- Recovery invariably occurs within 24 hours.

Carbamazepine

Clinical features

- Dry mouth, coma, convulsions, nystagmus, ataxia and incoordination occur. The pupils are often dilated, a divergent strabismus may be present, and complete external ophthalmoplegia has been reported.
- Hallucinations occur, particularly in the recovery phase.

Treatment

- **MDAC** (p. 663) increases the elimination of carbamazepine significantly.

Carbon monoxide

- Carbon monoxide combines with haemoglobin to form carboxyhaemoglobin (COHb), thereby reducing the total oxygen-carrying capacity of the blood and increasing the affinity of the remaining haem groups for oxygen. This shifts the oxyhaemoglobin dissociation curve to the left, impairing liberation of oxygen to the cells. Tissue hypoxia results.
- Carbon monoxide also inhibits cytochrome oxidase a_3.

Clinical features

- Symptoms of mild to moderate exposure to carbon monoxide may be mistaken for a viral illness with headache, dizziness, nausea and vomiting.
- A peak COHb concentration of $\leq 10\%$ is not normally associated with symptoms. Peak COHb concentrations of 10–30% may result only in headache and mild exertional dyspnoea.
- Higher concentrations of COHb are associated with coma, convulsions and cardiorespiratory arrest.
- Myocardial ischaemia, hypertonia and extensor plantar responses are relatively common in severe cases.
- Pulmonary oedema, retinal haemorrhages and papilloedema secondary to cerebral oedema also occur.

Kumar & Clark's Medical Management and Therapeutics

- Neuropsychiatric features (including amnesia, parkinsonism, chorea and choreoathetosis) may occur after apparent recovery from carbon monoxide intoxication but usually improve within a year of exposure.

Treatment

- In addition to removing the patient from carbon monoxide exposure, administer **high-flow oxygen** using a tight-fitting face mask.
- Mechanical ventilation may be required in those who are unconscious.
- Measure COHb concentrations every 2–4 hours until below 10%.
- Measure ABGs. Metabolic acidosis (p. 382) with normal oxygen tension but reduced oxygen saturation is characteristic.
- Monitor heart rhythm.
- The use of hyperbaric oxygen remains controversial, as the results of clinical trials are conflicting.
- Patients who survive severe carbon monoxide poisoning should be followed up for assessment of neurological recovery.

Chloroquine

Clinical features

- Hypotension is often the first clinical manifestation of poisoning. It may progress to cardiogenic shock, pulmonary oedema and cardiac arrest.
- Agitation and acute psychosis, convulsions and coma occur.
- Hypokalaemia is common and is due to chloroquine-induced potassium channel blockade.

Treatment

- Hypokalaemia should be corrected.
- There is some evidence that **mechanical ventilation**, the administration of **adrenaline (epinephrine)** and high doses of **diazepam** reduce morbidity and mortality.
- MDAC (p. 663) may enhance chloroquine elimination.

Cocaine

Clinical features

- After initial euphoria, cocaine produces agitation, tachycardia, hypertension, sweating, hallucinations, convulsions, metabolic acidosis, hyperthermia, rhabdomyolysis and ventricular arrhythmias.
- Dissection of the aorta, myocarditis, myocardial infarction, dilated cardiomyopathy, subarachnoid haemorrhage and cerebral haemorrhage also occur, which can be fatal.

Treatment

- Sedation with **diazepam** 10–20 mg IV, repeated as necessary, is effective in controlling agitation in adults.
- Active external cooling is required when the patient's temperature exceeds 41°C.
- Hypertension and tachycardia usually respond to sedation and cooling. If hypertension persists, give **IV nitrates** such as **glyceryl trinitrate** starting at 1–2 mg/hour and gradually increase the dose (maximum 12 mg/hour) until BP is controlled. **Calcium channel blockers** such as **nifedipine**, **verapamil** or **diltiazem** are an alternative as second-line therapy. The use of β-blockers is controversial.

- Early use of a **benzodiazepine** is often effective in relieving cocaine-associated non-cardiac chest pain. **Aspirin and nitrates** should be given to all patients with chest pain suspected of being cardiac in origin.
- Treat myocardial ischaemia/infarction (p. 433).

Copper

Copper sulfate is a fungicide (when mixed with lime it is called Bordeaux mixture). It is a common cause of deliberate self-harm in some developing countries.

Clinical features

- Vomiting, abdominal pain and diarrhoea (occasionally bloody due to corrosive damage) occur. Body secretions may turn blue/green.
- In severe poisoning hypotension, intravascular haemolysis, methaemoglobinaemia, jaundice, acute kidney injury, coma and convulsions are seen.

Treatment

- Adequate initial resuscitation is vital.
- Correct methaemoglobinaemia with methylthioninium chloride (methylene blue) 1–2 mg/kg, repeated as necessary.
- In severe poisoning chelation therapy with **DMPS** (2,3-dimercaptopropanesulfonate (unithiol) can be used. Seek expert advice from a poisons centre.

Corrosive ingestions

Exposure to strong acids and alkalis causes tissue injury from an exothermic chemical reaction in addition to a direct corrosive effect. Examples of strong alkalis include oven cleaners, some toilet cleaners and drain cleaners, while strong acids may be encountered in metal cleaners, battery acids or swimming pool cleaners.

Clinical features

- Ingestion causes immediate pain, with pharyngeal oedema and burns. Drooling is common. Features of pharyngeal involvement include hoarseness, stridor, respiratory distress and laryngeal and/or epiglottic oedema. Perforation of the oesophagus or stomach may occur and can lead to chemical peritonitis.
- Abdominal pain, vomiting, haematemesis and diarrhoea occur in severe poisoning. Systemic effects include circulatory collapse, metabolic acidosis, hypoxia, respiratory and acute kidney injury, intravascular coagulation and haemolysis.
- Later complications include stricture formation, achlorhydria, protein-losing gastroenteropathy and gastric or oesophageal carcinoma.

Treatment

- Establish a clear airway and adequate ventilation.
- There is no role for gastrointestinal decontamination or neutralization.
- The presence of laryngopharyngeal oedema requires expert assessment for the risk of airway compromise and need for intubation.
- Give adequate analgesia. **Opiates** are usually required.
- Early endoscopy by an expert endoscopist is essential to grade the severity of injury. If drooling, severe pain or stridor is present, endoscopy should be undertaken immediately.

Kumar & Clark's Medical Management and Therapeutics

- Early surgical intervention may prevent life-threatening haemorrhage and perforation, and is the treatment of choice in those with severe oesophageal or gastric burns.
- There is no evidence that corticosteroids have any role in the acute management of acid or alkaline burns, and they may be harmful because they may mask other clinical signs. Stricture formation is also unaffected by corticosteroids.
- Prophylactic antibiotics are not helpful.
- Follow-up to assess for stricture formation is necessary in all those with significant mucosal damage.

Cyanide

Cyanide reversibly inhibits cytochrome oxidase a_3 so that cellular respiration ceases.

Clinical features

- Inhalation of hydrogen cyanide gas may produce symptoms within seconds and death within minutes. In contrast, the ingestion of a cyanide salt may not produce features for 1 hour.
- After exposure initial symptoms are non-specific and include a feeling of constriction in the chest and dyspnoea. Coma, convulsions and metabolic acidosis may then supervene.

Treatment

- **Oxygen** should be administered, as it prevents inhibition of cytochrome oxidase a_3 and accelerates its reactivation.
- **Dicobalt edetate** or **hydroxocobalamin** should then be given; hydroxocobalamin is much more expensive than dicobalt edetate.
  - **Dicobalt edetate solutions** contain free cobalt, which complexes six times more cyanide than dicobalt edetate itself. Cobalt is toxic, however, and the use of this formulation in the absence of cyanide poisoning may cause cobalt toxicity. Dicobalt edetate 300 mg IV should therefore be administered only when the diagnosis is certain; the dose may be repeated in severe cases.
  - **Hydroxocobalamin** 5 g is given IV *over at least 15 mins*; a second dose (5 g) may be required in severe cases. It combines with cyanide to form cyanocobalamin, which is excreted in the urine.
- If these two preferred antidotes are not available, **sodium nitrite** 30 mg IV and **sodium thiosulphate** 12.5 mg IV should be administered (preferred treatment in the USA). Sodium nitrite produces methaemoglobinaemia; methaemoglobin combines with cyanide to form cyanmethaemoglobin. As the effect of sodium nitrite is relatively rapid and methaemoglobin formation slower, the benefit of sodium nitrite may also be from its vasodilator action and the consequent improved tissue perfusion. Sodium thiosulphate enhances endogenous cyanide detoxification mechanisms.

Digoxin

Toxicity occurring during chronic administration is common; acute poisoning is infrequent.

Clinical features

- These include nausea, vomiting, dizziness, anorexia and drowsiness. Rarely, confusion, visual disturbances and hallucinations occur. Sinus bradycardia is often marked and may be followed by supraventricular arrhythmias with or without heart block, ventricular premature beats and ventricular tachycardia.

- Hyperkalaemia occurs due to the inhibition of the sodium–potassium ATPase pump.

Treatment

- Sinus bradycardia, atrioventricular block and sinoatrial standstill are often reduced or abolished by **atropine** 1.2–2.4 mg IV.
- The indications for **digoxin-specific antibody therapy** are significant hyperkalaemia and marked arrhythmias, usually severe bradycardia compromising cardiac output and, more rarely, ventricular arrhythmias and asystole.
- In patients not prescribed digoxin, serum digoxin concentrations do not equate to the total body burden, as tissue distribution will not have occurred. Calculations using serum concentrations are therefore likely to result in too much antibody being administered. It is recommended that half the calculated dose (based on serum concentration or ingested dose) should be administered and the impact on clinical features observed.
- In patients who are prescribed digoxin and develop poisoning, the serum digoxin concentration will reflect the total body load. However, since such patients are receiving digoxin for therapeutic purposes, full neutralization is again not indicated. Half the calculated dose, based on serum concentration, should be administered.
- To calculate the total body burden of digoxin, multiply serum concentration in mcg/L (nmol/L × 1.28) × weight (kg) × volume of distribution (adults 8 L/kg, children 2–10 years 13 L/kg, infants 2–24 months 16 L/kg, neonates 10 L/kg). As one 40 mg vial of digoxin-specific antibody binds 0.6 mg of digoxin, the total calculated number of 40 mg vials required = total body burden/0.6. This number is then halved.
- In both circumstances, and if clinically indicated, digoxin-specific antibody fragments should be administered intravenously. If a clinical response is not seen within 1–2 hours, a further similar dose should be given.
- Be aware that most serum digoxin assays measure both antibody-bound and free drug and therefore the result is difficult to interpret after administration of antibody fragments.

Ecstasy (3,4-methylenedioxymethamfetamine; MDMA)

Clinical features

- Mild cases are characterized by agitation, tachycardia, hypertension, widely dilated pupils, trismus and sweating.
- Hyperthermia, hyponatraemia, cerebral oedema, seizures, disseminated intravascular coagulation, rhabdomyolysis, severe hepatic damage including fulminant hepatic failure (experimentally, hyperthermia potentiates ecstasy-induced hepatotoxicity), and acute kidney injury predominate in more severe cases.
- MDMA can cause life-threatening hyponatraemia due to inappropriate secretion of antidiuretic hormone, particularly when accompanied by excessive fluid ingestion.
- The **serotonin syndrome** has been reported.

Treatment

See treatment of amfetamines (p. 666).

Kumar & Clark's Medical Management and Therapeutics

Ethanol

Clinical features

- In children severe hypoglycaemia may accompany alcohol intoxication due to inhibition of gluconeogenesis. Hypoglycaemia is also observed in those who are malnourished or who have fasted in the previous 24 hours.
- In severe cases of intoxication, coma and hypothermia are often present and lactic acidosis, ketoacidosis and acute kidney injury occur.

Treatment

- Supportive measures are all that is required for most patients with acute ethanol intoxication, even if the blood ethanol concentration is very high. Particular care should be taken to protect the airway.
- In more severe cases, acid–base status should be determined 2-hourly.
- Lactic acidosis requires correction of hypoglycaemia, hypovolaemia and circulatory insufficiency, if present. An infusion of **sodium bicarbonate** 50–100 mmol will be necessary in those patients in whom a lactic acidosis persists.
- Blood sugar should be determined hourly and the rate of **IV glucose** adjusted accordingly. If blood sugar concentrations fall despite an infusion of 5–10% glucose, a 20% glucose solution 50 mL IV should be given; hypoglycaemia is usually unresponsive to glucagon.
- Haemodialysis or haemodiafiltration may be necessary if the blood ethanol concentration exceeds 7500 mg/L and if a severe metabolic acidosis is present, which has not been corrected by the measures outlined above.
- Fructose is of negligible clinical benefit in accelerating ethanol oxidation and may cause acidosis.

Ethylene and diethylene glycols

Clinical features

- The features observed are due to the metabolites predominantly, not the parent chemical. Ethylene glycol is oxidized by alcohol dehydrogenase to glycoaldehyde. Aldehyde dehydrogenase rapidly converts glycoaldehyde to glycolate. The conversion of glycolate to glyoxylate is slow. A small proportion of glyoxylate is metabolized to oxalate. Calcium ions chelate oxalate to form insoluble calcium oxalate monohydrate crystals. Diethylene glycol is metabolized by alcohol dehydrogenase to 2-hydroxyethoxyacetaldehyde and by aldehyde dehydrogenase to 2-hydroxyethoxyacetate (2-HEAA).
- Initially, the features of ethylene glycol (in antifreeze and windscreen de-icer) poisoning are similar to ethanol intoxication (though there is no ethanol on the breath). Coma and convulsions follow and a variety of neurological abnormalities, including nystagmus and ophthalmoplegias, may be observed. Severe metabolic acidosis, hypocalcaemia and the presence of calcium oxalate crystalluria are well-recognised complications.
- In diethylene glycol poisoning nausea and vomiting, headache, abdominal pain, coma, seizures, metabolic acidosis and acute kidney injury commonly occur. Pancreatitis and hepatitis, together with cranial neuropathies and demyelinating peripheral neuropathy, are also seen.

Treatment

- Supportive measures to combat cardiorespiratory depression should be employed and metabolic acidosis, hypocalcaemia and acute kidney injury should be treated conventionally.
- If the patient presents early after ingestion, the priority is to inhibit metabolism of ethylene or diethylene glycol using either **IV fomepizole or ethanol** (if fomepizole is not available). *Do not wait for confirmatory blood concentrations before starting treatment.*
- **Fomepizole** 15 mg/kg should be administered over 30 mins, followed by four 12-hourly doses of 10 mg/kg and then by 15 mg/kg 12-hourly until the glycol concentration is not detectable. If haemodialysis or haemodiafiltration is used, the frequency of dosing should be increased to 4-hourly, as fomepizole is dialysable.
- Alternatively, a loading dose of IV **ethanol** 50 g for an adult (50 mL of absolute ethanol in 1 L 5% glucose, i.e. a 5% ethanol solution) should be given, followed by an IV infusion of ethanol 10–12 g/hour (most easily given as 1 L 5% ethanol solution over 4–5 hours), to achieve a blood ethanol concentration of ~1000 mg/L. Administration of ethanol should be continued until the glycol is undetectable in the blood. If dialysis is used, greater amounts of ethanol (17–22 g/hour) must be given, because ethanol is readily dialysable. Ideally, glycol and ethanol concentrations should be measured frequently until recovery.
- **Haemodialysis and haemodiafiltration** remove glycol, glycolaldehyde and glycolate, but not oxalate, and will also correct acid–base disturbances; haemodialysis is 2–3 times more efficient than peritoneal dialysis. Haemodialysis or haemodiafiltration should be employed, particularly if presentation is late and marked metabolic acidosis is present. Dialysis should be continued until the glycol and glycolate are no longer detectable in the blood.

Gabapentin

Clinical features

- Drowsiness, vomiting, slurred speech, tremulousness and myoclonus may occur.
- Coma, respiratory depression, convulsions, hearing loss and hallucinations have been reported in severe cases.

Treatment

- Treatment is symptomatic and supportive.
- As elimination occurs renally, haemodialysis/haemodiafiltration may have a role in the management of severely poisoned patients with acute kidney injury.

Gamma-hydroxybutyrate (GHB)

Clinical features

- GHB is taken as a colourless liquid dissolved in water.
- Low doses cause mild agitation, excitement, nausea and vomiting with euphoria and possibly hallucinations at higher doses progressing to coma, bradycardia and respiratory depression in the most severely poisoned.
- The most unique aspect of GHB intoxication is its brief duration. Patients may progress from deep coma requiring intubation to self-extubation and full alertness over only a few hours.

- A **GHB withdrawal syndrome** can occur in chronic users, with clinical features occurring within 6–12 hours of the last dose. Features include insomnia, tremor and confusion, which may progress to delirium not dissimilar to the alcohol withdrawal syndrome.
- **Gamma-butyrolactone (GBL)**, a 'legal high', has similar clinical effects.

Treatment
- Supportive measures to maintain adequate ventilation and circulation should be employed and this is often all that is required.
- Monitor cardiac rhythm.
- Give **atropine** 0.6–1.2 mg IV for persistent symptomatic bradycardia.

Household products

The agents most commonly involved are bleach, cosmetics, toiletries, detergents, disinfectants and petroleum distillates such as paraffin and white spirit.

- If the ingestion of these products is accidental and in children ≤ 5 years old, features very rarely occur, except in the case of petroleum distillates (p. 687).
- Powder detergents, sterilizing tablets, denture cleaning tablets and industrial bleaches (which contain high concentrations of sodium hypochlorite) are corrosive to the mouth and pharynx if ingested (p. 673).
- Nail polish and nail polish remover contain acetone (p. 664).
- Inhalation by small children of substantial quantities of talcum powder has occasionally given rise to severe pulmonary oedema and death.

Iron

Unless > 60 mg of elemental iron per kg body weight is ingested, symptoms are unlikely to develop. As a result poisoning is seldom severe but deaths still occur, particularly in children. Iron salts have a direct corrosive effect on the upper gastrointestinal tract.

Clinical features
- The initial features are nausea, vomiting (the vomit may be grey or black in colour), abdominal pain and diarrhoea.
- Severely poisoned patients develop haematemesis, hypotension, coma and shock at an early stage.
- A small minority develop shock, metabolic acidosis, acute kidney injury and hepatocellular necrosis 12–48 hours after ingestion.
- Rarely, up to 6 weeks after ingestion of iron, strictures due to corrosive damage may occur.

Treatment
- The serum iron concentration should be measured some 4 hours after ingestion. If the concentration exceeds 5 mg/L (90 µmol/L), free iron is circulating and treatment with **desferrioxamine** 15 mg/kg/hour IV is used (total amount of infusion not usually to exceed 80 mg/kg in 24 hours).
- If a patient develops coma or shock, desferrioxamine (deferoxamine) should be given without delay.

- Adverse effects, including pulmonary oedema and ARDS, have been reported following excess desferrioxamine administration.
- Serum iron concentrations measure free and desferrioxamine-bound iron, so are not helpful following antidotal treatment.

Isopropanol

This is more toxic than ethanol and is the base for many hand washes.

Clinical features

- Coma and respiratory depression are the major sequelae following substantial use. Coma may be prolonged due to the relatively slow metabolism of isopropanol and the subsequent generation of acetone.

Treatment

- Activated charcoal does not bind isopropanol. Gastric lavage is unlikely to be of value, as its absorption is rapid.
- Isopropanol has a small volume of distribution (0.6–0.7 L/kg) and is responsible (together with its metabolite, acetone, p. 358) for toxicity. **Haemodialysis or haemodiafiltration** may therefore be helpful in severely poisoned patients in whom the plasma isopropanol concentrations are high. Acetone is also removed effectively by haemodialysis or haemodiafiltration.

Lamotrigine

Clinical features

- Mild toxicity causes nausea and vomiting, ataxia and drowsiness.
- More severely poisoned patients may develop coma, convulsions and hypertonia.
- Hypokalaemia and QRS interval prolongation have been reported.

Treatment

- Treatment is symptomatic and supportive.
- Perform an ECG and check the plasma potassium concentration.

Lead

Clinical features

- Mild poisoning causes lethargy and occasional abdominal discomfort, though abdominal pain, vomiting, constipation and encephalopathy (seizures, delirium, coma) may develop in more severe cases.
- A normochromic normocytic anaemia is typical in severe poisoning.
- Basophilic stippling is seen on the blood film and high hepatic transferase activities occur.
- Measure whole-blood lead concentrations in all suspected cases of poisoning. *Plasma samples must not be used, as they are misleading – lead accumulates in red cells.*

Treatment

- Identification of the source of lead exposure and prevention of further exposure are the priorities.
- The decision to use chelation therapy is based not only on the blood lead concentration but also on the presence of symptoms.
- Give either IV **sodium calcium edetate** 75 mg/kg/day or **oral dimercaptosuccinic acid (DMSA)** 30 mg/kg/day. These antidotes are of similar efficacy and the choice is usually determined by availability and whether an oral agent is feasible.

- Chelation therapy should be continued for 5 days, or until the 24-hour urine lead excretion is no longer substantially greater than pre-chelation urine lead excretion.
- During chelation, measure plasma electrolyte and creatinine concentrations daily, particularly with sodium calcium edetate, since transiently impaired renal function is a potential adverse effect of this agent.
- Measure serum zinc before, during and after chelation and give zinc sulphate supplements if necessary, as sodium calcium edetate may deplete body zinc stores. DMSA causes significantly less zinc depletion.
- Successive courses of chelation therapy are likely to be required once re-equilibration of lead from bone to blood has occurred.

Lithium

Clinical features

- Features of intoxication include thirst, polyuria, diarrhoea and vomiting.
- In more serious cases, tremor, nystagmus, impairment of consciousness, hypertonia, convulsions and irreversible neurological damage may occur.
- Measurement of the serum lithium concentration confirms the diagnosis. Chronic toxicity is usually associated with concentrations > 1.5 mmol/L (10.4 mg/L). Acute massive overdose may produce concentrations of 5 mmol/L (34.7 mg/L) without causing toxic features.

Treatment

- Since lithium is renally excreted unchanged, maximizing urine output with IV **sodium chloride 0.9%** is effective in increasing lithium elimination.
- **Haemodialysis** is far superior and is used if neurological features are present, if renal function is impaired and if chronic toxicity is the mode of presentation.

Mercury

Clinical features

- Acute mercury vapour inhalation causes headache, conjunctivitis, cough, nausea and vomiting, dyspnoea and chest pain. Chemical pneumonitis occurs and, in severe cases, renal and/or liver failure may occur.
- Repeated exposure to low mercury vapour concentrations presents typically with characteristic neurological features such as fine tremor, lethargy, memory loss, insomnia, personality changes and ataxia. Other features include stomatitis, gingivitis, hypersalivation and renal tubular damage. Mixed motor and sensory peripheral neuropathy may develop.
- There is no evidence that mercury from amalgam dental fillings causes mercury poisoning.
- Many inorganic mercury salts are corrosive, and substantial ingestion has led to fatalities from haemorrhagic gastroenteritis. Renal tubular damage predominates in those who survive this initial phase. Neurological features of mercury poisoning may follow chronic exposure.
- Methylmercury compounds have been used as fungicides, and poisoning has usually followed ingestion of contaminated foods. Features of mercury poisoning typically occur after a latent period of several weeks.

Treatment

- Send blood and urine for mercury concentration estimation.
- Assess U&E, creatinine and liver function.
- Perform an X-ray if elemental mercury has been injected or ingested, as elemental mercury is radiopaque.
- Remove the patient from exposure.
- Respiratory features following acute mercury vapour inhalation require only symptomatic and supportive measures.
- Soft-tissue deposits of elemental mercury usually require surgical excision, preferably under X-ray control.
- If there is analytical evidence of a substantial body burden of mercury and symptoms of mercury poisoning, chelation therapy with **IV DMPS 30 mg/kg/day (typically for 5 days)** is used. Where extracorporeal renal support is required for the management of acute kidney injury, there is some evidence that continuous venous–venous haemofiltration is more effective than haemodialysis at removing DMPS–mercury complexes.

Methanol

This is found in windscreen washer fluid, antifreeze and duplicator fluid.

Clinical features

- Patients often present after a delay of several hours, with nausea, vomiting, abdominal pain, tachypnoea, inebriation and drowsiness; after a latent period coma supervenes.
- Blurred vision and diminished visual acuity occur. The presence of dilated pupils that are unreactive to light suggests that permanent blindness is likely to occur.
- A severe metabolic acidosis may develop and be accompanied by hyperglycaemia and a raised serum amylase activity.
- Survivors may show permanent neurological sequelae, including parkinsonian-like signs as well as blindness.
- The mortality correlates well with the severity and duration of metabolic acidosis.
- A blood methanol concentration of > 500 mg/L (15.6 mmol/L) confirms severe poisoning.

Treatment

- Treatment is similar to that of ethylene glycol poisoning (p. 677).
- Correct metabolic acidosis.
- Inhibit methanol metabolism by the administration of **fomepizole** or **ethanol** (p. 677).
- **Folinic acid 30 mg** IV 6-hourly for 48 hours may protect against ocular toxicity by accelerating formate metabolism.

Mirtazapine

This is a $5HT_2$ and $5HT_3$ receptor agonist and a potent α_2-adrenergic blocker.

Clinical features

- Drowsiness is the most common feature.
- Confusion or agitation is possible and coma is recognized in more severely poisoned patients.

- Sinus tachycardia is common but mirtazapine does not typically cause the cardiac conduction abnormalities seen with tricyclic antidepressant poisoning.
- Mirtazapine appears to have a low potential to cause seizures.

Treatment
- Symptomatic and supportive measures are the mainstay of management.
- Ensure a clear airway and adequate ventilation.

Monoamine oxidase inhibitors

Clinical features
- Features after overdose may be delayed for 12–24 hours.
- They include excitement, restlessness, hyperpyrexia, hyper-reflexia, convulsions, opisthotonos, rhabdomyolysis and coma.
- Sinus tachycardia and either hypo- or hypertension are also observed.

Treatment
- Treatment is supportive, with control of convulsions and marked excitement; **diazepam** 10–20 mg IV in an adult should be given as necessary and repeated.
- **Dantrolene** 1 mg/kg IV is used if hyperpyrexia develops despite cooling measures.
- Hypotension should be treated with plasma expansion and hypertension by the administration of an α-adrenoceptor blocker such as **chlorpromazine**.

Neuroleptics and atypical neuroleptics

Older neuroleptics include the phenothiazines, the butyrophenones (benperidol, haloperidol), the substituted benzamides (sulpiride), diphenylbutylpiperidines (pimozide) and thioxanthenes (flupentixol).

More selective 'atypical' antipsychotic drugs are available and include amisulpride, aripiprazole, clozapine, olanzapine, quetiapine and risperidone.

Clinical features
- These include impaired consciousness, hypotension, respiratory depression, hypothermia or hyperthermia, antimuscarinic effects such as tachycardia, dry mouth and blurred vision, occasionally seizures, rhabdomyolysis, cardiac arrhythmias (both atrial and ventricular) and ARDS.
- Extrapyramidal effects, including acute dystonic reactions, may occur but are not dose-related.
- Most 'atypical' antipsychotics have less profound sedative actions than the older neuroleptics.
- QT interval prolongation and subsequent ventricular arrhythmias (including torsades de pointes) have occurred following overdose with the atypical neuroleptics.
- Unpredictable fluctuations in conscious level, with variations between agitation and marked somnolence, have been particularly associated with olanzapine overdose.

Treatment
- Symptomatic and supportive measures are the mainstay of management.

- Monitor body temperature, BP, cardiac rhythm, conscious level and urine output.
- Check ABGs if conscious level is impaired or pulse oximetry on room air is < 95%.
- Correct metabolic acidosis that persists despite fluid resuscitation and adequate ventilation with **50–100 mmol of sodium bicarbonate** (50–100 mL of 8.4% sodium bicarbonate). IV administration of 8.4% sodium bicarbonate must be through a wide-bore cannula that has been tested for patency since it will cause tissue necrosis if extravasation occurs. Alternatively, administer sodium bicarbonate through a central venous line.
- **Procyclidine 5–10 mg** IV or IM in an adult is occasionally required for the treatment of dyskinesia and oculogyric crisis.
- Single brief convulsions do not require treatment. If frequent or prolonged, control with **IV diazepam** 10–20 mg in an adult.
- If hypotension is severe and does not respond to IV fluids, a sympathomimetic amine such as **noradrenaline (norepinephrine)** may be required.
- After correcting acidosis with sodium bicarbonate, the preferred treatment for arrhythmias caused by antipsychotic drugs (usually **torsades de pointes**) is **IV magnesium** or cardiac pacing. **Lidocaine or phenytoin** may be effective if multi-focal ventricular arrhythmias occur.

Non-steroidal anti-inflammatory drugs (NSAIDs)

Clinical features
- Minor gastrointestinal disturbances are usually the only feature.
- In more severe cases, coma, convulsions, acute kidney injury and metabolic acidosis can occur.
- Poisoning with mefenamic acid commonly results in convulsions, though these are usually short-lived.

Treatment
- Treatment is symptomatic and supportive. Check acid-base status and renal function.

Opiates and opioids

Clinical features
- Cardinal signs of opiate poisoning are pinpoint pupils, reduced respiratory rate and coma.
- Hypothermia, hypoglycaemia and convulsions are occasionally observed in severe cases.
- In severe heroin overdose, ARDS has been reported.

Treatment
- **Naloxone 1.2 mg** IV in an adult (5–10 mcg body weight in a child) will reverse severe respiratory depression and coma, at least partially.
- In severe poisoning larger initial doses and/or repeat doses will be required.
- **N.B.** The duration of action of naloxone is invariably less than the drug taken in overdose and an **infusion of naloxone** may be required. For example, in chronic use the mean half-life of methadone is 25 hours. Naloxone infusions may be given undiluted or diluted in saline or dextrose.
- ARDS should be treated with assisted ventilation and PEEP.

Kumar & Clark's Medical Management and Therapeutics

Organophosphorus insecticides

These insecticides inhibit acetylcholinesterase, allowing accumulation of acetylcholine.

Clinical features

- Poisoning is characterized by anxiety, restlessness, headache, and muscarinic features such as nausea, vomiting, abdominal colic, diarrhoea, sweating, hypersalivation and chest tightness.
- Miosis may be present.
- Nicotinic effects include muscle fasciculation and flaccid paresis of limb muscles, respiratory and, occasionally, extra-ocular muscles.
- Respiratory failure occurs in severe cases and is exacerbated by the development of bronchorrhoea and pulmonary oedema.
- Coma and convulsions occur in severe poisoning.
- Diagnosis is confirmed by measuring the erythrocyte cholinesterase activity; plasma cholinesterase activity is less specific but may also be depressed.

Treatment

- Soiled clothing should be removed; contaminated skin should be washed with soap and water to prevent further absorption.
- **Atropine 2 mg** IV should be given to reduce bronchorrhoea. Repeat doses will be required in severe cases.
- Severely poisoned patients are also likely to require mechanical ventilation.
- In addition, **pralidoxime 30 mg/kg by slow IV injection** followed by an **infusion** of 8–10 mg/kg/hour should be given until symptoms resolve. Pralidoxime reactivates phosphorylated (inhibited) acetylcholinesterase; an alternative is **obidoxime**.

Paracetamol (acetaminophen)

Clinical features

- Following the ingestion of an overdose of paracetamol, patients usually remain asymptomatic or may have nausea and vomiting and abdominal pain.
- Liver damage is not usually detectable by routine LFTs until at least 18 hours after ingestion of the drug.
- Liver damage usually reaches a peak, as assessed by measurement of ALT/AST activity and prothrombin time (INR), at 72–96 hours after ingestion.
- Without treatment, a small percentage of patients will develop fulminant hepatic failure.
- Acute kidney injury due to acute tubular necrosis occurs in 25% of patients with severe hepatic damage and in a few without evidence of serious disturbance of liver function.

Treatment

- The treatment protocol is dependent on the time of presentation (Fig. 18.1) and this is summarized in Box 18.1. **IV acetylcysteine** is an effective protective agent, provided that it is administered within 8–10 hours of ingestion of the overdose.
- Some 10% of patients treated with **IV acetylcysteine** (20.25-hour regimen) develop rash, angio-oedema, hypotension and bronchospasm.

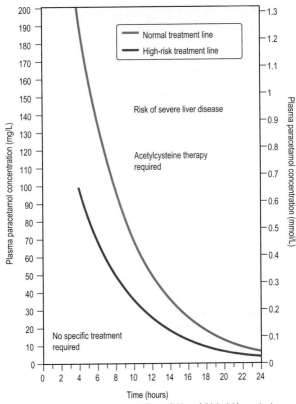

Fig. 18.1 Nomogram of paracetamol. For definition of 'high risk', see text. (*British National Formulary* 2009, with permission.)

- These reactions, which are related to the initial bolus, are seldom serious and temporarily discontinuing the infusion is usually all that is required.
- In more severe cases **chlorphenamine 10 mg** IV in an adult should be given.
- If liver or renal failure ensues, this should be treated conventionally, though there is evidence that a continuing infusion of **acetylcysteine** (continue 16-hour infusion until recovery) will improve the morbidity and mortality.
- Liver transplantation has been performed successfully in patients with paracetamol-induced fulminant hepatic failure using established criteria (p. 187).

Box 18.1 Management of patients with paracetamol poisoning

≤ 8 hours after ingestion

- Take blood for urgent estimation of the plasma paracetamol concentration as soon as 4 hours or more have elapsed since ingestion. Check INR, plasma creatinine and ALT activity
- Assess whether the patient is at increased risk of liver damage. Patients with pre-existing liver disease, those with a high alcohol intake *and* poor nutrition, those receiving enzyme-inducing drugs, and those suffering from anorexia nervosa and other eating disorders (including those who have starved for 2–3 days during an intercurrent illness) or HIV infection should be considered to be at greater risk and given treatment at plasma paracetamol concentrations lower than those normally used for interpretation, i.e. according to the 'high-risk line' (Fig. 18.1)
- If needed, give acetylcysteine 150 mg/kg over 15 min, then 50 mg/kg over the next 4 hours and then 100 mg/kg over the ensuing 16 hours *(total dose 300 mg/kg over 20.25 hours)*
- If the plasma paracetamol concentration is not available within 8 hours of the overdose and if > 150 mg/kg paracetamol has been ingested, treatment should be started at once and stopped if the plasma paracetamol concentration subsequently indicates that treatment is not required
- Check INR, plasma creatinine and ALT activity on completion of treatment and before discharge

8–15 hours after ingestion

- Urgent action is required because the efficacy of treatment declines progressively from 8 hours after overdose. If > 150 mg/kg paracetamol has been ingested, start treatment immediately
- Take blood for urgent estimation of the plasma paracetamol concentration, INR, plasma creatinine and ALT activity
- Assess whether the patient is at increased risk of liver damage
- The need for treatment should be determined by using Fig. 18.1
- In patients already receiving treatment, only discontinue if the plasma paracetamol concentration is below the relevant treatment line (Fig. 18.1), there is no abnormality of the INR, plasma creatinine or ALT activity, and the patient is asymptomatic. Do not discontinue the infusion if there is any doubt as to the timing of the overdose
- At the end of treatment, measure INR, plasma creatinine and ALT activity. If any test is abnormal or the patient is symptomatic, further monitoring is required and expert advice should be sought
- Patients with normal INR, plasma creatinine and ALT activity who are asymptomatic may be discharged

15–36 hours after ingestion

- Urgent action is required because the efficacy of treatment is limited more than 15 hours after overdose. Start treatment immediately if > 150 mg/kg paracetamol has been ingested

- In all patients, take blood for urgent estimation of the plasma paracetamol concentration, INR, plasma creatinine and ALT activity
- Assess whether the patient is at increased risk of liver damage
- Give acetylcysteine, if needed. The prognostic accuracy of the '200 mg/L line' after 15 hours is uncertain but a plasma paracetamol concentration above the extended treatment line should be regarded as carrying serious risk of severe liver damage
- At the end of treatment, check INR, plasma creatinine and ALT activity. If any test is abnormal or the patient is symptomatic, further monitoring is required and expert advice should be sought

>36 hours after ingestion
- Take blood for urgent plasma paracetamol concentration, INR, plasma creatinine and ALT activity. Wait for the results, a short delay in giving acetylcysteine does no harm. If the patient is jaundiced, treat.

Paraquat

Paraquat is a herbicide that has now been banned in many countries. Poisoning is common in Asia and Pacific and Caribbean areas.

Clinical features
- Mild poisoning follows the ingestion of < 20 mg of paraquat ion/kg body weight. Patients are asymptomatic or develop vomiting and diarrhoea. Full recovery occurs but there may be a transient fall in the gas transfer factor and vital capacity.
- Moderate to severe poisoning follows the ingestion of 20–40 mg of paraquat ion/kg body weight. Vomiting and diarrhoea occur and pulmonary fibrosis develops in all cases. In addition, kidney injury and, sometimes, hepatic dysfunction may supervene. Death occurs in the majority of cases but can be delayed for 2 or 3 weeks.
- Acute fulminant poisoning follows the ingestion of more than (usually considerably in excess of) 40 mg of paraquat ion/kg body weight. In addition to nausea and vomiting, there is marked ulceration of the oropharynx with multiple organ (cardiac, respiratory, hepatic, renal, adrenal, pancreatic, neurological) failure. The mortality is 100%. Death commonly occurs within 24 hours of ingestion and is never delayed for more than 1 week.

Treatment
- Treatment is supportive but does not change the outcome.

Petroleum distillates

Petroleum distillates are complex chemical mixtures derived from crude oil, which consist predominantly of aliphatic hydrocarbons with smaller amounts of aromatic hydrocarbons. The main hazard is aspiration pneumonitis following ingestion.

Clinical features

● After ingestion, nausea and vomiting are likely but systemic toxicity is not expected unless aspiration has occurred since absorption of petroleum distillates from the gastrointestinal tract is poor.
● Aspiration causes chemical pneumonitis. Signs and symptoms progress over 24–48 hours with wheeze, breathlessness, dyspnoea, tachypnoea, bronchospasm, hypoxia, cyanosis, fever and leucocytosis.
● Prolonged inhalation causes nausea, vomiting, headache, dizziness, respiratory tract irritation, shortness of breath, euphoria, delirium, ataxia and drowsiness. Severe cases may be complicated by ARDS, rhabdomyolysis, amnesia, coma, convulsions, ventricular arrhythmias and cardiopulmonary arrest.
● **CXR** may show shadowing in the mid- or lower zones.

Treatment

● Patients with significant respiratory compromise need urgent supportive measures (oxygen, bronchodilators).
● *Do not* do a gastric lavage due to the increased risk of aspiration.
● All patients with a definite history of ingestion should have a **CXR** since radiological abnormalities may be present even in asymptomatic patients. However, the X-ray should be delayed until at least 6 hours post ingestion in those who have no or only minimal symptoms at presentation.
● Measure ABGs.
● There is no good evidence that **prophylactic** corticosteroids (inhaled or systemic) and antibiotics are of benefit in the management of pulmonary complications of petroleum distillate toxicity.
● Patients may be discharged 6 hours after ingestion if asymptomatic, there are no signs in the chest and a CXR is normal.

Phenytoin

Clinical features

● Poisoning results in nystagmus, dysarthria, cerebellar ataxia (which may be persistent), drowsiness, coma and, rarely, hypoglycaemia.

Treatment

● Management is supportive.
● There is some evidence that **MDAC** (p. 663) increases phenytoin elimination.

Plant toxins

Yellow oleander (*Thevetia peruviana*)

This is a cause of poisoning in tropical and subtropical countries. Yellow oleander seeds contain highly toxic cardiac glycosides, including thevetins and peruvoside.

● Clinical features. Ingestion leads to severe glycoside toxicity (see digoxin poisoning, p. 675).
● Treatment
  • The role of MDAC is still debated.
  • Hypokalaemia or hyperkalaemia should be corrected.
  • Sinus bradycardia, atrioventricular block and sinoatrial standstill are often reduced or abolished by **atropine** 1.2–2.4 mg IV.

- **The administration of IV digoxin-specific antibody fragments** (see digoxin poisoning, p. 675) has been shown in an RCT to reverse yellow oleander-induced arrhythmias rapidly, restore sinus rhythm, and reverse bradycardia and hyperkalaemia rapidly.

Gloriosa superba

Poisoning due to ingestion of the tubers of *Gloriosa superba* (containing the alkaloid colchicine) occur in some rural areas of tropical countries. Colchicine inhibits mitosis and tissues that have a high cell turnover.

- Clinical features Severe abdominal pain, vomiting, diarrhoea (sometimes bloody), electrolyte imbalance, hypovolaemia and shock occur.
- Bone marrow depression with abnormal bleeding tendency, cardiac arrhythmias, hepatic toxicity and acute kidney injury can develop 24 hours after ingestion.
- Respiratory depression and coma can occur in severe poisoning, which is often fatal.
- Treatment This is supportive. Colchicine Fab fragments have been used but are not generally available.

Quinine

Quinine poisoning is relatively common in Western Europe, probably because of its use for the treatment of leg cramps. It is also ingested in overdose in the developing world, where it is employed as an antimalarial.

Clinical features

- In addition to the development of tinnitus and deafness, a substantial number of patients develop oculotoxicity and blindness, which may be irreversible.
- Ventricular arrhythmias, convulsions and coma are observed in severe cases.

Treatment

- In addition to supportive measures there is evidence that **MDAC** (p. 663) increases quinine elimination.

Salicylates

Clinical features

- After overdose, tachypnoea, sweating, vomiting, epigastric pain, tinnitus and deafness develop.
- Respiratory alkalosis and metabolic acidosis supervene and a mixed acid–base disturbance is observed commonly.
- Rarely, in severe cases, ARDS, coma and convulsions may ensue.

Treatment

- Give fluid and electrolyte replacement with potassium supplementation.
- Severe metabolic acidosis requires at least partial correction with the administration of **sodium bicarbonate** 50–100 mmol intravenously (p. 382).
- Mild cases of salicylate poisoning may be managed with parenteral fluid and electrolyte replacement only.
- Patients whose plasma salicylate concentrations are in excess of 500 mg/L (3.62 mmol/L) should receive **urine alkalinization** (p. 663).

- **Haemodialysis** is the treatment of choice for severely poisoned patients (plasma salicylate concentration > 700 mg/L (> 5.07 mmol/L)), particularly those with coma and metabolic acidosis.

Selective serotonin reuptake inhibitors (SSRIs)

Citalopram, fluoxetine, fluvoxamine, paroxetine and sertraline are antidepressants that inhibit serotonin reuptake. They lack the antimuscarinic actions of tricyclic antidepressants.

Clinical features

- Even large overdoses appear to be relatively safe unless potentiated by ethanol.
- Most patients will show no signs of toxicity but drowsiness, nausea, diarrhoea and sinus tachycardia have been reported.
- Rarely, junctional bradycardia, seizures, hypertension and the serotonin syndrome (p. 666) have been encountered.

Treatment

- Supportive measures are generally all that is required.
- Monitor cardiac rhythm if the 12-lead ECG shows a conduction abnormality.

Snake bites

Clinical features

- **Viperidae (Viperinae and Crotalinae)** Russell's viper causes most of the snake-bite mortality in India, Pakistan and Myanmar.
- There is local swelling at the site of the bite, which may become massive.
- Local tissue necrosis may occur, particularly with cobra bites.
- Evidence of systemic involvement (envenomation) occurs within 30 mins, including vomiting, evidence of shock and hypotension.
- Haemorrhage due to incoagulable blood can be fatal.
- **Elapidae** There is usually no swelling at the site of the bite, except with Asian cobras and African spitting cobras — here the bite is painful and is followed by local tissue necrosis.
- Vomiting occurs first, followed by shock and then neurological symptoms and muscle weakness, with paralysis of the respiratory muscles in severe cases. Cardiac muscle can be involved.
- **Hydrophiidae** Systemic features are muscle involvement, myalgia and myoglobinuria, which can lead to acute kidney injury. Cardiac and respiratory paralysis may occur.

Treatment

- A firm pressure bandage should be placed over the bite and the limb immobilized, which may delay the spread of the venom. Arterial tourniquets should *not* be used, and incision or excision of the bite area should not be performed.
- Local wounds often require little treatment. If necrosis is present, antibiotics should be given.
- Anti-tetanus prophylaxis must be given.
- Identify the type of snake if possible.
- In about 50% of cases no venom has been injected by the bite. Nevertheless, careful observation for 12–24 hours is necessary in case envenomation develops.

- General supportive measures include IV fluids with volume expanders for hypotension and **diazepam** 5–10 mg for anxiety.
- Treatment of acute respiratory, cardiac and acute kidney injury is instituted as necessary.
- Some forms of neurotoxicity, such as those induced by the death adder, have responded to therapy with **neostigmine** and **atropine**.
- Antivenoms are not generally indicated unless envenomation is present, as they can cause severe allergic reactions. They can rapidly neutralize venom, but only if an amount in excess of the amount of venom is given. Large quantities may be required. As antivenoms cannot reverse the effects of the venom, they must be given early to minimize some of the local effects and may prevent necrosis at the site of the bite. Antivenoms should be administered intravenously by slow infusion, the same dose being given to children and adults. **Side-effects**: allergic reactions are frequent, and **adrenaline (epinephrine)** 1 in 1000 solution should be available. In severe cases, the antivenom infusion should be continued, even if an allergic reaction occurs, with SC injections of adrenaline being given as necessary.

Sodium valproate

Clinical features

- These include fever, drowsiness, coma, sinus tachycardia, muscle spasms, seizures, hypocalcaemia, liver damage and thrombocytopenia.
- Cerebral oedema and optic atrophy are uncommon.
- Hyperammonaemia and metabolic acidosis have been reported.

Treatment

- Treat any seizures with IV benzodiazepines (e.g. **diazepam** 5–10 mg; repeat every 20 mins).
- Haemodialysis increases elimination of valproate and is used in severe poisoning.
- Early IV supplementation with **carnitine** (100 mg/kg, followed by 15 mg/kg every 4 hours) to reduce formation of hepatotoxic metabolites and ammonaemia, may improve survival in severe valproate-induced hepatotoxicity, although clinical benefit in terms of liver protection or hastening of recovery from unconsciousness has not been clearly established.

Theophylline

Clinical features

- Nausea, vomiting, hyperventilation, haematemesis, abdominal pain, diarrhoea, sinus tachycardia, supraventricular and ventricular arrhythmias, hypotension, restlessness, irritability, headache, hyperreflexia, tremors and convulsions have been observed.
- Hypokalaemia results from activation of Na^+/K^+ ATPase.
- A mixed acid–base disturbance is common.

Treatment

- There is good evidence that **MDAC** (p. 663) enhances the elimination of theophylline.
- However, protracted theophylline-induced vomiting may mitigate the benefit of this therapy. Vomiting may be suppressed by, for example, **ondansetron 8 mg IV** in an adult.

Kumar & Clark's Medical Management and Therapeutics

- Correct hypokalaemia to prevent or treat tachyarrhythmias.
- A non-selective β-adrenoceptor-blocking drug, such as **propranolol** 1–5 mg by slow IV infusion, is also useful in the treatment of tachy-arrhythmias secondary to hypokalaemia. It should not be given if the patient has chronic respiratory disease, e.g. asthma.
- Convulsions should be treated with **diazepam 10–20 mg** IV in an adult.

Tricyclic antidepressants (TCAs)

Clinical features

- Features of poisoning usually begin within 60 mins of ingestion and reach maximum intensity in 6–12 hours.
- Drowsiness, sinus tachycardia, dry mouth, dilated pupils, urinary retention, increased reflexes and extensor plantar responses are the most common features of mild poisoning.
- Severe intoxication leads to coma, often with divergent strabismus and convulsions. Plantar, oculo-cephalic and oculo-vestibular reflexes may be abolished temporarily.
- An ECG will often show a wide QRS interval and there is a reasonable correlation between the width of the QRS complex and the severity of poisoning. A QRS duration of > 160 ms suggests severe cardiotoxicity with a high risk of arrhythmia.
- Conduction block predisposes to supraventricular and/or ventricular arrhythmias.
- Metabolic acidosis, rhabdomyolysis and cardiorespiratory depression are observed in severe cases.

Treatment

- The majority of patients recover with supportive therapy alone (ingestion of < 20 mg/kg). Overdose of 35 mg/kg is a median lethal dose; > 50 mg/kg is likely to be fatal.
- Priority should be given to the correction of hypoxia, hypotension, electrolyte abnormalities and acidosis.
- Measure ABGs.
- Check plasma total creatine kinase activity and monitor urine output.
- Patients may deteriorate rapidly in the first few hours of poisoning and close cardiorespiratory monitoring is essential during this time.
- Ensure a clear airway and adequate ventilation. Mechanical ventilation may be necessary.
- Establish IV access and give a **crystalloid** bolus, e.g. 0.9% saline 500–1000 mL to an adult, if hypotension is present.
- Correct metabolic acidosis that persists despite fluid resuscitation and adequate ventilation with IV 50–100 mmol of **sodium bicarbonate** (e.g. 50–100 mL of 8.4% sodium bicarbonate).
- Alkalinization (IV 1–2 mmol of sodium bicarbonate/kg) to a systemic pH of 7.45–7.55 may reverse TCA-induced cardiotoxicity even in the absence of acidosis.
- **Avoid** conventional anti-arrhythmic agents, particularly class Ia (e.g. **procainamide**) and class Ic (e.g. **flecainide**), as these will exacerbate TCA-induced cardiotoxicity.
- There may be an occasional role for class Ib (lidocaine) or class II (**β-blockers**) agents (or **magnesium**) in refractory ventricular arrhythmias.

- Treat sustained convulsions with IV **diazepam 10–20 mg**. Phenytoin is best avoided in TCA overdose because, in common with TCAs, it blocks sodium channels and may increase the risk of cardiac arrhythmias.
- Treat hypotension that is unresponsive to fluids and sodium bicarbonate with **noradrenaline (norepinephrine)**.
- If cardiac arrest ensues prolonged resuscitation may be successful, particularly if the patient had no pre-existing cardiac morbidity, and should be continued for at least 1 hour.

Venlafaxine

This antidepressant is a serotonin–noradrenaline (norepinephrine) reuptake inhibitor (SNRI).

Clinical features
- Common features include drowsiness, tachycardia, dizziness and diaphoresis.
- Both hypertension and hypotension are recognized.
- Severely poisoned patients are at risk of convulsions and cardiac conduction abnormalities, particularly QRS and QT interval prolongation with the associated risk of ventricular arrhythmias including torsades de pointes.
- Complications include rhabdomyolysis, the serotonin syndrome and rarely hepatic necrosis, disseminated intravascular coagulation and cardiomyopathy.

Treatment
- Establish a clear airway and maintain adequate ventilation.
- Gastric lavage or the administration of oral activated charcoal 50–100 g to an adult is used if the patient presents within the first hour, although no clinical trials have confirmed the efficacy of either procedure.
- Perform a 12-lead ECG and commence cardiac monitoring in all symptomatic patients.
- Treat prolonged seizures with IV diazepam 5–10 mg.
- Measure ABGs.
- Correct metabolic acidosis that persists despite fluid resuscitation and adequate ventilation with IV 50–100 mmol of sodium bicarbonate (e.g. 50–100 mL of 8.4% sodium bicarbonate).
- Check plasma electrolytes, creatinine concentration and total creatine kinase activity and monitor urine output and core body temperature.
- Marked hypotension that does not resolve with fluid resuscitation may require IV inotropic support with, for example, noradrenaline (norepinephrine).

Warfarin (p. 245)

Clinical features
- Manifestations of excess anticoagulation may be delayed for some 15 hours after acute ingestion of warfarin as a medicine or as an anticoagulant rodenticide.
- Patients may have significant prolongation of the prothrombin time without evidence of bleeding.
- Common features include epistaxis, gingival bleeding, spontaneous bruising, haematomas, haematuria, menorrhagia and rectal bleeding.

Treatment

- Routine measurement of the INR (p. 246) is unnecessary in young children, as they invariably ingest only very small amounts of warfarin.
- In all other cases, the INR should be measured on presentation and 36–48 hours post exposure.
- If the *INR is normal* at this time, no further action is required.
- If *active bleeding* occurs, **prothrombin complex concentrate** (which contains factors II, VII, IX and X) 50 U/kg *or* fresh frozen plasma 15 mL/kg (if no concentrate is available) *and* **phytomenadione** 10 mg IV (100 mcg/kg body weight for a child) should be given, see p. 250 and Table 7.3.
- If there is no active bleeding and the *INR is ≤ 4.0*, treatment with **phytomenadione** is not required.
- If the *INR is ≥4.0*, **phytomenadione** 10 mg by slow intravenous injection (100 μg/kg body weight for a child) should be administered, unless the patient is anticoagulated for therapeutic reasons.
- If the patient is prescribed *anticoagulants and the INR is ≥ 8.0*, but there is no active bleeding or only minor bleeding, stop warfarin (restart when the INR ≤ 5.0), give **phytomenadione** 0.5 mg by slow intravenous injection and repeat the dose if the INR is ≥ 8.0 24 hours later.
- If the *INR is 6.0–8.0* and there is no active bleeding or only minor bleeding, warfarin should be discontinued and restarted when the INR is ≤ 5.0.
- In a patient taking warfarin therapeutically vitamin K may be harmful (see p. 250).

Further reading

Bailey B: Glucagon in β-blocker and calcium channel blocker overdoses: a systematic review, *J Toxicol Clin Toxicol* 41:595–602, 2003.

Barceloux D, McGuigan M, Hartigan-Go K, et al: Position paper: cathartics, *J Toxicol Clin Toxicol* 42:243–253, 2004.

Bateman DN: Digoxin-specific antibody fragments: how much and when? *Toxicol Rev* 23:135–143, 2004.

Bateman DN: Tricyclic antidepressant poisoning: central nervous system effects and management, *Toxicol Rev* 24:181–186, 2005.

Borron SW, Baud FJ, Barriot P, et al: Prospective study of hydroxocobalamin for acute cyanide poisoning in smoke inhalation, *Ann Emerg Med* 49:794–801, 2007.

Bradberry S, Sheehan T, Vale A: Use of oral dimercaptosuccinic acid (succimer; DMSA) in adult patients with inorganic lead poisoning, *QJM* 102:721–732, 2009.

Bradberry SM, Sheehan TMT, Barraclough CR, Vale JA: DMPS can reverse the features of severe mercury vapor-induced neurological damage, *Clin Toxicol* 47:894–898, 2009.

Bradberry SM, Thanacoody HKR, Watt BE, et al: Management of the cardiovascular complications of tricyclic antidepressant poisoning: role of sodium bicarbonate, *Toxicol Rev* 24:195–204, 2005.

Brent J: Fomepizole for ethylene glycol and methanol poisoning, *N Engl J Med* 360:2216–2223, 2009.

British Medical Association and Royal Pharmaceutical Society of Great Britain: *British National Formulary 58*. London, 2009, BMJ Group and RPS Publishing.

Buckley NA, Isbister GK, Stokes B, Juurlink DN: Hyperbaric oxygen for carbon monoxide poisoning: a systematic review and critical analysis of the evidence, *Toxicol Rev* 24:75–92, 2005.

Chyka PA, Seger D, Krenzelok EP, et al: Position paper: single-dose activated charcoal, *Clin Toxicol* 43:61–87, 2005.

DeWitt CR, Waksman JC: Pharmacology, pathophysiology and management of calcium channel blocker and beta-blocker toxicity, *Toxicol Rev* 23:223–238, 2004.

Flamminger A, Maibach H: Sulfuric acid burns (corrosion and acute irritation): evidence-based overview of management, *Cutan Ocul Toxicol* 25:55–61, 2006.

Hall AP, Henry JA: Acute toxic effects of 'ecstasy' (MDMA) and related compounds: overview of pathophysiology and clinical management, *Br J Anaesth* 96:678–685, 2006.

Hoffman RS: Cocaine and β-blockers: should the controversy continue? *Ann Emerg Med* 51:127–129, 2008.

Krenzelok EP, McGuigan M, Lheureux P, et al: Position paper: ipecac syrup, *J Toxicol Clin Toxicol* 42:133–143, 2004.

Kulig K, Vale JA: Position paper: gastric lavage, *J Toxicol Clin Toxicol* 42:933–943, 2004.

Lheureux PE, Zahir S, Gris M, et al: Bench-to-bedside review: hyperinsulinaemia/euglycaemia therapy in the management of overdose of calcium-channel blockers, *Crit Care* 10:212, 2006.

Lheureux PER, Hantson P: Carnitine in the treatment of valproic acid-induced toxicity, *Clin Toxicol* 47:101–111, 2009.

Morgan M, Hackett LP, Isbister GK: Olanzepine overdose: a series of analytically confirmed cases, *Int Clin Psychopharmacol* 22:183–186, 2007.

Proudfoot AT, Krenzelok EP, Brent J, Vale JA: Does urine alkalinization increase salicylate elimination? If so, why? *Toxicol Rev* 22:129–136, 2003.

Proudfoot AT, Krenzelok EP, Vale JA: Position paper on urine alkalinization, *J Toxicol Clin Toxicol* 42:1–26, 2004.

Tenenbein M, Lheureux P: Position paper: whole bowel irrigation, *J Toxicol Clin Toxicol* 42:843–854, 2004.

Vale JA, Krenzelok EP, Barceloux DG, et al: Position statement and practice guidelines on the use of multi-dose activated charcoal in the treatment of acute poisoning, *J Toxicol Clin Toxicol* 37:731–751, 1999.

Waring WS, Good AM, Bateman DN: Lack of significant toxicity after mirtazapine overdose: a five-year review of cases admitted to a regional toxicology unit, *Clin Toxicol* 45:45–50, 2007.

Further information

(+44) 844 892 0111
UK National Poisons Information Service (24 hours)

www.toxbasebackup.org/
UK NPIS Primary Clinical Toxicology Database

www.toxnet.nlm.nih.gov
US National Library of Medicine's Toxicology Data Network.

www.who.int/ipcs/poisons/centre/directory/en/
WHO World Directory of poisons centres

Environmental medicine 19

CHAPTER CONTENTS

HEAT

Body core temperature (T_{Core}) is maintained at 37°C by the thermoregulator centre in the hypothalamus.

- **Heat acclimatization.** This occurs over several weeks. The sweat volume increases and the sweat salt content falls. Increased evaporation of sweat results in a reduced T_{Core}.
- **Heat cramps.** Painful muscle cramps, usually in the legs, occur in fit people during exercise in hot weather. They respond to combined salt and water replacement, and in the acute stage to stretching and muscle massage. T_{Core} remains normal.
- **Heat illness (heat exhaustion).** At any environmental temperature (especially with T_{Env} of > 25°C), and with a high humidity, exercise in clothes that inhibit sweating can cause an elevation in T_{Core} in less than 15 mins. Heat illness with a T_{Core} > 37°C causes weakness, cramps and syncope, and may progress to heat injury.

Management

Reduce (T_{Env}) and cool the patient with sponging and fans. Give O_2 by mask.

Oral rehydration with both salt and water (25 g of salt per 5 L of water/day) is given initially, followed by normal daily fluids. In severe heat illness, IV 0.9% saline is given. Monitoring of serum sodium with correction of secondary potassium loss is required.

Heat injury (heat stroke)

Heat injury (heat stroke) is an acute life-threatening condition when T_{Core} rises above 41°C. Headache, nausea, vomiting and weakness, progressing to confusion, coma and death occur. The skin feels intensely hot to the touch, usually with absence of sweating.

Heat injury develops in unacclimatized people in hot, humid windless climates, often without exercise. Drugs and alcohol, e.g. antimuscarinics, diuretics and phenothiazines, contribute.

Prevention

- Acclimatization, fluids and appropriate clothing.

Management

Management is as above. Intensive care may be necessary for severe cases. Intravascular volume can remain normal and the use of IV fluids must be monitored with a CVP line.

Prompt treatment is essential, as complications of hypovolaemia, intravascular coagulation, cerebral oedema, rhabdomyolysis, and renal and hepatic failure can occur rapidly.

COLD

Hypothermia is defined as a core temperature of less than 32°C and is often lethal when T_{Core} falls below 30°C.

Hypothermia

- Hypothermia can occur when T_{Env} is below 8°C with inadequate heating and clothing. Drugs, e.g. hypnotics, alcohol, hypothyroidism or intercurrent illness also contribute. The elderly have diminished ability to sense cold and also have little insulating fat. Neonates and infants become hypothermic rapidly because of a relatively large surface area in proportion to subcutaneous fat.
- Hypothermia often occurs in climbers, skiers and polar travellers, and in wartime. Wet, cold conditions with wind chill, physical exhaustion, injuries and inadequate clothing are contributory.
- Serious hypothermia can develop following immersion for more than 1 hour in water temperatures of 15–20°C. In water temperatures below 12°C limbs rapidly become numb and weak. Recovery takes place gradually, often taking several hours.

Clinical features

Mild hypothermia (T_{Core} < 32°C) causes shivering and initially intense discomfort. As the T_{Core} falls below 32°C, severe hypothermia causes impaired judgement — including lack of awareness of cold. Drowsiness and coma, followed by death, occur.

Diagnosis

Someone who feels icy to the touch — abdomen, groin, axillae — is probably hypothermic. If the patent is clammy, uncooperative or sleepy, T_{Core} is almost certainly ≤ 32°C.

Pulse rate and systemic BP can fall. Cardiac output and cerebral blood flow are greatly affected by change in posture in hypothermia, and can fall further if the upright position is maintained or the thorax is restrained by a harness. Respiration becomes shallow and slow. Muscle stiffness develops; tendon reflexes become sluggish and/or lost.

In coma, pupillary and other brainstem reflexes are lost; pupils are fixed and may be dilated in severe hypothermia.

Reduction in the temperature of haemoglobin causes a falsely high arterial PO_2 and oxygen saturation. Using a pulse oximeter, the level of arterial oxygen saturation (Sa_{O_2}) will, however, be correct.

Bradycardia with 'J' waves (rounded waves above the isoelectric line at the junction of the QRS complex and ST segment (Fig. 19.1)) is pathognomonic of hypothermia. Prolongation of PR and QT intervals and of the QRS complex also occurs. Ventricular dysrhythmia (tachycardia/fibrillation) or asystole is the usual cause of death.

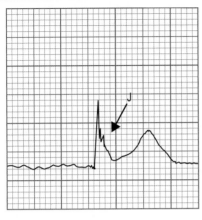

Fig. 19.1 ECG showing J waves.

Management

Maintain the patient in a horizontal position or slightly head-down, rewarm gradually, correct metabolic abnormalities, anticipate and treat dysrhythmias, and check for hypothyroidism (p. 570).

If the patient is awake, with a core temperature of more than 32°C (with a low-reading thermometer), place him/her in a warm room, use a foil wrap and give warm fluids orally. Outdoors, add extra dry clothing, huddle together and use a warmed sleeping bag. Rewarming may take several hours. Avoid alcohol; this adds to confusion, boosts confidence factitiously, causes peripheral vasodilatation and further heat loss, and can precipitate hypoglycaemia.

In **severe hypothermia**, people look dead. Always exclude hypothermia before diagnosing brainstem death (p. 561). Warm gradually, aiming at an increase in T_{Core} of 1°C per hour. Direct mild surface heat can be helpful. Monitor all vital functions.

Give warm IV fluids slowly and correct metabolic abnormalities. Hypothyroidism, if present, should be treated with **liothyronine**.

DROWNING AND NEAR-DROWNING

Drowning caused over 500 000 deaths worldwide in 2007. Exhaustion, alcohol, drugs and hypothermia all contribute to deaths following immersion. People can also drown after an epileptic seizure or a myocardial infarct whilst in water.

Dry drowning

Between 10 and 15% of drownings occur without water aspiration into the lungs. Laryngeal spasm develops acutely, followed by apnoea and cardiac arrest.

Wet drowning

Fresh- or sea-water aspiration destroys pulmonary surfactant, leading to alveolar collapse, ventilation/perfusion mismatch and hypoxaemia.

Kumar & Clark's Medical Management and Therapeutics

Aspiration of hypertonic seawater (5% NaCl) pulls additional fluid into the alveoli with further ventilation/perfusion mismatch. In practice, there is little difference between salt-water and fresh-water aspiration. In both, severe hypoxaemia develops rapidly. Severe metabolic acidosis develops in the majority of survivors.

Emergency treatment

CPR should be started immediately (p. 704). Patients have survived for up to 30 mins under water without suffering brain damage — and sometimes for longer periods if the temperature of the water (T_{Water}) is near 10°C.

Resuscitation should always be attempted, even with an absent pulse and fixed dilated pupils. All survivors should be admitted to hospital for intensive monitoring, as they are liable to develop acute lung injury during the subsequent 48 hours.

IONIZING RADIATION

- Ionizing radiation is either penetrating (X-rays, γ-rays or neutrons) or non-penetrating (α- or β-particles). Penetrating radiation affects the skin and deeper tissues, while non-penetrating radiation affects the skin alone.
- All radiation effects depend on the type of radiation, the distribution of dose and the dose rate.
- Dosage is measured in joules per kilogram (J/kg); 1 J/kg = 1 gray (1 Gy) = 100 rads.
- Radioactivity is measured in becquerels (Bq). 1 Bq is defined as the activity of a quantity of radioactive material in which one nucleus decays per second; 3.7×10^{10} Bq = 1 curie (Ci), the older, non-SI unit.
- Radiation differs in the density of ionization it causes. Therefore a dose-equivalent called a sievert (Sv) is used. This is the absorbed dose weighted for the damaging effect of the radiation. The annual background radiation is approximately 2.5 mSv. A CXR delivers 0.02 mSv, and CT of the abdomen/pelvis about 8–10 mSv.

Acute radiation sickness

Nausea, vomiting and malaise follow doses of approximately 1 Gy. Lymphopenia occurs within several days, followed 2–3 weeks later by a fall in all white cells and platelets. Higher doses cause:

- **Haematopoietic syndrome.** Absorption of 2–10 Gy is followed by transient vomiting in some individuals, while severe lymphopenia develops over several days. A decrease in granulocytes and platelets follows 14–21 weeks later, as no new cells are formed in the marrow. Bleeding and frequent overwhelming infections develop, with a high mortality.
- **Gastrointestinal syndrome.** Doses ≥ 6 Gy cause acute vomiting several hours after exposure. The vomiting usually then stops, only to recur some 4 days later accompanied by diarrhoea. The villous lining of the intestine becomes denuded. Intractable bloody diarrhoea follows, with dehydration, secondary infection and sometimes death.
- **CNS syndrome.** Exposures of ≥ 30 Gy are followed rapidly by nausea, vomiting, disorientation and coma. Death due to cerebral oedema can follow, usually within 36 hours.
- **Radiation dermatitis.** Skin erythema, purpura, blistering and secondary infection occur. Total loss of body hair is a bad prognostic sign and usually follows an exposure ≥ 5 Gy.

Late effects of radiation exposure

Risks of acute myeloid leukaemia and cancer, particularly of skin, thyroid and salivary glands, increase. Infertility, teratogenesis and cataract are also late sequelae, developing years after exposure.

For the sequelae of therapeutic radiation — early, early-delayed and late-delayed radiation — see p. 256).

Treatment

Prevention and treatment of infection, haemorrhage and fluid loss are the mainstays of treatment.

Accidental ingestion of, or exposure to, bone-seeking radioisotopes (e.g. ^{90}strontium and ^{137}caesium) is treated with chelating agents, e.g. EDTA and massive doses of oral calcium. Radio-iodine contamination should be treated immediately with potassium iodide to block radio-iodine absorption by the thyroid.

ELECTRIC SHOCK

- The common domestic electric shock is typically painful, and is rarely fatal or followed by serious sequelae. More serious effects are rare following accidents in the home or in industry.
- Ventricular fibrillation, muscular contraction and spinal cord damage can follow a major shock. These are typically seen following lightning strikes with exceedingly high voltage and amperage.
- Non-fatal lightning strikes can cause fern-shaped burns. Deeper injuries can also occur, with muscle and spinal cord damage.

BIOTERRORISM/BIOWARFARE

The potential of bacteria as weapons is illustrated by a suggestion that several kilograms of anthrax spores might kill as many people as a Hiroshima-sized nuclear weapon.

Potential pathogens

The US Centers for Disease Control in Atlanta, Georgia, have developed a classification of potential biological agents (Table 19.1).

Table 19.1 Critical biological agents

Category	Pathogens
A — Very infectious and/or readily disseminated organisms: high mortality with a major impact on public health	Smallpox, anthrax, botulism, plague
B — Moderately easy to disseminate organisms causing moderate morbidity and mortality	Q fever, brucellosis, glanders, food-/water-borne pathogens, influenza
C — Emerging and possible genetically engineered pathogens	Viral haemorrhagic fevers, encephalitis viruses, drug-resistant TB

(From Khan AS, et al 2000, with permission)

Smallpox

Smallpox is a highly infectious disease with a mortality ≥ 30%. There is no proven therapy but there is an effective vaccine. Universal vaccination was stopped in the early 1970s, with the result that most of the world's population is now unprotected.

Smallpox has an incubation period of around 12 days; the rash develops on the second or third day of the illness. Infection is transmitted by the airborne route; the patient becomes infectious to others 12–24 hours before the rash appears, thus allowing a potential infected volunteer to pass infection to others before being recognized as suffering from smallpox.

Anthrax

In late 2001, 22 individuals who were sent anthrax organisms through the US mail were infected; 11 developed pulmonary anthrax; 5 died despite ciprofloxacin therapy. The other 11 suffered from cutaneous anthrax.

Botulism

As a bioweapon, botulinum toxin could be transmitted in food or by air, e.g. from a crop-spraying light aircraft. The toxin is inactivated by chlorine in domestic water supplies. There is no vaccine available.

Plague

Plague (p. 38) could be transmitted as a bioweapon, either by airborne dissemination or by infected rats. Immunization is of limited value.

Further reading

Buchler JW, Berkelman RL, Hartley DM: Syndromic surveillance and bioterrorism-related epidemics, *Emerg Infect Dis* 10:1197–1204, 2003.

Khan AS, Morse S, Lillibridge S: Public-health preparedness for biological terrorism in the USA, *Lancet* 356:1179–1182, 2000.

Lazar HL: Editorial: The treatment of hypothermia, *New Engl J Med* 337:1545–1547, 1997.

Modell JH: Drowning, *New Engl J Med* 328:253–256, 1993.

Emergencies in medicine 20

CHAPTER CONTENTS

This chapter consists of algorithms which should be used in conjunction with the appropriate chapters to enable emergencies to be dealt with quickly and effectively.

An assessment and initial resuscitation of the critically ill patient should be undertaken (ABCDE):

- Airway — remove any obstructing material and make sure airway is clear.
- Breathing — look, listen and feel for signs of breathing.
- Circulation — check carotid and peripheral pulses and start external chest compression if cardiac arrest.
- Disability — conscious level — Glasgow Coma Scale (see Table 17.1, p. 624).
- Examination/exposure — to allow a full examination to be carried out.

Recent evidence emphasises that maintaining the circulation is the key factor overall. The order of resuscitation should be CAB, i.e. Circulation, Airways, Breathing.

DEFINITIONS

- An **emergency** is something dangerous or serious, such as an accident which happens suddenly or unexpectedly and needs fast action in order to avoid harmful results.
- **Urgent** cases need attention very soon (*Cambridge Advanced Learners Dictionary*).

BASIC LIFE SUPPORT

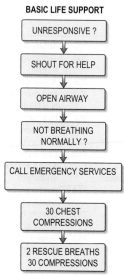

BASIC LIFE SUPPORT

UNRESPONSIVE ?

↓

SHOUT FOR HELP

↓

OPEN AIRWAY

↓

NOT BREATHING
NORMALLY ?

↓

CALL EMERGENCY SERVICES

↓

30 CHEST
COMPRESSIONS

↓

2 RESCUE BREATHS
30 COMPRESSIONS

Send or go for help as soon as possible according to guidelines

Fig. 20.1 Basic life support. (out of hospital). With permission from Resuscitation Council UK http://www.resus.org.uk
* Studies have shown that compression alone is as good as compression with rescue breaths. Compression should be at least 5 cm and performed at 100 compressions/min. The heel of one hand is placed over the centre of the chest, and the heel of the second hand is placed over the first, with the fingers interlocked.

SEVERE UPPER GASTROINTESTINAL BLEEDING

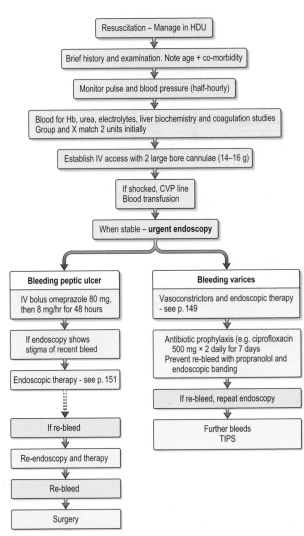

Fig. 20.4 Management of severe upper gastrointestinal bleeding (see also Box 5.3). TIPS, transjugular intrahepatic portocaval shunt. (Tool-Kit for upper GI bleeding see: http://aomrc.org.uk/projects/upper-gastrointestinal-bleeding-toolkit. html)

Kumar & Clark's Medical Management and Therapeutics

FULMINANT HEPATIC FAILURE

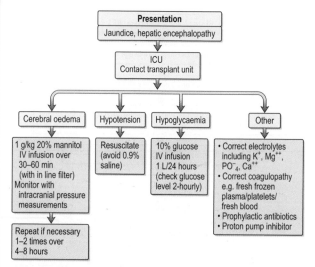

Fig. 20.5 Management of **fulminant hepatic failure**. See along with Boxes 6.2, 6.3 for referral to liver transplant unit.

FEBRILE NEUTROPENIC PATIENT

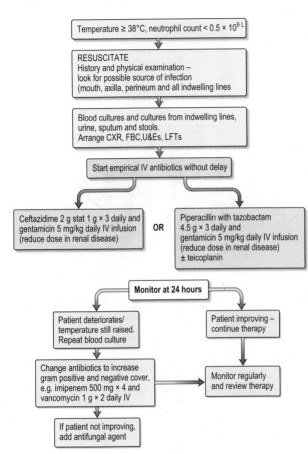

Fig. 20.6 Management of **febrile neutropenic patient**. See in conjunction with Box 8.5.

Kumar & Clark's Medical Management and Therapeutics

HOT SWOLLEN JOINT

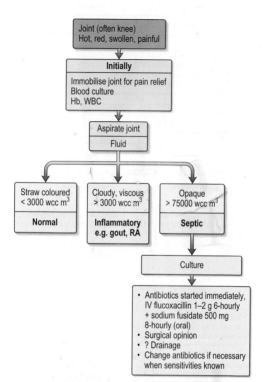

Fig. 20.7 Management of hot swollen joint (monoarthritis) (see also p. 321).

EXTREME HYPONATRAEMIA WITH A NORMAL EXTRACELLULAR VOLUME

Encephalopathy

↓

Serum Na⁺ < 125 mmol/L
(< 48 hours duration)
i.e. acute and therefore
can cause cerebral swelling

↓

Give 3% saline (hypertonic)
500 mL over 4–6 hours
via central vein

AIM

To increase Na by 2 mmol/L/hr
to correct the low sodium slowly
with reduction of symptoms. No
greater than 10 mmol in 24 hrs

Fig. 20.8 Treatment of **extreme hyponatraemia** with a normal extracellular volume (see also p. 372).

SEVERE ACUTE HYPERKALAEMIA

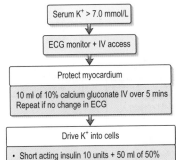

Serum K⁺ > 7.0 mmol/L

↓

ECG monitor + IV access

↓

Protect myocardium

10 ml of 10% calcium gluconate IV over 5 mins
Repeat if no change in ECG

↓

Drive K⁺ into cells

• Short acting insulin 10 units + 50 ml of 50%
  glucose IV over 10–15 mins.
  Repeat as necessary
• Correction of severe acidosis pH < 6.9
  give 1.2% sodium bicarbonate over 3–6 hours
• Monitor K⁺ and blood glucose repeatedly

LATER

Deplete body K⁺
• Polystyrene sulphonate resins
  15 g × 3 daily with laxative oral or rectally
• Dialysis

Fig. 20.9 Treatment of **severe acute hyperkalaemia** (see also p. 376).

CENTRAL CHEST PAIN — CARDIAC CAUSE LIKELY

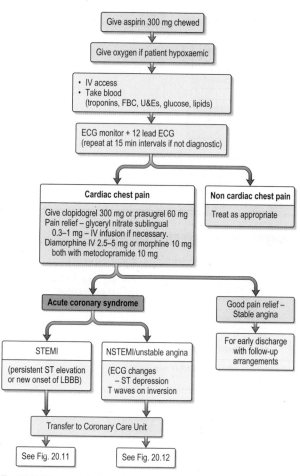

Fig. 20.10 Management of central chest pain — cardiac cause likely (see also p. 433).

ACUTE CORONARY SYNDROME—MANAGEMENT OF STEMI

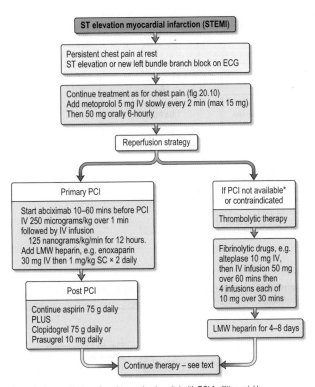

Fig. 20.11 Acute coronary syndrome—management of STEMI (ST elevation myocardial infarction). (see also p. 437).

*or patient cannot be transferred to another hospital with PCI facilities quickly

ACUTE CORONARY SYNDROME AND MANAGEMENT IN N-STEMI

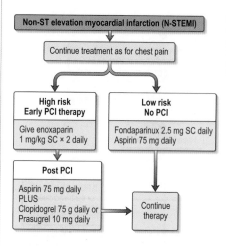

Fig. 20.12 Acute coronary syndrome and management in N-STEMI (non-ST elevation myocardial infarction).

HEIMLICH MANOEUVRE FOR TREATMENT OF INHALED FOREIGN BODIES

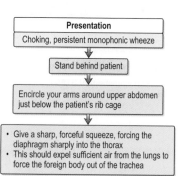

Fig. 20.13 Heimlich manoeuvre for treatment of inhaled foreign bodies.

PNEUMOTHORAX

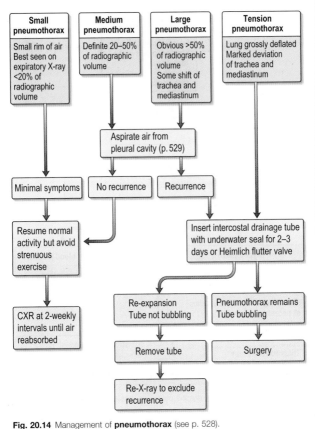

Fig. 20.14 Management of **pneumothorax** (see p. 528).

ACUTE MASSIVE PULMONARY EMBOLISM

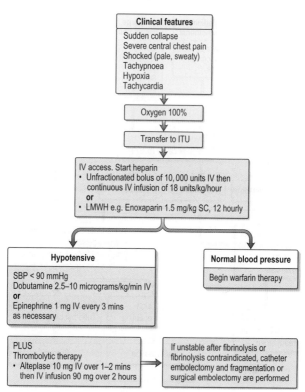

Fig. 20.15 Management of massive pulmonary embolism (see p. 522).

ACUTE SEVERE ASTHMA

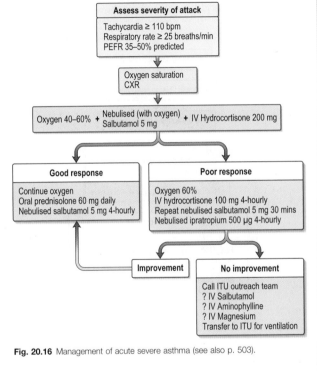

Fig. 20.16 Management of acute severe asthma (see also p. 503).

Kumar & Clark's Medical Management and Therapeutics

SHOCK

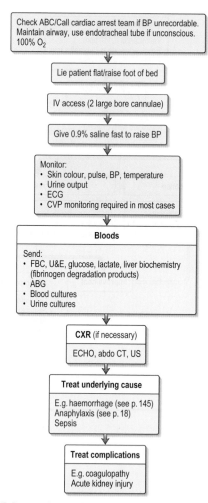

Check ABC/Call cardiac arrest team if BP unrecordable.
Maintain airway, use endotracheal tube if unconscious.
100% O$_2$

↓

Lie patient flat/raise foot of bed

↓

IV access (2 large bore cannulae)

↓

Give 0.9% saline fast to raise BP

↓

Monitor:
- Skin colour, pulse, BP, temperature
- Urine output
- ECG
- CVP monitoring required in most cases

↓

Bloods

Send:
- FBC, U&E, glucose, lactate, liver biochemistry (fibrinogen degradation products)
- ABG
- Blood cultures
- Urine cultures

↓

CXR (if necessary)

ECHO, abdo CT, US

↓

Treat underlying cause

E.g. haemorrhage (see p. 145)
Anaphylaxis (see p. 18)
Sepsis

↓

Treat complications

E.g. coagulopathy
Acute kidney injury

NB: Do not overload with fluids if in cardiogenic shock.
Fluid input – monitor with urine output, CVP and BP.
May require inotropes if patient remains hypotensive.
Do not sit patient up if hypotensive, even with breathing difficulties.

Fig. 20.17 Management of shock (see also p. 555).

SEVERE HYPERCALCAEMIA

```
┌─────────────────────────────────────┐
│         Clinical features:          │
├─────────────────────────────────────┤
│ Asymptomatic or variable symptoms,  │
│ e.g. abdominal pain, constipation,  │
│ anorexia, cardiac arrest            │
└─────────────────────────────────────┘
              ↓
   ┌───────────────────────────────┐
   │ Hypercalcaemia > 3 mmol/L     │
   │ (1 mg/dL above reference range)│
   └───────────────────────────────┘
              ↓
  ┌──────────────────────────────────┐
  │ Rehydrate  4–6 L 0.9% saline day 1│
  │            3–4 L 0.9% saline day 2–5│
  └──────────────────────────────────┘
              ↓
 ┌────────────────────────────────────┐
 │ Infuse IV pamidronate 60–90 mg in  │
 │ 0.9% saline/5% glucose over 2–4 hours│
 └────────────────────────────────────┘
              ↓
 ┌────────────────────────────────────┐
 │ Further treatment depends on cause │
 │ (e.g. prednisolone for sarcoidosis,│
 │ zoledronate for multiple myeloma)  │
 └────────────────────────────────────┘
```

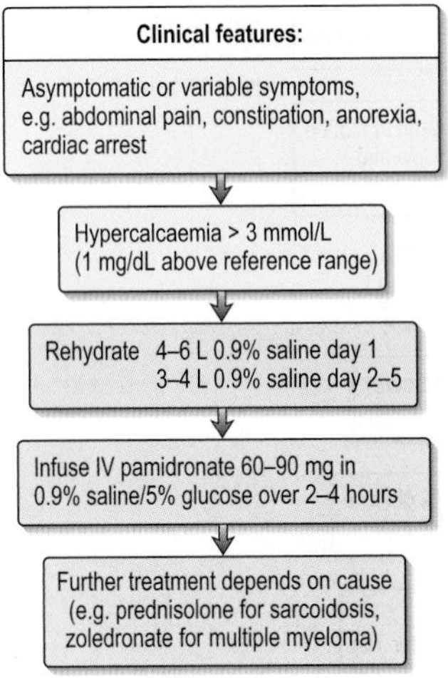

Fig. 20.18 Management of severe hypercalcaemia (see also p. 587).

ACUTE ADRENAL FAILURE

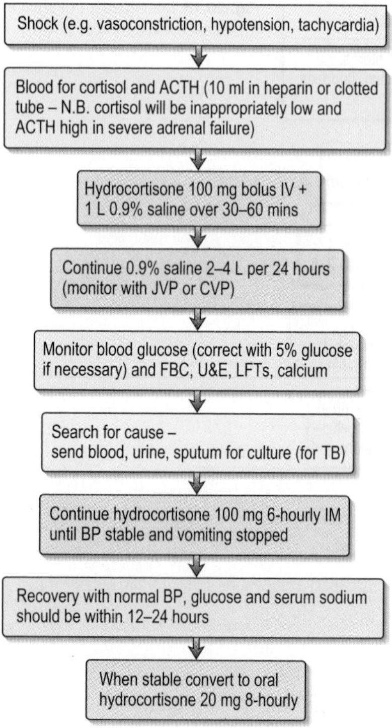

Shock (e.g. vasoconstriction, hypotension, tachycardia)

⬇

Blood for cortisol and ACTH (10 ml in heparin or clotted tube – N.B. cortisol will be inappropriately low and ACTH high in severe adrenal failure)

⬇

Hydrocortisone 100 mg bolus IV + 1 L 0.9% saline over 30–60 mins

⬇

Continue 0.9% saline 2–4 L per 24 hours (monitor with JVP or CVP)

⬇

Monitor blood glucose (correct with 5% glucose if necessary) and FBC, U&E, LFTs, calcium

⬇

Search for cause – send blood, urine, sputum for culture (for TB)

⬇

Continue hydrocortisone 100 mg 6-hourly IM until BP stable and vomiting stopped

⬇

Recovery with normal BP, glucose and serum sodium should be within 12–24 hours

⬇

When stable convert to oral hydrocortisone 20 mg 8-hourly

Fig. 20.19 Management of acute adrenal failure (see also p. 583).

STROKE

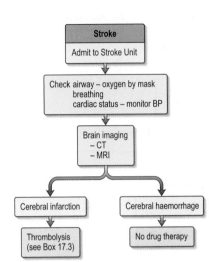

Fig. 20.20 Management of stroke (see also p. 628 and p. 631, Box 17.3).

THE COMATOSE PATIENT

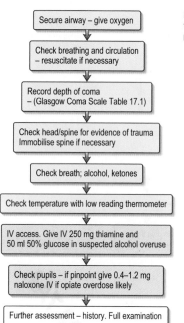

Fig. 20.21 Management of the comatose patient (see also p. 624, Box 17.1).

Secure airway – give oxygen

↓

Check breathing and circulation – resuscitate if necessary

↓

Record depth of coma – (Glasgow Coma Scale Table 17.1)

↓

Check head/spine for evidence of trauma Immobilise spine if necessary

↓

Check breath; alcohol, ketones

↓

Check temperature with low reading thermometer

↓

IV access. Give IV 250 mg thiamine and 50 ml 50% glucose in suspected alcohol overuse

↓

Check pupils – if pinpoint give 0.4–1.2 mg naloxone IV if opiate overdose likely

↓

Further assessment – history. Full examination

R

RA *see* Rheumatoid arthritis (RA)
RA (reactive arthritis), 312
Rabies, 56–57
  paralytic, 56–57
Radiation
  inpatient care, 7
  ionizing, 700–701
Radiation dermatitis, 700
Radiation-induced diffuse parenchymal lung disorders, 520
Radiation proctitis, 153
Radiation sickness, acute, 700–701
Radical prostatectomy, 257, 276
Radical radiotherapy *see* Radiotherapy
Radioactive ^{32}P, polycythaemia vera, 221
Radioactive iodine, 573
Radio-isotope imaging, 331
Radio-labelled red cell scan, 153
Radiology
  critical care, 535
  cystic fibrosis, 492
Radionuclide angiography, 418–419
Radionuclides, systemic, 256
Radionuclide ventilation/perfusion scan, 523–524
Radiotherapy, 255–257
  accelerated, 257
  adjuvant *see* Adjuvant radiotherapy
  administration, 255–257
  brachytherapy, 255–256
  breast cancer, 271
  chemoradiation, 257
  conformal external beam, 276–277
  external beam *see* External beam radiotherapy
  external beam radiotherapy, 255–256
  intensity-modulated radiotherapy, 276–277
  palliative, 256b, 257
  prostate cancer treatment, 277
  radical, 257
    non-small cell lung cancer treatment, 269
  side effects, 256b
  systemic radionuclides, 256

units of absorbed dose, 255
Raised intracranial pressure
  chemotherapy, 291
  malignant disease, 291
Raloxifene, 324t, 325
Raltegravir, 102t–105t, 108
Ramipril
  acute coronary syndrome therapy, 435t–436t
  heart failure management, 420t
  hypertension therapy, 465
Randomized controlled trials (RCTs), 12–13
Ranitidine, 537
Ranolazine, 447
Rapamycin (sirolimus), 362t
Rapidly progressive glomerulonephritis (RPGN), 344
  renal disease, 327t
  see also Nephritic syndrome
Rapid plasma reagin (RPR), 72
Rasagiline, 643t–644t
Rasburicase, 263
Rash, fever of unknown origin, 30–31
Rate/rhythm control, cardiovascular failure, 555
Raynaud's phenomenon/disease, 318
  systemic sclerosis, 318
RBBB (right bundle branch block), 394
RCC (renal cell carcinoma), 279–280, 363–364
R-CHOP (rituximab, cyclophosphamide, doxorubicin, vincristine, prednisolone) chemotherapy, 282
RCTs (randomized controlled trials), 12–13
Reactive arthritis (RA), 312
Reactive thrombocytosis, 234
Real-time polymerase chain reaction (RT-PCR), 34
Reassurance, severely disturbed patient, 21
Receiver operator characteristic (ROC) curve, 14

Recombinant DNAase, cystic fibrosis treatment, 494
Recombinant erythropoietin, 205
Recombinant humanized antibodies, 503
Rectal tumours, 273–274
  local trans-anal surgery, 273
  total mesorectal excision, 273
Recurrent urinary tract infection, 333
Red blood cell distribution width (RDW), 199–201
Red blood cells, storage effects, 539
Red cell transfusion, 223–224
  anaemias of chronic disease, 205
  aplastic anaemia, 208
  compatibility testing, 223–225
  idiopathic myelofibrosis, 222
  myelodysplastic syndromes, 209–210
  platelet function disorders, 234
  procedure, 223–225
  β-thalassaemia, 203–204
Red eye, 23–25
  red flags, 23b
Refeeding syndrome, 130–131
Reference nutrient intake (RNI), protein, 120
Refractory ischaemia, acute coronary syndromes, 443
Regurgitation, 139
Rehydration therapy
  Clostridium difficile associated diarrhoea, 61
  hyperosmolar hyperglycaemic state, 611
  oral, 136
Rejection, acute, renal transplants, 361
Relative risk (RR), 13
Remifentanil, 541t
Remission therapy, acute lymphoblastic leukaemia, 285
Renal angiography, 331
Renal biopsy
  acute kidney injury, 349
  chronic kidney disease, 354
  diabetic nephropathy, 340–341
  renal disease, 332

Appendix A

USEFUL WEBSITES FOR DRUGS AND THEIR USE IN DISEASE STATES AND PREGNANCY, AND FOR TOXICOLOGY

Pharmacotherapy moves at a very rapid pace and it is impossible for anyone to keep up to date. Never prescribe an unfamiliar drug without looking it up and checking the dose and route of administration. Never, ever, give a drug intrathecally unless you are absolutely sure that it can be given by this route. Always check on dosage when prescribing drugs for renal and liver disease. Do not prescribe in pregnancy unless the drug is essential and check website and company fact-sheets. Details of current prescribing advice can be found in:

- The **Summary of Product Characteristics (SmPCs)** produced by manufacturers but vetted by the UK drug regulatory authority (the Medicines and Healthcare Products Regulatory Agency).
- The **British National Formulary (BNF)** produced, jointly, by the British Medical Association and the Royal Pharmaceutical Society. Many countries have their own formularies.
- The **Technology Appraisals Guidance** series from the National Institute for Health and Clinical Excellence (NICE).

Advice on the management of individual conditions, in the form of clinical guidelines (systematically developed statements to assist practitioner and patient decisions about appropriate healthcare for specific clinical circumstances), can be accessed from:

- the National Institute for Clinical Excellence (NICE):
  http://www.nice-org.uk
- the Scottish Intercollegiate Guidelines Network (SIGN):
  http://www.sign.ac.uk/
- the National Guidelines Clearing House in the USA:
  http://www.guideline.gov.

Patient information leaflets (PILs) are supplied with all prescribed medication.

Other resources

World Health Organization: *WHO Model Formulary*, 2004: the equivalent of the *British National Formulary* for developing countries.

www.bnf.org
British National Formulary

www.clinicalevidence.com
A compendium of clinical evidence, BMJ learning

www.cochrane.co.uk
The Cochrane Collaboration

www.hpa.org.uk/infections/topics_az/antimicrobial_resistance/
guidance.htm
Antibiotic guidelines from the Health Protection Agency

http://mednet3.who.int/medicine/organization/par/edl/eml.shtml
The WHO limited list and formulary

www.nlm.nih.gov
National Library of Medicine

www.spib.axl.co.uk
National Poisons Information Centre

Websites for toxicology

www.toxbase.co.uk
Toxbase — database of the UK National Poisons Information Service

www.toxinz.com
Database of the New Zealand Poisons Centre

www.toxnet.nlm.nih.gov
National Library of Medicine's database

www.who.int/ipcs/poisons/centre/directory/en
Contact details of all poisons centres worldwide

www.wikitox.org
Home of the Clinical Toxicology Teaching Resource Project

Appendix B

NORMAL VALUES

(These vary. Please check with your local laboratory)

Haematology

Haemoglobin

    Male   13.5–17.7 g/dL

    Female   11.5–15.5 g/dL

Mean corpuscular haemoglobin (MCH)   27–32 pg

Mean corpuscular haemoglobin concentration (MCHC)   32–36 g/dL

Mean corpuscular volume (MCV)   80–96 fL

Packed cell volume (PCV) or haematocrit

    Male   0.40–0.54 L/L

    Female   0.37–0.47 L/L

White blood count (WBC) $4–11 \times 10^9/L$

    Basophil granulocytes $< 0.01–0.1 \times 10^9/L$

    Eosinophil granulocytes $0.04–0.4 \times 10^9/L$

    Lymphocytes $1.5–4.0 \times 10^9/L$

    Monocytes $0.2–0.8 \times 10^9/L$

    Neutrophil granulocytes $2.0–7.5 \times 10^9/L$

Platelet count $150–400 \times 10^9/L$

Serum B_{12} 160–925 ng/L (150–675 pmol/L)

Serum folate   4–18 mcg/L (5–63 nmol/L)

Red cell folate   160–640 mcg/L

Red cell mass

    Male   25–35 mL/kg

    Female   20–30 mL/kg

Reticulocyte count   0.5–2.5% of red cells ($50–100 \times 10^9/L$)

Erythrocyte sedimentation rate (ESR)   < 20 mm in 1 hour

Plasma viscosity   1.5–1.72 mPa.s

Coagulation

Bleeding time (Ivy method)   3–10 min

Activated partial thromboplastin time (APTT)   26–37 s

Prothrombin time   12–16 s

   International Normalized Ratio (INR)   1.0–1.3

D-dimer   < 500 ng/mL

BIOCHEMISTRY

(Serum/plasma in alphabetical order)

Alanine aminotransferase (ALT)   < 40 U/L

Albumin   35–50 g/L

Alkaline phosphatase   39–117 U/L

Amylase   25–125 U/L

Angiotensin-converting enzyme   10–70 U/L

α_1-Antitrypsin   2–4 g/L

Aspartate aminotransferase (AST)   12–40 U/L

Bicarbonate   22–30 mmol/L

Bilirubin   < 17 μmol/L (0.3–1.5 mg/dL)

Brain natriuretic peptide (BNP) threshold   100 pg/mL

Caeruloplasmin   1.5–2.9 μmol/L

Calcium   2.20–2.67 mmol/L (8.5–10.5 mg/dL)

Chloride   98–106 mmol/L

Complement

   C3   0.75–1.65 g/L

   C4   0.20–0.60 g/L

Copper   11–20 μmol/L (100–200 mg/dL)

C-reactive protein   < 5 mg/L

Creatinine   79–118 μmol/L (0.6–1.5 mg/dL)

Creatine kinase (CPK)

   Female   20–170 U/L

   Male   30–200 U/L

   CK-MB fraction   0–7 U/L (< 6% of total activity)

Ferritin

   Female   15–200 μg/L

   Post-menopausal   4–230 μg/L

   Male   30–300 μg/L

α-Fetoprotein   < 10 k U/L

Fructosamine   up to 285 μmol/L

Glucose (fasting)   4.5–5.6 mmol/L (70–110 mg/dL)

γ-Glutamyl transpeptidase (γ-GT)

   Male   11–58 U/L

   Female   7–32 U/L

Glycosylated (glycated) haemoglobin (HbA$_{1c}$)   3.7–5.1 %

Hydroxybutyric dehydrogenase (HBD)   72–182 U/L

Immunoglobulins (11 years and over)

   IgA   0.8–4 g/L

   IgG   5.5–16.5 g/L

   IgM   0.4–2.0 g/L

Iron   13–32 μmol/L (50–150 μg/dL)

Iron binding capacity (total) (TIBC)   42–80 μmol/L (250–410 μg/dL)

Lactate dehydrogenase   240–480 U/L

Magnesium   0.7–1.1 mmol/L

β_2-Microglobulin   1.0–3.0 mg/L

Osmolality   275–295 mOsm/kg

Phosphate   0.8–1.5 mmol/L

Potassium   3.5–5.0 mmol/L

Prostate-specific antigen (PSA)   up to 4.0 μg/L

Protein (total)   62–77 g/L

Sodium   135–146 mmol/L

Urate   0.18–0.42 mmol/L (3.0–7.0 mg/dL)

Urea   2.5–6.7 mmol/L (8–25 mg/dL)

Vitamin A   0.5–2.01 μmol/L

Vitamin D (seasonal variation)

   25-hydroxy   37–200 nmol/L (0.15–0.80 ng/L)

   1,25-dihydroxy   60–108 pmol/L (0.24–0.45 pg/L)

Zinc   11–24 μmol/L

Lipids and lipoproteins

Cholesterol   3.5–6.5 mmol/L (ideal < 5.2 mmol/L)

HDL cholesterol

   Male   0.8–1.8 mmol/L

   Female   1.0–2.3 mmol/L

LDL cholesterol   < 4.0 mmol/L (ideal < 2 mmol/L)

Lipids (total)   4.0–10.0 g/L

Lipoproteins

   VLDL   0.128–0.645 mmol/L

   LDL   1.55–4.4 mmol/L

   HDL (male)   0.70–2.1 mmol/L

   HDL (female)   0.50–1.70 mmol/L

Phospholipid   2.9–5.2 mmol/L

Triglycerides

   Male   0.70–2.1 mmol/L

   Female   0.50–1.70 mmol/L

Thyroid-stimulating hormone   0.3–3.5 mU/L

Blood gases (arterial)

Pa_{CO_2} 4.8–6.1 kPa (36–46 mmHg)

Pa_{O_2} 10–13.3 kPa (75–100 mmHg)

[H+]   35–45 nmol/L

pH   7.35–7.45

Bicarbonate   22–26 mmol/L

Urine values

Calcium   7.5 mmol per 24 hours or less (< 300 mg daily)

Copper   0.2–1.0 µmol per 24 hours (15–40 mg/24 hours)

Creatinine   0.13–0.22 mmol per kg body weight, per day

5-hydroxyindole acetic acid (5HIAA)   < 47 µmol daily; amounts lower in females than males

Protein (quantitative)   < 0.15 g per 24 hours

Sodium   60–180 mmol per 24 hours

Serum values

eGFR

    Male   90–140 mL/min

    Female   80–125 mL/min

Index

Kumar & Clark's Medical Management and Therapeutics